Resistance, Diagnostic and Therapeutic Applications of Drugs in Cancer

Resistance, Diagnostic and Therapeutic Applications of Drugs in Cancer

Edited by Sydney Bruce

STATES
ACADEMIC PRESS
www.statesacademicpress.com

States Academic Press,
109 South 5th Street,
Brooklyn, NY 11249, USA

Visit us on the World Wide Web at:
www.statesacademicpress.com

ISBN: 978-1-63989-470-3

Cataloging-in-Publication Data

Resistance, diagnostic and therapeutic applications of drugs in cancer / edited by Sydney Bruce.
p. cm.
Includes bibliographical references and index.
ISBN 978-1-63989-470-3
1. Cancer – Chemotherapy. 2. Cancer--Diagnosis. 3. Cancer--Treatment. 4. Chemotherapy. I. Bruce, Sydney.
RC271.C5 .R47 2022
616.994 061--dc23

Table of Contents

Preface

The usage of drugs to treat cancer is termed as chemotherapy. It is aimed at killing the cancer cells or stopping their growth and spread to other parts of the body. There are several mechanisms through which it can work such as by destroying both non-cancerous and cancerous cells, attacking only cancer cells, and fighting the genes of the cancer cells in order to kill them and stop their spread. The different types of chemotherapy drugs are alkylating agents, antimetabolites, mitotic inhibitors, topoisomerase inhibitors and steroids. The drugs given to cure cancer are selected on the basis of the type of cancer, whether the patient has a history of cancer, and other health issues such as kidney, liver or heart disease. This book attempts to understand the multiple drugs that are used to treat cancer and their diagnostic and therapeutic applications. The various studies that are constantly contributing towards advancing technologies and evolution of this field are examined in detail. The book is appropriate for students seeking detailed information in this area as well as for experts.

All of the data presented henceforth, was collaborated in the wake of recent advancements in the field. The aim of this book is to present the diversified developments from across the globe in a comprehensible manner. The opinions expressed in each chapter belong solely to the contributing authors. Their interpretations of the topics are the integral part of this book, which I have carefully compiled for a better understanding of the readers.

At the end, I would like to thank all those who dedicated their time and efforts for the successful completion of this book. I also wish to convey my gratitude towards my friends and family who supported me at every step.

Editor

Navigating the rapids: the development of regulated next-generation sequencing-based clinical trial assays and companion diagnostics

Saumya Pant, Russell Weiner and Matthew J. Marton*

Merck Research Laboratories, Molecular Biomarkers and Diagnostics, Rahway, NJ USA

Edited by:
Jan Trøst Jørgensen, Dx-Rx Institute, Denmark

Reviewed by:
William Douglas Figg, National Cancer Institute, USA
Federico Manuel Giorgi, Columbia University, USA
Hardik J. Patel, Memorial Sloan-Kettering Cancer Center, USA

***Correspondence:**
Matthew J. Marton, Merck Research Laboratories, Molecular Biomarkers and Diagnostics, 126 East Lincoln Avenue, Rahway, NJ 07065, USA
e-mail: matthew_marton@merck.com

Over the past decade, next-generation sequencing (NGS) technology has experienced meteoric growth in the aspects of platform, technology, and supporting bioinformatics development allowing its widespread and rapid uptake in research settings. More recently, NGS-based genomic data have been exploited to better understand disease development and patient characteristics that influence response to a given therapeutic intervention. Cancer, as a disease characterized by and driven by the tumor genetic landscape, is particularly amenable to NGS-based diagnostic (Dx) approaches. NGS-based technologies are particularly well suited to studying cancer disease development, progression and emergence of resistance, all key factors in the development of next-generation cancer Dxs. Yet, to achieve the promise of NGS-based patient treatment, drug developers will need to overcome a number of operational, technical, regulatory, and strategic challenges. Here, we provide a succinct overview of the state of the clinical NGS field in terms of the available clinically targeted platforms and sequencing technologies. We discuss the various operational and practical aspects of clinical NGS testing that will facilitate or limit the uptake of such assays in routine clinical care. We examine the current strategies for analytical validation and Food and Drug Administration (FDA)-approval of NGS-based assays and ongoing efforts to standardize clinical NGS and build quality control standards for the same. The rapidly evolving companion diagnostic (CDx) landscape for NGS-based assays will be reviewed, highlighting the key areas of concern and suggesting strategies to mitigate risk. The review will conclude with a series of strategic questions that face drug developers and a discussion of the likely future course of NGS-based CDx development efforts.

Keywords: companion diagnostics, disruptive technology, precision medicine, next-generation sequencing, clinical next-generation sequencing, molecular diagnostics, drug development strategy, mutation detection methods

INTRODUCTION

The concept of personalized medicine relies heavily on access to information on an individual's unique genetic characteristics to tailor therapy. However, the current paradigm of regulated molecular diagnostic (Dx) testing, in which individual Food and Drug Administration (FDA)-cleared Dx tests are employed to detect mutations in a single gene, sits uneasily in this framework of personalized medicine (1, 2). The advent of clinical next-generation sequencing (NGS) has begun to provide to the clinic a more expansive insight into genetic mutations in a broader set of genes, usually drawn from pathways implicated in and actionable by current therapeutics or by promising drug candidates in development (3). NGS-based diagnosis is specially promising for diseases that have a highly complex and heterogeneous genetic composition. The field of oncology is therefore very well positioned to benefit greatly from such an approach (4, 5). Since NGS-based technology permits a more complete view into a tumor's genetic composition, it is easy to foresee that treatment paradigms must

Abbreviations: ABRF, Association of Biomolecular Resource Facilities; ACMG, American College of Medical Genetics and Genomics; BRAF, v-Raf murine sarcoma viral oncogene homolog B; CAP, College of American Pathologists; CDER, Center for Drug Evaluation and Research; CDRH, Center for Devices and Radiological Health; CDx, companion diagnostic; CE Conformité Européenne, Conformity Marking for Relevant European Council Directives; CFTR, cystic fibrosis transmembrane conductance regulator; CLIA, Clinical Lab Improvement Amendment; CRO, contract research organization; CTA, clinical trial assay; ddNTPs, dideoxynucleotide triphosphates; DNA, deoxyribonucleic acid; dNTPs, deoxynucleotide triphosphates; Dx, diagnostic; EGFR, epidermal growth factor receptor gene; EMR, electronic medical records; ePCR, emulsion PCR; FDA, United States Food and Drug Administration; FFPE, formalin fixed paraffin embedded; gDNA, genomic DNA; IHC, immunohistochemistry; ISPs, ion sphere particles; IUO, investigational use only; IVD, *in vitro* diagnostic; KRAS, Kirsten rat sarcoma viral oncogene homolog gene; LDT, lab-developed test; MAQC, microarray quality control; NCI, National Cancer Institute; NGS, next-generation sequencing, NIST, National Institute of Standards and Technology; NTC, no template control; PacBio, Pacific Biosciences; PGM, Personal Genome Machine; PMA, pre-market approval; PT, proficiency testing; QC, quality control; qPCR, quantitative polymerase chain reaction; RNA, ribonucleic acid; RNA-Seq, RNA sequencing; RUO, research usage only; SMRT, single molecule real time sequencing; SNV, single nucleotide variant; TAT, turnaround time; UTR, untranslated region; VCF, variant calling file; ZMW, zero-mode waveguides.

change accordingly to allow treatment based on the molecular pathological fingerprint of the individual. As a result, the question is not technological ("Can it be done?"), but rather practical ("How can NGS technology be developed into a mainstream multi-gene or multi-transcript Dx fingerprint?") and regulative ("What are the barriers that must be overcome for this disruptive technology be approved as a general companion diagnostic (CDx) device for multiple therapeutics?"). It is clear the scientific community is rapidly embracing the technology as NGS-based tests are being employed across multiple disease areas, including oncological, metabolic, cardiovascular and neurosensory disorders, and in prenatal diagnoses (6–10) where genetic components are defined. As of late 2013, several dozen clinical labs offer over 50 different laboratory-developed tests (LDTs) using NGS (11). These tests are offered as single-gene assays or multi-gene or multi-transcript panels. Commercially available NGS-based cancer panels are already being used in clinical practice and as clinical trial assays (CTAs) to guide patients to most appropriate experimental treatment (8, 12, 13). Nonetheless, there are no FDA-approved NGS CDxs available today and there are significant challenges in developing such tests. We compare developing NGS-based Dx to navigating the rapids, an exercise full of challenges, continuously changing technologies, policies, and regulations as the field develops at a rapid pace, and yet the promise of personalized medicine is within reach and closer than ever before.

CURRENT PARADIGM IS UNSUSTAINABLE

Precision medicine has been defined as identifying the right drug, for the right patient, at the right dose, at the right time (14). Intrinsic to identifying the right patient is a Dx device. If it is linked to a specific therapeutic and if the test is required for the safe and effective use of the drug, then Dx device is termed a CDx. The current testing paradigm for precision medicine links a specific drug to the Dx (15, 16) and can be summarized as "one-drug/one-gene Dx." This is abundantly illustrated for FDA-approved Dxs, such as the one-gene tests approved for mutations in *EGFR*, *KRAS*, and *BRAF*. Yet, it is equally clear that the current paradigm is not sustainable (17, 18). First, cancer is an exceedingly complex molecular and epigenomic disorder, resulting from perhaps hundreds of different molecular defects, including somatic mutations, gene expression changes, and genome rearrangements. Furthermore, tumorigenesis and tumor progression are driven by altered gene regulation networks that are not always tractable to a clear and defined somatic mutation (19). Recent results from clinical studies support the emerging concept of the "mutation signature" or spectrum of correlated mutations in cancer (20, 21), which postulates that the combination of mutations present is more predictive of the response to treatment than individual gene mutation status. Thus, to ensure their patients are offered the best possible treatment, physicians will want to examine the tumor's whole cancer genome, both somatic mutation and transcriptional changes, to identify the most personalized therapy, and they will do so whether or not there is a FDA-sanctioned Dx for a particular drug. Instead, they will use LDTs, which the FDA believes should be regulated as *in vitro* diagnostics (IVDs) (75 FR 34463, 2010). Thus, the current situation is untenable since it is only a matter of time before more comprehensive tests will routinely be used to diagnose a patient's tumor. Second, not only do physicians need more molecular information, but patients want it too. In this age of internet medicine, many patients are well-informed and strongly advocate for more comprehensive testing, even to the point of paying for it themselves in order to get a more complete picture of their cancer (22). Their reasoning that more information is better is hard to argue against. Hospitals and for-profit companies have developed tests to meet this need, and advertisements for comprehensive genomic tumor assessment on television, radio, and internet are not uncommon. Furthermore, patients considering a clinical trial at a major hospital are beginning to expect molecular characterization of their tumor as a *quid pro quo* for participation in the clinical study. A third, more practical, reason why the current model is not sustainable is the limitation of tissue. A Dx tumor specimen block can only be sectioned into a limited number of sections. Sample is limiting and tests are not currently multiplexed; separate slides are usually required for different immunohistochemical (IHC)-, ribonucleic acid (RNA)-, or deoxyribonucleic acid (DNA)-based tests. In most cases, there is simply not enough material to test for every gene mutation that is available, and therefore a more efficient use of the patient's specimen is needed. For these reasons, it is clear the "one-drug/one-gene Dx" paradigm is unsustainable and that the drive toward precision medicine is changing clinical practice, and as it does, it will change the clinical testing paradigm for cancer treatment decisions.

DISRUPTIVE SHIFT

Next-generation sequencing is a classic disruptive technology (23). It may even change the way precision medicines are developed (24). Although these changes will impact the healthcare community and their patients, in this section we will only focus on the potential impact on drug developers and manufacturers of Dx tests. The crux of these changes is the shift from a "one-drug/one-gene Dx" model to a "multi-gene Dx/many drugs" paradigm (25, 26). An oversimplification of the interaction between the drug developer and the Dx company can be summarized as: the drug company develops a promising drug and discovers late in development that a Dx is needed to identify the appropriate patient population. Then it works with the Dx company to develop the test to detect and/or quantify the specific biomarker, and they are both tested in pivotal trials. Thus, the drug drives the device development. The use of a multi-gene or multi-transcript panel has the potential to change that. Instead of a single drug developer partnering to develop a single Dx test, what may happen is that the device manufacturer may design an assay able to detect a myriad of RNA or DNA biomarkers. That is, the device manufacturer may drive content on the device and may proactively seek FDA-clearance independent of a partnership with a drug maker. The implication of this disruptive shift is a set of challenges that will be discussed in a later section.

PRIMER ON NGS PLATFORMS

Several firms have developed small benchtop NGS sequencers for the clinical Dxs market. The current leading platforms are the MiSeq from Illumina, Inc. and the Personal Genome Machine (PGM) from Life Technologies, Inc., which together comprise >85% of market as of early 2014 (Bloomberg Businessweek,

January 2014). The recent agreement between Roche Molecular Diagnostics and Pacific Biosciences (PacBio) heralds the entry of the latter into the Dx arena. Qiagen has announced that it will release its benchtop GeneReader™ NGS platform in 2014. Key factors that influence clinical labs' adoption of a particular platform include sequencing quality, turnaround time (TAT), cost per sample, optimal ease of use for the operator, and sample multiplexing capability (recognizing that multiplexing is likely required to reduce cost). We provide a brief overview of the main clinical NGS technology platforms here and refer the reader to exhaustive reviews on NGS technology and instrumentation advances for further details on each (27–30).

ION TORRENT

Life Technologies' Ion Torrent semiconductor sequencing technology, which made its debut in 2011, is based on a sequencing-by-synthesis approach in which individual templated DNA molecules positioned in microwells on a semiconductor chip are sequentially incubated with each of the four deoxynucleotide triphosphates (dNTPs) to support DNA strand polymerization (31). Only the dNTP complementary to the template is incorporated at the end of each template strand. As each dNTP is incorporated, a proton is released, which acts as an indicator of base incorporation and the number of bases incorporated consecutively. The resulting pH changes are recorded as voltage changes that convey the sequence of bases for the flow. Advantages of this technology include optics-free readout, low input DNA requirement (which is critical for clinical practice), and longer read length with accurate base calling (32).

ILLUMINA

The Illumina technology also utilizes a sequencing-by-synthesis approach with bridge amplification (27). Clonally amplified DNA templates are immobilized to an acrylamide coating on the surface of a glass flowcell that serves as the reaction and sequencing substrate. Fluorescently labeled reversible-terminator dideoxynucleotide triphosphates (ddNTPs) are added one base at time in this sequencing technology. After the addition of each nucleotide, the clusters in the flowcell are imaged to determine which fluorescent dye was incorporated. In its current manifestation, Illumina's greatest strength is the easier workflow of the amplicon library preparation and reduced hands-on time as compared to other platforms. Data from research versions of the technology, such as the larger HiSeq platform, associates Illumina with greater accuracy of base calls and lower indel detection errors (29).

PACIFIC BIOSCIENCES

To compete in the clinical and Dx space, PacBio introduced the desktop RS machine in 2011. PacBio utilizes single molecule real time (SMRT) sequencing. DNA template bound to DNA polymerase molecules is attached to the bottom of 50 nm-width wells termed zero-mode waveguides (ZMWs). Each polymerase molecule carries out second strand DNA synthesis using γ-phosphate fluorescently labeled nucleotides present in the reaction mix. The ZMW width does not allow light to propagate, but energy penetration excites the nucleotide fluorophores in the vicinity of the polymerase at the bottom of the well. As DNA synthesis occurs, the incorporation of each base creates a distinctive pulse of fluorescence, which is detected and recorded in real time (33). In a platform comparison of the three technologies, Quail et al. noted the high fidelity of PacBio data and the ability to read long sequences (28), but added the caveat that very high read depth is required for achieving accuracy near that of MiSeq and PGM. Additionally, in the context of formalin fixed paraffin embedded (FFPE) and fragmented DNA material, PacBio's long read strength may not be of great advantage.

It must be noted that the rapid pace of performance improvement of both the Illumina and Life Technologies benchtop sequencers has been instrumental in making NGS-based Dxs within reach (34). Both platforms have incrementally increased the quantity and quality of base calling while reducing library preparation time and allowing on-instrument primary and secondary data analysis, which was considered the largest bottleneck to clinical and Dx NGS up to early 2011. For example, advances in library preparation have reduced processing times two-fold compared to older version kits available from both companies in 2011. On the instrumentation side, the new, smaller instruments (MiSeq and PGM), have enhanced output and accuracy of base calling compared to the earlier larger throughput NGS instruments (Illumina GAIIx, Illumina HiSeq 2000, and earlier versions of PGM) (28). An Ion Torrent 318 chip with 400 bp sequencing reads can easily produce >1 Gbp aligned data passing Q20 scores. Furthermore, the newer versions of chemistry have significantly improved the average error rates over the length of reads. Also, the design of the new emulsion PCR (ePCR) Ion One Touch 2 system released in late 2012 increased the uniformity of sequencing by enhancing inclusion of low length template Ion Sphere particles (ISPs) in the template and enhancing library templating for sequencing. Additionally, on-instrument analysis improvements significantly reduced the challenges and time constraints imposed by bioinformatic analysis. Although even more improvements are anticipated, these technical advances have made clinical NGS a reality.

OPERATIONAL CHALLENGES FOR NGS ASSAYS IN THE CLINIC

SPECIMEN TYPE AND AMOUNT

One of the key considerations with current clinical NGS tests with Dx aspirations is the reliance on FFPE material. DNA isolated from FFPE specimens presents unique challenges in being highly degraded and of poor quality compared to that from fresh frozen specimens (35). This places a limitation on the size of amplicons that can be reliably amplified from this material, with tests targeting amplicon targeted regions from around 120–180 bp (Ion Torrent AmpliSeq Cancer Hot Spot panel)[1] to ~175 bp (Illumina TruSeq and TruSight assays)[2]. Additionally, DNA derived from FFPE material undergoes cytosine deamination during the fixation process, which can complicate analyses in downstream Dx applications unless a downstream bioinformatic solution is able to address and compensate for such base alterations (36, 37). What is perhaps an equally great challenge is the amount of specimen required for the assay. Ion Torrent assays for cancer mutational hot spot panels

[1] www.iontorrent.com

[2] www.illumina.com

require about 10 ng input of FFPE DNA, the Illumina TruSight clinical assay panel requires 30–300 ng input DNA (as determined by quantitative polymerase chain reaction (qPCR)-based functional DNA assessment) and a majority of the established clinical NGS panels available as lab-developed tests require about 40 μm FFPE material or >100 ng input DNA, in addition to sections for pathology review and tumor markup. In contrast, individual Dx tests using either traditional Sanger sequencing or other PCR-based assays typically require at least 15 μm input per assay. This apparent drawback of large input NGS-based testing (particularly for Illumina assays) has led to methods to reduce sample requirements, such as Rubicon Genomics ThruPLEX kit, Illumina's Epistem technology, NuGen amplification products, and New England Biolabs NEBNext Ultra for low input NGS. Importantly, the assay manufacturers have themselves adopted steps to further decrease input amount for assays without compromising on test sensitivity. One final note: for NGS-based tests, the sample requirement for material is relatively independent of the number of genes in the assay since the test requires the input of a minimal number of amplifiable genomes only (38).

ASSAY TURN-AROUND TIME

A major hurdle in the adoption of a NGS-based test as a CTA is the logistics in terms of the length of time from sample collection to reporting of results. Most clinically applicable NGS-based tests require 7–14 business days TAT (39). In the case of hematological malignancies, such a long reporting time seems to be clinically untenable. Some clinicians are hesitant to use NGS tests for patient stratification and prospective enrollment in trials because patients may not be willing or able to wait 2 weeks for a test result, and thus will pursue other clinical trials in the meantime. As the NGS assay TAT continues to improve (discussed under analytical challenges) this is likely to be a smaller concern in the next few years.

AVAILABILITY OF CROs WITH CLIA NGS CAPABILITIES

Clinical trial sponsors typically prefer to perform clinical trial sample analysis in a single central lab to avoid potential liabilities of using multiple local hospital laboratories, which can compromise results or complicate interpretation due to the use of different tests, different instruments, different validation standards, and quality control (QC) processes, and different histopathological practices such as macrodissection (14, 40). Unfortunately, despite the potential commercial opportunity that available NGS-based multi-gene panels represent, only a few contract research organizations (CROs) or specialty testing labs have invested the effort to develop the expertise to offer NGS services as Clinical Lab Improvement Amendment (CLIA) laboratory tests suitable as CTAs. Thus, the majority of the technical expertise does not reside in traditional central labs and CROs (11), but rather in academic institutions and in large clinical hospitals, where medical practitioners have begun to use NGS-based mutational profiling screening to match their patients to the appropriate therapeutic (41). These factors represent a significant challenge for pharmaceutical companies interested in developing NGS-based CDxs.

The concern about using local laboratory for enrollment to clinical trials comes from several different areas. First, there may be variability due to different interpretation of the various guidelines, checklists, and recommendations available for NGS assays (42–44) since laboratory directors have some discretion and may interpret the rules differently in some cases. An example is the interpretation of the College of American Pathologists (CAP) NGS checklist that recommends orthogonal analytical confirmation of all encountered mutations from an assay before the mutation is reported as clinically actionable (43). This guidance seems to be interpreted differently in different labs based on the availability of subjects, which limits the probability of encountering samples with said mutations. Second, the current lack of standardization between hospital laboratories, especially in analytical and post-analytical processes, introduces risk in, for example, mutation calls for the same samples since they may utilize different platforms, assays, software, and algorithms to make mutation calls. This is even seen for simpler, non-NGS-based assays such as for *KRAS* mutation detection assays. In a retrospective study (29) in which specimens from colorectal cancer patients treated with panitumumab (an anti-epidermal growth factor receptor gene (EGFR) monoclonal antibody) were analyzed for the presence of activating *KRAS* mutations in both local hospital labs and a centralized testing facility at a CRO, the authors found that 6 of the 60 patients tested had mutations and should have been excluded from the study. The conclusion was that the LDTs in local hospital labs failed to detect the *KRAS* mutations, allowing ineligible patients to be enrolled, and thereby diluted the drug response rate since patients with *KRAS* mutations were not expected to respond to panitumumab treatment (45). That this can happen with a simple PCR-based mutation test illustrates the risk associated with complex assays such as NGS-based assays (43).

The challenge for the pharmaceutical company is how to run a clinical trial that maintains the homogeneity of the trial population in light of the paucity of CROs with CLIA NGS capabilities. Some have suggested to use the local lab test as a CTA for enrollment but confirm the result with a centralized assay or to use the local lab test as a screen to identify patients whose samples should be analyzed by the centralized CTA. Both of these suggestions are problematic. First, analyzing the patient specimen by two assays unnecessarily consumes limiting material. Second, discordant calls are inevitable, especially for assays as complex as NGS-based assays. Determining which of two discordant results is accurate will likely be time-consuming and expensive. Furthermore, the discordant data will likely raise concerns of any regulatory agency reviewing the clinical trial and it may call into question the accuracy of the CTA. Similarly, the idea to use local lab assays to screen patients for subsequent central lab testing will definitely introduce a patient population bias if the study only enrolls biomarker positive patients (12), and it may introduce a bias even if the study has both biomarker positive and negative arms. In general, it seems better to focus on reducing the TAT of sample analysis at the centralized laboratory than to rely on local laboratories for patient eligibility decisions.

A new paradigm in clinical NGS testing is the emergence of companies like Foundation Medicine (FM) and Personal Genome Diagnostics (PGD), which offer NGS-based panel tests as CTAs to support clinical trials as well as directly to physicians. Boston-based FM offers the Foundation One panel that reports on the mutational status of 285 genes that are found to be commonly mutated in cancers; it has also recently announced a similar panel for hematological malignancies (46). PGD, based out of Baltimore, offers a clinical targeted cancer gene panel cancer select for the detection of genetic alterations in 120 well-characterized cancer and pharmacogenomics genes (47). These companies thus offer an alternative to local laboratory testing for clinical trials. Companies can either use one of these commercial panels as a CTA or can establish a clinical trial protocol that enables recruitment of subjects that have already had the tests performed (13, 48, 49).

FDA-CLEARED INSTRUMENTATION

Although Illumina's MiSeqDx instrument received CE marking in June 2013, the lack of commercially available instrumentation was a major hurdle to CDx development prior to the FDA-clearance of Illumina's MiSeqDx platform as a class II device in November 2013 [510(k) number K123989]. In addition, the FDA also made the device and substantially similar devices exempt from the premarket notification requirements. At the same time, the FDA-cleared Illumina's cystic fibrosis carrier screening assay, an assay that detects all 139 variants in the cystic fibrosis transmembrane conductance regulator (CFTR) gene, as well as an assay for CF diagnosis by sequencing all the medically relevant regions of the CFTR gene assay (Source accessdata.fda.gov and illumina.com). The type of data required for these submissions provides the first documented and public view into the Center for Devices and Radiological Health's (CDRH) specific expectations for verification and validation of NGS-based Dx tests; see below for a section in which this is discussed in detail.

Life Technologies' has recently stated that its Ion Torrent PGM Dx System will be registered as a class II 510(k)-exempt device with the FDA, as opposed to applying for 510(k) clearance as was done for the Illumina MiSeqDx (50). This is apparently prompted by the FDA decision that the MiSeqDx instrument and substantially equivalent devices of that generic type will be classified into class II and be exempt from premarket notification requirements [510(k) K123989]. The Ion Torrent PGM Dx will be building on Life Technologies' expertise with Dx instruments such as the 510(k)-cleared 3500 Dx Genetic Analyzer. The PGM Dx instrument will be an open platform for NGS tests but without specific assays submitted to the FDA. Life Technologies has stated that Dxs manufacturers applying for tests on the PGM Dx will reference the master file as needed to support their submission to the FDA and those assays would be evaluated by the FDA through either the 510(k) or premarket approval (PMA) processes. The Ion Torrent system has one significant difference in that it includes two peripheral accessory instruments, the Ion OneTouch Dx for ePCR-based template preparation and the OneTouch ES Dx for magnetic bead-based ePCR library enrichment.

Pacific Biosciences RS II DNA Sequencing System's regulatory path is currently not clear. However, in a significant move recently, Roche Diagnostics and PacBio entered into an agreement to develop Dx sequencing systems and consumables utilizing PacBio's SMRT technology. Per this agreement Roche will become the exclusive worldwide distributor for PacBio's human IVD products (51).

TECHNICAL AND ANALYTICAL CHALLENGES FOR NGS ASSAYS IN THE CLINIC

DESIGN OF THE NGS ASSAY

The first challenge toward a successful NGS CDx is the assay design. Most current clinical NGS assays rely on a hybrid-capture or PCR amplicon-based approach to provide overlapping, high density coverage across regions of interest (52). When working with FFPE biopsy specimens, the number of amplicons needs to be judiciously optimized to allow efficient coverage of large regions while keeping amplicon size small to enable efficient amplification of formalin-damaged DNA (53). The choice of platform and the degree to which the assay needs to include promoter, 3′ untranslated region (UTR), splice sites, or introns also affects assay design. Currently, most commercially available panels only cover exonic regions. While Ion Torrent's hot spot mutation panels cover shorter fragment amplicons, Illumina's exon coverage-based design tends to favor longer amplicons. While overlapping longer amplicons may increase the fidelity of readout by utilizing multiple overlapping fragments per base, amplicon length must be judiciously balanced to enable FFPE fragmented DNA analysis.

Genomic complexity of the region of interest can impact accuracy and precision of an assay (54), so it is also important to understand and to give due consideration to the same in assay design. Since the genome has been shown to replicate at different times with variable error as a function of time of replication, the analytical parameters including error rate must be calculated accordingly for specific regions based on sequence context (55, 56). Knowing whether the region of interest is a region of lower intrinsic fidelity allows one to improve accuracy by compensating with higher read depth. Similarly, the degree to which samples will be multiplexed must be planned into the design to balance read depth (and thus higher confidence in calls) versus the cost of the assay, since higher read depth leads to lower multiplexing capacity and thus increased per sample assay cost (43, 57, 58). Ensuring that the assay design and bioinformatics analysis take into account the region's characteristics, it should be applicable to individual assay developers building Dx assays on other platforms as well. Finally, it is important to develop models that take into account the expected sample throughput, frequency of testing, the assay TAT, and the degree of batching to forecast the optimal multiplexing strategy. For batching samples there must exist guidelines for standard multiplexing and read depth to ensure equivalence of test results.

QUALITY CONTROL STANDARDIZATION

The lack of industry-wide standardization of critical components of QC also represents a challenge for CDx development. The current NGS technologies have higher error rates and novel error modes compared to traditional sequencing, which results in variability in mutation reporting (59–61). Thus, during test development it is essential to have a strategy to detect and reduce the frequency of false positives and then to establish QC procedures to assess test performance, yet there is no established or generally accepted approach (62, 63). This strategy will likely involve varying bioinformatics parameters of the variant calling software and establishing a method to confirm mutation calls with orthogonal methods. Investigating false positive calls is crucial during assay development and refinement. While Sanger sequencing is still considered the gold standard, its lower sensitivity of detection [around 17–25%; (64)] limits its use for confirming mutations at the low frequencies that are commonly detected with NGS. Multiple strategies for orthogonal validation are possible, such as using a different assay design on the same NGS platform to evaluate design robustness or employing an orthogonal NGS platform with similar sensitivity to identify any platform-specific artifacts. Orthogonal validation with non-NGS platforms such as Sequenom, COLD-PCR, and pyrosequencing may be a preferable approach and these are also gaining popularity as clinical NGS validation strategies (44, 46, 65). False negative calls are more difficult to detect but the utilization of variant call files (VCFs) that report read depth at every position allows for positive confirmation of a wildtype call and not just the absence of a variant call at that position. Second, standardized procedures for QC, including spike-in sequences are yet to be standardized. Some have proposed that spike-in samples should mimic the region of interest in terms of genomic region tertiary structure, interfering genomic regions competing for similar priming sites and, lastly, for genomic complexity, including but not limited to base distribution, presence of similarly presented homopolymeric regions or the known regions of ambiguity such as GC combinations that have been found to complicate variant analysis in a platform-specific manner (29). Recent forums for NGS standardization (43, 44) have discussed the needs for both artificial sequences, which will allow quality assessment of library preparation and analysis (66), and clinically relevant biological mimics, which can faithfully recapitulate biological variation induced by genome complexity as well as serve as a good benchmark for matrix-associated artifacts, e.g., FFPE matrix artifacts. Without industry-wide recommendations or guidance from regulatory authorities, this aspect of CDx development represents a challenge.

CLINICAL AND DIAGNOSTIC RNASeq ASSAY DESIGN CHALLENGES

The use of RNASeq for transcriptional profiling, gene expression studies, identification of variants, and pathological fusion or splicing events (67) is an area of great interest to the clinical genomics community. Clinical RNASeq brings to the fore the capacity to utilize gene expression signatures for highly informative disease sub-type classification or prognosis signature development, as has been demonstrated by gene expression based Dx tests like Agendia's MammaPrint test (68) or Genomic Health's OncotypeDX tests (69). Clinical RNASeq at the whole transcriptome level offers invaluable insight into a patient's transcriptome and associated gene expression changes informative of pre-disposition to cancer or patient stratification strategies. It is especially pertinent for conditions where alternative splicing and isoform selection can affect response to drugs or can predict selective outcomes in response to therapy. RNASeq analysis can be used to develop a robust molecular sub-type signature for a cancer as is apparent from recent studies utilizing gene expression signatures for prognostic and Dx assays (70, 71). In reality, as with issues facing the whole genome sequencing and whole exome sequencing field, it is more likely that targeted panels rather than whole transcriptome offerings will first show clinical utility.

Some of the issues that hinder the adoption of clinical RNASeq are the quality of the RNA from clinical biopsy materials, extremely complex bioinformatics and statistical analysis as well as design of the experiment and its execution in the clinic. The quality and quantification of RNA is critical for successful library preparation and QC controlled analysis of the sample. Clinical FFPE sample-derived RNA is likely to require pre-processing repairs or methodologies to enable low input amplification or enrichment based library preparation. Sample RNA preparation and RNASeq process reproducibility and accurate quantification will have to be highly validated to avoid issues such as prep based biases in quantification of GC-rich transcripts or small RNA species. It will also be important to assess the impact of factors such as RNA secondary structure, the presence of small RNAs in the sample or interfering substances (72). Any lack of read-out reproducibility in a gene-specific manner will hinder the establishment of fold change cut-offs for clinical decision-making (73). Qualifying adequate depth of coverage is critical because accurate quantification of transcripts in clinical RNAseq is dependent on read depth (74).

The bioinformatics analysis of RNASeq in the clinic is considerably more complex than pipelines for DNASeq. For one thing, normalization of data needs to be highly accurate for the technology to be quantitative for the measurement of relative expression values (75). As algorithms for non-clinical RNASeq are improved and as scientists employ better controlled experiments and statistical strategies (76), some of the issues that have plagued clinical RNASeq bioinformatics may be resolved in the near future. Definition and standardization of clinical databases and annotation pipelines is another critical requirement for clinical RNASeq. Currently, because of variability in gene models in different databases such as AceView and RefSeq as well as frequent changes to the databases, non-clinical RNASeq efforts encounter high variability in definition and annotation of regions. In addition, one of the key features of clinical RNASeq will be the ability to identify specific re-arrangements and spliced isoforms. Considering that detection of fusions and gene re-arrangements have high clinical relevance, it will be necessary to develop both bioinformatics methods and mate pair library construction protocols or similar technology but simpler workflows to detect re-arrangements and gene fusions (77). The design of targeted experiments should enable more hypothesis-free quantification of the staggering complexity of gene fusions and transcript re-arrangements possible as well (78). Without such a highly complex identification and quantification strategy the power of clinical RNASeq cannot be fully realized. Targeted RNASeq approaches, particularly with amplicon-based panels, would need to have highly plexed designs to allow a more discovery oriented capture approach while allowing highly sensitive quantification. Hybrid capture based panels would possibly offer more robust splice isoform coverage but suffer from more labor intensive protocols.

Reference materials, controls, and QC standards need to be defined for clinical grade RNASeq in the same way these are becoming standardized for clinical DNASeq. An advantage for the clinical RNASeq field is the availability of the highly qualified human reference MAQC-A and MAQC-B reference materials and the extensive data on tissue-specific expression of potential housekeeping genes from exhaustive microarray profiling (79).

This approach has been utilized to test and aid data correction in RNASeq in research settings and may find easy integration into clinical practice as well (80). Recently, the set of eukaryotic mRNA mimic Spike-In Control Mixes developed by the External RNA Control Consortium (ERCC) has been suggested as a clinically useful control option. These have pre-formulated quantified blends of 92 transcripts derived from National Institute of Standards and Technology (NIST)-certified DNA plasmids. The call for a MAQC-like platform comparison for RNASeq to identify issues and to evaluate platform-specific biases or strengths is being addressed by at least two consortia, the FDA's SEQC (MAQC-III) group and the Association of Biomolecular Resource Facilities – Next-Generation Sequencing (ABRF–NGS) group study. These results will be highly informative to the developers of clinical RNA sequencing (RNA-Seq) assays.

An emerging theme in the translational NGS community has been the utilization of RNASeq for detection of mutations (81, 82). Analysis pipelines that can account for factors like editing biases are not publicly available or are not sufficiently validated to allow such analysis in a clinical context, but once achieved these may offer a highly efficient method for capturing both mutational and expression level information in the same analysis (24, 83). Increasingly, studies that compare the benefits of both types of studies in combination with even epigenetic and microRNA signatures of the tumor for comprehensive profiling are likely to gain traction. The use of RNAseq instead of clinical DNASeq is likely to require a significant effort that includes matched RNAseq–DNAseq analysis and the development of sophisticated algorithms for analysis. Nonetheless, it appears likely that for at least certain molecular sub-types RNASeq-based gene expression profiling and analysis may provide a more predictive result than mutation based analysis alone.

POST-ANALYTICAL CHALLENGES

BIOINFORMATIC MUTATION CALLING ALGORITHMS

One of the major hurdles to adoption of NGS for CDxs is the current state of variability in the performance of variant calling software depending upon the bioinformatics pipeline used (84, 85). It is a routine occurrence that variations in mutation detection are observed from the same raw data set when utilizing different algorithms for variant calling, even with the assumption that similar pre-variant calling processing was performed on the final dataset (86). **Figure 1** is a high level schematic illustrating the basic steps in a bioinformatics pipeline to stress the number of steps and the complexity of variables that impact mutation detection. The initial sequencing data (DAT files) are derived from Illumina imaging data or Ion Torrent pH change related voltage data. Basecall (BCL) files contain data where the sequencing data (images or voltage) have been translated into a nucleotide call. Multiplexed data are then separated into per sample data via the sequencing index identity and FASTQ files are generated, which contain sequencing read data that include the sequence and an associated per base quality score, called a phred score or Q score (87,88). Reads are then aligned to a known reference sequence containing genomic coordinates and organized into BAM files (89). Variation analysis, or variant calling, refers to the assignment of

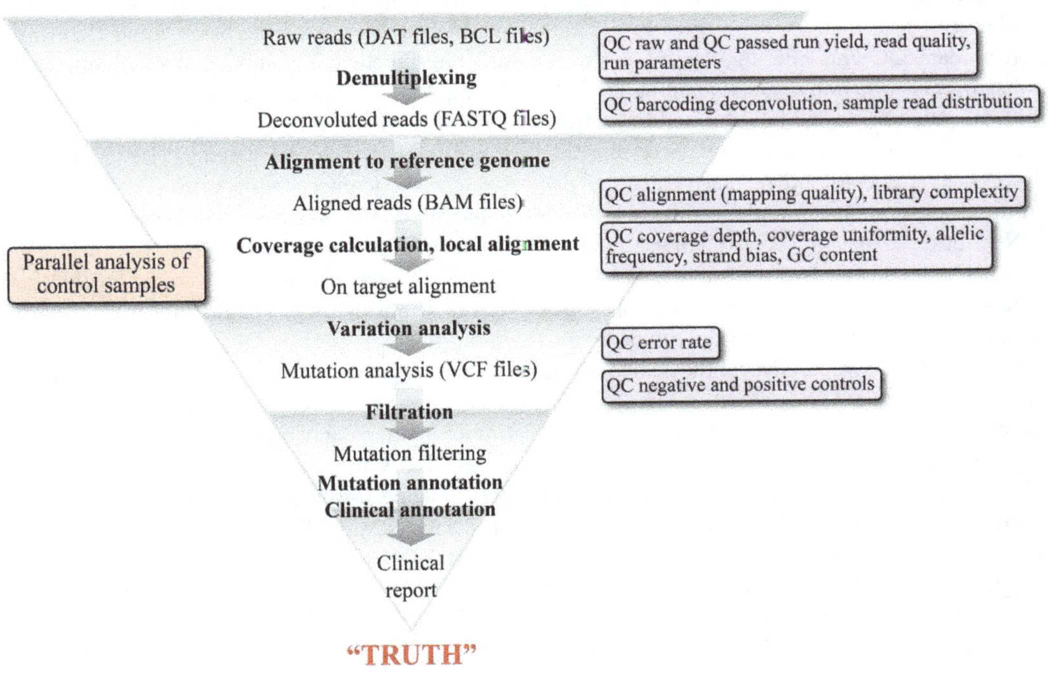

FIGURE 1 | Schematic representation of the various bioinformatics and statistical analysis steps of a typical clinical NGS variant detection data pipeline. The graphic illustrates the major modules of the pipeline and their output file types, beginning with raw reads (DAT files) and ending with a clinical report. The pipeline is highly tunable, as each of the steps can be optimized by adjusting parameters specific to each step. The triangular shape is intended to convey that each step acts as a filter to remove reads that do not represent variants. The key quality filters that can be applied are shown in the boxes to the right.

non-reference status (i.e., a mutation or a variant) to a specific queried position in the genome and generates a tab separated VCF. The variant calls are filtered to minimize false positives and false negatives while maintaining the sensitivity and specificity of the data by utilizing the phred quality scores, which vary on different platforms (63). To generate a clinically actionable report, the high confidence variants are unambiguously annotated based on clinical data showing a causal relationship between the variant and disease and with information about the variant in the literature (90, 91). A vast variety of software is available for each step of NGS data analysis, as are a number of bioinformatics suites designed specifically for Dx testing and which can be tailored to provide a streamlined, module locked analysis for Dx processing (63, 91). Some suites may also allow the user to change settings for test development purposes. Recently, the NIST spearheaded an effort (92) to develop a highly confident variant caller by encouraging the NGS community to share sequencing data of their NGS reference material NA12878 (v.2.15). This effort should greatly aid the standardization of analysis methodology and better QC for assessing false positives and false negatives (66, 92).

The traditional regulatory framework makes integration of the NGS data analysis software into the Dx device system imperative, with a fixed version of the analysis algorithm for the regulatory submission. This presents a challenge for the device developers since variant calling software applications are continually evolving, particularly in the ability to detect indels, in efforts to reduce analysis time and in the use of control set parallel analysis (41, 85, 86, 93). As new versions of variant calling software with better sensitivity and specificity become available, it is reasonable to assume, based on current precedent, that new 510(k) submissions will be required for these devices.

Standardization of data QC and filtering, variant detection and annotation of samples is imperative for developing Dx tests. Ideally, NGS-based data analysis should be subjected to rigorous internal and external QC with rules to accept or reject data akin to Westgard rules (94, 95) used for other analytical tests. The field is still open for discussions on how these rules should be implemented for NGS-based CTAs and Dx tests. For example, are traditional Westgard rules applicable to a quantitative parameter of NGS-based mutation detection tests such as mutation allele frequency? If not, then what type of quantitative rules can be used to establish in control processes? It is imperative for the field to define the type of control samples and the QC procedures to accept or reject runs. Some laboratories argue that internal control targets must also be met prior to a decision to report mutations (43, 85).

Another novel aspect of NGS mutation calling is that variants are rated based on the certainty of the call (87, 88). Phred quality values are assigned to specific steps in the process such as base calling and read alignment. Read depth, read quality, frequency of detection of the allele, strand bias, annotation as germline variant or variant of unknown significance, or lack of "actionability" all can be used to assign a confidence score to a particular call (57, 89, 96). Segregation of variants per characteristics of read depth, base quality, read quality, and strand bias are easily automatable with most Dx instruments available, but current software programs do not provide easy readout of mis-alignment-based read drops, reads that are exempted from final analysis by homopolymer-based inaccuracies, reference allele bias, or reference genome bias (60, 61, 97). These are post-analysis computing requirements that still need to be built into software to minimize operator involvement.

It is interesting to note that each sequencing platform has its particular advantages and drawbacks in terms of regional biases that complicate variant calling. In the past, Illumina MiSeq data have been associated with high accuracy but increased strand bias with GC-rich motifs, as well as low accuracy for homopolymer stretches beyond 20 bp (97, 98). In the November 2013 FDA 510(k) Decision Summary for the MiSeqDx instrument (Number k123989), Illumina specifically claims the ability to detect single nucleotide variants (SNVs) as well as deletions up to three bases. Based on a very limited data set, the instrument can also detect 1 bp insertions, but this is limited to non-homopolymer regions, since the MiSeqDx instrument was shown to have problems detecting 1 bp indels in homopolymer tracts, e.g., polyAs. The notification also states that Illumina's current MiSeqDx analysis software will automatically remove any homopolymer tracts of longer than eight continuous identical bases (R8 error). Interestingly, the MiSeqDx instrument claims to be a qualitative detection platform rather than quantitative. The MiSeq has generally been reported to have higher fidelity for indel calling than Ion Torrent (28, 61, 99). Ion Torrent homopolymer regions beyond 20 bp tend to be misaligned and discarded so that alignment algorithms must be optimized per region of interest to allow inclusion of misaligned regions (32, 61). The Ion Torrent Dx platform specifications will become clear when it is registered. Strand bias related inaccuracies and decreased depth of coverage or uneven coverage (due to allele dropout in case of sampling error or as a function of tumor heterogeneity) can also compound the problem of mutation calling inaccuracies. Accurate base calling algorithms for Dx assays must minimally utilize spike-in controls during technical feasibility experiments and raw data controls for software training that include mutation calls in regions of predicted poor base calling if those are part of the assay design (41, 43, 66). The use of a highly sequenced reference sample, such as NA12878 by NIST (v.2.15) for software training and algorithm development has been proposed in many forums such as the NIST "Genome in a Bottle" Consortium (92). Recently, the same was used by Illumina to demonstrate accuracy in its MiSeqDx platform 510(k) submission application. Additionally, it is reasonable to propose to include engineered mutations as part of spike-ins where inaccurate calls may result due to biases from GC-rich motifs, strand bias, reference allele bias, homopolymers, and regions of low coverage if down-sampling total calls for normalization, etc. For assessing the accuracy of the data pipeline, normal/reference sample pairs may be developed as proficiency testing (PT) material. Alternatively, specially designed artificial DNA mixtures that contain the majority of expected mutations (from literature and clinical findings) should be used as reference material in accuracy, sensitivity, and precision studies in the technical feasibility phase. The National Cancer Institute (NCI) initiative to make specific mutations available as plasmid constructs as well as the availability of characterized mutant DNA or recombinant tissues from companies like Horizon Dx are allowing test developers to devise such experiments with spike-in-based QC (43, 66). From its recent guidance on Personalized Medicine, the FDA also seems to acknowledge that testing of variant calling

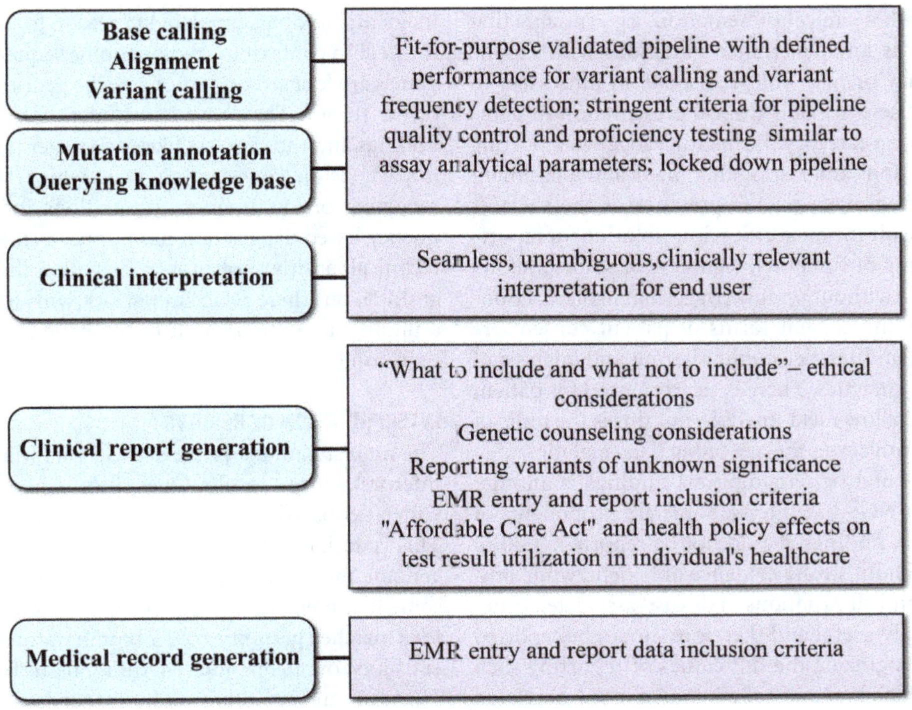

FIGURE 2 | Aspects and key considerations of clinical NGS data reporting. Main aspects of clinical data reporting are shown in ovals to the left; key considerations are shown in boxes to the right. The uppermost three aspects rely on the bioinformatic pipeline. What test results are reported in the clinical report (fourth oval) is influenced by socio-ethical considerations and may require genetic counseling and support systems. The evolving payer landscape and medical records guidance will affect how NGS clinical reports are captured in patient records.

for a specific set of mutations and the establishment of the platform's sensitivity and specificity may be sufficient for the clearance of a NGS-based regulated device. One novel aspect to the application of NGS-based tests is the need for a standardized set of raw data for mutation calling algorithm development. To meet this PT need, the NIST Genome in a Bottle Consortium as well as CAP have both been actively advocating availability of public data sets from extremely well studied samples as PT material to assess a particular pipeline's sensitivity and specificity in mutation detection to avoid lab to lab variation in mutation detection.

In addition to bioinformatics analysis for variant calling, there are several aspects of data interpretation and annotation that must be standardized for NGS tests to be adopted into clinical practice. These are graphically represented in **Figure 2** and are discussed below.

DATA REPORTING

If the FDA requirement for a NGS-based Dx approval is demonstration of accuracy and precision for each assayed base, it is possible that Dx developers may choose to limit the reportable content of a NGS panel by utilizing base masking in an effort to reduce the extent of analytical validation efforts. In the recent 510(k) application for the MiSeqDx instrument and the CFTR gene Dx test on the instrument, data showing the orthogonal validation of a subset of base positions was accepted, suggesting that the FDA may only require a sponsor to show performance data for the unmasked, reportable nucleotide positions on future submissions of panels or single-gene assays. It will be interesting to note the Agency's guidance on this topic since the masked data could potentially still be utilized for analysis to develop or enhance predictive mutation signatures on retrospective analysis.

Another key consideration for data reporting is the reporting of variants of unknown significance. The ACMG guidelines from 2008 (100) defined various cases of variants of unknown significance including: (1) previously unreported variations with possible ramifications for the disease being studied. This includes indels, frameshift mutations, and invariant splice site AG/GT nucleotides variants that can alter the reading frame and thus the expressed gene product. (2) Previously unreported variations that may or may not be causative of the condition. These are exemplified by missense changes, in-frame indels, and splice consensus sequence variants or cryptic splice sites that may affect regulatory processes, e.g., interruption of splicing enhancers or suppressor sites. In these cases, clarification of the clinical significance of variants is required and it may be important to flag them accordingly in a report. (3) Previously unreported variations that are probably not causative of disease, e.g., synonymous mutations that do not alter protein sequence or affect processing or regulatory pathways, or are found in addition to a variant known to be associated with pathologic change (in autosomal dominant disorders). (4) Previously reported sequence variations that are recognized as neutral variants with evidence available that the variation has been consistently observed in a normal population and does not associate with disease or predisposition to disease. (5) Sequence variation not known or expected to be causative of disease, but is found associated with a clinical presentation, e.g., variants that contribute to disease as low-penetrance mutations which alone or in combination may or may not predispose an individual to disease or modify the severity of a clinical presentation in complex disorders. For such a category the institute suggests reporting as not definitive mutations and stating that medical management decisions should not be made on the presence of the variants alone. This last is probably the most efficacious solution for reporting NGS-based variants of unknown significance since it allows capturing of the profile without unduly triggering medical actionability. Unfortunately, the current forms of patient consent are usually quite limiting and restrict public sharing and analysis of data utilizing big data analytics. There is clearly a need for patient consent agreements to allow meta-analysis, but this is the topic of the next section, data privacy in the age of big data analytics.

Reporting of incidental or serendipitous findings is another area of complexity for NGS-based tests. Some are proponents of the idea that incidental findings should not be reported at all in clinical sequencing without strong evidence of benefit, while others advocate that any and all variations in disease-associated genes are potentially medically useful and therefore should be reported (2, 17, 41, 44, 46). Recognizing the difficulties of reporting such secondary findings which are medically important but unrelated to the reason for test ordering, the ACMG constituted a special Working Group on Incidental Findings in Clinical Exome and Genome Sequencing to make recommendations for addressing such findings in pretest patient discussions, clinical testing, and the reporting of results (101). In the case of targeted oncology panels, this may not be an issue unless specific loci are associated with enhanced risk for other conditions or where particular polymorphisms can affect existing health care routines and drug regimens. Currently, the ACMG working group has only recommended reporting those incidental findings for which preventive measures or treatments are already available or for disorders in which patients are asymptomatic despite the presence of pathogenic mutations. Generally, the recommendation was to report pathogenic variants as incidental findings, e.g., those where the "sequence variation is previously reported and is a recognized cause of the disorder" or "sequence variation is previously unreported and is of the type, which is expected to cause the disorder" (100). These two were chosen no doubt because the group recognized that attempting to report and interpret variants of unknown significance as incidental findings would be particularly challenging. The report also stressed that identification of monogenic diseases via a clinical NGS panel as an incidental finding is highly improbable by current practice.

PRIVACY OF AND ACCESS TO PATIENT RESULTS

Ever since the report that individuals could be identified from anonymous NGS data (102), privacy groups have been justified in their concerns about having sensitive data made public as a result of inappropriately controlled data and reports. Privacy of patient results is also linked to maintaining the highest standards for patient consent to NGS-based testing, anonymized data generation, secure data storage, encryption, and transfer processes that meet the highest standards data (103). The converse of this concern relates to the data that reported back to the patient, especially incidental findings unrelated to reason for which the test was performed. In contrast to whole genome sequencing, oncology-based panels are focused on tumor specific genes assessed in the context of the tumor. They have less content with associated incidental findings and thus are less likely to trigger traditional socio-ethical impact (104). However, an issue which lacks resolution is the reporting of low frequency mutations for which the allele frequency based drug action has not been studied. For example, the technical sensitivity of an assay may allow the detection of a mutant at 0.1%, but there is no framework with which to interpret such a finding, and reporting it to the patient may cause more harm than good.

INTERPRETATION OF RESULTS

The mainstream adoption of NGS Dxs will rely heavily on easily interpretable test results. One critical aspect of data interpretation with NGS-based tests is the comparative reference human genome. This is an individual genome and may not be an ideal reference genome for most individuals in the population. For this reason, some commercial NGS providers have started stressing the need for a matched germline control comparator sample such as peripheral blood or normal adjacent tumor tissue from tested individuals. The constant evolution and enhanced annotation of the reference genome as sequencing-based studies continue to reveal new genomic complexities also confounds interpretation. In the example from the MiSeqDx 510(k) decision summary, it is interesting to note that a compound reference genome derived from two well-characterized samples was utilized in addition to human genome build 19 [NCBI Human reference February, 2009 (GRCh37/hg19) assembly] [FDA 510(k) K123989 decision summary]. For example, the two genomes differed in a particular homopolymer run, which was a run of 14 A's according human genome 19, while the sequence in the composite reference genome had a run of 15 A's. This was significant because it directly impacted interpretation of the MiSeqDx sequencing accuracy study, since all 13 samples analyzed were reported as having 1 bp insertions since 15 A's were detected in all 13 samples. As new variants and polymorphisms are identified, it may be warranted to re-annotated or re-issued reports to include the new data or its new interpretation.

OVERVIEW OF DIAGNOSTIC TEST REGULATORY APPROVAL PROCESS

As a prelude to the regulatory challenges, we digress to provide an overview of the Dx test regulatory approval process. The basic regulatory pathway options for Dx device development are summarized in **Figure 3**. This section describes a generic IVD submission process with the authors' comments on possible paths for NGS-based devices.

For any given test that is submitted for FDA consideration, the route to commercialization may be via a 510(k)/pre-market notification process or via a PMA application. The decision to take a NGS-based clinical test via the 510(k) or PMA process will depend largely upon the perceived risk associated with the Dx device. The 510(k) Dx IVD process relies on the presence of a predicate device or devices. However, FDA has utilized the *de novo* 510(k) pathway when the risks of the new device are consistent with other

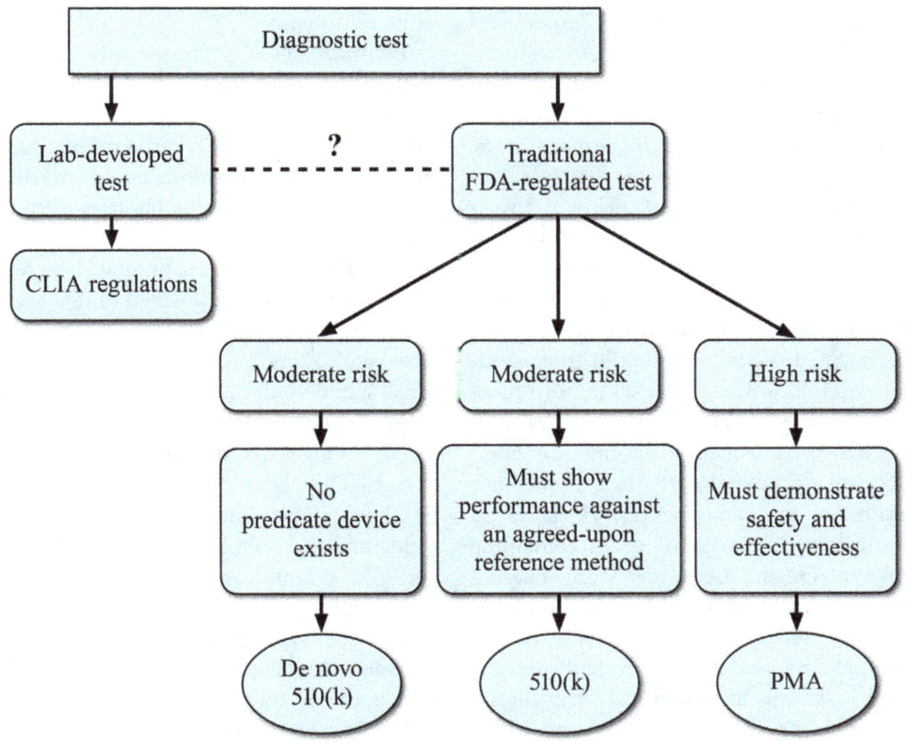

FIGURE 3 | Regulatory models for development of NGS-based diagnostics. The FDA device classification for a regulated NGS-based diagnostic device will depend on the perceived risk associated with the diagnostic device.

510(k)-cleared devices but a clear predicate is not available. The 510(k) process may be appropriate for those NGS-based tests that will be utilized for monitoring disease or for tests where the perceived risks are lower. Although the concept of a predicate device is woven into FDA's device regulation, the reality for the genetic tests that have been cleared or approved to date is the new system is not compared head-to-head with a previously cleared system. Rather, the new method is compared to a gold standard method, which is considered truth. For most DNA applications, the gold standard has been bi-directional Sanger sequencing. Applications which have relatively higher perceived risk to the patient, such as NGS-based oncology tests, will likely be required to go the PMA route to demonstrate safety and efficacy. In these cases, a reference method will also be used to demonstrate accuracy of the device.

A PMA submission for a CDx NGS test will entail coordinated review of the drug by the Center for Drug Evaluation and Research (CDER) and of the device by the CDRH (or CBER for certain disease indications). The IVD developer will have to demonstrate the safety and effectiveness of the *in vitro* Dx device when used as specified in the label. The Dx device must be considered as an entire Dx system including reagents, hardware, software, data analysis, and result reporting. Use of the device in the pharmaceutical clinical trial will provide important data to demonstrate clinical validation of the assay. Although NGS IVD submitters may have to undergo an advisory panel review regarding clinical, regulatory, scientific and statistical issues due to the novelty of the NGS platform and assay structure and readout, it seems doubtful since other CDx applications have not had this hurdle and FDA has seen fit to clear the Illumina platform with no such advisory panel requirement. For an approved PMA any modifications to the test or device, manufacturing process, its labeling, intended use or sensitivity or specificity would require FDA notification and prior approval. In general, it is imperative that NGS-based Dx stakeholders seek clarity utilizing pre-submission meetings with the CDRH, and specifically the Office of *In vitro* Diagnostics and Radiological Health (OIR), well in advance of trial planning. It is important to engage in such discussions early as FDA thinking is evolving rapidly.

Many of the regulatory challenges for CDxs are not unique to NGS. Although NGS tests may be more complex than other technologies, the same principles will apply. The FDA's expectations on the analytical validation and performance characteristics of NGS-based assays will differ somewhat for each individual assay. However, the 510(k) clearance of Illumina MiSeqDx reveals some aspects of the regulatory agency's viewpoint on validation. Since this is the crux of the regulatory challenge, we summarize in detail the main aspects of Illumina's 510(k) submission studies [510(k) summary, e.g., K124006, November 2013] as early pointers to the type of experiments FDA may expect.

510(k) CLEARANCE OF ILLUMINA MiSeqDx

With the MiSeqDx clearance, the FDA has given some indication the type of information that will be required for approval a NGS-based CDx for tumor mutation status. First, the 510(k) summary indicates that accuracy data for all claimed specimen types and nucleic acid types were required. Two sources of well-characterized samples (based on well validated sequencing methods) were queried with all of the claimed sequence variation types, types of sequencing and with the sequences located in varying sequence context (e.g., different chromosomes, GC-rich regions). The 510(k) summary indicates that sequence data generated with a sequencing technology platform and variant calling method independent of the device manufacturer is required for at least one of the reference samples. Percent agreement and percent disagreement with the reference sequences were described for all the regions that were queried by the instrument. Illumina performed accuracy testing in three studies. The first assessed overall accuracy over a wide portion of the genome by utilizing 13 very well-characterized samples from parent–child triads that had been sequenced by multiple laboratories and multiple sequencing technologies. Human reference genome 19 was used to assess accuracy across 24,434 bases on 19 chromosomes encompassing a variety of genes containing potentially clinically relevant exons. The second study assessed the accuracy of the MiSeqDx instrument at 17 highly confident variant calls in the NIST NA12878 standard reference material. The third accuracy study assessed the instrument's performance in detecting small insertions and deletions by analyzing six samples using the Cystic Fibrosis 139 Variant Assay, which included a subset of clinically significant indels in *CFTR*. The detected insertions and deletions were all confirmed with bidirectional Sanger sequencing as the reference method. Such accuracy studies helped Illumina define its performance specifications for homopolymer stretches, nucleotide repeat regions, and ability to detect indels.

For precision/reproducibility studies, the 510(k) summary indicates that data should be generated using on multiple instruments, with multiple operators and at multiple sites, and that performance data are required for all claimed specimen types, nucleic acid types, sequence variation types, and types of sequencing. As discussed in the Assay Design, a special emphasis was given to variants located in varying sequence context, such as different chromosomes and GC-rich regions, along with a requirement to utilize a high confidence reference sequence data. To this end, Illumina performed three precision studies. For the first study, 13 well-characterized sequenced samples were analyzed in 9 runs using 3 different MiSeqDx instruments and 3 different operators. Samples NA12877 and NA12878 were run in duplicate to assess repeatability. Ninety-four samples and two non-template controls were tested across three lots to establish lot-to-lot reproducibility of the Illumina universal reagents. Each lot was split into two 48-sample runs to test reagents and all possible index primer combinations. All sequencing runs were completed by a single operator and on a single MiSeqDx instrument to remove potential variance contribution from operator or instrument. The MiSeqDx Cystic Fibrosis 139 Variant Assay reproducibility study involved a blinded study with three trial sites and two operators per site. Two well-characterized panels of 46 samples each were used for testing. These contained a mix of genomic DNA (gDNA) from cell lines with known variants in the *CFTR* gene and variant containing cell lines spiked into leukocyte-depleted blood to assess variability from the gDNA extraction steps.

Illumina also addressed the issues of sample cross-contamination (carryover) and intra-run performance. For intra-run performance, a 48-sample library of two samples with unique variants arrayed in a checkerboard of an alternating high concentration (500 ng) and low concentration (100 ng) input was utilized. For inter-run carryover 2 libraries were prepared each with 47 replicates of a single gDNA sample and 1 no template control (NTC). The samples were unique in each library and continuous run assessment was performed to demonstrate absence of carryover. The reproducibility and accuracy of multiplexing was also tested with 12 indices (barcodes) per sample sequenced. Accuracy for all sample/index primer combinations was confirmed as 100% by Sanger bi-directional sequencing and PCR-based confirmation.

For testing the contribution of common interfering substances to variability, four endogenous interfering substances (bilirubin, hemoglobin, cholesterol, and triglycerides) were spiked in eight unique whole blood samples. Blood collection variability and gDNA sample preparation variability were also evaluated, along with sample input amounts, thermal cycler effects, and sample stability. DNA extraction methods were assessed using 168 specimens (14 samples × 2 operators/extraction method × 3 runs/operator × 2 replicates/extracted gDNA sample).

The MiSeqDx approval gives insight into some of the regulatory expectations for NGS-based assays and is summarized here with some general headers for reader clarity:

Specimen and processing-related validation:

(i) The specimen type(s) as source of nucleic acid.
(ii) The type(s) of nucleic acids (e.g., germline DNA, tumor DNA).
(iii) The nucleic acid extraction method(s).

Sequencing variation-related validation:

(i) Type(s) of sequence variations (e.g., SNVs, insertions, and deletions).
(ii) Type(s) of sequencing (e.g., targeted sequencing).
(iii) The read depth required for the sensitivity being claimed and the validation data that supports those claims.
(iv) Accuracy and precision of the test and the types of sequence variations that the test cannot detect with the claimed accuracy and precision (e.g., insertions or deletions larger than a certain size, translocations)
(v) The upper and lower limit of input nucleic acid to achieve the claimed accuracy and reproducibility.

The MiSeqDx instrument's current *de novo* classification is for qualitative assessment for profiling of peripheral whole blood samples, which tend to be of a higher quality. It is important to note new tests, including CDx devices, on the platform are likely to require PMA submissions, especially for tests utilizing heterogeneous samples like tumors. The current MiSeqDx clearance for qualitative results opens the discussion on what further validation strategies may be required to achieve quantitative detection of mutations (e.g., quantitative allele frequency), which may be one of the strengths of clinical NGS.

UNANSWERED ANSWERED REGULATORY QUESTIONS

HOW MANY MUTATIONS WILL HAVE TO BE CLINICALLY VALIDATED?

The FDA has hinted at possible accuracy requirements for complex, multi-analyte specific assays, genes, and panels at the DIA Meeting on Personalized Medicine and CDxs (November 6, 2013). This provides important insight for CDx applications involving tumor suppressor genes and certain oncogenes since actionable mutations may occur anywhere along the length of the gene. FDA has suggested three potential strategies:

- Sequence clinical samples from the intended use population and compare to reference method results.
- Sequence procured samples that span the relevant classes of variants and compare to reference method results.
- Sequence well-characterized reference sample(s) and compare to reference sequence.

CAN AN NGS MULTI-GENE OR MULTI-TRANSCRIPT PANEL BE APPROVED AS A DIAGNOSTIC PLATFORM, ALLOWING MULTIPLE CDx SUBMISSIONS?

At the 2012 Friends of Cancer Meeting the FDA publicly indicated their interest in reviewing NGS-based cancer panels similar to the panels that have been cleared as microbiology devices (i.e., devices that detect multiple viruses and bacteria in a single product) (105) (focr.org). Although the details of this type of submission would need to be worked out between FDA and an individual sponsor, it seems likely that some level of clinical evidence would be needed for each gene or mutation included on the panel. It is possible, similar to the cystic fibrosis assays, that this list could be developed based on medical input and literature. From that point, more specific claims about individual genes could be made on a gene-by-gene basis including CDx claims if the product has been used as part of a clinical trial investigating a particular drug. It is likely that any cancer panel would be subject to a PMA [rather than a 510(k)], and amendments to the original PMA with additional claims on a per panel member basis would be a rational approach to updating the claims for each new CDx.

HOW WILL EXISTING GENOMIC DIAGNOSTICS ALIGN WITH APPROVED NGS-BASED DIAGNOSTICS?

Currently, the intended use statement for each of the Dxs that have been approved in conjunction with a drug list the drug name in the intended use statement. It is reasonable to expect that this policy will continue and that in order for a drug and Dx to be co-marketed the drug and device will need to be linked. Even if there are multiple devices available for testing in conjunction with a specific drug, any of the approved devices will be allowed.

WHAT IS THE APPROPRIATE ORTHOGONAL TECHNOLOGY?

What is the true measure of truth when comparing discordant results? FDA has shown with the recent Illumina clearance that they expect NGS-based mutation calls to be confirmed by an orthogonal technology (in many cases bi-directional sequencing). However, disagreement exists within the NGS community as to what is true orthogonal validation of a NGS-based mutation call (17, 64, 106). The enhanced sensitivity of mutation detection down to 1–5% allele frequency implies that orthogonal validation will require a platform with similar sensitivity. While Sanger sequencing is being used to support mutation validation, for example in the Illumina MiSeqDx 510(k) clearance, it is not possible to use Sanger data to provide a definitive call when mutations in the range of 1–15%. Generally, if NGS and Sanger give discordant results labs tend to use tie breaker tests such as pyrosequencing or Sequenom-based sequencing on the MassArray system. Both of these technologies can detect mutant allele frequencies down to 5–10% frequency and are finding increasing usage in NGS validation. As Sequenom and pyrosequencing vendors create niche products tailored for NGS validation these will likely integrate into clinical NGS workflows. The FDA has shown flexibility in allowing use of these types of technology as orthogonal methods when Sanger is not sensitive enough. However, the FDA will insist on appropriate validation of these methods and will expect to review these validation packages as part of the review process.

Another approach, likely to be costlier but with the opportunity to have near equivalent sensitivity of detection, is the utilization of a second NGS technology for confirmation of assay results, e.g., utilizing both the Illumina and Ion Torrent platforms where the difference in underlying technology make a confirmation of positive results quite robust. The main issue to be cognizant of is the need to adjust analysis parameters to provide equivalent performance with respect to mutation call sensitivity, since each platform uses its unique quality score for data quality assessment. For example, while Ion Torrent recommends using a phred value of Q20 (99% specificity) for high confidence variant analysis, Illumina recommends at phred value of Q30 (99.9% specificity) for ensuring high confidence calls (61). The difference in acceptable phred scale values arises from differences in platform technology, related background signal and noise calculation algorithms (107).

STRATEGIC CHALLENGES FOR DRUG AND DIAGNOSTIC DEVELOPERS

Developing any CDx can be enormously challenging, as seen in the development of the *BRAF* mutation (108) and *ALK* gene fusion (109, 110) tests. A primary reason is that the device development timeline does not align with the drug development timeline, as illustrated in a development timeline chart (**Figure 4**) (15, 108, 111). Ideally, CDx development for the NGS assay would start with the initiation of early phase studies (Ph1/2a studies in **Figure 4**) to allow sufficient time for development of the Investigational Use Only (IUO) version of the device before start of the phase 3 pivotal trials. But this is not often the case, and compromises and work-around strategies are sometimes necessary. Thus, in another example of navigating the rapids, pharmaceutical and Dx companies face some unique challenges in NGS-based CDx development, which are summarized in the next sections.

DRUG DEVELOPMENT CHALLENGE 1 – IS A COMPANION DIAGNOSTIC NEEDED?

The first challenge is whether a co-Dx test is in fact required and how a multiplexed RNA- or DNA-based NGS panel would fit into the traditional CDxs scheme. While a CDx may uniquely position the drug in the marketplace, the overarching reason for developing

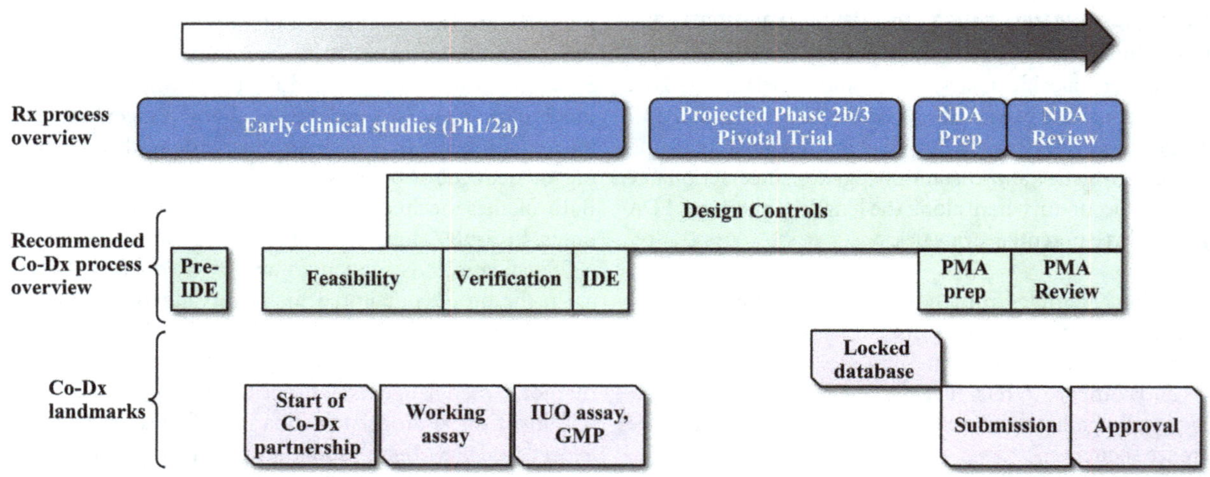

FIGURE 4 | Coordination of drug and device development for a successful companion diagnostic submission. Drug companies and diagnostic developers may work together in several different cost sharing and assay development landmark payment formats for the development of the final IVD product.

a CDx is because it is required for the drug approval. The current FDA guidance dictates that if the test is necessary for the safe and effective use of the drug, then a co-Dx is required. The key factor to determining whether a CDx is required is the efficacy of the drug in a biomarker negative population. If efficacy in the biomarker negative population is sufficient for drug approval, then a CDx may not be required, at least for an initial approval. Thus, this question should be answered early in drug development (12, 109). It appears that NGS-based CDxs will be more relevant in the near future in certain oncology indications where genetically targeted therapies are currently prevalent, such as lung cancer, breast cancer, and colorectal cancer.

DRUG DEVELOPMENT CHALLENGE 2 – USE A SINGLE-GENE ASSAY OR MULTI-GENE PANEL?

At one level, the question seems to challenge one of the guiding principles of Dx development: the simpler the better. Analytical validation of a multi-gene assay, as discussion elsewhere in this article, will undeniably be more work than validation of a single gene. Yet, it might be necessary to consider the pursuit of the multi-transcript or multi-gene panel in some cases such as if the predictive biomarker is a set of mutations in the genes on the panel, i.e., if the marker is a signature for response rather than a single Dx gene mutation. The multi-gene panel approach is predicated on two assumptions: (1) that the FDA will permit the sponsor to mask data from genes that are not required for safe and effective use of the companion therapeutic, and (2) that the FDA will permit different levels of rigor in the validation of genes on the panel, based on whether they are necessary for safe and effective use of the companion therapeutic. The authors firmly believe that the multi-gene panel is a step toward the "multi-gene Dx/many drugs" model even though the path there is not obvious. One of the reasons that the change from "one-drug/one-gene Dx" model to the "multi-gene Dx/many drugs" model will be so disruptive is that the test results from a multiplexed panel could actually lead to the use of a competitor's drug. This leads to the next challenge of how best to design clinical studies to best take advantage of all the content on the NGS assay.

DRUG DEVELOPMENT CHALLENGE 3 – OPTIMAL TRIAL DESIGN FOR NGS-BASED DIAGNOSTICS?

By definition precision medicine focuses on a subpopulation of patients expected to respond to a given therapeutic. Sometimes the population can be quite small, as in the case of metastatic lung cancer patients with the ALK gene fusion, for which crizotinib is indicated (112, 113). Only about 5% of lung cancer patients have the ALK gene fusion (113, 114), which means a great deal of screening was required to identify and enroll patients in the crizotinib studies. This was very inefficient compared to a "basket trial" design (115) in which patients are screened simultaneously for a large number of genetic aberrations using a multi-gene panel to determine their eligibility for a large number of clinical trials involving different therapeutic interventions. Some forward-looking models in this area propose a multi-institution collaboration that employs a multi-gene panel assay in which the cost of the screening assay (including validation) is shared by different drug development entities (49, 115, 116). While this approach would significantly reduce the cost of screening patients for rare subpopulations of patients in PhII and PhIII trials for each individual company, it presents the equally interesting question of whether drug developers will collaborate with competitors in such basket trials. The Friends of Cancer Research initiative for enrollment of patients with advanced NSCLC into trials matched by their tumor profile is one of the first examples of this kind of study (49). The trial seeks to utilize a NGS panel-based approach for enrolling patients into the most suitable trial using an adaptive trial design that allocates patients to suitable drugs from different pharmaceutical participants. It includes five drugs from five different companies and will employ the FM NGS-based panel assay to guide subject assignment and is expected to launch in spring 2014 (116). Overall, drug developers and Dx companies will have to work together to navigate this disorderly transition in testing paradigm (12).

DRUG DEVELOPMENT CHALLENGE 4 – WHEN TO COMMIT TO CO-DIAGNOSTIC DEVELOPMENT?

An important question arises as to when the pharmaceutical company should invest in the NGS co-Dx development process. The best guidance would dictate that CDx assay development must begin at least 18–24 months prior to the start of the registrational studies to allow sufficient time for development of the IUO assay for demonstration of clinical utility in the registrational trial. The Dx development plan depends on many factors such as complexity of the assay, cost of pre-investment, strength of the data confirming the biomarker hypothesis, as well as timeline of drug registration (e.g., whether a traditional Phase 2 to Phase 3 transition timeline is expected) (117). Therefore, variation to the ideal development timeline is often observed and drug companies and Dx developers utilize different developmental strategies to develop the final IVD product with significant investment by both parties (**Figure 4**). Development of a CDx test typically links the market uptake and return on investment of Dx device to the performance of the companion drug in pivotal clinical trials. As a consequence, the cost of development may require creative cost sharing and milestone payment agreements between the pharmaceutical and Dx partner. Some of the plausible developmental strategies possible for current NGS-based Dxs may be summarized as follows:

(i) Linear, risk-averse development model: in this model, development proceeds by a linear, logical flow, minimizing investment risk by delaying decisions as long as possible. CDx development is only begun after the need for a CDx is unequivocally established or until after initial data show the therapeutic has efficacy. Although avoiding pre-investment in Dx development until it is clearly needed may appear to be wise, in reality this may be a poor strategy because once it is clear that the drug is effective, there will be a great urgency to initiate the pivotal studies. The second aspect of risk aversion is the desire to avoid a bridging strategy for the Dx, i.e., starting the Ph3 studies with CTA instead of an IVD-ready version of the Dx (i.e., the IUO version of the assay) and then transitioning, i.e., bridging, to the IUO version by re-analyzing all (or nearly all) of the samples on the IUO version of the assay. This transition introduces significant risk into the process, so avoiding bridging is a good plan, but the cost is a significant delay in the start of the pivotal trial.

(ii) Pre-investment model: the Dx partnership is finalized and the IVD assay development starts prior to the initiation of the Phase 2 study, allowing sufficient time for development of the IUO assay to be completed prior to the Phase 3 start. In this case, the Dx development risk is low, but the Dx utility and therapeutic development risks are high. This is because the Dx development starts before the therapeutic is shown to be effective and before the Dx is shown to be required. Thus, the key risks are the uncertainty of biomarker's clinical utility and the therapeutic's clinical efficacy from Phase 2 data. Although the therapeutic sponsor partner may essentially partially fund Dx development as part of the Dx agreement, the therapeutic sponsor does not absorb all the risk. Dx companies have limited resources and have to select partnerships most likely to lead to a successful Dx product launch. In other words, one of the risks felt by the Dx company is opportunity cost if the program is canceled for any reason, including the failure of the therapeutic.

(iii) Bridging strategy + partial pre-investment. In cases where the traditional 18–24-month window for pivotal trial start is not possible, this model may be utilized to allow a pivotal trial start in a timely manner. This is a very expensive strategy with the drug sponsor absorbing most of the risk. IVD assay developments starts with a prototype assay (non-NGS or NGS-based) and bridging studies proceed as soon as an IUO version of NGS-based assay is ready. This strategy suffers from having high sample requirements as well as necessitating sample stability studies.

DRUG DEVELOPMENT CHALLENGE 5 – TYPE OF A CDx DEVICE: LDT OR KIT?

Many of the early leaders in precision medicine, realizing the possible complexity of the traditional PMA regulatory path for CDx kit development, may consider the LDT IVD model for their therapeutic that requires an *in vitro* Dx. This scenario could arise if the drug maker wants to avoid a large upfront investment in a CDx effort and has identified a reliable partner that can develop an acceptable assay, support clinical trials and provide worldwide access to the assay in their laboratory. The LDT route might also be selected if the company only recognizes it needs an IVD late in clinical development (i.e., in PhII) and wants to avoid a bridging strategy. Even though an LDT can receive FDA-clearance through the 510(k) process (118, 119), it seems likely that the FDA would require the LDT to go through the PMA process. Thus, the main advantage of the LDT route would be to avoid investment in a traditional kit and to avoid a delay related to the development of the IUO device. The current debate on stricter regulation of LDTs may play an important role in such decisions (75 FR 34463, 2010). Variability in LDT design and the increase in number of LDTs over 510(k)-cleared Dx devices is a growing concern (14), since it would take enormous efforts to standardize LDTs to achieve universally accepted tests. Standardization and strict regulation of CLIA NGS LDTs may be the practical scenario encountered most in next few years. As the FDA's guidance and recommendations for LDT regulation become clear and start getting enforced, the clinical NGS field will see standardization at many diverse levels, e.g., controls used in assays, reagents/panels, assay QC parameters and rules for accepting or failing data, bioinformatics pipelines and biostatistics modules, interpretation of data, reporting of data, etc. Key considerations must include early adoption of the Dx assay, preferably prior to pivotal studies. As discussed under time line constraints and in **Figure 4**, not many current NGS-based assays are suitable as Dxs or are ready to be developed into a regulated Dx.

DRUG DEVELOPMENT CHALLENGE 6 – HOW SHOULD CLINICAL ACTIONABILITY BE DEFINED?

While detection of low frequency mutations is one of the great promises of a NGS-based Dx, detection of very low frequency mutations in a Dx test requires several serious design considerations as well. For example, even if a test is technically able to detect a very low frequency mutation (e.g., $<1\%$), the presence of the mutation may not correlate with therapeutic response since the majority of the tumor (>99%) ultimately does not carry the said mutation. In this case, reporting of the detected mutation may require special consideration. For example, if the said mutation were present at 5% allele frequency, the Dx might report the mutation present and qualify the patient for treatment with the paired pharmaceutical, but if at 0.5%, it might not. In other words, a scenario is possible where patients with a low frequency mutation detected by a Dx test may be ineligible for a clinical trial due to mutation frequency actionability thresholds (41, 120). However, while not "pharmacologically" actionable, the 0.5% mutation detected would likely require reporting for follow-up. Ultimately clinical utility of low frequency mutations will be demonstrated by clinical response, which will provide clarity on what level of sensitivity of mutation detection is acceptable for drug labeling. Similarly, tumor heterogeneity may reveal mutations in a gene or transcriptional changes that are not yet clinically actionable.

DRUG DEVELOPMENT CHALLENGE 7 – WHAT IS THE EX-US REGULATORY ENVIRONMENT FOR NGS DIAGNOSTICS?

In some situations, the Dx that supports approval of a drug outside of the US will be different than the assay that is approved by FDA. This can be due to a number of factors including the US testing being a lab-based assay or the readiness of the Dx company to support distribution worldwide. Additionally, it is particularly important that the policies governing genetic data collection, reporting, and analysis be clear from the start of a Dx program in a territory. In the EU for example, a CDx is not specifically formally classified, though the regulations may change soon (121). However, the test must be CE marked under the EU IVDs Directive (122, 123). The clinical trial use of the test can then be included in the label following a European Commission approval.

DIAGNOSTIC DEVELOPMENT CHALLENGE 1 – ADDITIONAL REGULATORY GUIDANCE

Through the MiSeqDx decision summary, Dx companies are just now getting a glimpse into FDA thinking regarding NGS technology and the use of multi-gene panels. The FDA has indicated that a guidance on regulated NGS assays is due in 2014 and has proposed that individual companies request early pre-submission meetings with the Agency to discuss Dx development plans and trial design. It is encouraging that FDA officials have offered at public forums personal opinions that convey the Agency's enthusiasm about the technology and its application for therapy, as well as the recognition of the inevitability of usage of NGS-based tests in public health (focr.org). The FDA has encouraged early and open dialog on the NGS CDx process and has implied that the process, in spite of its complexity, is likely to be facilitated in a manner as similar as possible to that done for existing complex Dx assays.

DIAGNOSTIC DEVELOPMENT CHALLENGE 2 – COMPETITION FROM LDTs

The current environment is one in which NGS-based lab-developed tests are rapidly gaining popularity in the healthcare community and the growing use of NGS-based cancer genome profiling may be pushing the community toward a fast adoption of NGS-based tests. Although there are several sets of guidelines and recommendations (CLIA, CAP, and state guidances) (43, 44) describing the validation and use of existing NGS LDTs, the FDA has indicated that regulation may be necessary to stop the growth of less rigorously validated assays and to reduce the risk to patients. The oncology community's clamor for an information rich NGS Dx is possibly similar to the initial excitement around using microarrays as Dxs, with the goal of having a single comprehensive test that captures a large amount of relevant content. Tests that identify patients that benefit, or not benefit, from certain treatments represent new opportunities and a new market for some companies. Many different types of companies are building research usage only (RUO) cancer panels in the expectation that they could be adopted as LDTs. Other companies are setting up laboratories or expanding their current laboratory capabilities to offer LDT cancer panels and other NGS-based tests (47, 124). The latter represent a significant threat for Dx companies and may make them hesitant to invest heavily in developing an FDA-approved Dx product, especially as less regulated LDTs continue to increase their segment of the Dx market. For example, the recently FDA-approved molecular Dx BRAF V600E test was followed by the development and rapid uptake of cheaper LDTs. FDA recently issued a guidance document (Distribution of IVD Products labeled for Research Use Only or IUO) which may address some of the issues with RUO marketing in particular.

DIAGNOSTIC COMPANY CHALLENGE 3 – LDT VERSUS IVD KIT CONSIDERATIONS

Both LDTs and kit-based Dxs are considered to be *in vitro* Dxs by the FDA, and either can go through the PMA process. Thus, one of the major decisions for NGS-based Dxs developers will be choosing between development of a LDT (currently working under enforcement discretion from FDA regulation) or a commercialized kit-based FDA-approved product. In this context drug companies can choose to partner with "traditional Dx companies" which do not work with a LDT model (they don't have or want a CLIA service lab) or with "Lab-focused Dxs companies" which have a CLIA service lab and that could potentially offer an LDT-based Dx.

Currently, the NGS-based genetic tests on the market are all CLIA/CAP-regulated lab-developed tests (11). To date, none of these tests have been cleared or approved through FDA's stringent pre-marketing review process, which verifies the performance claims of the test. To date only a very small number of molecular genetic tests have FDA approval for marketing as CDxs. Examples of FDA-approved kitted CDxs are the Roche COBAS 4800 test for BRAF V600E mutation detection as a CDx for vemurafenib (Zelboraf) and the Abbott Vysis ALK Break Apart FISH Probe test to identify ALK-positive NSCLC patients for Pfizer's approved NSCLC therapy Xalkori (Crizotinib) (108, 109, 113, 125). There is a separate class of lab-based, FDA-cleared IVDs, e.g., the Agendia MammaPrint assay (126) and the XDx AlloMap assay (127). The largest class of genetic tests is currently unregulated clinical lab-developed tests. Clinical labs are overseen and regulated by the Centers for Medicare and Medicaid Services (CMS) with the CLIA certification process (40). Lab-developed test markets have grown mainly because the FDA approval process is time-consuming and very expensive (117). The extensive clinical validation and design control requirements expected in FDA-regulated IVD products are deterring many companies from submitting their NGS-based tests for the IVD process. At the same time, valid concerns about the lack of regulatory oversight that allows tremendous variability in test results from LDTs have led to a call for stricter regulation of the LDT (14). The FDA has sought more involvement in LDT regulation for a while now and there is increasing indication that LDT regulation will be on FDA's agenda as evident in FDA's Guidance on Personalized Medicine from October 2013. In 2010, FDA announced plans to expand its regulation to lab-developed genetic tests. This announcement led to heated debate within the industry (117). While this is yet to happen, it may impact the clinical LDT format of NGS assays should they become a specific CDx that requires FDA clearance or approval.

CONCLUDING THOUGHTS

We have provided a summary of the practical challenges to the widespread adoption of NGS-based CTAs and their further development as CDxs. For some challenges we suggested possible remedies that alleviate some of these concerns; for others we framed the relevant questions from a stakeholder's perspective.

It is certain that despite the challenges, in the near future NGS-based Dxs will be a major component of the highly remunerative personalized medicine and Dx industry. What was said about genome sequencing may also be true for clinical NGS-based Dx testing: that we may be overestimating the impact in the short run but we are probably underestimating the impact in the long run (original quote is attributed to renowned futurist Roy Amara). It is a certainty that the healthcare system will be transformed if the technology is embraced and implemented into clinical practice with its full potential. We project that a variety of NGS Dx associated companies or specializations will see exponential growth as they aid the simplification of NGS in the clinic, especially those that offer easy-to-use clinical interpretation interfaces or EMR data incorporation methodologies. It is also foreseeable that clinical NGS will be coupled with methods for minimally invasive monitoring utilizing bio-fluid-based assays instead of traditional tissue biopsies. It is also notable that as pharmaceutical companies and healthcare systems drive clinical NGS into practice, several models for global collaboration between pharmaceutical companies may arise which can help the field of personalized medicine move forward exponentially.

ACKNOWLEDGMENTS

We thank Steven Engel, Ken Emancipator, and Mya Thomae for reading the manuscript and making helpful suggestions. We acknowledge the NGS diagnostic teams at Illumina (Nitin Udar, Naomi O'Grady, and Alex Young) and Life Technologies (Jill Stefanelli and Brian Kelly) for helpful discussions around the CTA and diagnostic aspects of their platforms. We thank Gary Latham, Matt Hawryluk, Nazneen Aziz, Anup Madan, and Seth Crosby for stimulating discussions.

REFERENCES

1. Garraway LA. Genomics-driven oncology: framework for an emerging paradigm. *J Clin Oncol* (2013) **31**(15):1806–14. doi:10.1200/JCO.2012.46.8934
2. Williams ES, Hegde M. Implementing genomic medicine in pathology. *Adv Anat Pathol* (2013) **20**(4):238–44. doi:10.1097/PAP.0b013e3182977199
3. Aftimos PG, Barthelemy P, Awada A. Molecular biology in medical oncology: diagnosis, prognosis, and precision medicine. *Discov Med* (2014) **17**(92): 81–91.
4. Gerlinger M, Rowan AJ, Horswell S, Larkin J, Endesfelder D, Gronroos E, et al. Intratumor heterogeneity and branched evolution revealed by multiregion sequencing. *N Engl J Med* (2012) **366**(10):883–92. doi:10.1056/NEJMoa1113205
5. Sequist LV, Waltman BA, Dias-Santagata D, Digumarthy S, Turke AB, Fidias P, et al. Genotypic and histological evolution of lung cancers acquiring resistance to EGFR inhibitors. *Sci Transl Med* (2011) **3**(75):75ra26. doi:10.1126/scitranslmed.3002003
6. Valencia CA, Ankala A, Rhodenizer D, Bhide S, Littlejohn MR, Keong LM, et al. Comprehensive mutation analysis for congenital muscular dystrophy: a clinical PCR-based enrichment and next-generation sequencing panel. *PLoS One* (2013) **8**(1):e53083. doi:10.1371/journal.pone.0053083
7. de Ligt J, Willemsen MH, van Bon BW, Kleefstra T, Yntema HG, Kroes T, et al. Diagnostic exome sequencing in persons with severe intellectual disability. *N Engl J Med* (2012) **367**(20):1921–9. doi:10.1056/NEJMoa1206524
8. Subbiah V, Westin SN, Wang K, Araujo D, Wang WL, Miller VA, et al. Targeted therapy by combined inhibition of the RAF and mTOR kinases in malignant spindle cell neoplasm harboring the KIAA1549-BRAF fusion protein. *J Hematol Oncol* (2014) **7**(1):8. doi:10.1186/1756-8722-7-8
9. Li X, Buckton AJ, Wilkinson SL, John S, Walsh R, Novotny T, et al. Towards clinical molecular diagnosis of inherited cardiac conditions: a comparison of bench-top genome DNA sequencers. *PLoS One* (2013) **8**(7):e67744. doi:10.1371/journal.pone.0067744
10. Bianchi DW, Wilkins-Haug L. Integration of noninvasive DNA testing for aneuploidy into prenatal care: what has happened since the rubber met the road? *Clin Chem* (2014) **60**(1):78–87. doi:10.1373/clinchem.2013.202663
11. Rehm HL. Disease-targeted sequencing: a cornerstone in the clinic. *Nat Rev Genet* (2013) **14**(4):295–300. doi:10.1038/nrg3463
12. Simon R, Roychowdhury S. Implementing personalized cancer genomics in clinical trials. *Nat Rev Drug Discov* (2013) **12**(5):358–69. doi:10.1038/nrd3979
13. Drilon A, Wang L, Hasanovic A, Suehara Y, Lipson D, Stephens P, et al. Response to cabozantinib in patients with RET fusion-positive lung adenocarcinomas. *Cancer Discov* (2013) **3**(6):630–5. doi:10.1158/2159-8290.CD-13-0035
14. Hamburg MA, Collins FS. The path to personalized medicine. *N Engl J Med* (2010) **363**(4):301–4. doi:10.1056/NEJMp1006304
15. Jorgensen JT. A changing landscape for companion diagnostics. *Expert Rev Mol Diagn* (2013) **13**(7):667–9. doi:10.1586/14737159.2013.834799
16. McDermott U, Downing JR, Stratton MR. Genomics and the continuum of cancer care. *N Engl J Med* (2011) **364**(4):340–50. doi:10.1056/NEJMra0907178
17. Cronin M, Ross JS. Comprehensive next-generation cancer genome sequencing in the era of targeted therapy and personalized oncology. *Biomark Med* (2011) **5**(3):293–305. doi:10.2217/bmm.11.37
18. Moch H, Blank PR, Dietel M, Elmberger G, Kerr KM, Palacios J, et al. Personalized cancer medicine and the future of pathology. *Virchows Arch* (2012) **460**(1):3–8. doi:10.1007/s00428-011-1179-6
19. Imielinski M, Berger AH, Hammerman PS, Hernandez B, Pugh TJ, Hodis E, et al. Mapping the hallmarks of lung adenocarcinoma with massively parallel sequencing. *Cell* (2012) **150**(6):1107–20. doi:10.1016/j.cell.2012.08.029
20. Alexandrov LB, Nik-Zainal S, Wedge DC, Aparicio SA, Behjati S, Biankin AV, et al. Signatures of mutational processes in human cancer. *Nature* (2013) **500**(7463):415–21. doi:10.1038/nature12477
21. Stephens PJ, Tarpey PS, Davies H, Van Loo P, Greenman C, Wedge DC, et al. The landscape of cancer genes and mutational processes in breast cancer. *Nature* (2012) **486**(7403):400–4. doi:10.1038/nature11017
22. Bellcross CA, Page PZ, Meaney-Delman D. Direct-to-consumer personal genome testing and cancer risk prediction. *Cancer J* (2012) **18**(4):293–302. doi:10.1097/PPO.0b013e3182610e38
23. Christensen CM, Baumann H, Ruggles R, Sadtler TM. Disruptive innovation for social change. *Harv Bus Rev* (2006) **84**(12):94–101.
24. Carlson B. Next generation sequencing: the next iteration of personalized medicine: next generation sequencing, along with expanding databases like the cancer genome atlas, has the potential to aid rational drug discovery and streamline clinical trials. *Biotechnol Healthc* (2012) **9**(2):21–5.
25. Jorgensen JT. Companion diagnostics in oncology – current status and future aspects. *Oncology* (2013) **85**(1):59–68. doi:10.1159/000353454

26. Carlson B. In search of the perfect business model: as personalized medicine moves into the mainstream, makers of diagnostics must face a new economic reality. How to develop a value proposition in a healthcare market that is becoming increasingly elastic? *Biotechnol Healthc* (2012) **9**(1):20–3.
27. Loman NJ, Misra RV, Dallman TJ, Constantinidou C, Gharbia SE, Wain J, et al. Performance comparison of benchtop high-throughput sequencing platforms. *Nat Biotechnol* (2012) **30**(5):434–9. doi:10.1038/nbt.2198
28. Quail MA, Smith M, Coupland P, Otto TD, Harris SR, Connor TR, et al. A tale of three next generation sequencing platforms: comparison of Ion Torrent, Pacific Biosciences and Illumina MiSeq sequencers. *BMC Genomics* (2012) **13**:341. doi:10.1186/1471-2164-13-341
29. Metzker ML. Sequencing technologies – the next generation. *Nat Rev Genet* (2010) **11**(1):31–46. doi:10.1038/nrg2626
30. Meldrum C, Doyle MA, Tothill RW. Next-generation sequencing for cancer diagnostics: a practical perspective. *Clin Biochem Rev* (2011) **32**(4):177–95.
31. Rothberg JM, Hinz W, Rearick TM, Schultz J, Mileski W, Davey M, et al. An integrated semiconductor device enabling non-optical genome sequencing. *Nature* (2011) **475**(7356):348–52. doi:10.1038/nature10242
32. Merriman B; Ion Torrent R&D Team, Rothberg JM. Progress in Ion Torrent semiconductor chip based sequencing. *Electrophoresis* (2012) **33**(23):3397–417. doi:10.1002/elps.201200424
33. Koren S, Schatz MC, Walenz BP, Martin J, Howard JT, Ganapathy G, et al. Hybrid error correction and de novo assembly of single-molecule sequencing reads. *Nat Biotechnol* (2012) **30**(7):693–700. doi:10.1038/nbt.2280
34. Desai AN, Jere A. Next-generation sequencing: ready for the clinics? *Clin Genet* (2012) **81**(6):503–10. doi:10.1111/j.1399-0004.2012.01865.x
35. Fairley JA, Gilmour K, Walsh K. Making the most of pathological specimens: molecular diagnosis in formalin-fixed, paraffin embedded tissue. *Curr Drug Targets* (2012) **13**(12):1475–87. doi:10.2174/138945012803530125
36. Briggs AW, Heyn P. Preparation of next-generation sequencing libraries from damaged DNA. *Methods Mol Biol* (2012) **840**:143–54. doi:10.1007/978-1-61779-516-9_18
37. Latham GJ. Next-generation sequencing of formalin-fixed, paraffin-embedded tumor biopsies: navigating the perils of old and new technology to advance cancer diagnosis. *Expert Rev Mol Diagn* (2013) **13**(8):769–72. doi:10.1586/14737159.2013.845090
38. Sah S, Chen L, Houghton J, Kemppainen J, Marko AC, Zeigler R, et al. Functional DNA quantification guides accurate next-generation sequencing mutation detection in formalin-fixed, paraffin-embedded tumor biopsies. *Genome Med* (2013) **5**(8):77. doi:10.1186/gm481
39. Thomas A, Rajan A, Lopez-Chavez A, Wang Y, Giaccone G. From targets to targeted therapies and molecular profiling in non-small cell lung carcinoma. *Ann Oncol* (2013) **24**(3):577–85. doi:10.1093/annonc/mds478
40. Marton MJ, Weiner R. Practical guidance for implementing predictive biomarkers into early phase clinical studies. *Biomed Res Int* (2013) **2013**:891391. doi:10.1155/2013/891391
41. Cottrell CE, Al-Kateb H, Bredemeyer AJ, Duncavage EJ, Spencer DH, Abel HJ, et al. Validation of a next-generation sequencing assay for clinical molecular oncology. *J Mol Diagn* (2014) **16**(1):89–105. doi:10.1016/j.jmoldx.2013.10.002
42. Schrijver I, Aziz N, Farkas DH, Furtado M, Gonzalez AF, Greiner TC, et al. Opportunities and challenges associated with clinical diagnostic genome sequencing: a report of the association for molecular pathology. *J Mol Diagn* (2012) **14**(6):525–40. doi:10.1016/j.jmoldx.2012.04.006
43. Gargis AS, Kalman L, Berry MW, Bick DP, Dimmock DP, Hambuch T, et al. Assuring the quality of next-generation sequencing in clinical laboratory practice. *Nat Biotechnol* (2012) **30**(11):1033–6. doi:10.1038/nbt.2403
44. Rehm HL, Bale SJ, Bayrak-Toydemir P, Berg JS, Brown KK, Deignan JL, et al. ACMG clinical laboratory standards for next-generation sequencing. *Genet Med* (2013) **15**(9):733–47. doi:10.1038/gim.2013.92
45. André T, Blons H, Mabro M, Chibaudel B, Bachet JB, Tournigand C, et al. Panitumumab combined with irinotecan for patients with KRAS wild-type metastatic colorectal cancer refractory to standard chemotherapy: a GERCOR efficacy, tolerance, and translational molecular study. *Ann Oncol* (2013) **24**(2):412–9. doi:10.1093/annonc/mds465
46. Frampton GM, Fichtenholtz A, Otto GA, Wang K, Downing SR, He J, et al. Development and validation of a clinical cancer genomic profiling test based on massively parallel DNA sequencing. *Nat Biotechnol* (2013) **31**(11):1023–31. doi:10.1038/nbt.2696
47. Leary RJ, Kinde I, Diehl F, Schmidt K, Clouser C, Duncan C, et al. Development of personalized tumor biomarkers using massively parallel sequencing. *Sci Transl Med* (2010) **2**(20):20ra14. doi:10.1126/scitranslmed.3000702
48. Ross JS, Wang K, Gay L, Al-Rohil R, Rand JV, Jones DM, et al. New routes to targeted therapy of intrahepatic cholangiocarcinomas revealed by next-generation sequencing. *Oncologist* (2014) **19**(3):235–42. doi:10.1634/theoncologist.2013-0352
49. Fox JL. Master protocol for squamous cell lung cancer readies for launch. *Nat Biotechnol* (2014) **32**(2):116–8. doi:10.1038/nbt0214-116b
50. Heger M. *Life Tech Plans to Register PGM with FDA in Third Quarter [Genome Web]* (2014). Available from: www.genomeweb.com/print/1351426
51. Pacific Biosciences. *Pacific Biosciences Announces Agreement With Roche Diagnostics to Develop and Supply DNA Sequencing-Based Products for Clinical Diagnostics* (2013). Available from: http://investor.pacificbiosciences.com/releasedetail.cfm?ReleaseID=793199
52. Mamanova L, Coffey AJ, Scott CE, Kozarewa I, Turner EH, Kumar A, et al. Target-enrichment strategies for next-generation sequencing. *Nat Methods* (2010) **7**(2):111–8. doi:10.1038/nmeth.1419
53. Corless CL, Spellman PT. Tackling formalin-fixed, paraffin-embedded tumor tissue with next-generation sequencing. *Cancer Discov* (2012) **2**(1):23–4. doi:10.1158/2159-8290.CD-11-0319
54. Veal CD, Freeman PJ, Jacobs K, Lancaster O, Jamain S, Leboyer M, et al. A mechanistic basis for amplification differences between samples and between genome regions. *BMC Genomics* (2012) **13**:455. doi:10.1186/1471-2164-13-455
55. Pink CJ, Hurst LD. Timing of replication is a determinant of neutral substitution rates but does not explain slow Y chromosome evolution in rodents. *Mol Biol Evol* (2010) **27**(5):1077–86. doi:10.1093/molbev/msp314
56. Sleep JA, Schreiber AW, Baumann U. Sequencing error correction without a reference genome. *BMC Bioinformatics* (2013) **14**:367. doi:10.1186/1471-2105-14-367
57. Hadd AG, Houghton J, Choudhary A, Sah S, Chen L, Marko AC, et al. Targeted, high-depth, next-generation sequencing of cancer genes in formalin-fixed, paraffin-embedded and fine-needle aspiration tumor specimens. *J Mol Diagn* (2013) **15**(2):234–47. doi:10.1016/j.jmoldx.2012.11.006
58. Chin EL, da Silva C, Hegde M. Assessment of clinical analytical sensitivity and specificity of next-generation sequencing for detection of simple and complex mutations. *BMC Genet* (2013) **14**:6. doi:10.1186/1471-2156-14-6
59. Cordero F, Beccuti M, Donatelli S, Calogero RA. Large disclosing the nature of computational tools for the analysis of next generation sequencing data. *Curr Top Med Chem* (2012) **12**(12):1320–30. doi:10.2174/156802612801319007
60. Abnizova I, Leonard S, Skelly T, Brown A, Jackson D, Gourtovaia M, et al. Analysis of context-dependent errors for Illumina sequencing. *J Bioinform Comput Biol* (2012) **10**(2):1241005. doi:10.1142/S0219720012410053
61. Bragg LM, Stone G, Butler MK, Hugenholtz P, Tyson GW. Shining a light on dark sequencing: characterising errors in Ion Torrent PGM data. *PLoS Comput Biol* (2013) **9**(4):e1003031. doi:10.1371/journal.pcbi.1003031
62. Park MH, Rhee H, Park JH, Woo HM, Choi BO, Kim BY, et al. Comprehensive analysis to improve the validation rate for single nucleotide variants detected by next-generation sequencing. *PLoS One* (2014) **9**(1):e86664. doi:10.1371/journal.pone.0086664
63. Wang S, Xing J. A primer for disease gene prioritization using next-generation sequencing data. *Genomics Inform* (2013) **11**(4):191–9. doi:10.5808/GI.2013.11.4.191
64. Tsiatis AC, Norris-Kirby A, Rich RG, Hafez MJ, Gocke CD, Eshleman JR, et al. Comparison of Sanger sequencing, pyrosequencing, and melting curve analysis for the detection of KRAS mutations: diagnostic and clinical implications. *J Mol Diagn* (2010) **12**(4):425–32. doi:10.2353/jmoldx.2010.090188
65. Feliubadaló L, Lopez-Doriga A, Castellsagué E, del Valle J, Menéndez M, Tornero E, et al. Next-generation sequencing meets genetic diagnostics: development of a comprehensive workflow for the analysis of BRCA1 and BRCA2 genes. *Eur J Hum Genet* (2013) **21**(8):864–70. doi:10.1038/ejhg.2012.270
66. Zook JM, Samarov D, McDaniel J, Sen SK, Salit M. Synthetic spike-in standards improve run-specific systematic error analysis for DNA and RNA sequencing. *PLoS One* (2012) **7**(7):e41356. doi:10.1371/journal.pone.0041356
67. Wang Z, Gerstein M, Snyder M. RNA-Seq: a revolutionary tool for transcriptomics. *Nat Rev Genet* (2009) **10**(1):57–63. doi:10.1038/nrg2484

68. Sapino A, Roepman P, Linn SC, Snel MH, Delahaye LJ, van den Akker J, et al. Mammaprint molecular diagnostics on formalin-fixed, paraffin-embedded tissue. *J Mol Diagn* (2014) **16**(2):190–7. doi:10.1016/j.jmoldx.2013.10.008
69. Marchionni L, Wilson RF, Wolff AC, Marinopoulos S, Parmigiani G, Bass EB, et al. Systematic review: gene expression profiling assays in early-stage breast cancer. *Ann Intern Med* (2008) **148**(5):358–69. doi:10.7326/0003-4819-148-5-200803040-00208
70. Sturm D, Bender S, Jones DT, Lichter P, Grill J, Becher O, et al. Paediatric and adult glioblastoma: multiform (epi)genomic culprits emerge. *Nat Rev Cancer* (2014) **14**(2):92–107. doi:10.1038/nrc3655
71. Frattini V, Trifonov V, Chan JM, Castano A, Lia M, Abate F, et al. The integrated landscape of driver genomic alterations in glioblastoma. *Nat Genet* (2013) **45**(10):1141–9. doi:10.1038/ng.2734
72. Sinicropi D, Qu K, Collin F, Crager M, Liu ML, Pelham RJ, et al. Whole transcriptome RNA-Seq analysis of breast cancer recurrence risk using formalin-fixed paraffin-embedded tumor tissue. *PLoS One* (2012) **7**(7):e40092. doi:10.1371/journal.pone.0040092
73. Marioni JC, Mason CE, Mane SM, Stephens M, Gilad Y. RNA-Seq: an assessment of technical reproducibility and comparison with gene expression arrays. *Genome Res* (2008) **18**(9):1509–17. doi:10.1101/gr.079558.108
74. Tarazona S, García-Alcalde F, Dopazo J, Ferrer A, Conesa A. Differential expression in RNA-Seq: a matter of depth. *Genome Res* (2011) **21**(12):2213–23. doi:10.1101/gr.124321.111
75. Rapaport F, Khanin R, Liang Y, Pirun M, Krek A, Zumbo P, et al. Comprehensive evaluation of differential gene expression analysis methods for RNA-Seq data. *Genome Biol* (2013) **14**(9):R95. doi:10.1186/gb-2013-14-9-r95
76. Seyednasrollah F, Laiho A, Elo LL. Comparison of software packages for detecting differential expression in RNA-Seq studies. *Brief Bioinform* (2013). doi:10.1093/bib/bbt086
77. Ozsolak F, Milos PM. RNA sequencing: advances, challenges and opportunities. *Nat Rev Genet* (2011) **12**(2):87–98. doi:10.1038/nrg2934
78. Lilljebjorn H, Agerstam H, Orsmark-Pietras C, Rissler M, Ehrencrona H, Nilsson L, et al. RNA-Seq identifies clinically relevant fusion genes in leukemia including a novel MEF2D/CSF1R fusion responsive to imatinib. *Leukemia* (2013). doi:10.1038/leu.2013.324
79. Shi L, Campbell G, Jones WD, Campagne F, Wen Z, Walker SJ, et al. The microarray quality control (MAQC)-II study of common practices for the development and validation of microarray-based predictive models. *Nat Biotechnol* (2010) **28**(8):827–38. doi:10.1038/nbt.1665
80. Mane SP, Evans C, Cooper KL, Crasta OR, Folkerts O, Hutchison SK, et al. Transcriptome sequencing of the microarray quality control (MAQC) RNA reference samples using next generation sequencing. *BMC Genomics* (2009) **10**:264. doi:10.1186/1471-2164-10-264
81. Liu P, Barb J, Woodhouse K, Taylor JG, Munson PJ, Raghavachari N. Transcriptome profiling and sequencing of differentiated human hematopoietic stem cells reveal lineage-specific expression and alternative splicing of genes. *Physiol Genomics* (2011) **43**(20):1117–34. doi:10.1152/physiolgenomics.00099.2011
82. Jones SJ, Laskin J, Li YY, Griffith OL, An J, Bilenky M, et al. Evolution of an adenocarcinoma in response to selection by targeted kinase inhibitors. *Genome Biol* (2010) **11**(8):R82. doi:10.1186/gb-2010-11-8-r82
83. Cancer Genome Atlas Research Network. Integrated genomic analyses of ovarian carcinoma. *Nature* (2011) **474**(7353):609–15. doi:10.1038/nature10166
84. Gullapalli RR, Desai KV, Santana-Santos L, Kant JA, Becich MJ. Next generation sequencing in clinical medicine: challenges and lessons for pathology and biomedical informatics. *J Pathol Inform* (2012) **3**:40. doi:10.4103/2153-3539.103013
85. Guo Y, Ye F, Sheng Q, Clark T, Samuels DC. Three-stage quality control strategies for DNA re-sequencing data. *Brief Bioinform* (2013). doi:10.1093/bib/bbt069
86. O'Rawe J, Jiang T, Sun G, Wu Y, Wang W, Hu J, et al. Low concordance of multiple variant-calling pipelines: practical implications for exome and genome sequencing. *Genome Med* (2013) **5**(3):28. doi:10.1186/gm432
87. Ewing B, Green P. Base-calling of automated sequencer traces using phred. II. Error probabilities. *Genome Res* (1998) **8**(3):186–94. doi:10.1101/gr.8.3.175
88. Ewing B, Hillier L, Wendl MC, Green P. Base-calling of automated sequencer traces using phred. I. Accuracy assessment. *Genome Res* (1998) **8**(3):175–85. doi:10.1101/gr.8.3.175
89. Elsharawy A, Forster M, Schracke N, Keller A, Thomsen I, Petersen BS, et al. Improving mapping and SNP-calling performance in multiplexed targeted next-generation sequencing. *BMC Genomics* (2012) **13**:417. doi:10.1186/1471-2164-13-417
90. Carter H, Chen S, Isik L, Tyekucheva S, Velculescu VE, Kinzler KW, et al. Cancer-specific high-throughput annotation of somatic mutations: computational prediction of driver missense mutations. *Cancer Res* (2009) **69**(16):6660–7. doi:10.1158/0008-5472.CAN-09-1133
91. Van Allen EM, Wagle N, Levy MA. Clinical analysis and interpretation of cancer genome data. *J Clin Oncol* (2013) **31**(15):1825–33. doi:10.1200/JCO.2013.48.7215
92. Zook JM, Chapman B, Wang J, Mittelman D, Hofmann O, Hide W, et al. Integrating human sequence data sets provides a resource of benchmark SNP and indel genotype calls. *Nat Biotechnol* (2014) **32**(3):246–51. doi:10.1038/nbt.2835
93. Duzkale H, Shen J, McLaughlin H, Alfares A, Kelly MA, Pugh TJ, et al. A systematic approach to assessing the clinical significance of genetic variants. *Clin Genet* (2013) **84**(5):453–63. doi:10.1111/cge.12257
94. Crolla LJ, Westgard JO. Evaluation of rule-based autoverification protocols. *Clin Leadersh Manag Rev* (2003) **17**(5):268–72.
95. Westgard JO. Internal quality control: planning and implementation strategies. *Ann Clin Biochem* (2003) **40**(Pt 6):593–611. doi:10.1258/000456303770367199
96. Duncavage EJ, Abel HJ, Szankasi P, Kelley TW, Pfeifer JD. Targeted next generation sequencing of clinically significant gene mutations and translocations in leukemia. *Mod Pathol* (2012) **25**(6):795–804. doi:10.1038/modpathol.2012.29
97. Allhoff M, Schönhuth A, Martin M, Costa IG, Rahmann S, Marschall T. Discovering motifs that induce sequencing errors. *BMC Bioinformatics* (2013) **14**(Suppl 5):S1. doi:10.1186/1471-2105-14-S5-S1
98. ElSharawy A, Warner J, Olson J, Forster M, Schilhabel MB, Link DR, et al. Accurate variant detection across non-amplified and whole genome amplified DNA using targeted next generation sequencing. *BMC Genomics* (2012) **13**:500. doi:10.1186/1471-2164-13-500
99. Oyola SO, Otto TD, Gu Y, Maslen G, Manske M, Campino S, et al. Optimizing Illumina next-generation sequencing library preparation for extremely AT-biased genomes. *BMC Genomics* (2012) **13**:1. doi:10.1186/1471-2164-13-1
100. Richards CS, Bale S, Bellissimo DB, Das S, Grody WW, Hegde MR, et al. ACMG recommendations for standards for interpretation and reporting of sequence variations: revisions 2007. *Genet Med* (2008) **10**(4):294–300. doi:10.1097/GIM.0b013e31816b5cae
101. Green RC, Berg JS, Grody WW, Kalia SS, Korf BR, Martin CL, et al. ACMG recommendations for reporting of incidental findings in clinical exome and genome sequencing. *Genet Med* (2013) **15**(7):565–74. doi:10.1038/gim.2013.73
102. Gymrek M, McGuire AL, Golan D, Halperin E, Erlich Y. Identifying personal genomes by surname inference. *Science* (2013) **339**(6117):321–4. doi:10.1126/science.1229566
103. Bunnik EM, de Jong A, Nijsingh N, de Wert GM. The new genetics and informed consent: differentiating choice to preserve autonomy. *Bioethics* (2013) **27**(6):348–55. doi:10.1111/bioe.12030
104. Bunnik EM, Schermer MH, Janssens AC. Personal genome testing: test characteristics to clarify the discourse on ethical, legal and societal issues. *BMC Med Ethics* (2011) **12**:11. doi:10.1186/1472-6939-12-11
105. McCaughan M. *Landmark Trial for Personalized Medicine Coming Soon: NGS Approval May Be One Offshoot of Lung Cancer "Master Protocol"*. The RPM report. Bedford, NJ: Informa Business Information, Inc. (2013).
106. Miller JK, Buchner N, Timms L, Tam S, Luo X, Brown AM, et al. Use of sequenom sample ID plus(R) SNP genotyping in identification of FFPE tumor samples. *PLoS One* (2014) **9**(2):e88163. doi:10.1371/journal.pone.0088163
107. Torri F, Dinov ID, Zamanyan A, Hobel S, Genco A, Petrosyan P, et al. Next generation sequence analysis and computational genomics using graphical pipeline workflows. *Genes (Basel)* (2012) **3**(3):545–75. doi:10.3390/genes3030545
108. Cheng S, Koch WH, Wu L. Co-development of a companion diagnostic for targeted cancer therapy. *N Biotechnol* (2012) **29**(6):682–8. doi:10.1016/j.nbt.2012.02.002
109. Malik SM, Maher VE, Bijwaard KE, Becker RL, Zhang L, Tang SW, et al. U.S. food and drug administration approval: crizotinib for treatment of advanced or metastatic non-small cell lung cancer that is anaplastic lymphoma kinase positive. *Clin Cancer Res* (2014). doi:10.1158/1078-0432.CCR-13-3077

110. Thunnissen E, Bubendorf L, Dietel M, Elmberger G, Kerr K, Lopez-Rios F, et al. EML4-ALK testing in non-small cell carcinomas of the lung: a review with recommendations. *Virchows Arch* (2012) **461**(3):245–57. doi:10.1007/s00428-012-1281-4
111. Fridlyand J, Simon RM, Walrath JC, Roach N, Buller R, Schenkein DP, et al. Considerations for the successful co-development of targeted cancer therapies and companion diagnostics. *Nat Rev Drug Discov* (2013) **12**(10):743–55. doi:10.1038/nrd4101
112. Soda M, Choi YL, Enomoto M, Takada S, Yamashita Y, Ishikawa S, et al. Identification of the transforming EML4-ALK fusion gene in non-small-cell lung cancer. *Nature* (2007) **448**(7153):561–6. doi:10.1038/nature05945
113. Butrynski JE, D'Adamo DR, Hornick JL, Dal Cin P, Antonescu CR, Jhanwar SC, et al. Crizotinib in ALK-rearranged inflammatory myofibroblastic tumor. *N Engl J Med* (2010) **363**(18):1727–33. doi:10.1056/NEJMoa1007056
114. Kwak EL, Bang YJ, Camidge DR, Shaw AT, Solomon B, Maki RG, et al. Anaplastic lymphoma kinase inhibition in non-small-cell lung cancer. *N Engl J Med* (2010) **363**(18):1693–703. doi:10.1056/NEJMoa1006448
115. Willyard C. 'Basket studies' will hold intricate data for cancer drug approvals. *Nat Med* (2013) **19**(6):655. doi:10.1038/nm0613-655
116. Ong MBH. "Master protocol" to rely on biomarkers in testing multiple lung cancer agents. *Cancer Lett* (2013) **39**:43.
117. Weiss RL. The long and winding regulatory road for laboratory-developed tests. *Am J Clin Pathol* (2012) **138**(1):20–6. doi:10.1309/AJCP6OAULC3CMFEJ
118. Mansfield E, O'Leary TJ, Gutman SI. Food and drug administration regulation of in vitro diagnostic devices. *J Mol Diagn* (2005) **7**(1):2–7. doi:10.1016/S1525-1578(10)60002-5
119. Gutman S. Regulatory issues in tumor marker development. *Semin Oncol* (2002) **29**(3):294–300. doi:10.1053/sonc.2002.33140
120. Tougeron D, Lecomte T, Pagès JC, Villalva C, Collin C, Ferru A, et al. Effect of low-frequency KRAS mutations on the response to anti-EGFR therapy in metastatic colorectal cancer. *Ann Oncol* (2013) **24**(5):1267–73. doi:10.1093/annonc/mds620
121. Hanamura N, Aruga A. Global development strategy for companion diagnostics based on the usage and approval history for biomarkers in Japan, the USA and the EU. *Per Med* (2014) **11**(1):27–40. doi:10.2217/pme.13.100
122. Dati F. The new European directive on in vitro diagnostics. *Clin Chem Lab Med* (2003) **41**(10):1289–98. doi:10.1515/CCLM.2003.196
123. Howes K. Regulatory challenges for diagnostic development – a European perspective. *Expert Opin Med Diagn* (2007) **1**(2):153–7. doi:10.1517/17530059.1.2.153
124. Young G, Wang K, He J, Otto G, Hawryluk M, Zwirco Z, et al. Clinical next-generation sequencing successfully applied to fine-needle aspirations of pulmonary and pancreatic neoplasms. *Cancer Cytopathol* (2013) **121**(12):688–94. doi:10.1002/cncy.21338
125. Halait H, Demartin K, Shah S, Soviero S, Langland R, Cheng S, et al. Analytical performance of a real-time PCR-based assay for V600 mutations in the BRAF gene, used as the companion diagnostic test for the novel BRAF inhibitor vemurafenib in metastatic melanoma. *Diagn Mol Pathol* (2012) **21**(1):1–8. doi:10.1097/PDM.0b013e31823b216f
126. Krijgsman O, Roepman P, Zwart W, Carroll JS, Tian S, de Snoo FA, et al. A diagnostic gene profile for molecular subtyping of breast cancer associated with treatment response. *Breast Cancer Res Treat* (2012) **133**(1):37–47. doi:10.1007/s10549-011-1683-z
127. Fang KC. Clinical utilities of peripheral blood gene expression profiling in the management of cardiac transplant patients. *J Immunotoxicol* (2007) **4**(3):209–17. doi:10.1080/15476910701385570

2

Where is it and how does it get there – intracellular localization and traffic of P-glycoprotein

Dong Fu*

Faculty of Pharmacy, The University of Sydney, Sydney, NSW, Australia

Edited by:
Stefania Nobili, University of Florence, Italy

Reviewed by:
Brion William Murray, Pfizer Oncology Research Unit, USA
Amit K. Tiwari, Tuskegee University, USA

***Correspondence:**
Dong Fu, Faculty of Pharmacy, The University of Sydney, Building A15, Sydney, NSW 2006, Australia
e-mail: dong.fu@sydney.edu.au

P-glycoprotein (P-gp), an ATP-binding cassette, is able to transport structurally and chemically unrelated substrates. Over-expression of P-gp in cancer cells significantly decreases the intercellular amount of anticancer drugs, and results in multidrug resistance in cancer cells, a major obstacle in cancer chemotherapy. P-gp is mainly localized on the plasma membrane and functions as a drug efflux pump; however, P-gp is also localized in many intracellular compartments, such as endoplasmic reticulum, Golgi, endosomes, and lysosomes. P-gp moves between the intracellular compartments and the plasma membrane in a microtubule-actin dependent manner. This review highlights our current understanding of (1) the intracellular localization of P-gp; (2) the traffic and cycling pathways among the cellular compartments as well as between these compartments and the plasma membrane; and (3) the cellular factors regulating P-gp traffic and cycling. This review also presents a potential implication in overcoming P-gp-mediated multidrug resistance by targeting P-gp traffic and cycling pathways and impairing P-gp localization on the plasma membrane.

Keywords: P-glycoprotein, intracellular localization, traffic, recycling, cell polarization, multidrug resistance in cancer

INTRODUCTION

P-glycoprotein (P-gp), a 170 kDa membrane protein, is a member of sub-family B of the ATP-binding cassette (ABC) transporter superfamily, and is also called ABCB1. P-gp has two structurally identical halves. Its N-terminal half contains six transmembrane domains, followed by a large cytoplasmic domain with an ATP-binding site. Similarly, the C-terminal half also has six transmembrane domains and an ATP-binding site (1, 2). Plasma membrane located P-gp is able to transport many chemically and structurally unrelated substrates out of the cells, and acts as an efflux pump (1, 2). P-gp is primarily expressed in the liver, kidney, gastrointestinal tract, and blood brain barrier. P-gp is located on the canalicular apical membrane of hepatocytes in the liver; on the brush border of proximal tubule cells in the kidney; and on the apical membrane of mucosal cells in the small intestine (3). Given the transporting function of P-gp, these tissue distributions allow P-gp to excrete endogenous metabolites, exogenous substrates, and toxins into the urine, bile, and feces. Thus, P-gp can protect the organism as well as eliminate cellular wastes (3, 4). Furthermore, another essential localization of P-gp is on the luminal surface of capillary endothelial cells of the blood brain barrier which prevents cytotoxins from penetrating the endothelium and protects brain (5).

Although animal well-being, normal physiological function, and life span were not affected after P-gp was knocked out in mice, higher drug sensitivity and increased drug side effect/toxicity occurred (6). While knocking out P-gp appears to be less problematic, over-expression of P-gp causes major concerns in clinical oncology. The most notable consequence of over-expression of P-gp in clinic is to cause multiple drug resistance (MDR) in cancer chemotherapy (2). Given P-gp has a structurally broad range of substrates, the occurrence of MDR during chemotherapy is one of the big challenges for successful cancer treatment in clinic. MDR can be either intrinsic, occurring in cancers that have not been exposed to chemotherapy before but derived from tissue naturally expressing P-gp (e.g., liver, kidney, intestinal cancers), or required MDR, which develops after cancers are treated with chemotherapy (7). Nearly half of human cancers express P-gp at levels sufficient to develop MDR. The likelihood of failure in chemotherapy is increased when P-gp expression is upregulated during therapy (8).

INTRACELLULAR LOCALIZATION OF P-gp

P-glycoprotein is primarily localized on the plasma membrane for its efflux function, however, it is also localized intracellularly (9, 10). Using immunofluorescence and over-expression of P-gp-GFP fusion protein approaches, co-localization results revealed that P-gp is localized in many cellular organelles, including endoplasmic reticulum (ER) (9), Golgi (9), early endosome (11–13), recycling endosome (12), later endosome, lysosome (9, 11), and proteasome (14) (**Figure 1**). These intracellular localizations link to synthesis (ER), modification (Golgi), traffic/recycling (Golgi and endosomes), and degradation (lysosome and proteasome) sites for P-gp. Although one study suggests P-gp is also located in mitochondria in doxorubicin-resistant K562 human leukemia cells (15), others reveal that P-gp is not presented in mitochondria either in MCF-7 (ADR) human breast cancer and KB-V1 human cervix carcinoma drug resistant cell lines (16) or in primary rat hepatocytes (17). Furthermore, transient transfection of P-gp-GFP in cancer cells reveals that the ER and Golgi localization of P-gp appears to be transient, suggesting that P-gp can rapidly traffic to the endosomal compartment and the plasma membrane

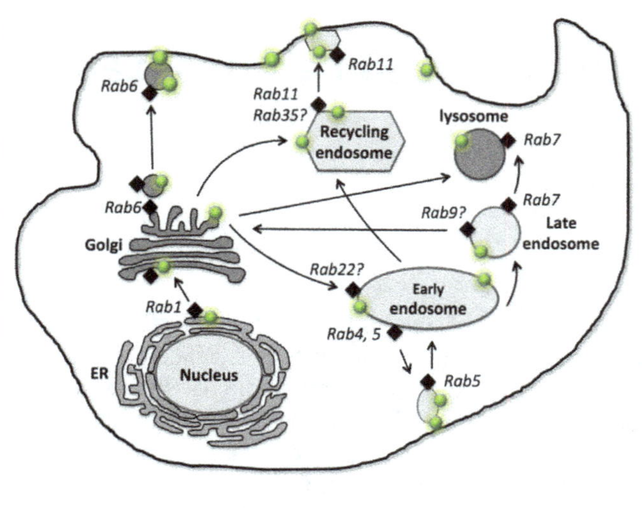

FIGURE 1 | Intracellular localization, traffic, and recycling of P-glycoprotein. P-gp is shown as "green dot ●." Different Rab GTPases that are involved in P-gp traffic and recycling are indicated as "black diamond ◆." Arrows represent the traffic and recycling path among the intracellular organelles and between the cellular organelles and the plasma membrane.

localization after it is synthesized in ER and modified in Golgi. This rapid transport to the membrane localization explains why less ER or Golgi localization can be observed in the stable cell line which is overexpressed with P-gp-GFP. It is possible that activity of P-gp synthesis remains at a relatively low level due to the very long half-life of P-gp (14–17 h) in the stable cell line (18). Similarly, the degradation localization (lysosome) also appears to be less common within the cells compared to the endosomal localization which is involved in constantly trafficking/recycling P-gp between the cellular pool and the plasma membrane (11).

INTRACELLULAR TRAFFIC AND RECYCLING OF P-gp

After synthesis in ER, P-gp first needs to be correctly folded before exit from ER and entry to Golgi for modification. Currently, very little information is available about the exact regulatory process for P-gp folding in ER. Glycoprotein glucosyl transferase (UGGT) is able to sense the folding states of glycoproteins, resulting in mis-folded glycoprotein rebinding calnexin (a chaperon for protein folding) and going through re-folding cycles or being rapidly degraded via endoplasmic-reticulum-associated protein degradation (ERAD) (19). Thus, UGGT may play a potential role in recognizing the folding of P-gp. Moreover, a study suggests that SPTLC1 (Serine palmitoyltransferase enzyme 1) is able to interact with ABCA1 and cause ER retention of ABCA1, revealing the role of SPTLC1 in ER exit of ABC transporters (20). Furthermore, the formation of disulfide bonds is a critical step in the maturation of the majority of the proteins inside ER (21). Studies showed that two other ABC transporters, ABCB6 and ABCC8, form the disulfide bonds between highly conserved cysteine, which is important for these ABC transporters to exit ER and traffic to the plasma membrane (22). We still lack direct evidence of how P-gp export at the ER – the first step of its trafficking along the biosynthetic secretory pathway. In mammalian cells, the ER export occurs via Coat Protein II (COPII)-coated vesicles. COPII vesicles bud from the ER and are able to fuse to ER-Golgi intermediated compartment (23). Studies reveal that COPII plays an essential role in exporting ABCB1 and ABCC7 (cystic fibrosis transmembrane conductance regulator, CFTR) from ER to Golgi (24, 25), suggesting COPII may regulate ER export of P-gp as well. Golgi is involved in the biosynthesis of glycan chains of glycoproteins, the 150 kDa P-gp is transported to the Golgi and glycosylated as the 170 kDa mature protein (26) (**Figure 1**).

After its modification in Golgi, the 170 kDa mature P-gp traffics to the plasma membrane. Membrane proteins can traffic to the plasma membrane via either the constitutive pathway which involves membrane protein-containing vesicles moving directly to the plasma membrane (27, 28) or the endosomal pathway in which protein-containing vesicles are first transported to endosomal compartments to establish the intracellular pool, and then traffic to the plasma membrane (29). In both cases, the cytoskeleton is needed for the traffic of these membrane protein vesicles (30). The *trans*-Golgi network (TGN) is a major sorting site for proteins trafficking to the plasma membrane and endosomal pathway. A study suggests that membrane proteins use *N*-glycan chains as sorting determinants (31); whether this also applies to P-gp needs to be investigated. However, some studies show that N-glycosylation at amino acid residue asparagine 596 at third extracellular loop is not necessary for ABCG2 traffic (32), and the immature core-glycosylated CFTR (ABCC7) can be transported to the plasma membrane and is functional (33).

In the non-polarized cancer cells, P-gp was reported localized in EEA1 and Rab5 positive early endosome which serves as an intracellular reservoir prior to P-gp moving to the plasma membrane (11), suggesting that P-gp can traffic to the plasma membrane via the indirect endosomal pathway. Furthermore, immunofluorescence study showed that P-gp is also localized in lysosome after transient expression of human P-gp-GFP in HeLa cells or in the human breast cancer MCF-7 cells, which are stably expressed with P-gp-GFP, suggesting P-gp can be moved to the lysosomal degradation compartment, presumably through the early and late endosome (12). However, an immunofluorescence study reveals that P-gp is not localized in Rab11 positive recycling endosomes in human breast cancer MCF-7 cells, which stably express P-gp-GFP (11). In the polarized WIFB9 cells as well as hepatocytes, apical ABC transporters (e.g., P-gp, ABCB11) move to the apical membrane via Rab11a recycling endosomes and recycle between the apical membrane and the Rab11a positive intracellular endosomal pool (29, 34) (**Figure 1**). These studies suggest that P-gp traffics and recycles via different endosomal pathways (early endosome vs. recycling endosome) in non-polarized cells (e.g., cancer cells) and polarized cells.

REGULATION OF P-gp TRAFFIC AND RECYCLING – ROLE OF Rab GTPases

Rab GTPases, the largest branch of small GTPase, are known to regulate vesicular transport in exocytosis, endocytosis, and recycling by controlling many steps in membrane trafficking such as vesicle formation, movement, uncoating, docking, and fusion (35). So far more than 70 Rab GTPases have been identified in humans (35). Each Rab protein is believed to be specifically associated with a particular organelle or pathway (35). Currently, few studies revealed the role of Rab proteins in P-gp trafficking, thus, the more general involvement of Rab proteins in ABC transporters trafficking and recycling will be discussed.

Rab1, 2, and 6 are localized in ER and Golgi and regulate vesicle transport along the ER-Golgi biosynthetic pathway. Rab1, 2 regulate vesicle movement from ER to Golgi (35, 36), while Rab6 is involved in Golgi to the cell surface for exocytosis of newly synthesized proteins and lipids (37). Study showed that P-gp was predominantly intracellular, largely in Rab6-containing Golgi vesicles and Golgi cisternae (7), suggesting Rab6 may regulate P-gp traffic directly from Golgi to the plasma membrane (**Figure 1**).

Along the endosomal trafficking pathway, Rab11 and Rab13 are involved in membrane protein traffic from Golgi to the recycling endosome (38–40). Rab11a was shown to regulate P-gp and ABCB11 traffic to the apical membrane in polarized WIFB9 cells (29, 34) (**Figure 1**). Furthermore, studies showed that Rab11a was also needed for both WT-CFTR and ΔF508-CFTR to undergo trafficking to the apical recycling compartment in polarized human airway epithelia cells (41) as well as polarized intestinal epithelial cells (42). These studies reveal that, in polarized cells, P-gp traffics to the apical membrane via the Rab11a positive recycling endosome. However, in non-polarized MCF-7 cells, stable expressed P-gp-EGFP did not co-localize with Rab11 positive recycling endosome (11), suggesting P-gp does not traffic to the cell surface via the Rab11a positive recycling endosome. Evidence indicates that membrane trafficking of CFTR is cell type-specific and it differs in polarized human airway epithelial cells such as CFBE41o- cells and in non-polarized fibroblasts such as BHK-21 cells (41). Thus, Rab11a may have a differential role in P-gp trafficking in non-polarized and polarized cells. Other Rab proteins, such as Rab17, Rab25, Rab35, and Rab40 are also localized in recycling endosome (36, 43). Rab35 is shown to play important role in insulin-stimulated GLUT4 (Glucose transporter type 4) translocation in adipocytes (44). Further studies are needed to investigate the role of Rab11 as well as other Rab proteins (e.g., Rab17, Rab25, Rab35, and Rab40) in P-gp traffic in both polarized and non-polarized cells.

Early endosomal pathway is shown to be involved in P-gp trafficking and recycling. Among many of the early endosomal Rab proteins, Rab4 and Rab5 are known to regulate P-gp trafficking and recycling in many cancer cells (12, 13, 45). Over-expression of dominant-negative Rab5 mutant (S34N-Rab5) results in large intracellular accumulation of P-gp-EGFP in non-polarized Hela cells, and similar cellular accumulation of wild type P-gp in multidrug resistant MCF-7/Adr cells, revealing that Rab5 regulates P-gp exocytosis from the endosome compartment (such as early endosome) to the plasma membrane in non-polarized cells (12). In contrast, another study in colon cancer cells LS174T, demonstrated that over-expression of wild-type Rab5 resulted in recycling P-gp from the plasma membrane into intracellular compartments, suggesting that Rab5 regulates P-gp endocytosis instead of exocytosis (13), however, this study did not investigate the polarization status of the cell culture of LS174T, which is shown to be polarized in normal culture condition (46). Thus, the differential role of Rab5 in P-gp trafficking and recycling in these cancer cells may be related to the difference in polarization (**Figure 1**).

Rab4 is also localized in early endosome and shown to regulate P-gp exocytosis in drug resistant leukemia cells, K562ADR (45). Cell surface expression of P-gp decreased after over-expression of GFP-Rab4 or constitutively active Rab4Q72L mutant, but not dominant-negative Rab4S27N mutant or Rab14 in the K562ADR cells, suggesting that Rab4 regulates P-gp trafficking to the plasma membrane from endosomal compartments (45). However, in HeLa cells, the intracellular localization of P-gp-EGFP was not affected when there was over-expression of either wild-type Rab4 or dominant-negative mutant N121I-Rab4 respectively (12), indicating Rab4 does not effect P-gp trafficking. The different cell lines used in these studies may be the reason for obtaining different results. Given many other Rab proteins, such as Rab10, 14, 15, 17, 22, and 23 are localized on early endosome (43), it is likely these Rab proteins can also regulate the trafficking and recycling of P-gp between the early endosomal compartment and the plasma membrane in a cell and tissue type-specific manner.

Transmembrane proteins can be transported from late endosome to lysosome which is responsible for degradation of the membrane proteins (47). P-gp is localized in Lamp-2 positive lysosome, revealing its lysosomal dependent degradation pathway (11). Rab7 is localized on late endosome and lysosome, and is essential for later endocytic membrane trafficking from late endosome to lysosome (48, 49), while Rab9 is localized on later endosome and responsible for transit from later endosome to the TGN (50). Although very little is known about the role of Rab7 and 9 on later endocytic membrane trafficking of P-gp, Rab7 and 9 are shown to regulate other ABC transporter trafficking (e.g., CFTR). Using over-expression of wild type and mutant Rab GTPases, a study revealed that CFTR could enter Rab7-dependent late endosomal traffic or Rab9-mediated translocation to the TGN (51), suggesting the role of both Rab7 and 9 in later endocytic trafficking of CFTR. However, the potential roles of Rab7 and 9 on P-gp trafficking need to be investigated (**Figure 1**).

CLINICAL IMPLICATIONS

P-glycoprotein plays an important role in drug excretion and is one of the main causes for MDR in cancer chemotherapy. Different generations of P-gp inhibitors are developed and enter into preclinical and clinical studies. The first generation of P-gp inhibitors, such as verapamil and cyclosporin A, are active substrates of P-gp. Both verapamil and cyclosporin A cause side effects in patients due to high dose of the drugs are need for their inhibition of P-gp (52, 53). The second generation of P-gp inhibitors include valspodar (PSC 833), dexverapamil, and dofequidar fumarate. However, these second generation inhibitors also inhibit drug metabolism enzymes and other ABC transporters, which results in impaired drug metabolism and elimination (54–56). The third generation of P-gp inhibitors, which are currently undergoing clinical trials, include zosuquidar (LY335979), elacridar (GF120918), CBT-1, and XR9576 (57–60). However, some of the trials are unsuccessful in improving therapeutic efficacy (61). For example, trial was stopped in patient with non-small-cell lung cancer due to chemotherapy-related toxicity after administration of XR9576 (60). Thus, there is an urgent need to develop innovative strategies to overcome P-gp-mediated MDR in cancer chemotherapy.

Given P-gp needs to be transported to the plasma membrane so as to efflux the anticancer drugs out of cells, blocking the trafficking of P-gp to its final destination – the plasma membrane location – can be an innovative approach to overcome MDR and improve therapy. There are multiple potential targets along the P-gp traffic pathway. Study revealed that inhibition of P-gp maturation resulted in accumulation of P-gp in Golgi, and this immature P-gp in Golgi was inactive and presumably led to degradation. Consequently there was an increased cellular accumulation of P-gp substrate (62). Experiments also reveal that blocking P-gp traffic to the plasma membrane by interrupting the cytoskeleton highway or modulating Rab activation can cause increased intracellular accumulation of P-gp, resulting in more intracellular retention of anticancer drug (9, 11, 12). Although the intracellular P-gp that is trapped on the way to the plasma membrane remains active, it is likely that intracellular P-gp do not contribute to drug resistance (63). It is essential to identify the regulatory effectors, such as specific Rab GTPases or Rab binding proteins for P-gp traffic and recycling, and to screen potential candidates for targeting these effectors. Therefore, more studies are needed to understand the molecular and cellular mechanisms of P-gp intracellular traffic/cycling and its regulatory factors.

REFERENCES

1. Endicott JA, Ling V. The biochemistry of P-glycoprotein-mediated multidrug resistance. *Annu Rev Biochem* (1989) **58**:137–71. doi:10.1146/annurev.bi.58.070189.001033
2. Gottesman MM, Pastan I, Ambudkar SV. P-glycoprotein and multidrug resistance. *Curr Opin Genet Dev* (1996) **6**:610–7. doi:10.1016/S0959-437X(96)80091-8
3. Thiebaut F, Tsuruo T, Hamada H, Gottesman MM, Pastan I, Willingham MC. Cellular localization of the multidrug-resistance gene product P-glycoprotein in normal human tissues. *Proc Natl Acad Sci U S A* (1987) **84**:7735–8. doi:10.1073/pnas.84.21.7735
4. Schinkel AH, Mayer U, Wagenaar E, Mol CA, van Deemter L, Smit JJ, et al. Normal viability and altered pharmacokinetics in mice lacking mdr1-type (drug-transporting) P-glycoproteins. *Proc Natl Acad Sci U S A* (1997) **94**:4028–33. doi:10.1073/pnas.94.8.4028
5. Cordon-Cardo C, O'Brien JP, Casals D, Rittman-Grauer L, Biedler JL, Melamed MR, et al. Multidrug-resistance gene (P-glycoprotein) is expressed by endothelial cells at blood-brain barrier sites. *Proc Natl Acad Sci U S A* (1989) **86**:695–8. doi:10.1073/pnas.86.2.695
6. Schinkel AH, Smit JJ, van Tellingen O, Beijnen JH, Wagenaar E, van Deemter L, et al. Disruption of the mouse mdr1a P-glycoprotein gene leads to a deficiency in the blood-brain barrier and to increased sensitivity to drugs. *Cell* (1994) **77**:491–502. doi:10.1016/0092-8674(94)90212-7
7. De Rosa MF, Sillence D, Ackerley C, Lingwood C. Role of multiple drug resistance protein 1 in neutral but not acidic glycosphingolipid biosynthesis. *J Biol Chem* (2004) **279**:7867–76. doi:10.1074/jbc.M305645200
8. Gottesman MM, Fojo T, Bates SE. Multidrug resistance in cancer: role of ATP-dependent transporters. *Nat Rev Cancer* (2002) **2**:48–58. doi:10.1038/nrc706
9. Fu D, Bebawy M, Kable EP, Roufogalis BD. Dynamic and intracellular trafficking of P-glycoprotein-EGFP fusion protein: implications in multidrug resistance in cancer. *Int J Cancer* (2004) **109**:174–81. doi:10.1002/ijc.11659
10. Fu D, Arias IM. Intracellular trafficking of P-glycoprotein. *Int J Biochem Cell Biol* (2012) **44**:461–4. doi:10.1016/j.biocel.2011.12.009
11. Fu D, Roufogalis BD. Actin disruption inhibits endosomal traffic of P-glycoprotein-EGFP and resistance to daunorubicin accumulation. *Am J Physiol Cell Physiol* (2007) **292**:C1543–52. doi:10.1152/ajpcell.00068.2006
12. Fu D, van Dam EM, Brymora A, Duggin IG, Robinson PJ, Roufogalis BD. The small GTPases Rab5 and RalA regulate intracellular traffic of P-glycoprotein. *Biochim Biophys Acta* (2007) **1773**:1062–72. doi:10.1016/j.bbamcr.2007.03.023
13. Kim H, Barroso M, Samanta R, Greenberger L, Sztul E. Experimentally induced changes in the endocytic traffic of P-glycoprotein alter drug resistance of cancer cells. *Am J Physiol* (1997) **273**:C687–702.
14. Katayama K, Noguchi K, Sugimoto Y. FBXO15 regulates P-glycoprotein/ABCB1 expression through the ubiquitin – proteasome pathway in cancer cells. *Cancer Sci* (2013) **104**:694–702. doi:10.1111/cas.12145
15. Munteanu E, Verdier M, Grandjean-Forestier F, Stenger C, Jayat-Vignoles C, Huet S, et al. Mitochondrial localization and activity of P-glycoprotein in doxorubicin-resistant K562 cells. *Biochem Pharmacol* (2006) **71**:1162–74. doi:10.1016/j.bcp.2006.01.006
16. Paterson JK, Gottesman MM. P-Glycoprotein is not present in mitochondrial membranes. *Exp Cell Res* (2007) **313**:3100–5. doi:10.1016/j.yexcr.2007.04.019
17. Fu D, Mitra K, Sengupta P, Jarnik M, Lippincott-Schwartz J, Arias IM. Coordinated elevation of mitochondrial oxidative phosphorylation and autophagy help drive hepatocyte polarization. *Proc Natl Acad Sci U S A* (2013) **110**:7288–93. doi:10.1073/pnas.1304285110
18. Muller C, Laurent G, Ling V. P-glycoprotein stability is affected by serum deprivation and high cell density in multidrug-resistant cells. *J Cell Physiol* (1995) **163**:538–44. doi:10.1002/jcp.1041630314
19. Dejgaard S, Nicolay J, Taheri M, Thomas DY, Bergeron JJ. The ER glycoprotein quality control system. *Curr Issues Mol Biol* (2004) **6**:29–42.
20. Tamehiro N, Zhou S, Okuhira K, Benita Y, Brown CE, Zhuang DZ, et al. SPTLC1 binds ABCA1 to negatively regulate trafficking and cholesterol efflux activity of the transporter. *Biochemistry* (2008) **47**:6138–47. doi:10.1021/bi800182t
21. Wedemeyer WJ, Welker E, Narayan M, Scheraga HA. Disulfide bonds and protein folding. *Biochemistry* (2000) **39**:7032. doi:10.1021/bi005111p
22. Fukuda Y, Aguilar-Bryan L, Vaxillaire M, Dechaume A, Wang Y, Dean M, et al. Conserved intramolecular disulfide bond is critical to trafficking and fate of ATP-binding cassette (ABC) transporters ABCB6 and sulfonylurea receptor 1 (SUR1)/ABCC8. *J Biol Chem* (2011) **286**:8481–92. doi:10.1074/jbc.M110.174516
23. Budnik A, Stephens DJ. ER exit sites – localization and control of COPII vesicle formation. *FEBS Lett* (2009) **583**:3796–803. doi:10.1016/j.febslet.2009.10.038
24. Tanaka AR, Kano F, Ueda K, Murata M. The ABCA1 Q597R mutant undergoes trafficking from the ER upon ER stress. *Biochem Biophys Res Commun* (2008) **369**:1174–8. doi:10.1016/j.bbrc.2008.03.018
25. Ameen N, Silvis M, Bradbury NA. Endocytic trafficking of CFTR in health and disease. *J Cyst Fibros* (2007) **6**:1–14. doi:10.1016/j.jcf.2006.09.002
26. Molinari A, Cianfriglia M, Meschini S, Calcabrini A, Arancia G. P-glycoprotein expression in the Golgi apparatus of multidrug-resistant cells. *Int J Cancer* (1994) **59**:789–95. doi:10.1002/ijc.2910590614
27. Kipp H, Arias IM. Newly synthesized canalicular ABC transporters are directly targeted from the Golgi to the hepatocyte apical domain in rat liver. *J Biol Chem* (2000) **275**:15917–25. doi:10.1074/jbc.M909875199
28. Kipp H, Pichetshote N, Arias IM. Transporters on demand: intrahepatic pools of canalicular ATP binding cassette transporters in rat liver. *J Biol Chem* (2001) **276**:7218–24. doi:10.1074/jbc.M007794200
29. Sai Y, Nies AT, Arias IM. Bile acid secretion and direct targeting of mdr1-green fluorescent protein from Golgi to the canalicular membrane in polarized WIF-B cells. *J Cell Sci* (1999) **112**(Pt 24):4535–45.
30. Musch A, Cohen D, Rodriguez-Boulan E. Myosin II is involved in the production of constitutive transport vesicles from the TGN. *J Cell Biol* (1997) **138**:291–306. doi:10.1083/jcb.138.2.291
31. Keller P, Simons K. Post-golgi biosynthetic trafficking. *J Cell Sci* (1997) **110**(Pt 24):3001–9.
32. Diop NK, Hrycyna CA. N-linked glycosylation of the human ABC transporter ABCG2 on asparagine 596 is not essential for expression, transport activity, or trafficking to the plasma membrane. *Biochemistry* (2005) **44**:5420–9. doi:10.1021/bi0479858
33. Gee HY, Noh SH, Tang BL, Kim KH, Lee MG. Rescue of DeltaF508-CFTR trafficking via a GRASP-dependent unconventional secretion pathway. *Cell* (2011) **146**:746–60. doi:10.1016/j.cell.2011.07.021

34. Wakabayashi Y, Dutt P, Lippincott-Schwartz J, Arias IM. Rab11a and myosin Vb are required for bile canalicular formation in WIF-B9 cells. *Proc Natl Acad Sci U S A* (2005) **102**:15087–92. doi:10.1073/pnas.0503702102
35. Hutagalung AH, Novick PJ. Role of Rab GTPases in membrane traffic and cell physiology. *Physiol Rev* (2011) **91**:119–49. doi:10.1152/physrev.00059.2009
36. Stenmark H. Rab GTPases as coordinators of vesicle traffic. *Nat Rev Mol Cell Biol* (2009) **10**:513–25. doi:10.1038/nrm2728
37. Grigoriev I, Splinter D, Keijzer N, Wulf PS, Demmers J, Ohtsuka T, et al. Rab6 regulates transport and targeting of exocytotic carriers. *Dev Cell* (2007) **13**:305–14. doi:10.1016/j.devcel.2007.06.010
38. Ullrich O, Reinsch S, Urbe S, Zerial M, Parton RG. Rab11 regulates recycling through the pericentriolar recycling endosome. *J Cell Biol* (1996) **135**:913–24. doi:10.1083/jcb.135.4.913
39. Schonteich E, Wilson GM, Burden J, Hopkins CR, Anderson K, Goldenring JR, et al. The Rip11/Rab11-FIP5 and kinesin II complex regulates endocytic protein recycling. *J Cell Sci* (2008) **121**:3824–33. doi:10.1242/jcs.032441
40. Nokes RL, Fields IC, Collins RN, Folsch H. Rab13 regulates membrane trafficking between TGN and recycling endosomes in polarized epithelial cells. *J Cell Biol* (2008) **182**:845–53. doi:10.1083/jcb.200802176
41. Swiatecka-Urban A, Brown A, Moreau-Marquis S, Renuka J, Coutermarsh B, Barnaby R, et al. The short apical membrane half-life of rescued {Delta}F508-cystic fibrosis transmembrane conductance regulator (CFTR) results from accelerated endocytosis of {Delta}F508-CFTR in polarized human airway epithelial cells. *J Biol Chem* (2005) **280**:36762–72. doi:10.1074/jbc.M508944200
42. Silvis MR, Bertrand CA, Ameen N, Golin-Bisello F, Butterworth MB, Frizzell RA, et al. Rab11b regulates the apical recycling of the cystic fibrosis transmembrane conductance regulator in polarized intestinal epithelial cells. *Mol Biol Cell* (2009) **20**:2337–50. doi:10.1091/mbc.E08-01-0084
43. Jean S, Kiger AA. Coordination between RAB GTPase and phosphoinositide regulation and functions. *Nat Rev Mol Cell Biol* (2012) **13**:463–70. doi:10.1038/nrm3379
44. Davey JR, Humphrey SJ, Junutula JR, Mishra AK, Lambright DG, James DE, et al. TBC1D13 is a RAB35 specific GAP that plays an important role in GLUT4 trafficking in adipocytes. *Traffic* (2012) **13**:1429–41. doi:10.1111/j.1600-0854.2012.01397.x
45. Ferrandiz-Huertas C, Fernandez-Carvajal A, Ferrer-Montiel A. Rab4 interacts with the human P-glycoprotein and modulates its surface expression in multidrug resistant K562 cells. *Int J Cancer* (2011) **128**:192–205. doi:10.1002/ijc.25310
46. Baas AF, Kuipers J, van der Wel NN, Batlle E, Koerten HK, Peters PJ, et al. Complete polarization of single intestinal epithelial cells upon activation of LKB1 by STRAD. *Cell* (2004) **116**:457–66. doi:10.1016/S0092-8674(04)00114-X
47. Settembre C, Fraldi A, Medina DL, Ballabio A. Signals from the lysosome: a control centre for cellular clearance and energy metabolism. *Nat Rev Mol Cell Biol* (2013) **14**:283–96. doi:10.1038/nrm3565
48. Feng Y, Press B, Wandinger-Ness A. Rab 7: an important regulator of late endocytic membrane traffic. *J Cell Biol* (1995) **131**:1435–52. doi:10.1083/jcb.131.6.1435
49. Bucci C, Thomsen P, Nicoziani P, McCarthy J, van Deurs B. Rab7: a key to lysosome biogenesis. *Mol Biol Cell* (2000) **11**:467–80. doi:10.1091/mbc.11.2.467
50. Barbero P, Bittova L, Pfeffer SR. Visualization of Rab9-mediated vesicle transport from endosomes to the trans-Golgi in living cells. *J Cell Biol* (2002) **156**:511–8. doi:10.1083/jcb.200109030
51. Gentzsch M, Chang XB, Cui L, Wu Y, Ozols VV, Choudhury A, et al. Endocytic trafficking routes of wild type and DeltaF508 cystic fibrosis transmembrane conductance regulator. *Mol Biol Cell* (2004) **15**:2684–96. doi:10.1091/mbc.E04-03-0176
52. Tan B, Piwnica-Worms D, Ratner L. Multidrug resistance transporters and modulation. *Curr Opin Oncol* (2000) **12**:450–8. doi:10.1097/00001622-200009000-00011
53. Thomas H, Coley HM. Overcoming multidrug resistance in cancer: an update on the clinical strategy of inhibiting p-glycoprotein. *Cancer Control* (2003) **10**:159–65.
54. Krishna R, Mayer LD. Multidrug resistance (MDR) in cancer. Mechanisms, reversal using modulators of MDR and the role of MDR modulators in influencing the pharmacokinetics of anticancer drugs. *Eur J Pharm Sci* (2000) **11**:265–83. doi:10.1016/S0928-0987(00)00114-7
55. Bates S, Kang M, Meadows B, Bakke S, Choyke P, Merino M, et al. A Phase I study of infusional vinblastine in combination with the P-glycoprotein antagonist PSC 833 (valspodar). *Cancer* (2001) **92**:1577–90. doi:10.1002/1097-0142(20010915)92:63.0.CO;2-H
56. Wandel C, Kim RB, Kajiji S, Guengerich P, Wilkinson GR, Wood AJ. P-glycoprotein and cytochrome P-450 3A inhibition: dissociation of inhibitory potencies. *Cancer Res* (1999) **59**:3944–8.
57. Morschhauser F, Zinzani PL, Burgess M, Sloots L, Bouafia F, Dumontet C. Phase I/II trial of a P-glycoprotein inhibitor, Zosuquidar.3HCl trihydrochloride (LY335979), given orally in combination with the CHOP regimen in patients with non-Hodgkin's lymphoma. *Leuk Lymphoma* (2007) **48**:708–15. doi:10.1080/10428190701190169
58. Kuppens IE, Witteveen EO, Jewell RC, Radema SA, Paul EM, Mangum SG, et al. A phase I, randomized, open-label, parallel-cohort, dose-finding study of elacridar (GF120918) and oral topotecan in cancer patients. *Clin Cancer Res* (2007) **13**:3276–85. doi:10.1158/1078-0432.CCR-06-2414
59. Shukla S, Wu CP, Ambudkar SV. Development of inhibitors of ATP-binding cassette drug transporters: present status and challenges. *Expert Opin Drug Metab Toxicol* (2008) **4**:205–23. doi:10.1517/17425255.4.2.205
60. Nobili S, Landini I, Giglioni B, Mini E. Pharmacological strategies for overcoming multidrug resistance. *Curr Drug Targets* (2006) **7**:861–79. doi:10.2174/138945006777709593
61. Palmeira A, Sousa E, Vasconcelos MH, Pinto MM. Three decades of P-gp inhibitors: skimming through several generations and scaffolds. *Curr Med Chem* (2012) **19**:1946–2025. doi:10.2174/092986712800167392
62. Loo TW, Clarke DM. The human multidrug resistance P-glycoprotein is inactive when its maturation is inhibited: potential for a role in cancer chemotherapy. *FASEB J* (1999) **13**:1724–32.
63. Larsen AK, Escargueil AE, Skladanowski A. Resistance mechanisms associated with altered intracellular distribution of anticancer agents. *Pharmacol Ther* (2000) **85**:217–29. doi:10.1016/S0163-7258(99)00073-X

3

In vitro development of chemotherapy and targeted therapy drug-resistant cancer cell lines: a practical guide with case studies

*Martina McDermott[1,2], Alex J. Eustace[1,3], Steven Busschots[4], Laura Breen[1], John Crown[1,5], Martin Clynes[1], Norma O'Donovan[1] and Britta Stordal[1,4]**

[1] National Institute for Cellular Biotechnology, Dublin City University, Dublin, Ireland
[2] Department of Drug Discovery and Biomedical Sciences, South Carolina College of Pharmacy, University of South Carolina, Columbia, SC, USA
[3] Department of Medical Oncology, Beaumont Hospital, Royal College of Surgeons in Ireland, Dublin, Ireland
[4] Department of Histopathology, St James' Hospital, Trinity College Dublin, Dublin, Ireland
[5] Department of Medical Oncology, St Vincent's University Hospital, Dublin, Ireland

Edited by:
Enrico Mini, University of Florence, Italy

Reviewed by:
Carine Michiels, University of Namur, Belgium
Marc Poirot, Institut National de la santé et de la Recherche Médicale, France

***Correspondence:**
Britta Stordal, Department of Histopathology, 1.18 Sir Patrick Dun Research Laboratory, St James' Hospital, Trinity College Dublin, Central Pathology Building, Dublin 8, Ireland
e-mail: stordalb@tcd.ie

The development of a drug-resistant cell line can take from 3 to 18 months. However, little is published on the methodology of this development process. This article will discuss key decisions to be made prior to starting resistant cell line development; the choice of parent cell line, dose of selecting agent, treatment interval, and optimizing the dose of drug for the parent cell line. Clinically relevant drug-resistant cell lines are developed by mimicking the conditions cancer patients experience during chemotherapy and cell lines display between two- and eight-fold resistance compared to their parental cell line. Doses of drug administered are low, and a pulsed treatment strategy is often used where the cells recover in drug-free media. High-level laboratory models are developed with the aim of understanding potential mechanisms of resistance to chemotherapy agents. Doses of drug are higher and escalated over time. It is common to have difficulty developing stable clinically relevant drug-resistant cell lines. A comparative selection strategy of multiple cell lines or multiple chemotherapeutic agents mitigates this risk and gives insight into which agents or type of cell line develops resistance easily. Successful selection strategies from our research are presented. Pulsed-selection produced platinum or taxane-resistant large cell lung cancer (H1299 and H460) and temozolomide-resistant melanoma (Malme-3M and HT144) cell lines. Continuous selection produced a lapatinib-resistant breast cancer cell line (HCC1954). Techniques for maintaining drug-resistant cell lines are outlined including; maintaining cells with chemotherapy, pulse treating with chemotherapy, or returning to master drug-resistant stocks. The heterogeneity of drug-resistant models produced from the same parent cell line with the same chemotherapy agent is explored with reference to P-glycoprotein. Heterogeneity in drug-resistant cell lines reflects the heterogeneity that can occur in clinical drug resistance.

Keywords: chemotherapy, cancer, drug-resistance, cell lines, selection strategy

INTRODUCTION AND HISTORICAL PERSPECTIVE

The development of chemotherapy drug-resistant cancer cell lines is a long established approach for investigating the mechanisms of cytotoxicity and resistance to chemotherapy agents. One of the first publications to describe the development of an anti-cancer drug-resistant *in vitro* model, which exhibited acquired resistance to a chemotherapy drug, was published in 1970 (1). Resistant cell lines were developed from parental Chinese hamster cells using a stepwise increase in treatment dose with actinomycin D. This induced 2500-fold greater resistance to the drug than that observed in the parental cells. These resistant cell lines were also cross resistant to other chemotherapy drugs such as vinblastine and daunorubicin. Some earlier drug-resistant cell lines were developed in the 1950 and 1960s using *in vivo* mouse models, including models resistant to methotrexate (2, 3), vinblastine, terephthalanilide (4), and the guanine analog, 8-azaguanine (5).

Publications in this research field usually place little emphasis on how the drug-resistant cell lines were established in the laboratory. The development of drug-resistant cell lines can take anything from 3 to 18 months in the laboratory and many decisions are taken along this journey. This review summarizes the major methodological approaches for developing drug-resistant

Abbreviations: 5-FU, fluorouracil; ADR, adriamycin; AUC, area under concentration time curve; CHL, chlorambucil; CIS, cisplatin; CR, complete response; CSC, cancer stem cells; CYC, cyclophosphamide; DNR, daunorubicin; DOCE, docetaxel; DOX, doxorubicin; EPI, epirubicin; ETO, etoposide; GFR, glomerular filtration rate; IC_{50}, 50% inhibitory concentration; IFO, ifosfamide; IV, intravenous; MEL, melphalan; MTT, 3-(4,5-dimethylthiazol-2-yl)-2,5-diphenyltetrazolium bromide; NR, no response; OX, oxaliplatin; PARP, poly (ADP-ribose) polymerase; PD, progressive disease; P-gp, P-glycoprotein; PR, partial response; PRED, prednimustine; RAD, radiation; SCLC, small cell lung cancer; TAX, paclitaxel; THI, thiotepa; UNK, unknown; VINC, vincristine; VIND, vindesine.

cell lines *in vitro* with reference to the literature and includes several case studies from our experience.

IC_{50} VALUES AND FOLD RESISTANCE

Drug-resistant cell models are developed in the laboratory by repeatedly exposing cancer cells growing in cell culture to drugs. The surviving daughter resistant cells are then compared to the parental sensitive cells using combination cell viability/proliferation assays such as the MTT (6), acid phosphatase (6), or clonogenic assays (7). The sensitivity of these paired cell lines is usually determined by exposing them to a range of drug concentrations and then assessing cell viability. The IC_{50} (drug concentration causing 50% growth inhibition) for these paired cell lines can be used to determine the increase in resistance known as fold resistance by the following equation:

$$\text{Fold Resistance} = IC_{50} \text{ of Resistant Cell Line}/IC_{50} \text{ of Parental Cell Line}$$

WHAT IS A CLINICALLY RELEVANT LEVEL OF RESISTANCE?

To determine the level of drug resistance that occurs in the clinical treatment of cancer we can compare cell lines that have been established from cancer patients before and after chemotherapy (**Table 1**) (8–14). The majority of cell lines listed in **Table 1** developed from patients post-chemotherapy show a two- to five-fold increase in resistance to the agents the patients were treated with, based on a comparison of IC_{50} values. Three cell lines had higher levels of resistance but these were still relatively low-level at ~8–12-fold higher than the parental cells (PEO4, SK-3, and GLC-16).

CLINICALLY RELEVANT VS. HIGH-LEVEL LABORATORY MODELS

For the purposes of this review we will divide drug-resistant cell models into two categories: clinically relevant models or high-level laboratory models. Both types of models have their advantages and disadvantages for research.

Clinically relevant models are developed with the aim of trying to mimic the conditions cancer patients experience during chemotherapy. Doses of drug are lower, and a pulsed treatment strategy is often used where the cells recover in drug-free media. This mimics the cycles of chemotherapy a patient receives in the clinic. Disadvantages to clinically relevant models can include unstable resistance, very low-level resistance, and small molecular changes to detect and analyze. Based on the cell lines derived from the patients before and after chemotherapy shown in **Table 1**; we have defined clinically relevant resistance as a two- to five-fold increase from the IC_{50} value of the parent cell line. Examples of clinically relevant models are shown in **Table 2** (15–21).

High-level laboratory models are developed with the aim of understanding potential mechanisms of toxicity and resistance to chemotherapy agents. Doses of drug are often high and treatment doses are escalated over time. Cells are frequently grown continually in the presence of drug or highly drug-resistant clones are selected from a mixed population. In some earlier drug-resistant models, mutagenesis was also induced prior to drug treatment (22,

Table 1 | Cell lines established from cancer patients before and after chemotherapy.

Cancer type	Parent cell line (established)	Chemotherapy received	Resistant cell line (established)	Fold resistance to chemotherapy received	Reference
Lung	EBC-2 (18th September 1997)	CIS, IFO, VIND	EBC-2/R (4th October 1997)	CIS – 2.3, IFO[a] – 3.2, VIND – 0.77	(8)
	SK-1 (August 1986)	CYC, ADR, ETO, VINC, RAD	SK-2 (March 1987)	ADR – 1.2, ETO – 1.2, CYC[b] – 1.3	(10)
		CIS, ETO	SK-3 (May 1987)	CIS – 8.6, ETO – 6.2	
	TM1 (April 1987)	CYC, ADR, ETO, VINC	TM2 (September 1987)	CYC[b] – 5.4, ADR – 3.0, ETO – 3.5	
	GLC-14 (December 1984)	CYC, DOX, ETO	GLC-16 (October 1985)	DOX – 3.18, ETO – 12.1	(11)
Neuroblastoma	KP-N-AY (October 1984)	ADR, CIS, CYC, VINC	KP-N-AYR (December 1985)	ADR – 3.0, CIS – 2.7	(9)
Ovarian	PEO1 (February 1982)	CIS, CHL, 5-FU	PEO4 (November 1982)	CIS – 8.72	(12, 13)
		CIS, CHL, 5-FU	PEO6 (February 1983)	CIS – 4.64	(12, 13)
	PEA1	CIS, PRED	PEA2	CIS – 4.30	(13, 14)
	PEO14	CIS, CHL	PEO23	CIS – 4.48	(13, 14)

ADR, adriamycin; CIS, cisplatin; CHL, chlorambucil; CYC, cyclophosphamide; DOX, doxorubicin; ETO, etoposide; 5-FU, fluorouracil; IFO, ifosfamide; RAD, radiation; PRED, prednimustine; VINC, vincristine; VIND, vindesine.

[a] *Used 4-hydroperoxy ifosfamide (the active form of ifosfamide).*

[b] *Used 4-hydroperoxycyclophosphamide (the active form of cyclophosphamide).*

Table 2 | Different selection strategies and classification of resulting drug-resistant cell lines.

Cancer type	Parent cell line	Selecting agent	Exposure	Dose	Population	Resistant cell line	Fold resistance to selecting agent	Development time (months)	Classification	Reference
Cervical	KB-3-1	CIS	Continuous	Stepwise and	Whole	KBCP10	1152	UNK	High-level lab	(22, 23)
		COL		mutagenesis	Cloned	KB-8-5-11	40	UNK	High-level lab	(24)
Leukemia	CCRF-CEM	EPI	Pulse	Constant	Whole	CEM/E25	7	UNK	Clinically relevant	(15, 16)
			Continuous	Stepwise	Whole	CEM/E1000	94	8 from E25	High-level lab	
	K562	DNR	Pulse	Stepwise	Whole	K562/DNR	3	2	Clinically relevant	(17)
Lung	DLKP	ADR	Continuous	Stepwise	Whole	DLKP-A	322	18	High-level lab	(25)
	A549	PAC	Pulse	Constant	Whole	A549-txl	5.5	2.5	Clinically relevant	(18)
	SKLU1					SKLU1-txl	5.0		Clinically relevant	
	SKMES1	PAC				SKMES1-txl	24.7		High-level lab	
		DOCE				SKMES1-Txt	29.1		High-level lab	
	DMS53	PAC				DMS53-txl	6.3		Clinically relevant	
		DOCE				DMS53-Txt	1.8		Clinically relevant	
	DLRP	DOCE				DLRP-Txt	4.1		Clinically relevant	
	H69	CIS	Pulse	Constant	Whole	H69CIS200	1.5–2	8	Clinically relevant	(19, 20)
		OX				H69OX400				
Ovarian	IGROV-1	CIS	Pulse	Stepwise	Whole	IGROVCDDP	8.41		Clinically relevant	(21)

ADR, adriamycin; CIS, cisplatin; DNR, daunorubicin; DOCE, docetaxel; EPI, epirubicin; OX, oxaliplatin; UNK, unknown.

23). High-level models are often more stably resistant and therefore easier to maintain in culture for an ongoing research project. Levels of resistance are often higher and as such molecular changes associated with the mechanism of resistance are larger and easier to identify. The disadvantage of these models is the higher the level of resistance the less relevant the model becomes to the clinic. Examples of high-level laboratory models are shown in **Table 2** (15, 16, 18, 22–25).

PLANNING A SELECTION STRATEGY FOR DRUG-RESISTANT CELL LINES

CHOICE OF PARENTAL CELL LINE

Choosing a parental cell line is very important as it is the basis of all the subsequent experiments. The parental cell line should be very easy to maintain in cell culture as resistant variants usually become more challenging to grow. Ideally, the researchers performing the drug-resistant selection in the laboratory should be very familiar with growing the parental cells. Researchers experienced in growing a particular cell line will have more of an idea of when the cells need to be subcultured and when it is best to leave them. This experience is important when deciding when to subculture cells recovering from the drug treatment.

It is also important to consider the patient from whom the cell line is derived. If possible, it is good to choose a chemotherapy and radiation naïve cell line. Previous treatment with chemotherapeutic agents and radiation may have already caused changes in resistance pathways, and increased expression of drug resistance markers that may not be relevant to the agent being studied. However, chemotherapy and radiation naïve cell lines are relatively rare. As an alternative to a chemotherapy naïve cell line, choose a cell line with a relatively low baseline IC_{50} value for the drug of interest as a two- to five-fold increase in resistance will result in an IC_{50} of the daughter resistant cell line remaining within the clinically relevant range. **Table 3** shows the clinical characteristics of some commonly used ovarian cancer cell lines as an example of the kind of information that is available for cell lines [(12, 14, 26–38); Sikic, personal communication]. In the case of ovarian cancer, the majority of cell lines commonly used in research are derived from metastatic ascites, and are not chemonaïve (**Table 3**).

EXPOSURE TO CHEMOTHERAPY AGENT

The researcher needs to decide what kind of model they are trying to develop, a clinically relevant model or a high-level laboratory model. A clinically relevant model is informed by data gathered from the clinical administration of drug and usually has minimal escalation of the treatment dose. The sky is the limit for a high-level laboratory model where dose escalation is used extensively to achieve a large fold resistance. However, the solubility of the selecting agent will be final limiting factor in how much drug can be applied to cancer cells. Doses that approach the limit of solubility will not be in the clinically relevant range.

The reality is that most selection strategies start out with a clinically relevant strategy and then are escalated within the clinical range and escalated further again beyond the clinical dose range to make a high-level model. The main reasons for this approach are the stability of the resistance phenotype produced and that the resistance established in the daughter cell line is statistically significant when compared to the parent cell line.

Table 3 | Clinical characteristics of ovarian tumors from which ovarian cell lines were established.

Cell line	Original tumor histology	Isolated from	Treatment received pre-isolation	Response	Reference
59M	Endometrioid/clear cell	Ascites	None	N/A	(26)
EFO27	Mucinous	Solid metastasis	None	N/A	(27)
ES2	Serous/clear cell	Primary tumor	None	N/A	[(28); Sikic, personal communication]
FUOV1	Serous	Primary tumor	None	N/A	(29)
HEY	Serous	Peritoneal deposit and xenograft	Radiotherapy, radium	CR	(26, 30)
HOC1	Serous	Ascites	MEL, CIS, ADR, CYC	PR, PR	(31, 39)
HOC8	Serous	Ascites	MEL	PR	(32, 33)
IGROV-1	Endometrioid/clear cell	Primary tumor	None	N/A	(34)
OAW28	Adenocarcinoma	Ascites	CIS, MEL	NR, NR	(26)
OAW42	Serous	Ascites	CIS	CR	(26)
OC316	Serous	Ascites	CIS, ETO, CYC, TAX	PD, SD	(35)
OVCAR3	Serous	Ascites	CYC, CIS, DOX	Unknown	(26, 36, 37)
PEA1	Adenocarcinoma	Pleural effusion	None	N/A	(14)
PEO1	Serous	Ascites	CIS, CHL, 5-FU	CR	(12, 14)
PEO14	Serous	Ascites	None	N/A	(14)
SKOV3	Adenocarcinoma	Ascites	THI	Unknown	(26)
SNU251	Endometrioid	Ascites	CYC, ADR, CIS	Unknown	(38)

ADR, adriamycin; CIS, cisplatin; CHL, chlorambucil; CR, complete response; CYC, cyclophosphamide; DOX, doxorubicin; ETO, etoposide; MEL, melphalan; N/A, not applicable; NR, no response; PD, progressive disease; PR, partial response; TAX, paclitaxel; THI, thiotepa.

Cell lines are frequently cultured in the presence of antibiotics in many laboratories. When establishing a new drug-resistant model, we recommend not using antibiotics as this does not mimic the clinical situation, cancer patients are not continually treated with antibiotics. Resistance mechanisms produced in the presence of antibiotics may not reflect clinical drug resistance.

Pharmacokinetics and drug stability

In order to produce a clinically relevant model of drug resistance, it is important to research how the chemotherapy agent is administered in the clinical treatment of cancer. The amount of chemotherapy administered intravenously (IV) is often expressed in the units milligrams per square meter. These can be converted to micrograms per milliliter or micromolar by consulting pharmacokinetic studies on the drug where the concentration achieved in the bloodstream is measured.

Chemotherapy administered by IV is often given in cycles where the patient receives the drug on a weekly or monthly basis. A pulsed-selection strategy where the cells are treated with drug and then the surviving population are allowed to recover in drug-free media mimics this clinical scenario. Pharmacokinetic studies will give a broad range of doses achieved in the bloodstream, the highest immediately after the bolus of drug is administered to the patient, this then drops over the next hours and days depending on the rate of excretion of the drug. This gives a broad dose range to define the clinical relevance of the dose of drug used in the development of a drug-resistant model. A higher dose for several hours could model the bolus of drug, a lower dose for a several days could model the longer excretion of the drug. Following an intravenous bolus injection of 100 mg/m^2 cisplatin a peak-plasma level of ~6 μg/mL is reached but this quickly drops to <2 μg/mL after 2 h (40) Clearance of cisplatin from the body is triphasic where the distribution half-life is 13 min, the elimination half-life is 43 min, and the terminal half-life is 5.4 days (41). After 24 h, 25% of the initial cisplatin dose has been eliminated from the body with renal clearance accounting for 90%.

Carboplatin has a similar mechanism of action to cisplatin but needs a 20–40-fold higher dose to exhibit the same cytotoxicity as cisplatin. However, only a 10-fold increase in carboplatin dose is required to reach similar intracellular platinum concentrations (42). After intravenous bolus injection of 375 mg/m^2 carboplatin peak-plasma levels of ~39 μg/mL are achieved, which drops to 9 μg/mL within 2 h (43). Clearance of carboplatin has a distribution half-life of 22 min, an elimination half-life of 116 min, and a terminal half-life of 5.8 days (44). Clearance of carboplatin from the body is primarily by the urine as unchanged drug. After 24 h, 90% clearance is achieved. Carboplatin does not have significant excretion from the renal tubules as seen for cisplatin, instead the glomerular filtrate accounts for the vast majority of elimination. For this reason, glomerular filtration rate (GFR) is linearly related to total renal clearance giving relatively simple pharmacokinetics for carboplatin. Even at high doses evidence suggests that carboplatin has linear pharmacokinetics (45). A formula called the "Calvert formula" has been derived, which is based on the GFR and is used to provide a suitable dose for patients in relation to an area under concentration time curve (AUC) value. AUC is the ratio of the amount of drug that reaches the systemic circulation and the clearance of the drug, which correlates to its clinical efficiency and toxicity. This formula has been validated in a perspective study (46). Conventional doses of carboplatin administered to patients generally are aimed at giving an AUC value of between 5 and 7 mg/mL/min.

The amount of chemotherapy administered orally is usually expressed in the unit milligrams per day. Again pharmacokinetic studies can be used to convert this to a concentration in the bloodstream. A continuous treatment strategy where the cells are cultured constantly in the presence of drug can be clinically relevant for an oral drug given daily or twice daily as a relatively constant amount of the drug is present. Olaparib is a member of the poly (ADP-ribose) polymerase (PARP) inhibitor class of drugs and is administered orally. The maximum tolerated dose of olaparib is 400 mg twice daily. Absorption is rapid and its peak-plasma concentration is reached within 1–3 h. Plasma levels then decline biphasically and it has a terminal elimination half-life of ~5–7 h (47). A phase 1 study on Japanese patients found that peak-plasma values for a single dose of 400 mg olaparib was ~7 μg/mL, which dropped below 0.1 μg/mL after 50 h. For a dose of 400 mg administered twice daily for 15 days, peak-plasma concentrations were found to be similar. The half-life of olaparib was recorded to be between 7 and 11 h across doses ranging from 100 to 400 mg (48).

The chemical stability of drugs used in establishing drug-resistant cell line models is also an important consideration when designing a selection strategy. For example, temozolomide an alkylating agent used in the treatment of glioblastoma and metastatic melanoma when in its active state, has a half-life of 25 and 60 min for the first and second phases (49) whilst docetaxel a microtubule destabilizing agent has a half-life of 12 h (50). Lapatinib, a dual EGFR HER2 inhibitor used in the treatment of HER2-positive breast cancer has a half-life of 24 h (51) whilst the monoclonal HER2 antibody trastuzumab also used in HER2-positive breast cancer has a half-life of over 5 days (52). Drugs with a shorter half-life will have to be dealt with carefully to ensure that cancer cells receive the maximal benefit from drug dosing. Also drugs with a long half-life should be removed from cells long before the models are to be used in experiments. This ensures that residual drug will not remain in the cells and effect proliferation assays comparing survival between the parental and resistant cells.

Optimization of treatment dose in parental cell line

The dose of drug used must be optimized for the parental cell line selected for use in developing the resistant model. A cytotoxicity assay in the parental cell line can be used to determine a suitable dose range. This dose range can then be compared to the pharmacokinetic information for the drug of interest. The rate of recovery from drug treatment is just as important as the IC_{50}; as the rate of recovery can be different between agents even if an equivalently cytotoxic dose is administered to cells. **Figure 1** shows the recovery of two ovarian cancer cell lines (OVCAR8 and UPN251) from equivalently cytotoxic doses of carboplatin and paclitaxel. The recovery from paclitaxel is much faster than carboplatin.

The chemotherapeutic drug paclitaxel is frequently given at a dose of 175 mg/m^2 as a single agent (53, 54). Pharmacokinetic studies for this dose show peak-plasma concentrations as high as 10,000 ng/mL but drop off quickly after 24 h to 50 ng/mL and below (55, 56). In the development of platinum/taxane-resistant OVCAR8 and UPN251 ovarian cancer cells, treatment doses were chosen trailed over the range of IC_{20}–IC_{80}, and were consistent with doses used in the clinical setting. Paclitaxel doses tested for OVCAR8 and UPN251 were from a range of 2.3–14 and 10–100 ng/mL. Carboplatin doses tested for OVCAR8 and UPN251 were 2.3–18.5 and 0.7–2 μg/mL, respectively. The final chosen

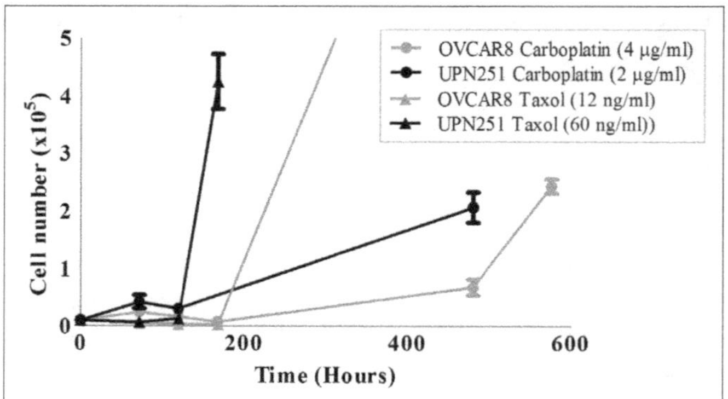

FIGURE 1 | Recovery of OVCAR8 and UPN251 from carboplatin or paclitaxel treatment. 1 × 10^4 cells were treated for 3 days with the indicated doses of either carboplatin or paclitaxel and recovery monitored as described in Section "Methods."

doses of paclitaxel and carboplatin displayed an initially large percentage cell death or growth inhibition compared to a control grown in drug-free media. Carboplatin doses of 4 and 2 μg/mL and paclitaxel doses of 12 and 60 ng/mL were chosen for OVCAR8 and UPN251, respectively (**Figure 1**). After treatment with the selected doses and removal of the drug, the cells were able to return to logarithmic growth ensuring the selection of resistant cell sub populations.

In the development of platinum-resistant H69 small cell lung cancer (SCLC) cells, treatment doses were chosen in the range of IC_{10}–IC_{40}, and were consistent with doses used in the clinical setting (19). Two exposure times and doses were used for cisplatin and oxaliplatin reflecting differing pharmacokinetic phases of the administration of platinum drugs; 2-h treatments at 1–8 μg/mL and 4-day treatments at 0.2–1.6 μg/mL. The lowest drug concentration treatments all produced 20–30% cell death and growth arrest in H69 cells. Drug-treated cells increased in size and did not aggregate in typical SCLC clumping morphology. Surviving cultures were then retreated when their normal growth rate and clumping morphology had returned, ~3–4 weeks later.

POPULATION DYNAMICS

In most selection strategies the whole population of cells remains as one group throughout the selection, no cloning or other separation methods are used. If a pulse of drug is given, a small percentage of cells remain, which repopulates the flask. This new population of cells is then retreated with the next pulse (18, 19). Alternatively a low-level of drug is present continuously, the cells adapt to growing in the presence of the drug and then the dose of drug is slowly increased (25).

It is well known that tumors are heterogeneous (57–59). Consequently, the cancer cell lines derived from tumors are also heterogeneous. For example, breast tumors from patients who are BRCA1/2 carriers have been shown to be heterogeneous, where not all cells have lost the second BRCA1/2 allele (60). Selection with chemotherapy agents therefore often result in the isolation of a cell population that already exists in the culture. Indeed, this has been demonstrated for many drug-resistant models, particularly in projects, which examine cancer stem cells (CSCs). CSCs are thought to be responsible for tumor regeneration after chemotherapy. Drug-resistant cell lines are often enriched for markers of stem cells. The stem-cell marker CD133 was found to be enriched in a panel of cisplatin-resistant lung cancer cell lines, with a 5-fold increase in both A549CisR and MORCisR, and a 12-fold increase in H460CisR cells (61).

There are other physical methods of separation available to select different populations from a cell line such as limited dilution or cell sorting by flow cytometry. This can isolate cells which may be more resistant to chemotherapy than other populations within the same cell line (62). The advantage of clonal populations as drug-resistant models for is that there is no drug treatment is required and the resulting model is more stable. The disadvantages however are that many clones must be established and there is no guarantee that the clonal populations derived will display any difference in drug resistance.

Clonal populations can be established by limited dilution. This relies on the ability of the cells to grow independently of each other, and as such may not be suitable for all cell lines. It involves seeding cells at a very low density to result in one cell per well of a 96-well plate. Once the cells grow to confluency, they can be tested as a clonal population. Another method to obtain clonal populations is cloning rings (62). Standard toxicity testing on the clonal populations generated will show whether they display an inherent resistance to the agent of interest.

A combination of drug treatment and cloning of cells has also been used to produce resistant models. KB-8-5-11 colchicine-resistant cells were developed from parental KB-3-1 cells by selecting clones after three stepwise increases in colchicine drug treatment (24). Clones 8, 5, and 11 were the successful clones picked each round of the selection strategy.

Cloning can also be used to investigate heterogeneity within a developed drug-resistant model. A human colon cancer cell line (LoVo) was treated with cisplatin using a continuous exposure ranging from 0.005 to 20.0 μg/mL over 20 months in culture (63). At the end of the treatment, two morphologically distinct subpopulations were observed; these were then cloned by limiting dilution. The subclones showed different patterns of cross resistance to chemotherapy agents. The first clone overexpressed the ABC efflux transporter P-glycoprotein (P-gp) and the other clone did not. Heterogeneity was also seen in cisplatin-resistant models developed from a human pancreatic cancer cell line with a mutation in DNA repair protein BRCA2. Fourteen cisplatin-resistant clones were obtained. In 7 of 14 clones, the functionality of BRCA2 had been restored by secondary mutations, the remaining clones still had a non-functional BRCA2 protein (64).

RISK-REDUCTION STRATEGIES: COMPARATIVE SELECTION

It is reasonably common to have difficulties developing resistance or to produce drug-treated daughter cell lines which have not increased in resistance relative to the parental cell line. Selection strategies which do not produce drug resistance are interesting from a clinical perspective as this is what we want to achieve for cancer patients. Unfortunately, failures to develop drug resistance are generally not reported in the literature.

As a risk-reduction strategy, a comparative selection strategy should be performed, where selection of multiple cell lines or multiple chemotherapeutic agents are performed in parallel in the laboratory. **Figure 2A** shows a strategy where two parental cell lines are each treated with two chemotherapy agents, producing four different daughter cell lines. **Figure 2B** shows one parental cell line being treated with two chemotherapy agents, in two different doses or intervals producing four different daughter cell lines. By using a comparative development strategy, it is hoped that at least one of them will successfully produce a stable drug-resistant model. It can be interesting to observe which strategies produced resistance and which did not. These may be useful observations for the clinical treatment of cancer.

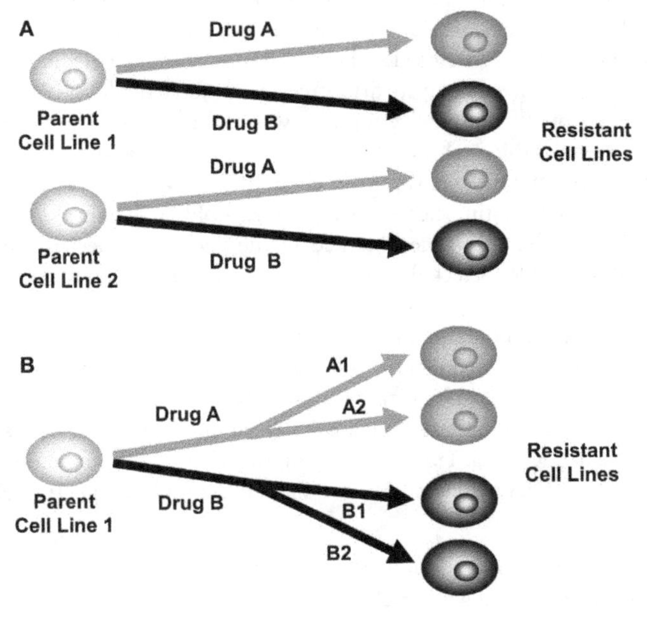

FIGURE 2 | Comparative selection of drug-resistant cell lines. (A) Plan for selection of two parent cell lines with two different drugs to produce four drug-resistant daughter cell lines. **(B)** Plan for selection of one parent cell line with two drugs at different doses or treatment intervals, producing four drug-resistant daughter cell lines.

An example of a comparative selection strategy used H69 SCLC cells treated with cisplatin or oxaliplatin for two time periods, 2 h or 4 days. The 4-day pulse selection produced more stable resistance than the 2-h pulse (19) (**Table 2**). Had only the 2-h pulsed treatment been tested in this model drug resistance would have not been developed. The comparative nature of the selection also led to the finding that oxaliplatin resistance developed faster than cisplatin resistance in H69 cells (19).

A large study by Tegze et al. aimed to develop 40 drug-resistant models from MCF-7 and MDA-MB-231 breast cancer cells using doxorubicin and paclitaxel as selecting agents. They succeeded in making 29 drug-resistant models, 10 doxorubicin and 4 paclitaxel-resistant MCF-7 cell lines, and 6 doxorubicin and 9 paclitaxel-resistant MDA-MB-231 cell lines. From this study it appears that paclitaxel resistance was easier to develop in MDA-MB-231 (ER-negative) cells and doxorubicin resistance was easier to develop in MCF-7 (ER-positive) cells.

A study by our group (18) developed resistance to paclitaxel and carboplatin in large cell lung cancer cell lines (H1299 and H460). Cells at low confluence in 75cm^2 flasks were exposed to 50 µg/mL carboplatin and 150 ng/mL (H1299) or 50 ng/mL (H460) paclitaxel for 4 h. After this period, the drug was removed and the flasks were rinsed and fed with fresh complete media. The cells were then grown in drug-free media for 6 days, replenishing the media every 2–3 days. This was repeated once a week for 10 weeks. **Table 4** shows the IC_{50}s of the platinum and taxane-resistant cell lines to a variety of chemotherapy agents. Resistance in the carboplatin-selected cells (1.5–2.3-fold) was considerably less than the resistance obtained in the paclitaxel-selected cells (2.4–4.4-fold). Selected cell lines show no obvious cross resistance pattern except within families of drugs, e.g., paclitaxel and docetaxel; carboplatin and cisplatin. The TAX-selected cells were also found to be resistant to vincristine, which is unsurprising since both agents affect microtubules. Both carboplatin-selected cell lines had a modest but statistically significant increased resistance to paclitaxel. The different patterns of resistance in cell lines selected under similar conditions show the complicated nature of multiple-drug resistance. For example, H1299-cpt became sensitive to vincristine, while after identical drug treatment, H460-cpt developed significant resistance to vincristine (2.9-fold). Overall, the low-level resistance (two- to five-fold) observed in these selected cell lines may be more clinically relevant to study than higher levels of resistance and this study highlights the importance to studying mechanisms in multiple models to identify relevant pathways.

Table 4 | Fold resistance of H1299 and H460 resistant variants compared with their parental cell lines.

Chemotherapeutic agent	H1299-cpt	H1299-txl	H460-cpt	H460-txl
Carboplatin	2.0**	1.7***	2.3*	0.8*
Cisplatin	1.5*	1.5	1.6	0.7
5-FU	1.0	1.8**	0.9	1.1
VP-16	1.4**	1.1	0.9	1
Vincristine	0.8*	2.3*	2.9***	2.5
Adriamycin	0.9	1	1	0.9
Paclitaxel	1.2*	4.4***	1.6***	2.4***
Docetaxel	0.6	2.5***	2.3	2.8***

**p*-Value <0.05; ***p*-value <0.01; ****p*-value <0.005.

If a selection strategy fails to develop resistance, the treatment conditions can be altered in an attempt to produce higher levels of resistance. If the cells are growing very well after drug treatment, consider dose escalation. In some cases this may push the dose used above clinically relevant levels but it will increase the chance of resistance developing. Alternatively, the length of time the cells are exposed to drug can be increased or a pulsed-selection strategy could be converted to a continuous selection strategy. This may make the model less clinically relevant but may produce resistance that can be studied in the laboratory.

CASE STUDIES OF DRUG-RESISTANT CELL LINES

The following section presents two case studies of drug-resistant cell lines developed in our laboratory, the reasons that selection conditions were chosen and the drug resistance outcomes of the developed cell lines. A case study using continuous selection is presented for lapatinib in breast cancer. A case study using pulsed selection is presented for temozolomide-resistant melanoma.

LAPATINIB-RESISTANT BREAST CANCER CELLS – CONTINUOUS SELECTION

Of the published models of acquired lapatinib resistance there is very little commonality in the procedures used to condition the cells, in either the concentrations of lapatinib used or in the determination of resistance status (**Table 5**) (65–72). For instance, the procedures used to develop models of acquired lapatinib resistance

Table 5 | Published cell line models of acquired lapatinib resistance, the method and concentration used to condition the cells and the proposed mechanism of lapatinib resistance.

Parent cell line	Conditioning method	Lapatinib concentration	Profiling technique	Resistance mechanism	Reference
BT474	Single cell cloning	5 µM[a]	Affymetrix array	Upregulation of ER signaling	(65)
BT474, SKBR3	Single cell cloning	5 µM[a]	Affymetrix array	Activation of RelA	(66)
SUM190	Continuous exposure	(0.25–2.5 µM)	Immunoblotting	Overexpression of XIAP	(67)
BT474	Single cell cloning	3 µM[a]	phospho-tyrosine immunoblotting	Overexpression of AXL	(68)
HCT116	Continuous exposure	10 µM[a]	Immunoblotting	Increased expression of MCL-1	(69)
HCC1954, BT474	Continuous exposure	(0.1–1 µM)	Immunoblotting	Increased expression of β1-integrin	(70)
SKBR3, MDA-MB-361, UACC893, BT474, HCC1954, SUM190	Continuous exposure	Increasing concentration up to 1 or 2 µM	Phospho-proteomic profiling	Increased SRC kinase activity	(71)
BT474, UACC812	Continuous exposure	(0.1–1 µM)	Immunoblotting	Upregulation of ER signaling	(72)

[a]*Denotes greater than peak-plasma concentration (2.5 µM).*

included a single cell cloning technique (65, 68) fixed dose conditioning (69) and dose escalation conditioning (67, 71, 72). There was significant variation in the concentrations of lapatinib used to condition the cells; many studies began with a low dose of lapatinib (e.g., 100 nM) which was dose-escalated to upwards of 2 μM. Fixed concentration conditioning was performed with concentrations of lapatinib ranging from 3 to 10 μM. The length of conditioning required to achieve resistance varied from study to study with the majority of studies taking ~12 weeks to achieve resistance, whereas other studies took up to 1 year to achieve resistance. Another variation in different models of lapatinib resistance was the definition of lapatinib resistance. Most of the studies defined their conditioned cell lines as resistant based on their ability to grow in the presence of the concentration of lapatinib used to condition the cells, only one study used an IC_{50} method while a number of studies did not quantify the level of resistance. In contrast to the previously published models of acquired lapatinib resistance, the resistant models developed by us use a relatively low dose of lapatinib relative to the IC_{50} of the resulting cell line. To our knowledge our model of acquired lapatinib resistance, HCC1954-L are the first to show that extended exposure to low dose lapatinib results in significant lapatinib resistance, with resulting lapatinib IC_{50} values significantly higher than the concentration used for conditioning.

HCC1954 cells overexpress HER2 (73) and therefore represent a cell line model of HER2-positive breast cancer. Lapatinib is a tyrosine kinase inhibitor that targets the intracellular domain of HER2 and EGFR and is approved for the treatment of HER2-positive breast cancer (74, 75). HCC1954 are moderately sensitive to lapatinib with an IC_{50} of 0.43 ± 0.03 μM (**Figure 3A**). Lapatinib is administered to cancer patients orally with a dose of 1000–1250 mg given daily (76). The median peak-plasma concentration of lapatinib reported in patients receiving 1200 mg lapatinib (once daily) was 1.2 μg/mL (2.1 μM) and the median steady-state trough concentration was 0.3 μg/mL (0.5 μM), with a range of 0.2–0.5 μg/mL (77). Therefore a continuous selection strategy is clinically relevant for lapatinib. To optimize the dose of drug used for selection, a lapatinib dose response assay was performed in order to determine the concentration of lapatinib which would result in 70% growth inhibition over a 4-day treatment. Treatment of HCC1954 cells with 1 μM lapatinib inhibited the growth of the cells by $71.5 \pm 1.2\%$ compared to untreated controls ($p = 0.004$) (**Figure 3B**). Therefore a selection strategy of continuous exposure of HCC1954 to 1 μM lapatinib was initiated with the media replenished every 4 days with fresh drug. The selection strategy was conducted in duplicate with "A" and "B" flasks as a backup in case there were problems with one flask.

HCC1954 cells were seeded into two flasks; 1×10^6 cells per $75cm^2$ flask. One flask was left untreated but was passaged alongside the treatment flask and named HCC1954-par, the cells treated with 1 μM lapatinib were named HCC1954-L. It is important to passage the untreated parental cells alongside the treated cells as a control as continuous cell culture can result in alterations in cellular characteristics, including drug resistance. The morphology of both cell lines and the sensitivity of the cell lines to lapatinib were monitored throughout the selection. After 3 months of treatment, the morphology of HCC1954-L was not altered (**Figure 3C**). For all cytotoxicity assays the HCC1954-L cells were grown in drug-free media for 5 days prior to testing. The lapatinib IC_{50} value for the HCC1954-par cells was 0.42 ± 0.01 μM, which is similar to the original HCC1954 cells. The lapatinib IC_{50} value for the HCC1954-L cells was 0.75 ± 0.07 μM (**Figure 3D**). This represents 1.8-fold increase in resistance to lapatinib. At this stage of the treatment process the lapatinib IC_{50} of HCC1954-L cells had not yet exceeded the treatment dose however they had begun to actively proliferate in the presence of lapatinib. The concentration of lapatinib was therefore increased from 1 to 1.25 μM and conditioning continued with this concentration for a further 3 months.

After 6 months of lapatinib conditioning, the sensitivity of the cells was again tested. Both the "A" and "B" flasks of HCC1954-L cells developed equivalent amounts of resistance, and the "As" were chosen for all subsequent experiments and the "Bs" frozen as a backup. The lapatinib IC_{50} value for the HCC1954-par cells was 0.42 ± 0.02 μM whereas the lapatinib IC_{50} for HCC1954-L cells was 2.67 ± 0.08 μM ($p = 0.01$) (**Figure 3E**). This represents 6.1-fold increase in resistance to lapatinib. HCC1954-L cells were deemed to be resistant to lapatinib as the lapatinib IC_{50} was above the 1 μM threshold for lapatinib sensitivity (78). The resistant cells also exhibited distinct morphological alterations compared to the parental cell line. These differences were indicated by more distinct colony boundaries and a flatter cell shape (**Figure 3F**).

In order to assess the stability of acquired resistance in the HCC1954-L cell line, sensitivity to lapatinib was assessed after freezing and thawing and following drug withdrawal. To establish a reliable cell line model of lapatinib resistance the phenotype must be stable when the cell line is frozen and re-thawed. To assess this, frozen stocks of the HCC1954-par and HCC1954-L cells were prepared in fetal calf serum containing 5% DMSO. After a minimum of 48 h in liquid nitrogen the frozen stocks were thawed and the viability of the stocks assessed by microscopy. The cells were then passaged a minimum of 3 times before lapatinib sensitivity assays were repeated (**Figure 3G**). The lapatinib IC_{50} was 0.44 ± 0.02 μM in the parental cells while the lapatinib IC_{50} in HCC1954-L cells was 2.73 ± 0.05 μM. This indicates that the HCC1954-L cells retain their resistant phenotype following a freeze/thaw cycle.

In order to access the long-term stability of the resistant phenotype, drug withdrawal assays were performed. Lapatinib was removed from the HCC1954-L cells and the sensitivity of the cells to lapatinib was tested at 4-week intervals for a period of 12 weeks, the results at each interval are illustrated in (**Figure 3G**). Following 12 weeks growth in the absence of lapatinib the lapatinib IC_{50} of the parental cells was 0.43 ± 0.05 μM while the lapatinib IC_{50} of HCC1954-L cells was 2.63 ± 0.16 μM. There was no significant difference between the initial lapatinib IC50 for either the parental or resistant cell line and the lapatinib IC50 for the cell lines after 12 weeks growth in the absence of lapatinib (**Figure 3H**).

Therefore, we successfully established a stable cell line of acquired lapatinib resistance (HCC1954-L) induced by long-term continuous treatment with sub-peak-plasma concentrations of lapatinib. The mechanisms of acquired resistance to lapatinib are being investigated in this model using proteomics and genomic techniques.

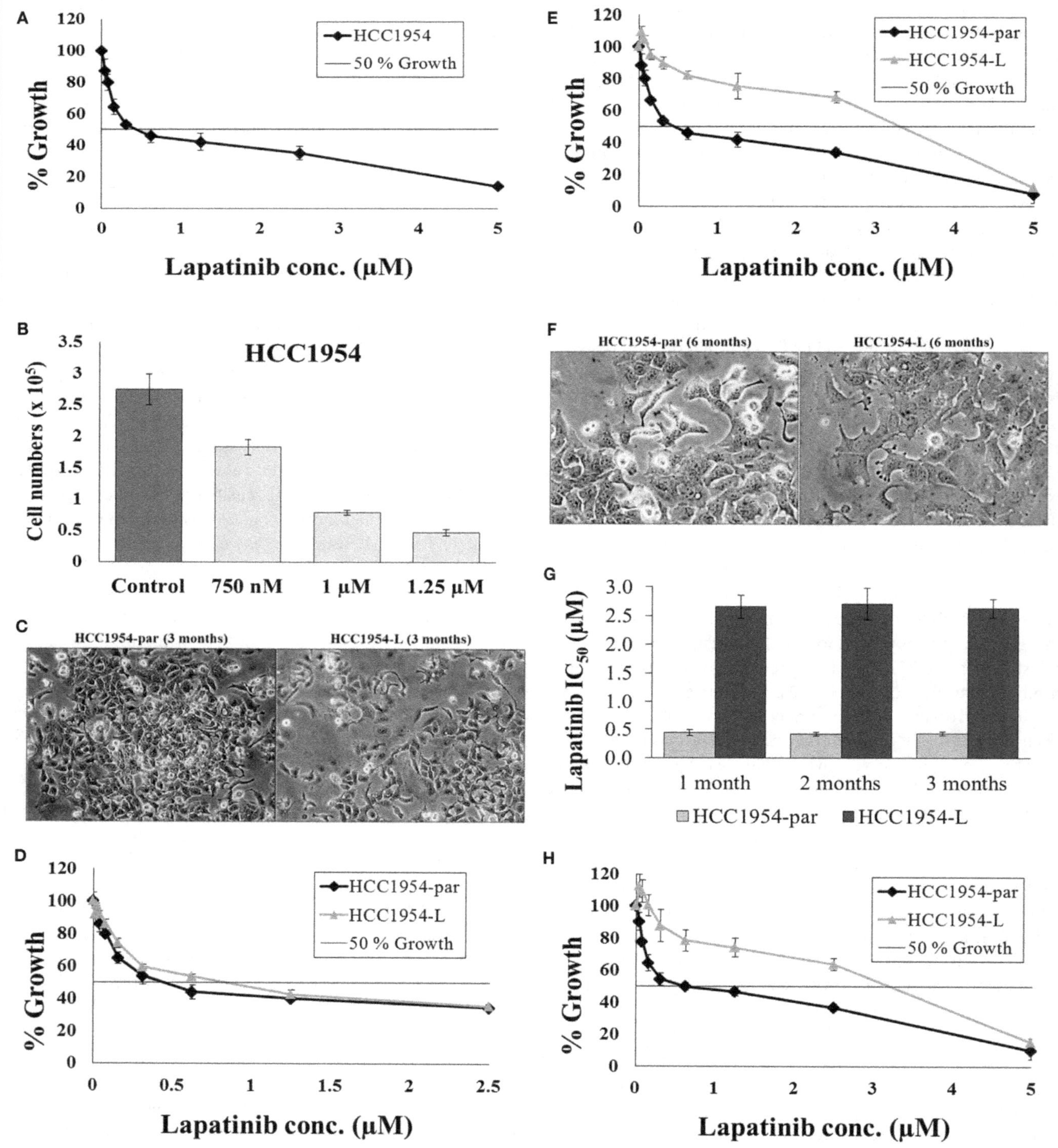

FIGURE 3 | Continuous selection of HCC1954 with lapatinib. **(A)** Proliferation of HCC1954 cells following a 5-day treatment with lapatinib. **(B)** HCC1954 cells treated with varying concentrations of lapatinib over a 4-day period. Cell counts were performed using ViaCount reagent and Guava Software and expressed relative to control untreated cells. **(C)** Images of HCC1954-par and HCC1954-L cells after 3 months of lapatinib conditioning at 100× magnification. **(D)** After 3 months conditioning with 1 μM lapatinib, the proliferation of HCC1954-par and HCC1954-L cells was measured. **(E)** After 6 months conditioning with lapatinib, the proliferation of HCC1954-par and HCC1954-L was assessed. **(F)** Images of HCC1954-par and HCC1954-L cells after 6 months of lapatinib conditioning at 200× magnification. **(G)** Sensitivity of HCC1954-par and HCC1954-L cells to lapatinib following a freeze-thaw cycle. Growth is expressed relative to untreated control cells. **(H)** Lapatinib IC_{50} values for HCC1954-par and HCC1954-L cells following 1, 2, and 3 months growth in the absence of lapatinib. All growth rates and IC_{50}s were calculated following a 5-day lapatinib treatment. Growth is expressed relative to untreated control cells. All error bars represent the standard deviation of triplicate experiments. Student's *t*-test was performed to determine significant differences: $*p < 0.05$; $**p < 0.01$.

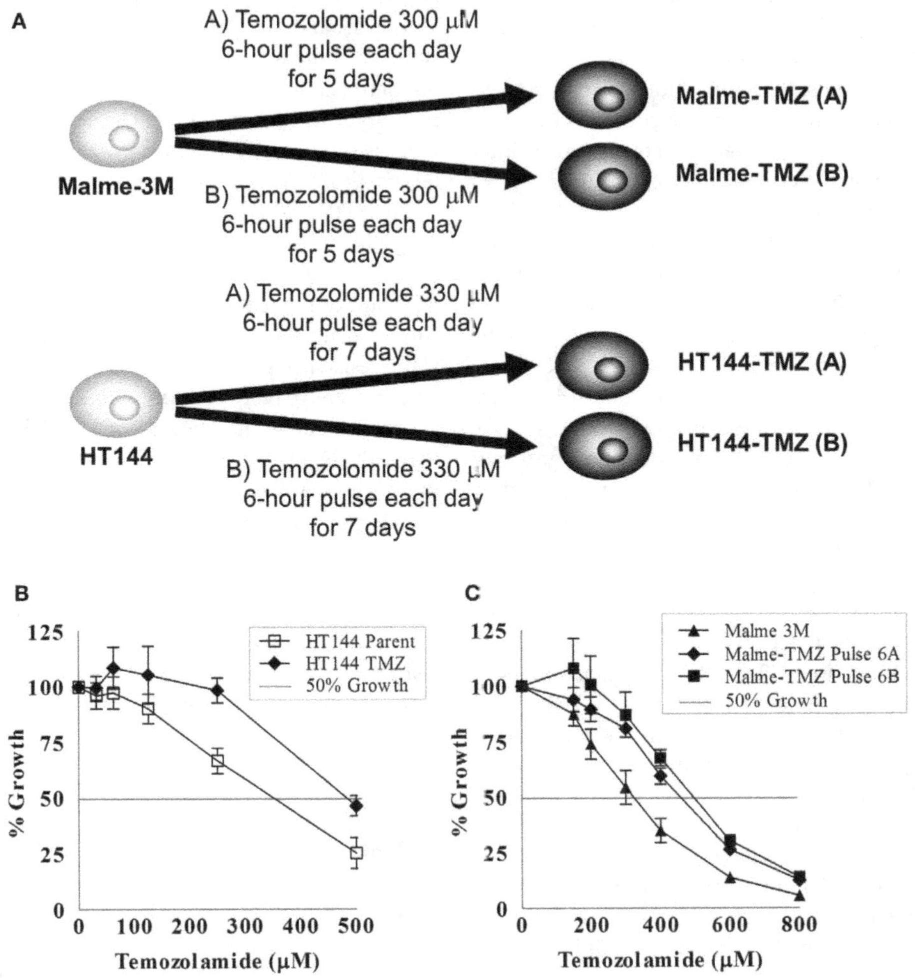

FIGURE 4 | Pulse selection of Malme-3M and HT144 with temozolomide. **(A)** Selection strategy of Malme-3M and HT144, each treatment of temozolomide was performed in duplicate. Effect of temozolomide in Malme-3M and HT144 and temozolomide "pulse selected" resistant variants. **(B)** Malme-TMZ(A) and Maleme-TMZ(B) vs. Malme-3M cells **(C)**. HT144-TMZ vs. HT144 cells. Error bars represent the standard deviation of triplicate assays.

TEMOZOLOMIDE-RESISTANT MELANOMA CELL LINES – PULSED SELECTION

Temozolomide is frequently used to treat metastatic melanoma. No dosing schedule of temozolomide has been clinically proven to be more effective than a single administration of temozolomide (79); however current treatments favor a 5-day treatment schedule (80). We found that the IC_{50} concentrations of temozolomide were in the high micromolar range in melanoma cell lines. Previous studies in two melanoma cell lines demonstrated temozolomide IC_{50} concentrations of ~800 μM (81), which is consistent with the values observed in our cell line panel of six melanoma cell lines (temozolomide IC_{50} ranged from 250 to 800 μM). However, in the clinical setting plasma levels of temozolomide only reach concentrations approaching 80 μM (82) The half-life of temozolomide is <2 h (83), which would reduce the efficacy of the drug in patients and may also explain the high IC_{50} values observed *in vitro*. A pulsed selection of drug was chosen to mimic these pharmacokinetic properties of temozolomide.

Malme-3M or HT144 melanoma cell lines were seeded at a density of 2.5×10^4 cells in a 75 cm^2 flask. The entire selection strategy was conducted in duplicate; two flasks of each cell line were set up for untreated control flasks and two for temozolomide selection (**Figure 4A**). Cells were allowed to attach for 24 h prior to treatment with chemotherapy. For Malme-3M cells, after each treatment cells were allowed to grow until confluent, then trypsinised and reseeded at a density of 2.5×10^4 cells per flask for the next round of selection. For HT144 cells, cells were grown in the flask for the 5 days of their treatment, then left to grow to confluence. After cells recovered they were trypsinised reseeded at 2.5×10^4 cells per flask for the next round of selection.

The Malme-3M cells were pulse treated with 300 μM temozolomide for 6 h and then the drug containing medium removed and replaced with fresh drug-free medium. This single pulse treatment was repeated six times. HT144 cells were treated for 6 h daily with 330 μM temozolomide for 5 days. After the five daily treatments the drug was removed and replaced with fresh drug-free media.

This treatment was repeated four times. This treatment schedule was used to replicate that of the clinical setting, where temozolomide is administered daily for 5 days, followed by a period of no treatment (84). The pulse selection strategy used in these cells allowed us to compare differences between the clinical daily administration and the lab based pulse selection to observe if either regimen resulted in increased levels of resistance acquired.

The IC_{50} for temozolomide in Malme-3M parent cells is $306 \pm 29\,\mu M$. Malme-TMZ(A) and Malme-TMZ(B) display significantly increased IC_{50}s for temozolomide of $440 \pm 21\,\mu M$ [1.44-fold increase ($p = 0.004$)] and $515 \pm 45\,\mu M$ [1.68-fold increase ($p = 0.04$)] (**Figure 4B**). The IC_{50} for temozolomide in HT144 cells is $338 \pm 25\,\mu M$. In HT144-TMZ(A), the pulse-selected variant of HT144, the IC_{50} increased to $490 \pm 15\,\mu M$, which represents a 1.45-fold increase in resistance to TMZ ($p = 0.002$) (**Figure 4C**). HT144(B) did not develop significant resistance to temozolomide, and so was not used in further studies.

During drug selection of cell lines, cells can acquire altered sensitivity to other chemotherapeutic drugs. The two temozolomide-selected cell lines from each parent cell line with the highest levels of resistance [Malme-TMZ(B) and HT144(A)] were tested with four drugs to examine the chemosensitivity between the parent and the resistant cell lines (**Table 6**). The melanoma cell line HT144 and the temozolomide-selected variant HT144-TMZ display similar sensitivity to cisplatin and epirubicin whilst the resistant cell line is significantly more sensitive to mitoxantrone ($p = 0.02$). Malme-3M and the pulse-selected cell line Malme-TMZ have similar IC_{50}s for EPI and mitoxantrone. Malme-TMZ is significantly more resistant to cisplatin ($p = 0.001$) and both HT144-TMZ and Malme-TMZ are significantly more resistant to docetaxel than the parent cell lines Malme-3M and HT144 ($p = 0.02$; $p = 0.02$), although the IC_{50} values are still in the very low nanomolar range.

Two temozolomide-resistant cell lines [Malme-TMZ(B) and HT144(A)] were established using two different selection methods. Duplicate selection proved useful in this selection strategy as one of the variants HT144-TMZ(B) did not develop resistance. Although the level of resistance induced was relatively low, these two cell lines provide unique clinically relevant models to study acquired temozolomide resistance in melanoma (85). The temozolomide-resistant variants were cross resistant to cisplatin. As temozolomide and cisplatin are both DNA damaging agents, there may be common mechanisms of resistance to the DNA damage induced by these agents.

Table 6 | Fold resistance of HT144 and Malme-3M resistant variants compared with their parental cell lines.

Chemotherapeutic agent	HT144-TMZ	Malme-TMZ
Cisplatin (nM)	1.4	2.0*
Epirubicin (nM)	1.3	0.8
Mitoxantrone (nM)	0.2*	1.3
Docetaxel (nM)	1.4*	1.2*

**Indicates a p-value <0.05 as calculated by Student's t-test.*

MAINTAINING DRUG-RESISTANT CELL LINES FOR RESEARCH

Once resistance has been established with the selection strategy the stability of the resistance needs to be determined. One important test of the stability of the model is the recovery of the drug-resistant phenotype from the frozen stocks. If the phenotype is lost or resistance is significantly lower on freeze thaw then the model will not be practical to use in the laboratory. If the resistance is not stable on freeze thaw then the drug-resistant cells need to be treated for longer, possibly with a higher dose of chemotherapeutic.

The long-term stability of resistance also needs to be examined. Resistant cell models that have been selected by continuous exposure to drug should be grown for several months to determine if the resistance phenotype remains present. Some cell lines may be completely stably resistant (**Figure 5A**) and are grown in the absence of chemotherapeutic, such as DLKP-A or IGROVCDDP (21, 25). Regular monitoring by cytotoxicity assay is required to make sure that the resistance phenotype of the cell lines persists.

Alternatively, the cells can be grown continuously in chemotherapeutic, either at the dose used in selection or a lower maintenance dose. This may be if the cells are not stably resistant on removal of the chemotherapeutic or if the researchers wish to ensure consistency of experiments. KB-CP20 cisplatin-resistant cells which were selected with increasing concentrations of cisplatin up to $20\,\mu g/mL$ over a period of 6 months. The

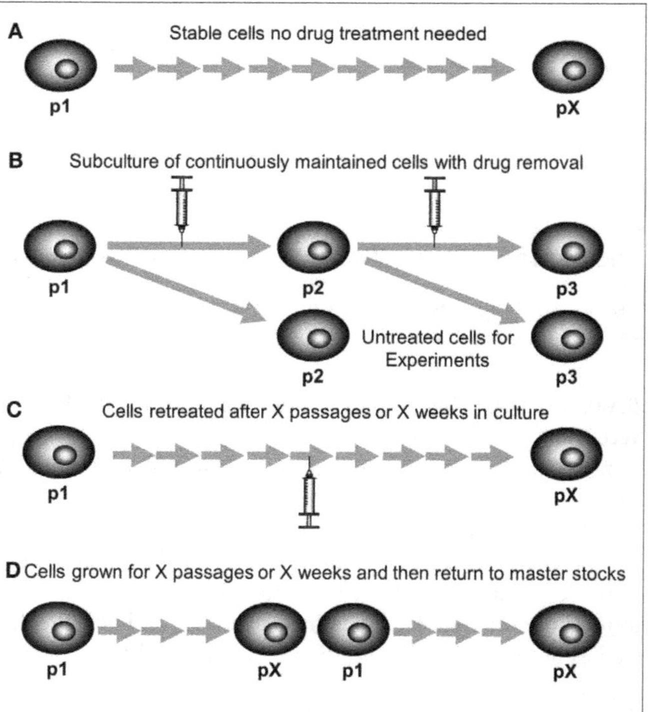

FIGURE 5 | Maintaining drug-resistant cell lines in cell culture.
(A) Stable cell lines require no drug treatment to maintain their resistant phenotype. **(B)** Some cell lines are grown continually in the presence of chemotherapy, chemotherapy needs to be removed for one subculture prior to using for experiments. **(C)** Some models are repeat pulse treated after a certain number of passages or weeks in culture once their resistant phenotype begins to fade. **(D)** Some models are discarded and new cells grown from master stocks after a certain number of passages or weeks in culture once their resistant phenotype begins to fade.

resistance was then maintained in media containing 5 µg/mL cisplatin (22). KB-5-8-11 colchicine-resistant cells are also maintained in 100 ng/mL of colchicine (24). Resistant cell models which are maintained in chemotherapy drug need to be grown in drug-free media for a passage prior to conducting experiments (86). This is so that the drug-free controls of experiments are cells not exposed to drug, rather than cells grown in the maintenance dose of chemotherapy. **Figure 5B** shows a subculture schematic for this technique. Another approach to maintaining stability is growing cells in drug-free media but using a pulse treatment at regular intervals (**Figure 5C**). This can be used even if the cell model was originally developed by continuous exposure. The CEM/E25 and CEM/E1000 epirubicin-resistant variants of CCRF-CEM leukemia cells were established by continuous exposure then grown without drug and resistance was maintained by repeat pulse treatment every 6 weeks with the selecting doses of epirubicin 25 and 1000 ng/mL, respectively (15, 16).

Resistant models that are selected by pulse selection are often less stable than their continuously selected counterparts. However, IGROVCDDP is a stably resistant cell line established by pulse selection using dose escalation (21). Pulse-selected cell lines which lose their resistant phenotype can also be maintained by re-treatment with the selecting dose (**Figure 5C**) such as K562/DNR resistant leukemia cells (17). Alternatively, instead of repeating the pulse treatment, resistant cells can be grown for a certain number of weeks or passages and then new stocks are defrosted of an earlier passage with the resistant phenotype present (**Figure 5D**). H69CIS200 and H69OX400 cisplatin and oxaliplatin-resistant cells were 1.5–2-fold resistant to platinums for 5–6 weeks in drug-free culture and then the resistance phenotype faded over the next 6–8 weeks in culture (20). This technique is also often used with resistant models regardless of selection strategy to ensure consistency, so that cells within a limited range of passage numbers are used for all experiments.

A REPRODUCIBLE EXPERIMENT?

Many mechanisms of resistance exist for each chemotherapy drug. The chemotherapeutic drug cisplatin has been studied in drug-resistant cell models for many years and mechanisms of resistance include decreased accumulation of drug, inactivation by glutathione and increased DNA repair (87). These mechanisms need not all occur in the same drug-resistant model. Over time more common mechanisms will be identified by their occurrence in many drug-resistant models.

A comparative selection strategy could involve parallel selections of the same parental cell line with the same chemotherapy agent, under the same treatment conditions. Similar or different mechanisms could develop in these independent treatments. This is the randomness of natural selection. A study by Tegze et al. developed multiple drug-resistant cell lines from MCF-7 and MDA-MB-231 breast cancer cells (88). The parent cell lines were split and new cell lines were generated in parallel by treatment with gradually increasing concentration of doxorubicin or paclitaxel. The study aimed to produce 10 resistant sublines for each agent in each parent cell line. Using a continuous treatment strategy they produced 29 resistant models over an 18-month period. There were 10 doxorubicin and 4 paclitaxel-resistant MCF-7 cell lines and 6 doxorubicin and 9 paclitaxel-resistant MDA-MB-231 cell lines. The fold resistance values compared to the parental cell lines show up to 46- and 28-fold resistance to doxorubicin and paclitaxel, respectively. The cell lines turned out to be highly heterogeneous for the mechanisms of drug resistance present, and in general only a few mechanisms are activated in one cell line to achieve drug resistance. Of note, the expression of P-gp did not correlate with resistance in the cell line models, despite the development of models with two P-gp substrates. This suggests that in some of the models P-gp was activated early in the selection process and became a dominant mechanism, in others this did not occur.

Two models of cisplatin resistance were developed from H69 SCLC cells in the same research group in successive years (19, 89). These models were developed independently rather than in parallel. H69-CP and H69CIS200 were developed with 100 or 200 ng/mL of cisplatin, respectively. Both cell models were two-to four-fold resistant to cisplatin, and had decreased expression of p21 which may increase the cell's ability to progress through the cell cycle in the presence of DNA damage. Both the H69-CP and H69CIS200 cells showed no decrease in cellular cisplatin accumulation. However, the H69-CP cells have increased levels of cellular glutathione and are cross resistant to radiation whereas the H69CIS200 cells have neither of these changes.

The cell line IGROV-1 has been used to develop cisplatin drug-resistant models by many research groups. IGROVCDDP cisplatin-resistant cells have an unusual resistant phenotype; they are cross resistant to paclitaxel as they overexpress P-gp (90). It is unusual but not unprecedented to see a model of acquired cisplatin resistance overexpress P-gp (63, 91–94). This most likely represents a generalized stress response to long-term cisplatin treatment as cisplatin is not a P-gp substrate (95). IGROVCDDP cells do not have increased total cellular glutathione but the way glutathione is recycled within and from outside the cell is enhanced, increased enzyme activity of glutathione reductase and gamma-glutamyltransferase 1 (GGT1) was present (90). In contrast, IGROV-1/Pt0.5 and IGROV-1/Pt1, platinum-resistant cell lines are sensitive to P-gp substrates, have increased cellular glutathione and decreased GGT1 (96) which is the reverse pattern to that seen in the IGROVCDDP platinum/taxane-resistant cells. However, it should be noted, that different research groups can of course have different sub clones of a parent cell line and this can be a factor for the differences in the resistant models produced.

These examples demonstrate that the same cell line, treated with the same chemotherapy agent leads to the development of a heterogeneous range of drug-resistant models. Therefore, the development of drug-resistant models should be regarded as a process rather than an experiment that can be repeated in biological triplicate. If parallel models of the same treatment are produced the heterogeneity between drug-resistant cell lines should be examined with interest rather than dismissed as a non-reproducible experiment.

CONCLUSION

We have provided a detailed guide to the decision-making process for the development and ongoing maintenance of drug-resistant cancer cell lines. There is no one right way to make drug-resistant cell lines. The case studies from our laboratories highlight how we have successfully developed models in a variety of ways for use in research projects.

METHODS

CELL CULTURE

H1299, H460, HCC1954, Malme-3M, OVCAR8, UPN251, and cells and their drug-resistant variants were grown in antibiotic and chemotherapy-free RPMI (Sigma #R8758). HT144 cells and their resistant variants were grown in antibiotic and chemotherapy-free McCoys 5A medium (Sigma). HT144, HCC1954, Malme-3M, OVCAR8, and UPN251 and their resistant variants were supplemented with 10% FCS (Lonza, Belgium). H1299, H460, and their resistant variants were supplemented with 5% FCS. All cell lines were maintained in a humidified atmosphere with 5% CO2 at 37°C. All cultures were tested routinely and were *mycoplasma*-free.

GROWTH CURVES FOR OPTIMIZATION OF SELECTION DOSES

OVCAR8 or UPN251 cells were plated in duplicate into 6-well plates at a cell density of 1×10^4 cells/mL in 1 mL media. A control plate was set up separately with duplicate wells. On day 2 1 mL of media with drug was added to all plates excluding the control, which received drug-free media to the same volume. On day 5 media was changed on all plates and replaced with drug-free media. The control plate and one drugged plate were taken down and cell counted. Cell counts for the control were compared to the drug treatment. A percentage cell survival was calculated in order to see the effects of drug treatment on cell growth/survival.

$$\text{Percentage cell survival} = \frac{\text{Average cell number of drugged cells}}{\text{Average control cell number}} \times 100$$

Over subsequent days one plate for each drug dose was observed under a light microscope to see when normal growth had returned. When cells were deemed to have returned to confluence this plate was cell counted to confirm recovery. Percentage cell survival will now be above or climbing to 100%. The time taken for cells to resume growth and return to confluence was recorded.

CYTOTOXICITY ASSAYS

To determine the cytotoxicity of chemotherapy drugs, cell growth/viability was measured using an acid phosphatase assay; $1.5–3 \times 10^3$ cells were seeded in flat-bottomed 96-well plates and incubated overnight prior to addition of drug. Chemotherapeutics were obtained from St Vincent's University Hospital, Dublin, Ireland. Lapatinib was purchased from Sequoia. Temozolomide was obtained from the National Cancer Institute. Other inhibitors and modulators were obtained from Sigma. Drug-free controls were included in each assay. Plates were incubated for a further 5 (HCC1954, Malme-3M and HT144) or 7 days (H1299 and H460) at 37°C in a humidified atmosphere with 5% CO_2 and cell viability was determined using an acid phosphatase assay (97). Growth of drug-treated cells was calculated relative to control untreated cells in biological triplicate.

STATISTICS

All experiments were performed at minimum in triplicate. Two-sample, two-tailed Student's t-tests were used to determine significant differences using $p < 0.05$ as a cut off.

AUTHOR CONTRIBUTIONS

Britta Stordal conceived the need for a review of methods of development of drug-resistant cell lines and wrote the manuscript. Martina McDermott, Alex J. Eustace, Steven Busschots, Laura Breen contributed their expertise in drug-resistant cell line development, contributed data for case studies and assisted with locating references, and drafting the manuscript. Norma O'Donovan, John Crown and Martin Clynes mentored the development of the drug-resistant cell lines used in the case studies, as well as contributing their expertise in drug-resistant cell line development. All authors approved the final version of the manuscript.

ACKNOWLEDGMENTS

This study was funded by an Irish Research Council for Science Engineering and Technology (post-graduate fellowship) (Martina McDermott); Ireland's Higher Educational Authority Program for Research in Third Level Institutions (PRTLI) Cycle 3 (Alex J. Eustace and Laura Breen); The Cancer Clinical Research Trust (Alex J. Eustace/Norma O'Donovan/John Crown), PhD Scholarship from the Royal City of Dublin Hospital Trust (Steven Busschots); Science Foundation Ireland Strategic Research Cluster (08/SRC/B1410) (Norma O'Donovan). Irish Cancer Society Postdoctoral Fellowship and a Marie Curie Re-integration Grant from the European Union P7 programme (Britta Stordal).

REFERENCES

1. Biedler JL, Riehm H. Cellular resistance to actinomycin D in Chinese hamster cells in vitro: cross-resistance, radioautographic, and cytogenetic studies. *Cancer Res* (1970) **30**(4):1174–84.
2. Roberts D, Wodinsky I, Hall TC. Studies on folic reductase. *Cancer Res* (1965) **25**(11 Pt 1):1899–903.
3. Burchenal JH, Robinson E, Johnston SF, Kushida MN. The induction of resistance to 4-amino-N10-methyl-pteroylglutamic acid in a strain of transmitted mouse leukemia. *Science* (1950) **111**(2875):116–7. doi:10.1126/science.111.2875.116
4. Kessel D, Botterill V, Wodinsky I. Uptake and retention of daunomycin by mouse leukemic cells as factors in drug response. *Cancer Res* (1968) **28**(5):938–41.
5. Law LW. Resistance in leukemic cells to a guanine analog, 8-azaguanine. *Proc Soc Exp Biol Med* (1951) **78**(2):499–502. doi:10.3181/00379727-78-19118
6. Martin A, Clynes M. Comparison of 5 microplate colorimetric assays for in vitro cytotoxicity testing and cell proliferation assays. *Cytotechnology* (1993) **11**(1):49–58. doi:10.1007/BF00749057
7. Franken NAP, Rodermond HM, Stap J, Haveman J, van Bree C. Clonogenic assay of cells in vitro. *Nat Protoc* (2006) **1**(5):2315–9. doi:10.1038/nprot.2006.339
8. Kawai H, Kiura K, Tabata M, Yoshino T, Takata I, Hiraki A, et al. Characterization of non-small-cell lung cancer cell lines established before and after chemotherapy. *Lung Cancer* (2002) **35**(3):305–14. doi:10.1016/S0169-5002(01)00430-5
9. Kuroda H, Sugimoto T, Ueda K, Tsuchida S, Horii Y, Inazawa J, et al. Different drug sensitivity in two neuroblastoma cell lines established from the same patient before and after chemotherapy. *Int J Cancer* (1991) **47**(5):732–7. doi:10.1002/ijc.2910470518
10. Hida T, Ueda R, Takahashi T, Watanabe H, Kato T, Suyama M, et al. Chemosensitivity and radiosensitivity of small cell lung cancer cell lines studied by a newly developed 3-(4,5-dimethylthiazol-2-yl)-2,5-diphenyltetrazolium bromide (MTT) hybrid assay. *Cancer Res* (1989) **49**(17):4785–90.
11. Berendsen HH, de Leij L, de Vries EGE, Mesander G, Mulder NH, de Jong B, et al. Characterization of three small cell lung cancer cell lines established from one patient during longitudinal follow-up. *Cancer Res* (1988) **48**(23):6891–9.

12. Sakai W, Swisher EM, Jacquemont C, Chandramohan KV, Couch FJ, Langdon SP, et al. Functional restoration of BRCA2 protein by secondary BRCA2 mutations in BRCA2-mutated ovarian carcinoma. *Cancer Res* (2009) **69**(16):6381–6. doi:10.1158/0008-5472.CAN-09-1178
13. Stronach EA, Chen M, Maginn EN, Agarwal R, Mills GB, Wasan H, et al. DNA-PK mediates AKT activation and apoptosis inhibition in clinically acquired platinum resistance. *Neoplasia* (2011) **13**(11):1069–80.
14. Langdon SP, Lawrie SS, Hay FG, Hawkes MM, McDonald A, Hayward IP, et al. Characterization and properties of nine human ovarian adenocarcinoma cell lines. *Cancer Res* (1988) **48**(21):6166–72.
15. Cullen KV, Davey RA, Davey MW. Verapamil-stimulated glutathione transport by the multidrug resistance-associated protein (MRP1) in leukaemia cells. *Biochem Pharmacol* (2001) **62**(4):417–24. doi:10.1016/S0006-2952(01)00681-5
16. Davey RA, Longhurst TJ, Davey MW, Belov L, Harvie RM, Hancox D, et al. Drug resistance mechanisms and MRP expression in response to epirubicin treatment in a human leukaemia cell line. *Leuk Res* (1995) **19**(4):275–82. doi:10.1016/0145-2126(94)00159-8
17. Locke VL, Davey RA, Davey MW. Altered drug sensitivity in response to idarubicin treatment in K562 human leukaemia cells. *Br J Haematol* (1999) **106**(1):86–91. doi:10.1046/j.1365-2141.1999.01494.x
18. Breen L, Murphy L, Keenan J, Clynes M. Development of taxane resistance in a panel of human lung cancer cell lines. *Toxicol In vitro* (2008) **22**(5):1234–41. doi:10.1016/j.tiv.2008.04.005
19. Stordal BK, Davey MW, Davey RA. Oxaliplatin induces drug resistance more rapidly than cisplatin in H69 small cell lung cancer cells. *Cancer Chemother Pharmacol* (2006) **58**(2):256–65. doi:10.1007/s00280-005-0148-7
20. Stordal B, Peters G, Davey R. Similar chromosomal changes in cisplatin and oxaliplatin-resistant sublines of the H69 SCLC cell line are not associated with platinum resistance. *Genes Chromosomes Cancer* (2006) **45**(12):1094–105. doi:10.1002/gcc.20373
21. Ma J, Maliepaard M, Kolker HJ, Verweij J, Schellens JH. Abrogated energy-dependent uptake of cisplatin in a cisplatin-resistant subline of the human ovarian cancer cell line IGROV-1. *Cancer Chemother Pharmacol* (1998) **41**(3):186–92. doi:10.1007/s002800050727
22. Liang XJ, Shen DW, Garfield S, Gottesman MM, Liang XJ, Shen DW, et al. Mislocalization of membrane proteins associated with multidrug resistance in cisplatin-resistant cancer cell lines. *Cancer Res* (2003) **63**(18):5909–16.
23. Shen DW, Akiyama S, Schoenlein P, Pastan I, Gottesman MM. Characterisation of high-level cisplatin-resistant cell lines established from a human hepatoma cell line and human KB adenocarcinoma cells: cross-resistance and protein changes. *Br J Cancer* (1995) **71**(4):676–83. doi:10.1038/bjc.1995.134
24. Akiyama S, Fojo A, Hanover JA, Pastan I, Gottesman MM. Isolation and genetic characterization of human KB cell lines resistant to multiple drugs. *Somat Cell Mol Genet* (1985) **11**(2):117–26. doi:10.1007/BF01534700
25. Clynes M, Redmond A, Moran E, Gilvarry U. Multiple drug-resistance in variant of a human non-small cell lung carcinoma cell line, DLKP-A. *Cytotechnology* (1992) **10**(1):75–89. doi:10.1007/BF00376102
26. Hills CA, Kelland LR, Abel G, Siracky J, Wilson AP, Harrap KR. Biological properties of ten human ovarian carcinoma cell lines: calibration in vitro against four platinum complexes. *Br J Cancer* (1989) **59**(4):527–34. doi:10.1038/bjc.1989.108
27. Kunzmann R, Hozel F. Karyotype alterations in human ovarian carcinoma cells during long-term cultivation and nude mouse passage. *Cancer Genet Cytogenet* (1987) **28**(2):201–12. doi:10.1016/0165-4608(87)90206-8
28. *CRL-1978™ (ES-2) ATCC Datasheet* (2012). Available from: http://www.lgcstandards-atcc.org
29. Emoto M, Oshima K, Ishiguro M, Iwasaki H, Kawarabayashi T, Kikuchi M. Establishment and characterization of a serous papillary adenocarcinoma cell line of the human ovary in a serum-free culture. *Pathol Res Pract* (1999) **195**(4):238–43. doi:10.1016/S0344-0338(99)80040-5
30. Hamidovic A, Hahn K, Kolesar J. Clinical significance of ABCB1 genotyping in oncology. *J Oncol Pharm Pract* (2010) **16**(1):39–44. doi:10.1177/1078155209104380
31. Mackillop WJ, Trent JM, Stewart SS, Buick RN. Tumor progression studied by analysis of cellular features of serial ascitic ovarian carcinoma tumors. *Cancer Res* (1983) **43**(2):874–8.
32. Filmus JE, Buick RN. Stability of c-K-ras amplification during progression in a patient with adenocarcinoma of the ovary. *Cancer Res* (1985) **45**(9):4468–72.
33. Filmus J, Trent JM, Pullano R, Buick RN. A cell line from a human ovarian carcinoma with amplification of the K-ras gene. *Cancer Res* (1986) **46**(10):5179–82.
34. Benard J, Da Silva J, De Blois MC, Boyer P, Duvillard P, Chiric E, et al. Characterization of a human ovarian adenocarcinoma line, IGROV1, in tissue culture and in nude mice. *Cancer Res* (1985) **45**(10):4970–9.
35. Alama A, Barbieri F, Favre A, Cagnoli M, Noviello E, Pedullá F, et al. Establishment and characterization of three new cell lines derived from the ascites of human ovarian carcinomas. *Gynecol Oncol* (1996) **62**(1):82–8. doi:10.1006/gyno.1996.0194
36. Schilder RJ, Hall L, Monks A, Handel LM, Fornace AJ Jr, Ozols RF, et al. Metallothionein gene expression and resistance to cisplatin in human ovarian cancer. *Int J Cancer* (1990) **45**(3):416–22. doi:10.1002/ijc.2910450306
37. Hamilton TC, Young RC, McKoy WM, Grotzinger KR, Green JA, Chu EW, et al. Characterization of a human ovarian carcinoma cell line (NIH:OVCAR-3) with androgen and estrogen receptors. *Cancer Res* (1983) **43**(11):5379–89.
38. Yuan Y, Kim WH, Han HS, Lee JH, Park HS, Chung JK, et al. Establishment and characterization of human ovarian carcinoma cell lines. *Gynecol Oncol* (1997) **66**(3):378–87. doi:10.1006/gyno.1997.4785
39. Buick RN, Pullano R, Trent JM. Comparative properties of five human ovarian adenocarcinoma cell lines. *Cancer Res* (1985) **45**(8):3668–76.
40. Himmelstein KJ, Patton TF, Belt RJ, Taylor S, Repta AJ, Sternson LA. Clinical kinetics of intact cisplatin and some related species. *Clin Pharmacol Ther* (1981) **29**(5):658–64. doi:10.1038/clpt.1981.91
41. Vermorken JB, van der Vijgh WJ, Klein I, Hart AA, Gall HE, Pinedo HM. Pharmacokinetics of free and total platinum species after short-term infusion of cisplatin. *Cancer Treat Rep* (1984) **68**(3):505–13.
42. Los G, Verdegaal E, Noteborn HP, Ruevekamp M, de Graeff GA, Meesters EW, et al. Cellular pharmacokinetics of carboplatin and cisplatin in relation to their cytotoxic action. *Biochem Pharmacol* (1991) **42**(2):357–63. doi:10.1016/0006-2952(91)90723-I
43. Oguri S, Sakakibara T, Mase H, Shimizu T, Ishikawa K, Kimura K, et al. Clinical pharmacokinetics of carboplatin. *J Clin Pharmacol* (1988) **28**(3):208–15. doi:10.1002/j.1552-4604.1988.tb03134.x
44. Elferink F, van der Vijgh WJ, Klein I, Vermorken JB, Gall HE, Pinedo HM. Pharmacokinetics of carboplatin after i.v. administration. *Cancer Treat Rep* (1987) **71**(12):1231–7.
45. Newell DR, Siddik ZH, Gumbrell LA, Boxall FE, Gore ME, Smith IE, et al. Plasma free platinum pharmacokinetics in patients treated with high dose carboplatin. *Eur J Cancer Clin Oncol* (1987) **23**(9):1399–405. doi:10.1016/0277-5379(87)90126-X
46. Calvert AH, Newell DR, Gumbrell LA, O'Reilly S, Burnell M, Boxall FE, et al. Carboplatin dosage: prospective evaluation of a simple formula based on renal function. *J Clin Oncol* (1989) **7**(11):1748–56.
47. Pohl G, Ho CL, Kurman RJ, Bristow R, Wang TL, Shih IM. Inactivation of the mitogen-activated protein kinase pathway as a potential target-based therapy in ovarian serous tumors with KRAS or BRAF mutations. *Cancer Res* (2005) **65**(5):1994–2000. doi:10.1158/0008-5472.CAN-04-3625
48. Yamamoto N, Nokihara H, Yamada Y, Goto Y, Tanioka M, Shibata T, et al. A phase I, dose-finding and pharmacokinetic study of olaparib (AZD2281) in Japanese patients with advanced solid tumors. *Cancer Sci* (2012) **103**(3):504–9. doi:10.1111/j.1349-7006.2011.02179.x
49. Kim HK, Lin CC, Parker D, Veals J, Lim J, Likhari P, et al. High-performance liquid chromatographic determination and stability of 5-(3-methyltriazen-1-yl)-imidazo-4-carboximide, the biologically active product of the antitumor agent temozolomide, in human plasma. *J Chromatogr B Biomed Sci Appl* (1997) **703**(1–2):225–33. doi:10.1016/S0378-4347(97)00431-3
50. Bruno R, Sanderink GJ. Pharmacokinetics and metabolism of Taxotere (docetaxel). *Cancer Surv* (1993) **17**:305–13.
51. Paul B, Trovato JA, Thompson J. Lapatinib: a dual tyrosine kinase inhibitor for metastatic breast cancer. *Am J Health Syst Pharm* (2008) **65**(18):1703–10. doi:10.2146/ajhp070646
52. Goldenberg MM. Trastuzumab, a recombinant DNA-derived humanized monoclonal antibody, a novel agent for the treatment of metastatic breast cancer. *Clin Ther* (1999) **21**(2):309–18. doi:10.1016/S0149-2918(00)88288-0
53. du BA, Luck HJ, Buser K, Meerpohl HG, Sessa C, Klaassen U, et al. Extended phase II study of paclitaxel as a 3-h infusion in patients with ovarian cancer previously treated with plantinum. *Eur J Cancer* (1997) **33**(3):379–84. doi:10.1016/S0959-8049(97)89009-0

54. Varma MVS, Sateesh K, Panchagnula R. Functional role of P-glycoprotein in limiting intestinal absorption of drugs: contribution of passive permeability to P-glycoprotein mediated efflux transport. *Mol Pharm* (2005) **2**(1):12–21. doi:10.1021/mp0499196
55. Mross K, Holländer N, Hauns B, Schumacher M, Maier-Lenz H. The pharmacokinetics of a 1-h paclitaxel infusion. *Cancer Chemother Pharmacol* (2000) **45**(6):463–70. doi:10.1007/s002800051020
56. Joerger M, Huitema AD, van den Bongard DH, Schellens JH, Beijnen JH. Quantitative effect of gender, age, liver function, and body size on the population pharmacokinetics of paclitaxel in patients with solid tumors. *Clin Cancer Res* (2006) **12**(7 Pt 1):2150–7. doi:10.1158/1078-0432.CCR-05-2069
57. Marusyk A, Polyak K. Tumor heterogeneity: causes and consequences. *Biochim Biophys Acta* (2010) **1805**(1):105–17. doi:10.1016/j.bbcan.2009.11.002
58. Gerlinger M, Swanton C. How Darwinian models inform therapeutic failure initiated by clonal heterogeneity in cancer medicine. *Br J Cancer* (2010) **103**(8):1139–43. doi:10.1038/sj.bjc.6605912
59. Cooke SL, Ng CKY, Melnyk N, Garcia MJ, Hardcastle T, Temple J, et al. Genomic analysis of genetic heterogeneity and evolution in high-grade serous ovarian carcinoma. *Oncogene* (2010) **29**(35):4905–13. doi:10.1038/onc.2010.245
60. Martins FC, De S, Almendro V, Gonen M, Park SY, Blum JL, et al. Evolutionary pathways in BRCA1-associated breast tumors. *Cancer Discov* (2012) **2**(6):503–11. doi:10.1158/2159-8290.CD-11-0325
61. Barr MP, Gray SG, Hoffmann AC, Hilger RA, Thomale J, O'Flaherty JD, et al. Generation and characterisation of cisplatin-resistant non-small cell lung cancer cell lines displaying a stem-like signature. *PLoS One* (2013) **8**(1):e54193. doi:10.1371/journal.pone.0054193
62. Breen L, Keenan J, Clynes M. Generation of lung cancer cell line variants by drug selection or cloning. *Methods Mol Biol* (2011) **731**:125–33. doi:10.1007/978-1-61779-080-5_11
63. Yang LY, Trujillo JM, Siciliano MJ, Kido Y, Siddik ZH, Su YZ. Distinct P-glycoprotein expression in two subclones simultaneously selected from a human colon carcinoma cell line by cis-diamminedichloroplatinum (II). *Int J Cancer* (1993) **53**(3):478–85. doi:10.1002/ijc.2910530321
64. Sakai W, Swisher EM, Karlan BY, Agarwal MK, Higgins J, Friedman C, et al. Secondary mutations as a mechanism of cisplatin resistance in BRCA2-mutated cancers. *Nature* (2008) **451**(7182):1116–20. doi:10.1038/nature06633
65. Xia W, Bacus S, Hegde P, Husain I, Strum J, Liu L, et al. A model of acquired autoresistance to a potent ErbB2 tyrosine kinase inhibitor and a therapeutic strategy to prevent its onset in breast cancer. *Proc Natl Acad Sci U S A* (2006) **103**(20):7795–800. doi:10.1073/pnas.0602468103
66. Xia W, Bacus S, Husain I, Liu L, Zhao S, Liu Z, et al. Resistance to ErbB2 tyrosine kinase inhibitors in breast cancer is mediated by calcium-dependent activation of RelA. *Mol Cancer Ther* (2010) **9**(2):292–9. doi:10.1158/1535-7163.MCT-09-1041
67. Aird KM, Ghanayem RB, Peplinski S, Lyerly HK, Devi GR. X-linked inhibitor of apoptosis protein inhibits apoptosis in inflammatory breast cancer cells with acquired resistance to an ErbB1/2 tyrosine kinase inhibitor. *Mol Cancer Ther* (2010) **9**(5):1432–42. doi:10.1158/1535-7163.MCT-10-0160
68. Liu L, Greger J, Shi H, Liu Y, Greshock J, Annan R, et al. Novel mechanism of lapatinib resistance in HER2-positive breast tumor cells: activation of AXL. *Cancer Res* (2009) **69**(17):6871–8. doi:10.1158/0008-5472.CAN-08-4490
69. Martin AP, Miller A, Emad L, Rahmani M, Walker T, Mitchell C, et al. Lapatinib resistance in HCT116 cells is mediated by elevated MCL-1 expression and decreased BAK activation and not by ERBB receptor kinase mutation. *Mol Pharmacol* (2008) **74**(3):807–22. doi:10.1124/mol.108.047365
70. Huang C, Park C, Hilsenbeck S, Ward R, Rimawi M, Wang YC, et al. Beta1 integrin mediates an alternative survival pathway in breast cancer cells resistant to lapatinib. *Breast Cancer Res* (2011) **13**(4):R84. doi:10.1186/bcr2936
71. Rexer BN, Ham A-JL, Rinehart C, Hill S, de Matos Granja-Ingram N, Gonzalez-Angulo AM, et al. Phosphoproteomic mass spectrometry profiling links Src family kinases to escape from HER2 tyrosine kinase inhibition. *Oncogene* (2011) **30**(40):4163–74. doi:10.1038/onc.2011.130
72. Wang YC, Morrison G, Gillihan R, Guo J, Ward R, Fu X, et al. Different mechanisms for resistance to trastuzumab versus lapatinib in HER2-positive breast cancers – role of estrogen receptor and HER2 reactivation. *Breast Cancer Res* (2011) **13**(6):R121. doi:10.1186/bcr3067
73. Gazdar AF, Kurvari V, Virmani A, Gollahon L, Sakaguchi M, Westerfield M, et al. Characterization of paired tumor and non-tumor cell lines established from patients with breast cancer. *Int J Cancer* (1998) **78**(6):766–74. doi:10.1002/(SICI)1097-0215(19981209)78:6<766::AID-IJC15>3.0.CO;2-L
74. Xia W, Mullin RJ, Keith BR, Liu LH, Ma H, Rusnak DW, et al. Anti-tumor activity of GW572016: a dual tyrosine kinase inhibitor blocks EGF activation of EGFR/erbB2 and downstream Erk1/2 and AKT pathways. *Oncogene* (2002) **21**(41):6255–63. doi:10.1038/sj.onc.1205794
75. Geyer CE, Forster J, Lindquist D, Chan S, Romieu CG, Pienkowski T, et al. Lapatinib plus capecitabine for HER2-positive advanced breast cancer. *N Engl J Med* (2006) **355**(26):2733–43. doi:10.1056/NEJMoa064320
76. Prescribing information for Tykerb. GlaxoSmithKline (2013). Available from: http://us.gsk.com/products/assets/us_tykerb.pdf
77. Burris HA, Hurwitz HI, Dees EC, Dowlati A, Blackwell KL, O'Neil B, et al. Phase I safety, pharmacokinetics, and clinical activity study of lapatinib (GW572016), a reversible dual inhibitor of epidermal growth factor receptor tyrosine kinases, in heavily pretreated patients with metastatic carcinomas. *J Clin Oncol* (2005) **23**(23):5305–13. doi:10.1200/JCO.2005.16.584
78. O'Brien NA, Browne BC, Chow L, Wang Y, Ginther C, Arboleda J, et al. Activated phosphoinositide 3-kinase/AKT signaling confers resistance to trastuzumab but not lapatinib. *Mol Cancer Ther* (2010) **9**(6):1489–502. doi:10.1158/1535-7163.MCT-09-1171
79. Brock CS, Newlands ES, Wedge SR, Bower M, Evans H, Colquhoun I, et al. Phase I trial of temozolomide using an extended continuous oral schedule. *Cancer Res* (1998) **58**(19):4363–7.
80. Quirt I, Verma S, Petrella T, Bak K, Charette M. Temozolomide for the treatment of metastatic melanoma: a systematic review. *Oncologist* (2007) **12**(9):1114–23. doi:10.1634/theoncologist.12-9-1114
81. Azzabi A, Hughes AN, Calvert PM, Plummer ER, Todd R, Griffin MJ, et al. Phase I study of temozolomide plus paclitaxel in patients with advanced malignant melanoma and associated in vitro investigations. *Br J Cancer* (2005) **92**(6):1006–12. doi:10.1038/sj.bjc.6602438
82. Friedman HS, Kerby T, Calvert H. Temozolomide and treatment of malignant glioma. *Clin Cancer Res* (2000) **6**(7):2585–97.
83. Dhodapkar M, Rubin J, Reid JM, Burch PA, Pitot HC, Buckner JC, et al. Phase I trial of temozolomide (NSC 362856) in patients with advanced cancer. *Clin Cancer Res* (1997) **3**(7):1093–100.
84. Middleton MR, Grob JJ, Aaronson N, Fierlbeck G, Tilgen W, Seiter S, et al. Randomized phase III study of temozolomide versus dacarbazine in the treatment of patients with advanced metastatic malignant melanoma. *J Clin Oncol* (2000) **18**(1):158.
85. Jordan E, Eustace A, Collins DM, O'Donovan N, Crown J. Src inhibition as a method to overcome temozolomide resistance in melanoma. ESMO Congress 2012. (2012). Available from: http://oncologypro.esmo.org/Meeting-Resources/ESMO-2012/Src-inhibition-as-a-method-to-overcome-temozolomide-resistance-in-melanoma
86. Liang XJ, Yin JJ, Zhou JW, Wang PC, Taylor B, Cardarelli C, et al. Changes in biophysical parameters of plasma membranes influence cisplatin resistance of sensitive and resistant epidermal carcinoma cells. *Exp Cell Res* (2004) **293**(2):283–91. doi:10.1016/j.yexcr.2003.10.012
87. Stordal B, Davey M. Understanding cisplatin resistance using cellular models. *IUBMB Life* (2007) **59**(11):696–9. doi:10.1080/15216540701636287
88. Tegze B, Zallasi Z, Haltrich I, Penzvalto Z, Toth Z, Liko I, et al. Parallel evolution under chemotherapy pressure in 29 breast cancer cell lines results in dissimilar mechanisms of resistance. *PLoS One* (2012) **7**(2):e30804. doi:10.1371/journal.pone.0030804
89. Locke VL, Davey RA, Davey MW. Modulation of drug and radiation resistance in small cell lung cancer cells by paclitaxel. *Anticancer Drugs* (2003) **14**(7):523–31. doi:10.1097/00001813-200308000-00004
90. Stordal B, Hamon M, McEneaney V, Roche S, Gillet JP, O'Leary JJ, et al. Resistance to paclitaxel in a cisplatin-resistant ovarian cancer cell line is mediated by P-glycoprotein. *PLoS One* (2012) **7**(7):e40717. doi:10.1371/journal.pone.0040717
91. Yang X, Page M. P-glycoprotein expression in ovarian cancer cell line following treatment with cisplatin. *Oncol Res* (1995) **7**(12):619–24.
92. Yang H, Zou W, Li Y, Chen B, Xin X. Bridge linkage role played by CD98hc of anti-tumor drug resistance and cancer metastasis on cisplatin-resistant ovarian cancer cells. *Cancer Biol Ther* (2007) **6**(6):942–7. doi:10.4161/cbt.6.6.4190
93. Xu H, Choi SM, An CS, Min YD, Kim KC, Kim KJ, et al. Concentration-dependent collateral sensitivity of cisplatin-resistant gastric cancer cell sublines. *Biochem Biophys Res Commun* (2005) **328**(2):618–22. doi:10.1016/j.bbrc.2005.01.015
94. Parekh H, Simpkins H. Cross-resistance and collateral sensitivity to natural product drugs in cisplatin-sensitive and -resistant rat lymphoma and human

ovarian carcinoma cells. *Cancer Chemother Pharmacol* (1996) **37**(5):457–62. doi:10.1007/s002800050412

95. Hamaguchi K, Godwin AK, Yakushiji M, O'Dwyer PJ, Ozols RF, Hamilton TC. Cross-resistance to diverse drugs is associated with primary cisplatin resistance in ovarian cancer cell lines. *Cancer Res* (1993) **53**(21):5225–32.
96. Perego P, Romanelli S, Carenini N, Magnani I, Leone R, Bonetti A, et al. Ovarian cancer cisplatin-resistant cell lines: multiple changes including collateral sensitivity to Taxol. *Ann Oncol* (1998) **9**(4):423–30. doi:10.1023/A:1008265012435
97. Martin A, Clynes M. Acid phosphatase: endpoint for in vitro toxicity tests. *In vitro Cell Dev Biol* (1991) **27A**(3 Pt 1):183–4. doi:10.1007/BF02630912

4

Co-development of diagnostic vectors to support targeted therapies and theranostics: essential tools in personalized cancer therapy

Nicholas C. Nicolaides, Daniel J. O'Shannessy *, Earl Albone and Luigi Grasso

Department of Translational Medicine and Diagnostics, Morphotek Inc., Exton, PA, USA

Edited by:
Jan Trøst Jørgensen, Dx-Rx Institute, Denmark

Reviewed by:
Hu Liu, Anhui Medical University, China
Alex Zhavoronkov, Federal Research Clinical Center for Pediatric Hematology, Oncology and Immunology, Russia

****Correspondence:***
Daniel J. O'Shannessy, Department of Translational Medicine and Diagnostics, Morphotek Inc., 210 Welsh Pool Road, Exton, PA 19341, USA
e-mail: doshannessy@morphotek.com

Novel technologies are being developed to improve patient therapy through the identification of targets and surrogate molecular signatures that can help direct appropriate treatment regimens for efficacy and drug safety. This is particularly the case in oncology whereby patient tumor and biofluids are routinely isolated and analyzed for genetic, immunohistochemical, and/or soluble markers to determine if a predictive biomarker signature (i.e., mutated gene product, differentially expressed protein, altered cell surface antigen, etc.) exists as a means for selecting optimal treatment. These biomarkers may be drug-specific targets and/or differentially expressed nucleic acids, proteins, or cell lineage profiles that can directly affect the patient's disease tissue or immune response to a therapeutic regimen. Improvements in diagnostics that can prescreen predictive response biomarker profiles will continue to optimize the ability to enhance patient therapy via molecularly defined disease-specific treatment. Conversely, patients lacking predictive response biomarkers will no longer needlessly be exposed to drugs that are unlikely to provide clinical benefit, thereby enabling patients to pursue other therapeutic options and lowering overall healthcare costs by avoiding futile treatment. While patient molecular profiling offers a powerful tool to direct treatment options, the difficulty in identifying disease-specific targets or predictive biomarker signatures that stratify a significant fraction within a disease indication remains challenging. A goal for drug developers is to identify and implement new strategies that can rapidly enable the development of beneficial disease-specific therapies for broad patient-specific targeting without the need of tedious predictive biomarker discovery and validation efforts, currently a bottleneck for development timelines. Successful strategies may gain an advantage by employing repurposed, less-expensive existing agents while potentially improving the therapeutic activity of novel, target-specific therapies that may otherwise have off-target toxicities or less efficacy in cells exhibiting certain pathways. Here, we discuss the use of co-developing diagnostic-targeting vectors to identify patients whose malignant tissue can specifically uptake a targeted anti-cancer drug vector prior to treatment. Using this system, a patient can be predetermined in real-time as to whether or not their tumor(s) can specifically uptake a drug-linked diagnostic vector, thus inferring the uptake of a similar vector linked to an anti-cancer agent. If tumor-specific uptake is observed, then the patient may be suitable for drug-linked vector therapy and have a higher likelihood of clinical benefit while patients with no tumor uptake should consider other therapeutic options. This approach offers complementary opportunities to rapidly develop broad tumor-specific agents for use in personalized medicine.

Keywords: companion diagnostics, CDx, co-development, TM601, theranostics, nanoparticles, naturally occurring proteins, personalized medicine

PERSONALIZED MEDICINE IN THE ERA OF TARGETED THERAPEUTIC STRATEGIES

Personalized medicine is generally considered as the precise use of drug(s) that can specifically target a patient's diseased tissue. This is typically achieved by using a diagnostic biomarker or biomolecular signature that can predict clinical response in patients before they are treated (1). In the broadest sense, an example of personalized medicine can be found in the therapeutic management of type 1 diabetes. Patients with this condition are identified initially by abnormal blood glucose levels, whereby glucose serves as a biomarker. Once confirmed by follow-up testing, the disease can be managed by drugs capable of modulating active insulin levels.

In more complex diseases such as cancer, an array of genetic and altered gene product expression changes may be required to determine or predict a patient's specific response(s) to therapy. Anti-cancer therapeutic strategies include: (i) binding to a specific molecular target of an altered pathway or a sequence-specific gene product that in turn results in selective killing of malignant but not normal cells; (ii) inducing a host immune response against malignant cells; and (iii) enhancing specific uptake of an agent(s) in target cells for disease suppression. Based on their chemical or biochemical nature, targeted anti-cancer agents can be classified into small chemical entities (SCE) capable of disrupting cellular processes such as enzymatic reactions, tubulin polymerization and DNA replication; nucleic acids that can specifically bind a gene product involved in tumor growth and metastasis; and cellular- and protein-based therapies that can specifically target tumor-associated cell surface proteins or soluble ligands (2). All these agents exert their pharmacologic activity by specifically suppressing growth and survival in malignant vs. normal cells.

For targeted cancer therapies, it is important that the compound can specifically bind to a gene product (e.g., ligands/receptors, transcription factors, or enzymes) or a molecular target within a pathway unique to a tumor cell or cells located within the tumor microenvironment that support tumor growth. These agents may include cell and protein-based vaccines, peptides, recombinant proteins, antibodies, antibody fragments, nucleic acid, and target-specific SCEs (2). The development of novel SCEs targeting tumor-altered gene products involved in driving the underlying cause of transformation is expanding across the industry as a result of recent approvals of compounds in this class (3). These include the anti BCR–ABL fusion protein tyrosine kinase inhibitor imatinib (4) and the more recently approved translocated ALK inhibitor, crizotinib (5), and mutant BRAF inhibitor, vemurafenib (6). While this class has shown robust clinical activity in patients containing the altered gene product, the low target frequency of the latter two compounds has minimized their utility in the greater patient population. Other classes of targeted therapies include antibody and protein-based agents that can specifically bind cell surface proteins on tumor cells and in turn block or activate receptor signaling, induce programed cell death and/or induce immune-mediated cytotoxicity. In all cases, patients may be prescreened to determine if their tumor expresses an agent-specific molecular target. These examples provide support for the validity of discovering modified disease-specific gene products that can serve as drug targets and be used to prescreen patients via diagnostic platforms capable of identifying those eligible for target-specific therapy.

Other personalized platforms include those that monitor gene expression profiles or soluble markers contained within biofluids (serum, plasma, urine, sputum, or whole cells) that may serve as surrogates for predictive response to a therapeutic regimen. While the example of type 1 diabetes fits into this category, broader discovery approaches are being pursued in oncology. These include biomarker signature profiles within disease tissue that may predict response to certain chemotherapeutic regimens as well as modifier genes that may predict response to a targeted therapy (7). The use of tumor-specific biomarker signature profiles has been widely pursued in breast cancer based on early successful prognostic and therapeutic paradigms that relied on tumor stage and grade, as well as HER2, estrogen (ER), and progesterone (PR) receptor expression status. Subsequent efforts have further refined breast cancer marker profiling to guide best course of therapy (8). This was achieved by development of a molecular signature panel comprising 21 genes, called Oncotype DX® (9), and subsequently MammaPrint™ (10), which comprises a 70 gene set. In both cases, surrogate gene expression profiles are measured to predict a patient's prognosis and guidance for use of existing therapies. More recently, a similar product for patient prognosis in colorectal cancer (OncoDX) has been developed (11). While these molecular signatures have value in predicting an individual's prognosis, they cannot predict potential clinical responses after specific targeted therapy. Despite their success and widespread use in breast or colorectal cancer for clinical follow-up after initial diagnosis, the generation and validation of these gene product signatures has taken a significant amount of time and effort before achieving clinical utility in managing personalized treatment for cancer patients.

There are currently 19 FDA approved companion diagnostic (CDx) assays, 18 of which are approved in oncology (**Table 1**). Ten of the 18 CDx assays are various qualitative assays for detecting HER2 expression or amplification in breast cancer; 2 are qualitative assays for BRAF V600E mutations; along with qualitative assays for ALK translocations, KRAS mutations and c-KIT; and 3 qualitative assays for EGFR mutations. The relative paucity of FDA approved CDx assays might reflect the difficulty and complexity in requirements for approval of such assays but might also be a reflection of a lack of in-depth knowledge of the underlying biology of cancer and/or the drug target interaction. Further, it is interesting to note that only 3 of the 18 (17%) oncology CDx assays are quantitative in format. While quantitative assays are not necessarily required, this undoubtedly speaks to the differences in regulatory requirements for quantitative relative to qualitative assays, at least with respect to CDx assays.

Interestingly, many more molecular diagnostic (Dx) assays are in drug labels (**Table 2**) – not as companion diagnostics but recommended or even required prior to prescribing therapy or for therapeutic monitoring – and some of these have been cleared by the FDA through the 510(k) process (**Table 3**). Complex pharmacogenomics signatures such as Oncotype DX® and even BRCA mutation analyses (12) are routinely used in clinical oncology but are performed under the CLIA regulation (Clinical Laboratory Improvement Amendments of 1988) and are classified as Laboratory Developed Tests (LDTs). This class of Dx does not go through the rigor of regulatory submissions such as 510(k) or PMA (Pre-Market Approval; a CDx requires a PMA) nor the post-marketing requirements of such assays. The FDA is currently reviewing and is expected to make recommendations in the near future regarding the oversight of LDTs, which may (significantly) change the present landscape.

ANTIBODY-DRUG CONJUGATES AND RADIOIMMUNOTHERAPIES

Recent clinical success of monoclonal antibody (mAb) drug conjugates (ADCs) has spurred the field of highly toxic chemotherapeutic drugs for targeted therapy. The development of ADCs offers dual benefits: the ability to preselect patients whose disease expresses the target antigen for tumor-specific delivery and the opportunity to deliver highly toxic (novel or repurposed) compounds to antigen positive tumors while avoiding toxic off-target effects commonly found with non-targeted SCEs or radionuclides

Table 1 | FDA approved companion diagnostics (CDx).

Drug trade name (generic name)	Device trade name	Device manufacturer	Approved	Technology/indication
Erbitux (cetuximab)	therascreen KRAS RGQ PCR Kit	Qiagen	2012	Qualitative RT-PCR/CRC
Erbitux (cetuximab); Vectibix (panitumumab)	DAKO EGFR PharmDx Kit	Dako	2006	Qualitative IHC/CRC
Exjade (deferasirox)	Ferriscan	Resonance Health Analysis Services	2013	FerriScan R2-MRI/thalassemia
Gilotrif (afatinib)	Therascreen EGFR RGQ PCR Kit	Qiagen	2013	Qualitative RT-PCR/NSCLC
Gleevec/glivec (imatinib mesylate)	Dako C-KIT PharmDx	Dako	2012	Qualitative IHC/GIST
Herceptin (trastuzumab)	INFORM HER2/neu	Ventana Medical Systems	2000	Qualitative FISH/breast cancer
	PathVysion HER2 DNA Probe Kit	Abbott Molecular	2013	Qualitative FISH/breast cancer
	PATHWAY anti-HER2/neu	Ventana Medical Systems	2013	Semi-quantitative IHC/breast cancer
	InSite HER2/neu Kit	BioGenex Laboratories	2005	Semi-quantitative IHC/breast cancer
	SPOT-Light HER2 CISH Kit	Life Technologies	2012	Quantitative CISH/breast cancer
	Bond Oracle Her2 IHC System	Leica Biosystems	2012	Semi-quantitative IHC/breast cancer
	HER2 CISH PharmDx Kit	Dako	2013	Quantitative ISH/breast cancer
	INFORM HER2 Dual ISH DNA Probe Cocktail	Ventana Medical Systems	2013	Two-color ISH/breast cancer
Herceptin (trastuzumab) Perjeta (pertuzumab)	HercepTest	Dako	2013	Semi-quantitative IHC/breast cancer, metastatic gastric, or gastroesophageal junction adenocarcinoma
KADCYLA (ado-trastuzumab emtansine)	HER2 FISH PharmDx Kit	Dako	2013	Quantitative FISH/breast cancer, metastatic gastric, or gastroesophageal junction adenocarcinoma
Mekinist (tramatenib); Tafinlar (dabrafenib)	THxID™ BRAF Kit	bioMérieux	2013	Qualitative RT-PCR/melanoma
Tarceva (erlotinib)	Cobas EGFR Mutation Test	Roche Molecular Systems	2013	Qualitative RT-PCR/NSCLC
Xalkori (crizotinib)	Vysis ALK Break Apart FISH Probe Kit	Abbott Molecular	2013	Qualitative FISH/NSCLC
Zelboraf (vemurafenib)	Cobas 4800 BRAF V600 Mutation Test	Roche Molecular Systems	2013	Qualitative RT-PCR/melanoma

Source: http://www.fda.gov/MedicalDevices/ProductsandMedicalProcedures/InVitroDiagnostics/ucm301431.htm.

(hereon referred to as cytotoxins) (13). Enhanced technologies that enable robust linkage of a targeting agent to a cytotoxin such as radionuclides, chemotherapeutic SCEs, and gene silencing nucleic acids has led to the establishment of a wide array of next generation targeted therapies (14). The targeting moieties themselves have varied from full-length antibodies to recombinant proteins, small polypeptides, and nanoparticles (NPs). A diversity of linkage chemistries that allow conjugation of a cytotoxin to the targeting agent have been implemented depending upon where in the tissue it is most desirable to have the cytotoxin delivered and, if required, liberated from the targeting agent. With the early success of antibody–cytotoxin conjugates using radionuclides (referred to as radioimmunotherapy, RIT), such as yttrium-90 (^{90}Y)-labeled-ibritumomab tiuxetan (15) and iodine-131 (^{131}I)-labeled tositumomab (16) in treating refractory lymphoma, as well as the recently approved ADC trastuzumab-DM1 (T-DM1, Kadcyla®) (17), and brentuximab vedotin (SGN35, Adcetris®) (18), significant progress in personalized medicine has been attained (19). Part of this advancement is due to the improved therapeutic activity over the parental agents (the cytotoxic or targeting agent alone) resulting in a better clinical outcome while minimizing toxicity. Rituximab is a chimeric mouse–human IgG1 mAb directed to the CD20 cell surface protein and approved for treatment of B-cell lymphomas. ^{90}Y-labeled-ibritumomab

Table 2 | Molecular diagnostics (Dx) in US drug labels.

Drug	HUGO symbol	Referenced subgroup	Labeling sections
Ado-trastuzumab emtansine	ERBB2	HER2 protein overexpression or gene amplification positive	Indications and usage, warnings and precautions, adverse reactions, clinical pharmacology, clinical studies
Afatinib	EGFR	EGFR exon 19 deletion or exon 21 substitution (L858R) mutation positive	Indications and usage, dosage and administration, adverse reactions, clinical pharmacology, clinical studies, patient counseling information
Anastrozole	ESR1, PGR	Hormone receptor positive	Indications and usage, clinical pharmacology, clinical studies
Arsenic trioxide	PML/RARα	PML/RARα [t(15;17)] gene expression positive	Boxed warning, clinical pharmacology, indications and usage, warnings
Bosutinib	BCR/ABL1	Philadelphia chromosome [t(9;22)] positive	Indications and usage, adverse reactions, clinical studies
Brentuximab vedotin	TNFRSF8	CD30 positive	Indications and usage, description, clinical pharmacology
Busulfan	Philadelphia chromosome	Ph chromosome negative	Clinical studies
Capecitabine	DPYD	DPD deficient	Contraindications, warnings and precautions, patient information
Cetuximab	EGFR	EGFR protein expression positive	Indications and usage, warnings and precautions, description, clinical pharmacology, clinical studies
	KRAS	KRAS codon 12 and 13 mutation negative	Indications and usage, dosage and administration, warnings and precautions, adverse reactions, clinical pharmacology, clinical studies
Cisplatin	TPMT	TPMT intermediate or poor metabolizers	Clinical pharmacology, warnings, precautions
Crizotinib	ALK	ALK gene rearrangement positive	Indications and usage, dosage and administration, drug interactions, warnings and precautions, adverse reactions, clinical pharmacology, clinical studies
Dabrafenib	BRAF	BRAF V600E mutation positive	Indications and usage, dosage and administration, warnings and precautions, clinical pharmacology, clinical studies, patient counseling information
	G6PD	G6PD deficient	Warnings and precautions, adverse reactions, patient counseling information
Dasatinib	BCR/ABL1	Philadelphia chromosome [t(9;22)] positive; T315I mutation posit	Indications and usage, clinical studies, patient counseling information
Denileukin diftitox	IL2RA	CD25 antigen positive	Indications and usage, warnings and precautions, clinical studies
Erlotinib	EGFR	EGFR protein expression positive EGFR exon 19 deletion or exon 21 substitution (L858R) positive	Clinical pharmacology Indications and usage, dosage and administration, clinical pharmacology, clinical studies
Everolimus	ERBB2	HER2 protein overexpression negative	Indications and usage, boxed warning, adverse reactions, use in specific populations, clinical pharmacology, clinical studies
Everolimus	ESR1	Estrogen receptor positive	Clinical pharmacology, clinical studies
Exemestane	ESR1	Estrogen receptor positive	Indications and usage, dosage and administration, clinical studies, clinical pharmacology

(Continued)

Table 2 | Continued

Drug	HUGO symbol	Referenced subgroup	Labeling sections
Fluorouracil	DPYD	DPD deficient	Warnings
Fulvestrant	ESR1	Estrogen receptor positive	Indications and usage, clinical pharmacology, clinical studies, patient counseling information
Ibritumomab tiuxetan	MS4A1	CD20 positive	Indications and usage, clinical pharmacology, description
Imatinib	KIT BCR/ABL1 PDGFRβ	c-KIT D816V mutation negative Philadelphia chromosome [t(9;22)] positive PDGFR gene rearrangement positive	Indications and usage, dosage and administration clinical pharmacology, clinical studies
	FIP1L1/PDGFRα	FIP1L1/PDGFRα fusion kinase (or CHIC2 deletion) positive	Indications and usage, dosage and administration, clinical studies
Irinotecan	UGT1A1	UGT1A1*28 allele carriers	Dosage and administration, warnings, clinical pharmacology
Lapatinib	ERBB2	HER2 protein overexpression positive	Indications and usage, clinical pharmacology, patient counseling information
Letrozole	ESR1, PGR	Hormone receptor positive	Indications and usage, adverse reactions, clinical studies, clinical pharmacology
Mercaptopurine	TPMT	TPMT intermediate or poor metabolizers	Dosage and administration, contraindications, precautions, adverse reactions, clinical pharmacology
Nilotinib	BCR/ABL1	Philadelphia chromosome [t(9;22)] positive	Indications and usage, patient counseling information
Nilotinib	UGT1A1	UGT1A1*28 allele homozygotes	Warnings and precautions, clinical pharmacology
Ofatumumab	MS4A1	CD20 positive	Indications and usage, clinical pharmacology
Omacetaxine	BCR/ABL1	BCR-ABL T315I	Clinical pharmacology
Panitumumab	EGFR KRAS	EGFR protein expression positive KRAS codon 12 and 13 mutation negative	Indications and usage, warnings and precautions, clinical pharmacology, clinical studies Indications and usage, clinical pharmacology, clinical studies
Pazopanib	UGT1A1	(TA)7/(TA)7 genotype (UGT1A1*28/*28)	Clinical pharmacology, warnings and precautions
Pertuzumab	ERBB2	HER2 protein overexpression positive	Indications and usage, warnings and precautions, adverse reactions, clinical studies, clinical pharmacology
Ponatinib	BCR/ABL1	Philadelphia chromosome [t(9;22)] positive, BCR–ABL T315I mutation	Indications and usage, warnings and precautions, adverse reactions, use in specific populations, clinical pharmacology, clinical studies
Rasburicase	G6PD	G6PD deficient	Boxed warning, contraindications
Rituximab	MS4A1	CD20 positive	Indication and usage, clinical pharmacology, description, precautions

(Continued)

Table 2 | Continued

Drug	HUGO symbol	Referenced subgroup	Labeling sections
Tamoxifen	ESR1, PGR F5 F2	Hormone receptor positive Factor V Leiden carriers Prothrombin mutation G20210A	Indications and usage, precautions, medication guide Warnings
Thioguanine	TPMT	TPMT poor metabolizer	Dosage and administration, precautions, warnings
Tositumomab	MS4A1	CD20 antigen positive	Indications and usage, clinical pharmacology
Trametinib	BRAF	BRAF V600E/K mutation positive	Indications and usage, dosage and administration, adverse reactions, clinical pharmacology, clinical studies, patient counseling information
Trastuzumab	ERBB2	HER2 protein overexpression positive	Indications and usage, warnings and precautions, clinical pharmacology, clinical studies
Tretinoin	PML/RARA	PML/RARα [t(15;17)] gene expression positive	Clinical studies, indications and usage, warnings
Vemurafenib	BRAF	BRAF V600E mutation positive	Indications and usage, warning and precautions, clinical pharmacology, clinical studies, patient counseling information

Source: http://www.fda.gov/Drugs/ScienceResearch/ResearchAreas/Pharmacogenetics/ucm083378.htm

tiuxetan and I^{131}-labeled tositumomab, both of which also target CD20, showed statistically significant clinical responses in patients as compared to rituximab or chemotherapy alone and were approved for use in rituximab-refractory patients. Unfortunately, the application of these RITs in clinical practice has been limited by the complexity of handling β-emitting radionuclide-labeled mAbs before and after patient treatment. These limitations have fostered the generation of alternate molecules, including alpha emitting RITs (20) as well as non-radioactive cytotoxins that can be more practically conjugated to mAb, protein, or peptide-based targeting agents, without affecting their pharmacokinetic or pharmacodynamic properties (i.e., diminished ability to maximally and specifically access its target expressed by the diseased tissue). While therapeutic improvements have been reported in cancers using RITs and ADCs vs. non-conjugated agents, not all patients treated with RIT or ADC agents have shown enhanced benefit, suggesting diagnostic opportunities for improving the therapeutic use of conjugates (21). **Table 4** provides an overview of approved ADCs and RITs.

As indicated above, continued improvement and development of targeted therapies, using ADCs, RITs, or other technologies, is required but not sufficient to realize the maximal therapeutic potential of personalized medicine. Tailoring of a therapy to an individual's cancer requires knowledge of the underlying biology of that cancer and may involve utilizing surrogate molecular signatures, drug target expression profiles, and/or degree of targeted conjugate uptake for predicting patient response. The heterogeneity described for individual tumors (22) only adds to the complexity of defining the biomolecular characteristics of a patient's malignant tissue and selecting a therapy, or combination of therapies, most likely to be effective for the individual patient. In turn, such tumor heterogeneity adds to the complexity of development of the requisite surrogate Dx or CDx that is required to maximize the benefit of targeted therapies. It is generally accepted that the more complex the diagnostic platform, the more intricate is the regulatory path for approval, especially if the diagnostic is a CDx. A CDx is considered high risk by most regulatory authorities as it specifically dictates therapeutic intervention, in contrast to Oncotype Dx, MammaPrint, or OncoDX type diagnostic tools that merely supply information relative to prognosis and guide the therapeutic intervention. The development, analytical, and clinical validation of complex multi-marker diagnostic biomarker signatures is both time consuming and expensive. In addition, the alignment of therapeutic-diagnostic development timelines is challenging at best, especially if such signatures are not discovered until *post hoc* analysis of Phase 2 clinical trials. The recent clearance by the US FDA of next generation sequencing (NGS) instrumentation for cystic fibrosis is an important step for the use of new technologies to support complex assay developments, particularly as they relate to oncology where such complex signatures are likely required (23). However, as noted, biomarker signatures for predicting response to a given therapy may not simply involve gene expression or mutation profiles but, rather, complex gene product expression profiles.

TARGETED CYTOTOXIC AGENTS – TCAs

Despite the successful demonstration that targeted cytotoxic agents (TCAs), such as ADCs and RITs, can provide added clinical benefit for certain cancers, a number of challenges still remain for their clinical success across a broad spectrum of cancer indications. The effectiveness of targeted cytotoxin conjugates depends in part on the inherent features of the conjugate used. Some of the

Table 3 | FDA 510(k) cleared molecular diagnostics (Dx).

Disease state	Device	Year	Device manufacturer	Comments
AML	Vysis EGR1 FISH Probe Kit	2011	Abbott Molecular	Deletions in EGR1; bone marrow specimens; aid in prognosis
B-cell CLL	Vysis CLL FISH Probe Kit	2011	Vysis	Deletions in TP53, ATM, and D13S319 and gain in D12Z3; peripheral blood; aid in prognosis
	CEP 12 DNA Probe	1997	Vysis	FISH; specific for centromere 12; peripheral blood; prognosis
Bladder cancer	Vysis UroVysion Bladder Cancer Recurrence Kit	2004	Vysis	Aneuploidy of chromosomes 3, 7, 17 and loss of 9p21 locus; urine specimens; TCC; monitor recurrence
Breast cancer	MammaPrint	2011	Agendia	Gene expression profile; fresh frozen tissue; assess risk for distant metastasis and prognosis
	GeneSearch Breast Lymph Node (BLN) Test Kit	2009	Veridex	Gene expression panel; metastasis in lymph nodes; aids in the decision to excise additional lymph nodes and staging
	Dako TOP2A FISH PharmDx Kit	2012	Dako	FISH to detect copy number changes of TOP2A; FFPE; prognosis in high risk breast cancer patients
Cystic fibrosis	eSensor CF Genotyping Test	2009	Osmetech Molecular Diagnostics	Detects a panel of mutations and variants in CFTR; genomic DNA; genetic carrier screening
	xTAG Cystic Fibrosis 60 Kit v2	2009	Luminex Molecular Diagnostics	Detects and identifies a panel of mutations and variants the CFTR; genetic carrier and newborn screening
Prostate cancer	NADiA ProsVue	2011	Iris Molecular Diagnostics	Determines rate of change of total PSA; serum; an aid in identifying those patients at reduced risk for recurrence of prostate cancer
	PROGENSA PCA3 Assay	2012	Gen-Probe	PCA3 and PSA RNA ratio; urine; aids physicians in determining the need for repeat prostate biopsies in men who have had a previous negative biopsy
Tissue of origin	Pathwork Tissue of Origin Test Kit – FFPE	2012	Pathwork Diagnostics	Compares RNA expression patterns in a patient's FFPE tumor with those in a database; tissue; aid in determining origin of cancer
	Pathwork Tissue of Origin Test	2008	Pathwork Diagnostics	Compares RNA expression patterns in a patient's fresh/frozen tumor with those in a database; tissue; aid in determining origin of cancer

Source: http://www.fda.gov/MedicalDevices/ProductsandMedicalProcedures/InVitroDiagnostics/ucm330711.htm

TCA properties that can be optimized include: (1) tumor recognition and penetration; (2) serum half-life to minimize liberation of the cytotoxin in serum that may result in off-target effects; (3) targeting epitopes on a cell surface antigen that can support maximal conjugate internalization; (4) ability of the targeting agent to retain its target specificity in the conjugated form; and (5) large-scale conjugation of the cytotoxin to the targeting moiety for GMP manufacturing at a reasonable cost-of-goods. Smaller molecular weight targeting conjugates that employ antibody fragment or peptide platforms offer the opportunity to improve TCA tumor penetration (21), enhance binding specificities (24) and internalization (25), as well as lower serum half-lives to avoid prolonged circulation (26). Furthermore, smaller sized TCAs offer the ability to employ alternative manufacturing approaches to minimize cost-of-goods in contrast to mammalian cell fermentation that is required for manufacturing of full-length monoclonal antibodies. While antibody and antibody fragment conjugates appear to offer additional benefits for developing disease-specific therapies, the limited frequency in which a cell surface target is strictly expressed across heterogeneous disease vs. normal tissue remains a major drawback. In cancer, several cell surface targets have been identified that appear to be tumor-specific but the frequency of expression is quite variable from one tumor type to another thereby limiting the breadth by which an approved TCA can be used across different cancer indications (27). Furthermore, recent studies have demonstrated that the expression levels and/or distribution of cell surface targets on tumor cells or tumor-associated stromal cells can vary within the same specimen (28). Hence, the development of high affinity and high specificity targeting agents to maximize tumor recognition in cases of low and heterogeneous target expression is needed. The number of broadly expressed molecular targets that are present on a diseased cell and not on normal tissues that can be selectively targeted by a TCA is low. Nevertheless, several disease-specific antigens have been identified as a result of epigenetic mechanisms, alternative splicing, gene rearrangement, and overexpression that

Table 4 | Examples of approved antibody-drug conjugates (ADCs) and radioimmunotherapeutics (RIT's) in oncology.

Trade name (generic)	Manufacturer	Target	Conjugate	Approved	Indication	Comments
ANTIBODY-DRUG CONJUGATES (ADCs)						
Mylotarg Gemtuzumab ozogamicin	Pfizer/Wyeth	CD33	Calecheamicin	2001	Recurrent AML (age 60+)	Voluntarily withdrawn in 2010, due to product safety issues and lack of clinical benefit
Adcetris Brentuximab vedotin	Seattle Genetics	CD30	Mono-methyl auristatin E (MMAE)	2011	Refractory Hodgkin's lymphoma Refractory systemic anaplastic large cell lymphoma	
Kadcyla Trastuzumab emtansine	Genentech/ Roche	Her2/ neu	Maytansinoid DM1	2013	HER2-positive metastatic breast cancer	Approved for patients who have received prior treatment with Herceptin® (trastuzumab) and a taxane chemotherapy
Trade name (generic)	**Manufacturer**	**Target**	**Isotope**	**Approved**	**Indication**	**Comments**
RADIOIMMUNOTHERAPEUTICS (RITs)						
Zevalin Ibritumomab tiuxetan	Biogen-Idec/ Spectrum pharmaceuticals	CD20	^{90}Y	2002	Recurrent, low-grade or follicular B-cell non-Hodgkin's lymphoma	
Bexxar Iodine (131I) tositumomab	Corixa/GSK	CD20	^{131}I	2003	CD20 positive, follicular NHL, refractory to rituximab and relapsed following chemotherapy	Manufacture discontinued in 2014 due to poor sales

support the potential use of this class for maximizing the therapeutic potential of targeted agents (27). As efforts continue across the industry to identify more disease-specific targets via a variety of genomic and proteomic discovery approaches (discussed below), more broadly expressed disease-associated targets and disease targeting agents have been identified from the screening of naturally occurring pathogenic proteins, intra-protein domains, and NPs scaffolds (29–31). These platforms offer the potential to employ theranostics: the co-development of a TCA along with the same targeting vector linked to a diagnostic agent to determine effective targeting and patient selection (32). Moreover, the use of TCA formats enables the potential repurposing of pharmacologically defined cytotoxic agents on the market, which may lead to faster development timelines of TCA by leveraging prior clinical experience, or the salvaging of compounds that showed anti-tumor activity in clinical trials but failed due to off-target toxicities. One should also bear in mind that, while the expression of the target is required, it may not be sufficient for long-lasting responses. In fact, due to the inherent heterogeneity of tumors and potential escape mechanisms [as seen for example with BRAF inhibitors (33)], theranostics and the TCA strategy in general would likely benefit from being combined with other drugs that have different mode of action and/or target.

NANOPARTICLES AND APTAMERS

Over the past two decades, the use of NPs has shown promise in delivering therapeutic drugs to malignant cells. Early NP-derived agents were primarily designed by optimizing particle size, chemical composition (lipids, silica, nucleic acids), and charge in an attempt to deliver tumor-specificity (34). Next generation NP technologies incorporated the use of disease-specific ligands, such as antibodies and aptamers, which could bind to disease-associated cell surface receptors and deliver therapeutic SCEs. Unfortunately, as mentioned above, the discovery of widely expressed disease-specific receptors that can mediate robust internalization are infrequent. More recently, aptamer-bound NPs have been found to be useful in delivering cytotoxic agents to cancers by targeting disease-specific epitopes on cell surface tumor antigens (35). Peptide aptamers are combinatorial protein molecules usually consisting of short peptides inserted within a scaffold protein resulting in conformational assortment that creates a target-binding diversity. Nucleic acid-based aptamers can achieve similar levels of conformational diversity and target specificity as peptide-based aptamers. Since nucleic acids are also being explored as NP to carry, deliver, and release chemotherapeutic agents, they may represent unique building blocks for both aptamers and NPs manufacturing. The use of aptamers expands the ability to identify subtle differences in the topographical structure of cell surface tumor antigen motifs that are not as easily recognized by traditional proteomic platforms. In light of their size, aptamer-guided NPs have been further engineered as theranostics, whereby the NP contains the targeting aptamer, a cytotoxic agent and an imaging agent that can monitor tumor uptake directly in the patient (36). Patients showing tumor-specific uptake are then deemed suitable for NP-cytotoxic therapy while those that do not can pursue other therapeutic options. Again, despite these promising results, challenges still remain in aptamer-guided NP theranostics including non-specific NP tissue binding, systemic stability, GMP manufacturing, and broad-based application to multiple cancer types. It is worth noting that the successful development of targeted NPs will be demonstrated through a combination of target specificity, a high tumor-to-normal tissue ratio and affinity that will enable the agent to "find and bind" low target expression to deliver their cytotoxic payload. Similarly, these properties are required for their use in diagnostic modalities including patient selection and monitoring of therapeutic efficacy. **Table 5** contains a list of marketed and clinical stage NPs being developed for oncology.

NATURAL AGENTS TARGETING TUMORS

Several natural agents are able to target differentially expressed or conformation-specific cell surface antigens that are not easily identified by nucleic acid or proteomic analyses nor are easily targeted using traditional protein/antibody approaches. In particular, proteins, toxins or metabolites contained within plants, insects, arthropods, reptiles, viruses, and bacteria have yielded a number of agents capable of binding to specific host cell surface and intracellular proteins as a means to defend against predators and/or suppress their immune system as well as paralyze or even kill their prey (37, 38). Biochemical studies using natural agents from these sources have found them to have disparate activities. These include those that bind and are retained on the cell surface to suppress the activity of enzymes and channels while others have been shown to internalize upon binding to cell type-specific cell surface proteins to suppress intracellular functions. Naturally occurring polypeptides (NOP) from these sources include the following agents: vacuolating toxin A (VacA), which enters human cells via sphingomyelin (39); hepatitis C viral coat protein, which enters cells via claudin-1 (40); *Clostridium perfringens* enterotoxin, which binds to claudin-4 and causes cytotoxicity in cancer cells (41); crotamine, a toxin from rattlesnake venom that enters cells via heparin sulfate proteoglycans (42); and cholorotoxin, which binds to activated epithelial cells and internalizes via the annexin A2 complex (43, 44). Upon further experimental validation of tumor selectivity, any of these agents may serve as potential targeting moieties in the context of a TCA and could also be incorporated into theranostics platforms.

A critical factor for a therapeutic conjugate to provide clinical benefit is the ability to be systemically maintained at a certain molar level in order for the drug to effectively reach the target cells and accumulate at a concentration sufficient for the cytotoxin to exert its pharmacologic effect. Potential drawbacks of using NPs are their relative short serum and intracellular half-lives making extensive dosing and formulation studies critical for their success (45). Alternatively, NOPs have been selected by nature for their ability to impact cellular targets and maintain their function upon exposure. Moreover, their structures have evolved to withstand systemic degradation and immune responses by the host's serum proteolytic and host defense systems. These features along with

Table 5 | Examples of clinical stage nanoparticles and naturally occurring proteins in development for oncology.

Organization	Compound name	Compound description	Target/active agent	Development stage
Alnylam Pharmaceuticals	ALN-VSP	Liposomal based nanoparticle containing siRNA	KSD and VEGF/siRNA	Phase 1
BIND Biosciences	Bind-014	Polylactide–polyethylene glycol biopolymer nanoparticle containing a chemotoxin and targeting ligand	PSMA/docetaxel	Phase 2
Celgene	Nab-paclitaxel	Albumin based nanoparticle	Paclitaxel	Approved (Abraxane®)
Cerulean Pharma	CRLX-101	Cyclodextrin-based nanoparticle encapsulating a chemotoxin	Camptothecin	Phase 1/2
Janssen Pharmaceuticals	Pegylated liposomal doxorubicin	Pegylated liposomal nanoparticle containing a chemotoxin	Doxorubicin	Approved (Doxil®)
Morphotek	TM601	36 Amino acid peptide from scorpion venom that binds transformed cells and tumor endothelial cells via annexin A2 complex	Annexin A2 complex	Phase 1 (naked peptide format)
University of Illinois at Chicago	NSC745104	28 Amino acid fragment of the protein cupredoxin azurin from pseudomonas aeruginosa that increases intracellular p53 concentrations	p53	Phase 1

KSD, kinesin spindle protein; PSMA, prostate-specific membrane antigen; VEGF, vascular endothelial growth factor.

their small molecular size warrant exploring NOP potential applications in theranostics platforms and large-scale manufacturing for development. Furthermore, NOPs could find applications in immunohistochemistry and potentially in biofluid-based assays for soluble ligands or in the detection of specific circulating tumor cells (CTCs).

Screening of natural peptides and cell penetrating peptides may offer an advantage for rapid development of targeted therapy by using cell-specific uptake as a predictive marker for therapeutic benefit. This approach may offer a more rapid approach for developing personalized medicines over traditional molecular association, pharmacogenomic, and/or gene signature platforms that may require longer timelines for discovery and validation. However, the use of the latter can be combined during development once biomarker signature profiles have been reproducibly validated for predictive responses to treatment for a disease or disease-specific targeting agent. **Table 5** contains a list of some NOPs being developed for oncology.

EXAMPLE OF NATURALLY OCCURRING POLYPEPTIDE: CHLOROTOXIN

Chlorotoxin (CTX) is one of several NOPs that may be utilized for development of theranostics. Protein fractions of the venom from the Israeli scorpion, *Leirius quinquestriatus* were screened for the ability to selectively suppress tumor cell growth while leaving normal epithelial cells unaffected (46). This effort identified a 36 amino acid peptide (CTX) that is able to preferentially bind tumor vs. normal epithelial cells and perturb cell growth. Molecular studies have suggested that CTX binds and internalizes into a wide range of tumor types via the annexin A2 complex, a ubiquitously expressed intracellular protein in normal cells that is found expressed in complexes on the exterior surface of extracellular membranes of transformed cells (44). Preclinical studies have shown the ability of CTX to deliver radionuclides, complex dyes, as well as NPs preferentially to tumor cells *in vitro* and *in vivo* (47). In addition, preclinical studies have also shown CTX to have antiangiogenic activity as a naked peptide (48). Synthetic CTX has been tested in clinical trials and has shown the ability to deliver specifically conjugated ^{131}I-radionuclide to tumors after local or systemic delivery with no detectable uptake observed in normal tissues (49) as well as affect angiogenesis as a naked peptide in a Phase 1 trial. The platform is currently being expanded for diagnostic applications (49) and for delivery of cytotoxic compounds including radionuclides to tumors (unpublished observations). The preclinical and clinical studies reported to date suggest a natural compound like CTX could be formatted as a theranostic agent to support personalized medicine. This would be beneficial in light of the broad presence of cell surface annexin A2 complexes in transformed vs. normal cells.

Several studies have provided examples of how CTX could potentially be used as a theranostic agent for cancer. These include imaging studies demonstrating CTX conjugate localization to tumors vs. normal tissues. In one format, CTX has been developed as an imaging bioconjugate composed of CTX and Cy5.5, a fluorescent agent that emits photons in the near-IR spectrum (49). The bioconjugate has been shown to be useful in detecting cancer foci and metastases non-invasively under surgical operating conditions. Systemically, a CTX radionuclide conjugate has been shown to detect metastatic lesions in cancer patients with peripheral and CNS disease (50). Ongoing efforts are aimed at selecting the payload(s) with theranostic features as well as optimizing conjugation chemistry for delivering both a cytotoxin and a tracer to the tumor site.

THERANOSTICS CHALLENGES AND OPPORTUNITIES: USE OF CO-DEVELOPING DIAGNOSTIC AND THERAPEUTIC TARGETING VECTORS

The definition of theranostics (the merging of the words therapeutics with diagnostics) can be very broad. In its most traditional sense of diagnostics-guided therapy, the concept of theranostics can be identified in the previously cited example, whereby glucose blood levels are measured to determine the timing of the treatment as well as which patients will benefit the most from a hormone (insulin)-based therapy. Nowadays, detecting BRAF mutation is equivalent to measuring blood glucose in that it allows identifying which cancer patients would benefit from an anti-cancer agent targeting a specific kinase (e.g., targeted theranostics against mutated BRAF). In both examples, the diagnostic tool and the therapeutic agent are completely different because they share no molecular components. On the other hand, these two examples differ at least in one regard: while glucose levels represent a "non-targeted" biomarker of the disease state (the true therapeutic target being insulin receptor), detection of BRAF mutation underpins the very presence of the target against which the targeted therapeutic agent has an inhibitory effect. The mutated BRAF constitutes both a therapeutic target as well as a disease biomarker. In another incarnation of targeted theranostics, the targeting agent could be employed in both the diagnostics and therapeutics strategy. In this instance, the diagnostic and the therapeutic agents do share at least one molecular component. Let us call it "leveraged theranostics." Hence, we can describe at least three different theranostics classes: non-targeted, targeted, and leveraged (**Figure 1**).

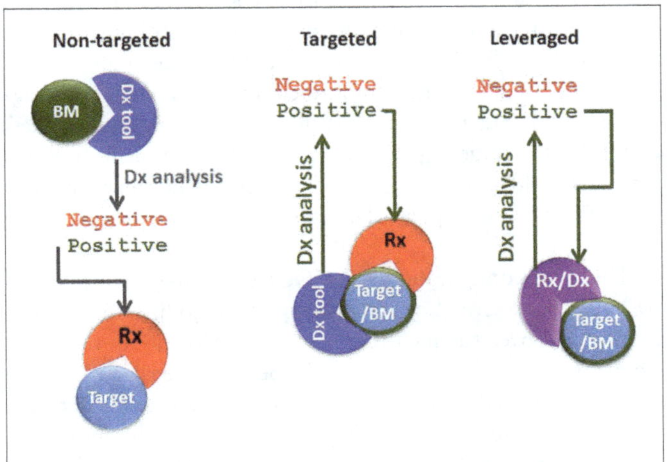

FIGURE 1 | Types of theranostic agents. In non-targeted theranostics (left panel), the biomarker (BM), the diagnostics (Dx) tool, the target, and the therapeutic agent (Rx) are separate entities. In the targeted theranostics (middle panel), the target and the biomarker are one and the same, but the Dx tool and the Rx are separate entities. In the leveraged theranostics (right panel), the diagnostic and the therapeutic agent share molecular components.

Monoclonal antibodies, antibody fragments, NPs, or NOPs may be armed with payloads and deployed in a leveraged theranostic strategy through the clever use of chemical linkers or couplers. One can envision three basic configurations for a leveraged theranostic compound: (1) one payload for therapy and one for diagnostics, with these payloads conjugated on different batches of the same targeting molecule; this configuration involves a single manufacturing process for the targeting moiety, and possibly one process for the linker attachment, but two separate processes for the conjugation of the two payload types; (2) one payload for therapy and one for diagnostics co-conjugated on the same targeting moiety; this implies a single compound and manufacturing process and represents a more ideal scenario; and finally (3) a single payload that can be cytotoxic as well as used for tumor uptake monitoring; this configuration allows for a single compound, manufacturing and conjugation process represents the most ideal scenario. An example of the first configuration (**Figure 2A**) is offered by the use of specific radionuclides. A radionuclide could be optimal for cytotoxicity but suboptimal for imaging, or vice versa. However, even by using currently available radionuclides, a single targeting agent such as CTX could be "functionalized" using a single chelator (hence a single manufacturing process for the targeting, functionalized moiety), and conjugated to Indium-111 for patient selection and Yttrium-90 for delivering cytotoxicity to the tumor by using two separate conjugation processes. Indium-111, while an excellent imaging agent, is not useful for therapy due to its low tissue penetration characteristic. These properties are reversed in Yttrium-90. Other radionucleotide pairs could be selected to satisfy the desired pharmacological as well as pharmacodynamic properties of the theranostic agent being pursued.

In the second configuration (**Figure 2B**), one where both payloads are co-attached on the same targeting molecule, one needs to be mindful of stereochemical interferences. For example, multiple payloads can disrupt the tumor cell binding activity of small targeting peptides such as CTX (36 amino acids). Structure–activity relationship analysis would need to be conducted to identify the best chemistry and attachment sites on both the targeting and payload molecules. NPs inherently offer the opportunity to carry multiple payloads to the tumor, including cytotoxins and diagnostic agents, but may not be sufficiently tumor-specific unless coupled with a targeting moiety. Another challenge using multiple payloads could be achieving a defined chemical homogeneity necessary for regulatory approval using a cost-effective manufacturing process.

The third configuration type (**Figure 2C**) has been achieved over the past several years by employing iodine-131, which, as noted above, suffers from the complexity of its handling. Therefore, this configuration could be improved by the selection of optimized radionuclides, their improved manufacturing processes, storage, and handling procedures, and by more sensitive whole-body radio-imaging devices. A new candidate for this mono-payload theranostic strategy is lutetium-177 (51). This radionuclide is a medium-energy β-emitter with a maximal tissue penetration of 2 mm, hence capable of delivering its cytotoxic energy through several cell layers, while potentially having less off-target toxicity than yttrium-90 (12 mm penetration range). Lutetium-177 also emits low-energy γ-rays allowing both imaging and dosimetry (quantitation of delivered or residual dose). Mono-payload, radiolabeled compounds could be used theranostically, whereby: (i) low, diagnostic (non-therapeutic) doses are used for initial assessment of *in vivo* targeting; (ii) sub-therapeutic doses are administered for dosimetry, allowing precise dose selection, and for monitoring potential toxic effect; and (iii) higher, therapeutic doses are administered to continue to monitor toxicity in conjunction with tumor burden (efficacy, acquired resistance) and tumor uptake (disease modifications, such as loss of target). This strategy is already being implemented when using BEXXAR®, an iodine-131-labeled antibody targeting CD20 positive B-lymphoma cells. Using dosimetry, physicians can use a low dose (5 mCi) and directly measure this TCA clearance rate. Patients with high tumor burden, splenomegaly, or bone marrow involvement tend to have faster clearance. Hence, the therapeutic dose (up to 90 mCi) can be prospectively individualized by using an equation (52).

By allowing patient selection and efficacy as well as toxicity monitoring, the potential success of pivotal trials using these theranostic strategies will allow the technological advancement and clinical benefit improvement of personalized medicine. **Table 6**

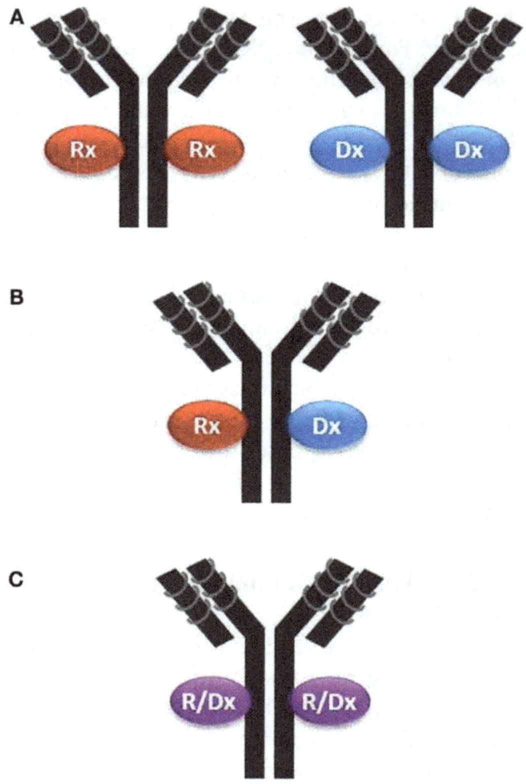

FIGURE 2 | Configurations of theranostic agents: (A) two separate batches of the same targeting moiety (in this example a mAb) are conjugated with either a therapeutic agent (Rx) such as a cytotoxin, or a diagnostic agent (Dx) such as a radionuclide; (B) the same batch of a mAb is conjugated with *both* Rx and Dx agents on the same targeting molecule; and (C) the same batch of a mAb is conjugated with an agent having both Rx and Dx properties (R/Dx), such as Lutetium-177, on the same targeting molecule.

Table 6 | Clinical stage theranostics.

Organization	Rx compound	Dx compound	Targeting moiety	Target	Configuration type	Development stage
Endocyte	Vinca alkaloid	Technetium-99m	Folate	Folate receptors	Figure 2A	Phase 3
Morphotek	Iodine-131	Iodine-131	Chlorotoxin	Annexin A2	Figure 2C	Phase 2
GlaxoSmithKline	Iodine-131	Iodine-131	Tositumomab (murine IgG2a)	CD20	Figure 2C	Approved (Bexxar®)
Institut Jules Bordet	Lutetium-177	Gallium-68	Octreotide (somatostatin analog)	Somatostatin receptor	Figure 2A	Phase 2
Peregrine	Neutralizing mAb	F(ab')2-indium-124	Bavituximab	Phosphatidylserine	Figure 2A[a]	Phase 1[b]/Phase 3[c]
Memorial Sloan-Kettering Cancer Center	Iodine-131	indium-124	8H9 (murine IgG1)	B7-H3	Figure 2A	Phase 1
University Medical Centre Groningen	Neutralizing mAb	Zirconium-89	Trastuzumab	HER2	Figure 2A[a]	Phase 1/2
Institut Jules Bordet/Roche	Maytansine	Zirconium-89	Trastuzumab	HER2	Figure 2A	Phase 2
Areva Med LLC	Lead-212	Lead-212	Trastuzumab	HER2	Figure 2C	Phase 1

[a] *Rx compound is a naked chimera IgG with target-neutralizing activity;*
[b] *Dx compound;*
[c] *Rx compound.*

contains a list of clinical stage theranostics being developed for oncology.

CONCLUSION AND FUTURE DIRECTIONS

The use of personalized medicine has many attributes that make the practice invaluable to patients, the pharmaceutical industry, and the healthcare system. The ability to predefine patients with a high likelihood to respond to a given therapy will provide benefit to all parties. For patients, the ability to predict response will improve therapeutic outcome while avoiding unnecessary treatment with ineffective, potentially toxic drugs and thereby lead to a better quality of life, if not a cure. For the pharmaceutical industry, predictive biomarkers (i.e., informative CDx) may improve the probability of success that a drug will provide meaningful clinical results in trials leading to higher approval rates by regulatory authorities and value-creation for the industry and patients alike. For the healthcare system, the ability to avoid futile, potentially toxic therapies will reduce not only drug costs but overall healthcare costs and potentially improve patient health by identifying agents that have a higher probability of success in treating their specific disease. While these attributes are compelling, the ability to implement platforms to support personalized medicine remains challenging. Attempts to identify disease-specific targets or molecular signatures that can provide predictive response outcomes are ongoing across the pharmaceutical industry and academia alike for many indications. While a few successful examples have been achieved, the majority of development programs are handicapped by the paucity of targets associated with disease as well as the time and effort required to validate molecular signatures that can unequivocally and reproducibly predict patient response to non-targeted SCEs.

As the industry refines its technologies and methods to improve upon personalized medicine, a few platforms exist today that may support this initiative in real-time clinical trials. Of particular note is the use of NPs and NOPs that can be conjugated to a therapeutic agent to improve disease-specific uptake of cytotoxic agents and patient response. As discussed above, the use of theranostic strategies employing, for example, a TCA and its co-developed diagnostic vector for *in vivo* prescreening of patients for tumor-specific uptake, offers the opportunity to identify patients with the highest likelihood of benefiting from the TCA therapy. Real-time theranostic imaging strategies may offer an alternative or supplemental approach to the more time consuming pharmacogenomics and/or molecular marker signature analyses for predicting response, although these approaches may yet prove complementary rather than mutually exclusive. Moreover, the application of NP or NOP containing vectors that enable their use for therapy in a broader range and higher frequency of cancers may offer better options than antibody-based therapies whose target is likely restricted to a few indications or across several indications at a low frequency. Other targeting agents in addition to NP and NOPs have also been formatted to support theranostic therapies. Studies in several cancers have found that cell surface proteins such as the folate receptor alpha (FOLR1), a highly expressed protein on ovarian and other epithelial derived cancers can be exploited in a theranostic context (53–55). Strategies to develop conjugates that can be selectively taken up via FOLR1 have been pursued in clinical trials whereby results from these studies have shown that patients whose tumors with uptake of an imaging-folate diagnostic conjugate have enhanced clinical response to a folate–vinblastine therapeutic conjugate compared to patients who do not have folate diagnostic vector uptake (56). Similar approaches to develop conjugate-imaging/conjugate-therapeutic vector pairs have suggested improved patient selection and therapeutic responses. Other examples of diagnostic and therapeutic targeting vector pairs have employed NP technologies to co-develop complexes containing diagnostic agents and an anti-cancer agent, including siRNAs (57). In all cases, the use of TCA and a co-developed targeting diagnostic vector offer alternative methods for delivering personalized therapies to patients in need of new treatments. The key, therefore, for the successful and continued evolution toward personalized medicine is co-development of both the therapeutic and the diagnostic agents as well as diagnostic modalities beginning at the time of target discovery and preclinical studies and continuing through clinical validation and regulatory approvals.

REFERENCES

1. Woodcock J. Assessing the clinical utility of diagnostics used in drug therapy. *Clin Pharmacol Ther* (2010) **88**:765–773. doi:10.1038/clpt.2010.230
2. Nicolaides NC, Sass PM, Grasso L. Advances in targeted therapeutic agents. *Expert Opin Drug Discov* (2010) **5**:1123–40. doi:10.1517/17460441.2010.521496
3. Eifert C, Powers RS. From cancer genomes to oncogenic drivers, tumour dependencies and therapeutic targets. *Nat Rev Cancer* (2012) **12**:572–8. doi:10.1038/nrc3299
4. Druker BJ, Guilhot F, O'Brien SG, Gathmann I, Kantarjian H, Gattermann N, et al. Five-year follow-up of patients receiving imatinib for chronic myeloid leukemia. *N Engl J Med* (2006) **355**:2408–17. doi:10.1056/NEJMoa062867
5. Mologni L. Inhibitors of the anaplastic lymphoma kinase. *Expert Opin Investig Drugs* (2012) **21**:985–94. doi:10.1517/13543784.2012.690031
6. Chapman PB, Hauschild A, Robert C, Haanen JB, Ascierto P, Larkin J, et al. Improved survival with vemurafenib in melanoma with BRAF V600E mutation. *N Engl J Med* (2011) **364**:2507–16. doi:10.1056/NEJMoa1103782
7. Towse A, Ossa D, Veenstra D, Carlson J, Garrison L. Understanding the economic value of molecular diagnostic tests: case studies and lessons learned. *J Pers Med* (2013) **3**:288–305. doi:10.3390/jpm3040288
8. van't Veer LJ, Dai H, van de Vijver MJ, He YD, Hart AA, Hart AA, et al. Gene expression profiling predicts clinical outcome of breast cancer. *Nature* (2002) **415**:530–6. doi:10.1038/415530a
9. National Comprehensive Cancer Network. Guidelines for Patients. Available from: http://www.nccn.org/patients/guidelines/cancers.aspx#breast
10. Paik S, Tang G, Shak S, Kim C, Baker J, Kim W, et al. Gene expression and benefit of chemotherapy in women with node-negative, estrogen receptor-positive breast cancer. *J Clin Oncol* (2006) **24**:3726–34. doi:10.1200/JCO.2005.04.7985
11. Park YY, Lee SS, Lim JY, Kim SC, Kim SB, Sohn BH, et al. Comparison of prognostic genomic predictors in colorectal cancer. *PLoS One* (2013) **8**:e60778. doi:10.1371/journal.pone.0060778
12. O'Shaughnessy J, Osborne C, Pippen J, Yoffe M, Patt D, Monoghan G, et al. Efficacy of BSI-201, a poly (ADP-ribose) polymerase-1 (PARP1) inhibitor, in combination with gemcitabine/carboplatin (G/C) in patients with metastatic triple-negative breast cancer (TNBC): results of a randomized phase II trial. *J Clin Oncol* (2009) **27**:18s.
13. Trail PA, Willner D, Lasch SJ, Henderson AJ, Hofstead S, Casazza AM, et al. Cure of xenografted human carcinomas by BR96-doxorubicin immunoconjugates. *Science* (1993) **261**:212–5. doi:10.1126/science.8327892
14. Junutula JR, Raab H, Clark S, Bhakta S, Leipold DD, Weir S, et al. Site-specific conjugation of a cytotoxic drug to an antibody improves the therapeutic index. *Nat Biotechnol* (2008) **26**:925–32. doi:10.1038/nbt.1480
15. Witzig TE, Gordon LI, Cabanillas F, Czuczman MS, Emmanouilides C, Joyce R, et al. Randomized controlled trial of yttrium-90-labeled ibritumomab tiuxetan radioimmunotherapy versus rituximab immunotherapy for patients with relapsed or refractory low-grade, follicular, or transformed B-cell non-Hodgkin's lymphoma. *J Clin Oncol* (2002) **20**:2453–63. doi:10.1200/JCO.2002.11.017
16. Kaminski MS, Zelenetz AD, Press OW, Saleh M, Leonard J, Fehrenbacher L, et al. Pivotal study of iodine I 131 tositumomab for chemotherapy-refractory low-grade or transformed low-grade B-cell non-Hodgkin's lymphomas. *J Clin Oncol* (2001) **19**:3918–28.
17. Burris HA, Rugo HS, Vukelja SJ, Vogel CL, Borson RA, Limentani S, et al. Phase II study of the antibody drug conjugate trastuzumab-DM1 for the treatment of human epidermal growth factor receptor 2 (HER2)-positive breast cancer after prior HER2-directed therapy. *J Clin Oncol* (2011) **29**:398–405. doi:10.1200/JCO.2010.29.5865
18. Foyil KV, Bartlett NL. Brentuximab vedotin for the treatment of CD30+ lymphomas. *Immunotherapy* (2011) **3**:475–85. doi:10.2217/imt.11.15
19. Trail PA. Antibody drug conjugates as cancer therapeutics. *Antibodies* (2013) **2**:113–29. doi:10.3390/antib2010113
20. Abbas N, Heyerdahl H, Bruland OS, Borrebæk J, Nesland J, Dahle J. Experimental α-particle radioimmunotherapy of breast cancer using 227Th-labeled p-benzyl-DOTA-trastuzumab. *EJNMMI Res* (2011) **1**:1–12. doi:10.1186/2191-219X-1-18
21. Adams GP, Schier R, McCall AM, Simmons HH, Horak EM, Alpaugh RK, et al. High affinity restricts the localization and tumor penetration of single-chain Fv antibody molecules. *Cancer Res* (2001) **61**:4750–5.
22. Burrell RA, McGranahan N, Bartek J, Swanton C. The causes and consequences of genetic heterogeneity in cancer evolution. *Nature* (2013) **501**:338–45. doi:10.1038/nature12625
23. FDA Press Release. *FDA Allows Marketing of Four "Next Generation" Gene Sequencing devices: Two Devices Aid in Screening and Diagnosis of Cystic Fibrosis* (2013). Available from: http://www.fda.gov/newsevents/newsroom/pressannouncements/ucm375742.html
24. Holliger P, Winter G. Diabodies: small bispecific antibody fragments. *Cancer Immunol Immunother* (1997) **45**:128–30. doi:10.1007/s002620050414
25. Jain M, Chauhan SC, Singh AP, Venkatraman G, Colcher D, Batra SK. Penetratin improves tumor retention of single-chain antibodies: a novel step toward optimization of radioimmunotherapy of solid tumors. *Cancer Res* (2005) **65**:7840–6.
26. Batra SK, Jain M, Wittel UA, Chauhan SC, Colcher D. Pharmacokinetics and biodistribution of genetically engineered antibodies. *Curr Opin Biotechnol* (2002) **13**:603–8. doi:10.1016/S0958-1669(02)00352-X
27. Kavak E, Ünlü M, Nistér M, Koman A. Meta-analysis of cancer gene expression signatures reveals new cancer genes, SAGE tags and tumor associated regions of co-regulation. *Nucleic Acids Res* (2010) **20**:7008–21. doi:10.1093/nar/gkq574
28. Cottu PH, Asselah J, Lae M, Pierga JY, Diéras V, Mignot L, et al. Intratumoral heterogeneity of HER2/neu expression and its consequences for the management of advanced breast cancer. *Ann Oncol* (2008) **19**:595–7. doi:10.1093/annonc/mdn021
29. Olivera BM, Rivier J, Clark C, Ramilo CA, Corpuz GP, Ramilo CA, et al. Diversity of *Conus* neuropeptides. *Science* (1990) **249**:257–63. doi:10.1126/science.2165278
30. Snyder EL, Dowdy SF. Recent advances in the use of protein transduction domains for the delivery of peptides, proteins and nucleic acids in vivo. *Expert Opin Drug Deliv* (2005) **2**:43–51. doi:10.1517/17425247.2.1.43
31. Petros RA, DeSimone JM. Strategies in the design of nanoparticles for therapeutic applications. *Nat. Rev. Drug Discov* (2010) **9**:615–27. doi:10.1038/nrd2591
32. Ozdemir V, Williams-Jones B, Glatt SJ, Tsuang MT, Lohr JB, Reist C. Shifting emphasis from pharmacogenomics to theragnostics. *Nat Biotechnol* (2006) **24**:942–6. doi:10.1038/nbt0806-942
33. Wagle N, Emery C, Berger MF, Davis MJ, Sawyer A, Pochanard P, et al. Dissecting therapeutic resistance to RAF inhibition in melanoma by tumor genomic profiling. *J Clin Oncol* (2011) **29**:3085–96. doi:10.1200/JCO.2010.33.2312
34. Kim JK, Choi KJ, Lee M, Jo MH, Kim S. Aptamer theragnostic. *Biomaterials* (2012) **33**:207–17. doi:10.1016/j.biomaterials.2011.09.023
35. Farokhzad OC, Jon S, Khademhosseini A, Tran TN, Lavan DA, Langer R. Nanoparticle aptamer bioconjugates: a new approach for targeting prostate cancer cells. *Cancer Res* (2004) **64**:7668–72. doi:10.1158/0008-5472.CAN-04-2550
36. Bates PJ, Laber DA, Miller DM, Thomas SD, Trent JO. Discovery and development of the G-rich oligonucleotide AS1411 as a novel treatment for cancer. *Exp Mol Pathol* (2009) **86**:151–64. doi:10.1016/j.yexmp.2009.01.004

37. De Luca V, Salim V, Atsumi SM, Yu F. Mining the biodiversity of plants: a revolution in the making. *Science* (2012) **336**:1658–61. doi:10.1126/science.1217410
38. Escoubas P, King GF. Venomics as a drug discovery platform. *Expert Rev Proteomics* (2009) **6**(221–224):2009. doi:10.1586/epr.09.45
39. Gupta VR, Wilson BA, Blanke SR. Sphingomyelin is important for the cellular entry and intracellular localization of *Helicobacter pylori*. *Cell Microbiol* (2010) **12**:1517–33. doi:10.1111/j.1462-5822.2010.01487.x
40. Evans MJ, von Hahn T, Tscherne DM, Syder AJ, Panis M, Wölk B, et al. Claudin-1 is a hepatitis C virus co-receptor required for a late step in entry. *Nature* (2007) **446**:801–5. doi:10.1038/nature05654
41. Michl P, Buchholz M, Rolke M, Kunsch S, Löhr M, McClane B, et al. Claudin-4: a new target for pancreatic cancer treatment using *Clostridium perfringens* enterotoxin. *Gastroenterology* (2001) **121**:678–84. doi:10.1053/gast.2001.27124
42. Nascimento FD, Hayashi MAF, Kerkis A, Oliveira V, Oliveira EB, Rádis-Baptista G, et al. Crotamine mediates gene delivery into cells through the binding to heparan sulfate proteoglycans. *J Biol Chem* (2007) **282**:21349–60. doi:10.1074/jbc.M604876200
43. DeBin JA, Maggio JE, Strichartz GR. Purification and characterization of chlorotoxin, a chloride channel ligand from the venom of the scorpion. *Am J Physiol* (1993) **264**:C361–9.
44. Kesavan K, Ratliff J, Johnson EW, Dahlberg W, Asara JM, Misra P, et al. Annexin A2 is a molecular target for TM601, a peptide with tumor-targeting and anti-angiogenic effects. *J Biol Chem* (2010) **285**:4366–74. doi:10.1074/jbc.M109.066092
45. Neuberger T, Schöpf B, Hofmann H, Hofmann M, von Rechenberg B. Superparamagnetic nanoparticles for biomedical applications: possibilities and limitations of a new drug delivery system. *J Magn Magn Mater* (2005) **293**:483–96. doi:10.1016/j.jmmm.2005.01.064
46. Lyons SA, O'Neal J, Sontheimer H. Chlorotoxin, a scorpion-derived peptide, specifically binds to gliomas and tumors of neuroectodermal origin. *Glia* (2002) **39**:162–73. doi:10.1002/glia.10083
47. Kievit FM, Veiseh O, Fang C, Bhattarai N, Lee D, Ellenbogen RD, et al. Chlorotoxin labeled magnetic nanovectors for targeted gene delivery to glioma. *J Drug Tar* (2012) **20**:67–75. doi:10.1021/nn1008512
48. Lima e Silva R, Shen J, Gong YY, Seidel CP, Hackett SF, Kesavan K, et al. Agents that bind annexin A2 suppress ocular neovascularization. *J Cell Physiol* (2010) **225**:855–64. doi:10.1002/jcp.22296
49. Mamelak AN, Jacoby DB. Targeted delivery of antitumoral therapy to glioma and other malignancies with synthetic chlorotoxin (TM-601). *Expert Opin Drug Deliv* (2007) **4**:175–86. doi:10.1517/17425247.4.2.175
50. Veiseh M, Gabikian P, Bahrami SB, Veiseh O, Zhang M, Hackman RC, et al. Tumor paint: a chlorotoxin:Cy5.5 bioconjugate for intraoperative visualization of cancer foci. *Cancer Res* (2007) **67**:6882–8. doi:10.1158/0008-5472.CAN-06-3948
51. Gribbin TE, Senzer N, Raizer JJ, Shen S, Nabors LB, Wiranowska M, et al. A phase I evaluation of intravenous (IV) 131I-chlorotoxin delivery to solid peripheral and intracranial tumors. *J Clin Oncol* (2009) **27**:e14507.
52. Kam BL, Teunissen JJ, Krenning EP, de Herder WW, Khan S, van Vliet EI, et al. Lutetium-labelled peptides for therapy of neuroendocrine tumours. *Eur J Nucl Med Mol Imaging* (2012) **39**:S103–12. doi:10.1007/s00259-011-2039-y
53. Seldin DW. Techniques for using BEXXAR for the treatment of non-Hodgkin's lymphoma. *J Nucl Med Technol* (2002) **30**:109–14.
54. Ebel W, Routhier EL, Foley B, Jacob S, McDonough JM, Patel RK, et al. Preclinical evaluation of MORAb-003, a humanized monoclonal antibody antagonizing folate receptor-alpha. *Cancer Immun* (2007) **7**:6–14.
55. O'Shannessy DJ, Somers EB, Albone E, Cheng X, Park YC, Tomkowicz BE, et al. Characterization of the human folate receptor alpha via novel antibody-based probes. *Oncotarget* (2011) **2**:1227–43.
56. Naumann RW, Coleman RL, Burger RA, Sausville EA, Kutarska E, et al. PRECEDENT: a randomized phase II trial comparing vintafolide (EC145) and pegylated liposomal doxorubicin (PLD) in combination versus PLD alone in patients with platinum-resistant ovarian cancer. *J Clin Oncol* (2013) **31**:4400–6. doi:10.1200/JCO.2013.49.7685
57. Medarova Z, Pham W, Farrar C, Petkova V, Moore A. In vivo imaging of siRNA delivery and silencing in tumors. *Nat Med* (2007) **13**:372–7. doi:10.1038/nm1486

5

Drug-diagnostics co-development in oncology: Part 1

Richard Simon*

Biometric Research Branch, National Cancer Institute, Bethesda, MD, USA

Edited by:
Jan Trøst Jørgensen, Dx-Rx Institute, Denmark

Reviewed by:
Olivier Micheau, Institut National de la Santé et de la Recherche Médicale, France
Fernando Rodríguez-Serrano, University of Granada, Spain

****Correspondence:***
Richard Simon, Biometric Research Branch, National Cancer Institute, 9609 Medical Center Drive, Bethesda, MD 20892-9735, USA
e-mail: rsimon@nih.gov

Developments in genomics are providing a biological basis for the heterogeneity of clinical course and response to treatment that have long been apparent to clinicians. The ability to molecularly characterize human diseases presents new opportunities to develop more effective treatments and new challenges for the design and analysis of clinical trials. In oncology, treatment of broad populations with regimens that benefit a minority of patients is less economically sustainable with expensive molecularly targeted therapeutics. The established molecular heterogeneity of human diseases requires the development of new paradigms for the design and analysis of randomized clinical trials as a reliable basis for predictive medicine. We review prospective designs for the development of new therapeutics and predictive biomarkers to inform their use. We cover designs for a wide range of settings. At one extreme is the development of a new drug with a single candidate biomarker and strong biological evidence that marker negative patients are unlikely to benefit from the new drug. At the other extreme are phase III clinical trials involving both genome-wide discovery of a predictive classifier and internal validation of that classifier. We have outlined a prediction based approach to the analysis of randomized clinical trials that both preserves the type I error and provides a reliable internally validated basis for predicting which patients are most likely or unlikely to benefit from a new regimen.

Keywords: predictive biomarker, clinical trial design, adaptive design, companion diagnostic, enrichment trial

INTRODUCTION

This dominant paradigm for oncology drug development has been rapidly changing. The paradigm for development of cytotoxics involved large phase III clinical trials to find relatively small, but statistically significant, average treatment effects for target populations defined in terms of primary site and stage. The primary analysis was relatively simple, consisting of a single statistical test of the null hypothesis of no average treatment effect for the intent to treat population with regard to a single primary endpoint. Any claim of treatment benefit based on subset analysis without an overall statistically significant intent to treat analysis was viewed with suspicion.

Randomized clinical trials have made important contributions to modern medicine and public health, but they have also led to the over-treatment of broad populations of patients, most of whom don't benefit from the increasingly expensive drugs and procedures shown to have statistically significant average treatment effects in increasingly large clinical trials. With the recognition of the molecular heterogeneity of cancer and the development of molecularly targeted drugs whose effects depend strongly on the genomic alterations and genetic background of the tumor, the broad eligibility primary site oriented clinical trial is playing a less dominant role. Increasingly sophisticated and cost effective biotechnology platforms are providing the tools to develop diagnostics that identify the patients most likely to benefit from molecularly targeted drugs.

Tumors of a primary site in many represent a heterogeneous collection of diseases that differ in pathophysiology, natural history, and sensitivity to treatment. These diseases differ with regard to the mutations that cause them and drive their invasion. The heterogeneous nature of tumors of the same primary site offers new challenges for drug development and clinical trial design. Physicians have always known that cancers of the same primary site were heterogeneous with regard to natural history and response to treatment. This understanding sometimes led to conflicts with statisticians over the use of subset analysis in the analysis of clinical trials. Although most statisticians expressed concern about the potential for false positive findings results from *post hoc* subset analysis, some practitioners rejected the results of clinical trials whose conclusions were based on average effects. Today we have better tools for characterizing the tumors biologically and using this characterization in the design and analysis of clinical trials that utilize this information prospectively.

Most oncology drugs are being developed for defined molecular targets. In some cases the targets are well understood and there is a compelling biological basis for restricting development to the subset of patients whose tumors are characterized by deregulation of the drug target. For other drugs there are multiple targets and more uncertainty about how to measure whether a drug target is driving tumor invasion in an individual patient (1). It is clear that the primary analysis of the new generation of oncology clinical trials must consist of more than just treating broad patient populations and testing the null hypothesis of no average effect. But it is also clear that the tradition of *post hoc* data dredging subset analysis is not an adequate basis for predictive oncology. For establishing practice standards and for drug approvals we need prospective analysis plans that provide for both preservation of the type I experiment-wise error rate and for focused predictive analyses that can be used to reliably select patients in clinical practice for use of the new regimen (2–4). These two primary objectives involve co-development of a drug and a companion diagnostic.

In the following sections we summarize some of the designs that are available for the co-development of a drug and companion diagnostic. Developing new treatments with companion diagnostics or predictive biomarkers for identifying the patients who benefit does not make drug development simpler, quicker, or cheaper as is sometimes claimed. Actually it makes drug development more complex and probably more expensive. But for many new oncology drugs it should increase the chance of success. It may also lead to more consistency in results among trials and increase the proportion of patients who benefit from the drugs they receive. This approach also has great potential value for controlling societal expenditures on health care.

The ideal approach to co-development of a drug and companion diagnostic involves: (i) identification of a predictive biomarker based on understanding the mechanism of action of the drug and the role of the drug target in the pathophysiology of the disease. This biological understanding should be validated and refined by pre-clinical studies and early phase clinical trials. The predictive biomarkers for successful cancer drugs have generally involved a single gene or protein rather than a multivariate classifier. Multivariate classifiers have been found some use as prognostic indicators that reflect a combination of the pace of the disease and the effect of standard therapy. Multivariate classifiers have rarely been used as predictive biomarkers for response to specific drugs because their use often reflects an incomplete understanding of the mechanism of action of the drug or the role of its molecular target. (ii) Development of an analytically validated test for measurement of that biomarker. Analytically validated means that the test accurately measures what it is supposed to measure, or if there is no gold-standard measurement, that the test is reproducible and robust. (iii) Use of that test to design and analyze a new clinical trial to evaluate the effectiveness of that drug and how the effectiveness relates to the biomarker value.

In the enrichment and stratified designs described below, biomarker discovery and determination of the threshold of positivity is performed prior to the phase III trial. Cancer biology is complex, however, and it is not always possible to have everything sorted out in this way before launching the phase III clinical trials. We will also discuss designs and prospective analysis plans that permit one to adaptively determine the best threshold of positivity for the biomarker and designs that incorporate multiple candidate biomarkers.

TARGETED (ENRICHMENT) DESIGNS

Designs in which eligibility is restricted to those patients considered most likely to benefit from the experimental drug are called "targeted designs" or "enrichment designs." With an enrichment design, the analytically validated diagnostic test is used to restrict eligibility for a randomized clinical trial comparing a regimen containing a new drug to a control regimen. This approach has now been used for pivotal trials of many drugs whose molecular targets were well understood in the context of the disease. Several authors (5–9) studied the efficiency of this approach relative to the standard approach of randomizing all patients without using the biomarker test at all. The efficiency of the enrichment design depends on the prevalence of test positive patients and on the effectiveness of the new treatment in test negative patients. When fewer than half of the patients are test positive and the new treatment is relatively ineffective in test negative patients, the number of randomized patients required for an enrichment design is dramatically smaller than the number of randomized patients required for a standard design. For example, if the treatment is completely ineffective in test negative patients, then the ratio of number of patients required for randomization in the enrichment design relative to the number required for the standard design is approximately $1/\gamma^2$ where γ denotes the proportion of patients who are test positive. The treatment may have some effectiveness for test negative patients either because the assay is imperfect for measuring deregulation of the putative molecular target or because the drug has off-target anti-tumor effects. Even if the new treatment is half as effective in test negative patients as in test positive patients, however, the randomization ratio is approximately $4/(\gamma+1)^2$. This equals about 2.56 when $\gamma = 0.25$, i.e., 25% of the patients are test positive, indicating that the enrichment design reduces the number of required patients to randomize by a factor of 2.56.

The enrichment design was very effective for the development of trastuzumab even though the test was imperfect and has subsequently been improved. Simon and Maitournam (5, 6) also compared the enrichment design to the standard design with regard to the number of screened patients. We have made the methods of sample size planning for the design of enrichment trials available on line at http://brb.nci.nih.gov. The web-based programs are available for binary and survival/disease-free survival endpoints. The planning takes into account the performance characteristics of the tests and specificity of the treatment effects. The programs provide comparisons to standard non-enrichment designs based on the number of randomized patients required and the number of patients needed for screening to obtain the required number of randomized patients.

The enrichment design is appropriate for contexts where there is a strong biological basis for believing that test negative patients will not benefit from the new drug. In such cases, including test negative patients may raise ethical concerns and may confuse the interpretation of the clinical trial. As described in the section on "stratification designs," if test negative patients are to be included then one should ensure that a sufficient number of test positive patients are included to provide an adequately powered evaluation. Often this is not done and instead one sees a mixed population of patients in an inadequately sized trial leading to ambiguous conclusions.

The enrichment design does not provide data on the effectiveness of the new treatment compared to control for test negative patients. Consequently, unless there is compelling biological or phase II data that the new drug is not effective in test negative patients, the enrichment design may not be adequate to support approval of the test. If the biological rationale or phase II data is strong, however, then the test can be approved for identifying a subset of patients for whom an effective drug exists, rather than for distinguishing patients who do and do not benefit from the new drug.

In oncology, sequencing of tumor DNA to test for point or structural alterations in genes whose protein products are druggable is rapidly becoming part of the standard diagnostic workup at advanced cancer centers. Regulatory body approvals of drugs for populations defined by such tests will require that the tests be shown to have good analytical performance (10).

BIOMARKER STRATIFIED DESIGN

When a predictive classifier has been developed but there is not compelling biological or phase II data that test negative patients do not benefit from the new treatment, it is generally best to include both classifier positive and classifier negative in the phase III clinical trials comparing the new treatment to the control regimen. In this case it is essential that an analysis plan be pre-defined in the protocol for how the predictive classifier will be used in the analysis. The analysis plan will generally define the testing strategy for evaluating the new treatment in the test positive patients, the test negative patients, and overall. The testing strategy must preserve the overall type I error of the trial and the trial must be sized to provide adequate statistical power for these tests. It is not sufficient to just stratify, i.e., balance, the randomization with regard to the classifier without specifying a complete analysis plan. The main value of "stratifying" (i.e., balancing) the randomization is that it assures that only patients with adequate test results will enter the trial. Pre-stratification of the randomization is not necessary for the validity of inferences to be made about treatment effects within the test positive or test negative subsets. If an analytically validated test is not available at the start of the trial but will be available by the time of analysis, then it may be preferable not to pre-stratify the randomization process.

The purpose of the pivotal trial is to evaluate the new treatment overall and in the subsets determined by the pre-specified classifier (generally biomarker plus cut-point for positivity). The purpose is not to modify or optimize the classifier unless an adaptive design is used. Several primary analysis plans have been described (10–12) and a web-based tool for sample size planning for some of these analysis plans is available at http://brb.nci.nih.gov For example, If one has moderate strength evidence that the treatment, if effective at all, is likely to be more effective in the test positive cases, one might first compare treatment versus control in test positive patients using a threshold of significance of 5%. Only if the treatment versus control comparison is significant at the 5% level in test positive patients, will the new treatment be compared to the control among test negative patients, again using a threshold of statistical significance of 5%. This sequential approach controls the overall type I error at 5%. To have 90% power in the test positive patients for detecting a 50% reduction in hazard for the new treatment versus control at a two-sided 5% significance level requires about 88 events of test positive patients. If at the time of analysis the event rates in the test positive and test negative strata are about equal, then when there are 88 events in the test positive patients, there will be about $88(1-\gamma)/\gamma$ events in the test negative patients where γ denotes the proportion of test positive patients. If 25% of the patients are test positive, then there will be approximately 264 events in test negative patients. This will provide approximately 90% power for detecting a 33% reduction in hazard at a two-sided significance level of 5%. In this case, the trial will not be delayed compared to the enrichment design, but a large number of test negative patients will be randomized, treated, and followed on the study rather than excluded as for the enrichment design. This will be problematic if one does not, *a priori*, expect the new treatment to be effective for test negative patients. In this case it will be important to establish an interim monitoring plan to terminate accrual of test negative patients when interim results and prior evidence of lack of effectiveness makes it no longer viable to enter them.

In the situation where one has more limited confidence in the predictive marker it can be effectively used for a "fall-back" analysis. In Simon and Wang (13), we proposed an analysis plan in which the new treatment group is first compared to the control group overall. If that difference is not significant at a reduced significance level such as 0.03, then the new treatment is compared to the control group just for test positive patients. The latter comparison uses a threshold of significance of 0.02, or whatever portion of the traditional 0.05 not used by the initial test. If the trial is planned for having 90% power for detecting a uniform 33% reduction in overall hazard using a two-sided significance level of 0.03, then the overall analysis will take place when there are 297 events. If the test is positive in 25% of patients and the event rates in test positive and test negative patients are about equal at the time of analysis, then when there are 297 overall events there will be approximately 75 events among the test positive patients. If the overall test of treatment effect is not significant, then the subset test will have power 0.75 for detecting a 50% reduction in hazard at a two-sided 0.02 significance level. By delaying the treatment evaluation in the test positive patients power 0.80 can be achieved when there are 84 events and power 0.90 can be achieved when there are 109 events in the test positive subset. Wang et al. have shown that the power of this approach can be improved by taking into account the correlation between the overall significance test and the significance test comparing treatment groups in the subset of test positive patients (14). So if, for example a significance threshold of 0.03 has been used for the overall test, the significance threshold for used for the subset can be somewhat >0.02 and still have the overall chance of a false positive claim of any type limited to 5%. Real world experience with stratification and enrichment designs are described by Freidlin et al. (15) and by Mandreakar and Sargent (16). Freidlin et al. (17) describe a randomized phase II design for providing information for the design of the phase III trial in cases where there is not a strong biological rationale for the enrichment approach.

INTERIM MONITORING OF TEST NEGATIVE PATIENTS

Interim monitoring of outcome for the test negative patients is very important in clinical trials where there is preliminary evidence that efficacy of the new regimen may be limited to the test positive patients. One approach is to perform an interim analysis focused on the test negative patients using a standard futility monitoring statistical plan for the primary endpoint of the clinical trial. Such methods are usually either based on the standardized treatment effect or the conditional power of rejecting the null hypothesis at the end of the trial. One simple approach is to compute the standardized treatment effect in the test negative patients at a time when half of the events in test negative patients projected to occur by the end of the trial have occurred. If the treatment effect is going in the wrong direction, then accrual to the test negative stratum ceases. This type of futility analysis is designed to be conservative enough that the power at the end of the trial for detecting a treatment effect is minimally reduced. This type of futility monitoring is used in the design proposed by Wang et al. (14) but in many cases it provides very limited protection for test negative patients for use in biomarker driven designs. Depending on the accrual rate and survival distributions, by the time half of the primary endpoint events have occurred for the test negative patients, the accrual of test negative patients may be close to complete.

An alternative approach would be to base the futility monitoring of the test negative patients on an intermediate endpoint rather than on the primary endpoint of the trial. There would be no assumption that the intermediate endpoint is a true surrogate for the primary endpoint, only that if there is no treatment effect on the intermediate endpoint, then there is unlikely to be a treatment effect for the primary endpoint. With this limited assumption, made for most phase II trials, the futility analysis can be performed at an earlier time so that a finding of futility will limit the number of test negative patients accrued.

In Karuri and Simon (18) we introduced a phase III design for this setting in which futility monitoring of the test negative patients is performed based on a joint prior joint distribution for the treatment effects in test negative and test positive patients. That prior distribution enables the trial investigator to represent the prior evidence that treatment effect will be reduced for test negative patients and use that information in monitoring the clinical trial. Although the formulation is Bayesian, the rejection region based on posterior probability is calibrated so that type I errors satisfy the usual frequentist requirements.

BIOMARKER ADAPTIVE THRESHOLD DESIGN

In Jiang et al. (19) we reported on a "Biomarker Adaptive Threshold Design" for situations where a biomarker is available at the start of the trial, but a cut-point for converting the value to a binary classifier is not established. For example, this design could be used with a FISH assay for EGFR positivity without pre-specification of the threshold of positivity. Tumor specimens are collected from all patients at entry, but the value of the biomarker is not used as an eligibility criteria. Their analysis plan does not stipulate that the assay for measuring the index needs to be performed in real time. Two analysis plans were described. Analysis plan A begins with comparing outcomes for all patients receiving the new treatment to those for all control patients. If this difference in outcomes is significant at a pre-specified reduced significance level α_1 (e.g., 0.03) then the new treatment is considered effective for the eligible population as a whole. Otherwise, a second stage test is performed using significance threshold $\alpha_2 = 0.05 - \alpha_1$. The second stage test involves finding the cut-point s^* for the biomarker score which leads to the largest treatment effect in comparing T to C restricted to patients with score greater than s^*. Jiang et al. employed a log-likelihood measure of treatment effect and let L^* denote the log-likelihood of treatment effect when restricted to patients with biomarker level above s^*. The null distribution of L^* was determined by repeating the analysis after permuting the treatment and control labels a thousand or more times, recomputing s^* and L^* each time. If the permutation statistical significance of L^* is $<0.05 - \alpha_1$ (e.g., 0.02), then treatment T is considered superior to C for the subset of the patients with biomarker level above s^*.

The advantage of procedure A is its simplicity and that it explicitly separates the test of treatment effect in the broad population from the subset selection. However, the procedure takes a conservative approach in adjusting for multiplicity of combining the overall and subset tests. An alternative analysis plan B proposed by Jiang et al. does not use a first stage comparison of treatment groups overall. Consequently, plan B is more appropriate to settings in which there is greater expectation that treatment effect will be limited to a marker defined subset. With analysis plan B they determine the cut-point value b at which $w(b)S(b)$ is maximized, where $w(b)$ is a pre-defined weight function. The weight function is used to give greater emphasis to the $b = 0$ subset, that is, the subset containing all patients (marker value is initially normalized to the 0–1 interval). Let $T(b) = w(b)S(b)$ denote the value of the maximized weighted partial log-likelihood. The statistical significance of $T(b)$ is determined by generating the null distribution by repeating the optimization procedure for many cases of randomly permuted data. With either procedure A or B, a confidence interval for the optimal cut-point b is generated by bootstrap re-sampling of the maximum likelihood estimate of the cut-point based on a proportional hazards model with an unknown cut-point and an unknown treatment effect for patients with biomarker values above the cut-point. Since the treatment is presumed effective only for patients with biomarker above the threshold b, the confidence coefficient associated with a given biomarker value x can be interpreted as the probability that a patient with marker value x benefits from the new treatment.

In Jiang et al. (19) we also provided an approach to sample size planning for the biomarker adaptive threshold design. With analysis strategy A, sample size is determined in the traditional manner for overall comparison of the treatment arms but powering the trial for using a reduced significance level a_1, e.g., 0.03. With analysis plan B a larger sample size is used to provides good power for establishing the statistical significance of treatment effects restricted to patients with biomarker values above an initially unknown cut-point.

ADAPTIVE ENRICHMENT DESIGNS

The adaptive threshold design described above (19) enables one to conduct the phase III clinical trial without pre-specifying the cut-point for the biomarker. It provides for a valid statistical significance test that has good statistical power against alternative hypotheses that the treatment effect is limited to patients with biomarker values above some unknown level, and it provides a confidence interval for estimation of the cut-point. These analyses are, however, performed at the end of the trial and accrual during the trial is not restricted by biomarker value. In Simon and Simon (20), we introduced a very general class of adaptive enrichment designs in which the eligibility criteria are adaptively adjusted during the course of the trial in order to exclude patient subsets unlikely to benefit from the new regimen. Others have also studied adaptive enrichment designs (21–23). Wang et al. (21) and Simon and Simon (20) provide general frameworks for adaption and identify statistical significance tests that provide protection of the study-wise type I error under broad conditions. In Simon and Simon (20) we applied this framework to the setting of adaptive threshold enrichment of a single biomarker.

DESIGNS THAT EVALUATE A SMALL NUMBER OF BIOMARKERS

Because of the complexity of cancer biology, there are many cases in which the biology of the target is not sufficiently well understood at the time that the phase III trials are initiated to restrict attention to a single predictive biomarker. The analysis plan used in the adaptive threshold design (19) is based on computing a global test based on a maximum test statistic. For the adaptive threshold design, the maximum is taken over the set of cut-points of a biomarker score. The idea of using a global maximum test statistic is much more broadly applicable, however. For example, suppose multiple candidate binary tests, $B_1, \ldots, B_K$ are available at the start of the trial. These tests may or may not be correlated with each other. Let L_k denote the log-likelihood of treatment effect for comparing T to C when restricted to patients positive for biomarker k. Let L^* denote the largest of these values and let k^* denote the test for which the maximum is achieved. As for the adaptive threshold design, the null distribution of L^* can be determined by repeating the analysis after permuting the treatment and control labels a thousand or more times. If the permutation statistical significance of L^* is $<0.05 - \alpha_1$ (e.g., 0.02), then treatment T is considered superior to C for the subset of the patients positive for biomarker test k^*. The stability of the indicated set of patients who benefit from T (i.e., k^*) can be evaluated by repeating the computation of k^* for bootstrap samples of patients. This approach can be useful when the number of candidate biomarkers is small, as it should be by the time a phase III trial is initiated. Some of the adaptive enrichment designs (20) can also be employed in that setting with multiple biomarker candidates with or without known cut-points of positivity.

ADAPTIVE CLASSIFICATION BASED ON SCREENING CANDIDATE BIOMARKERS

Designs such as the "adaptive signature design" have been developed for adaptive multivariate classifier development and internal validation based on high dimensional genomic tumor characterization (24). This design employs a "learn and confirm" structure in which a portion of the patients are used to select the biomarker hypothesis, i.e., to develop an "indication classifier" which identifies the target population of patients in which the test treatment is most likely to be effective, and to use the remainder of the patients to test the treatment effect in that subset. The adaptive signature design does not modify eligibility criteria. It is adaptive in the sense that the treatment effect is tested in a single subset determined based on the clinical trial data but in a manner that separates classifier development from testing of treatment effect. This is dramatically different than the current practice of *ad hoc* analysis in multiple subsets with no control of type I error or in using the full dataset to both develop a classifier and to classify patients for purpose of hypothesis testing. Since the adaptive signature design does not use the patients on which the classifier was developed for the testing of the treatment effect, it thus avoids the inflation of type I error described by Wang et al. (25) for other approaches. Scher et al. described the use of the adaptive signature design for planning a pivotal trial in advanced prostate cancer (26). The key idea of the adaptive signature approach is to replace multiple significance testing based subset analysis with development and internal validation of a single "indication classifier" that informs treatment selection for individual patients based on their entire vector of covariate values.

The adaptive signature design approach is very general with regard to the methodology applied to the training set for identifying the single candidate subset in which treatment effect will be tested in the validation set. In many cases this can be accomplished by developing a model for predicting outcome as a function of treatment, selected biomarkers and treatment by biomarker interactions. In the original adaptive signature design paper this was accomplished by screening all the candidate biomarkers using predictive models that include the main effect of treatment, main effect of a single biomarker, and the corresponding interaction of that biomarker with treatment. Candidate markers which exhibited an interaction nominally significant at a pre-specified level were included in a final multivariate predictive model. A machine learning weighted voting model was used in the original paper to classify patients as either likely to benefit from the new treatment or not likely to benefit from the new treatment. The tuning parameters for this classifier were optimized by cross-validation in the training set. The multivariate model was then used to classify the patients in the validation set, and the treatment effect was evaluated in the subset of the patients in the validation set that were classified as likely to benefit from the new treatment based on the classifier developed in the training set.

Many other methods of classifier development can be employed using the training set. It is important to recognize, however, that one is not developing a prognostic classifier. The classifier is used to classify patients as likely to benefit from the new treatment. One could develop prognostic classifiers separately for the treatment and control groups using standard penalized regression methods and then classify patients based on which prognostic classifier predicts the better outcome. More commonly, however, single predictive models have been used based on screening candidate markers based on their univariate interaction with treatment. Matsui et al. (27) used their model to predict a continuous score reflecting the expected benefit for the new treatment relative to the control rather than just classifying patients into one of two subsets. Gu et al. (28) have developed a two-step strategy for developing a model for predicting outcome as a function of treatment and selected biomarkers. The biomarkers are selected using a group lasso approach in which the main effects of a biomarker are grouped with the interactions of that marker with treatments and can be used with two or more treatments.

Freidlin et al. (29) described further extensions of the adaptive signature approach. They use cross-validation to replace sample splitting of the trial into a training set and test set in order to increase the statistical power.

CONCLUSION

Recognition of the molecular heterogeneity of human diseases such as cancers of a primary site and the tools for characterizing this heterogeneity presents new opportunities for the development of more effective treatments and challenges for the design and analysis of clinical trials. In oncology, treatment of broad populations with regimens that do not benefit most patients is less economically sustainable with expensive molecularly targeted therapeutics and less likely to be successful. The established molecular heterogeneity of human diseases requires the development of new approaches to use randomized clinical trials to provide a reliable basis predictive medicine (3, 4). This paper has attempted to review here some prospective phase III designs for the co-development of new therapeutics with companion diagnostics.

REFERENCES

1. Sawyers CL. The cancer biomarker problem. *Nature* (2008) **452**:548–52. doi:10.1038/nature06913
2. Simon RM. *Genomic Clinical Trials and Predictive Medicine.* Cambridge: Cambridge University Press (2013).
3. Simon R. An agenda for clinical trials: clinical trials in the genomic era. *Clin Trials* (2004) **1**:468–70. doi:10.1191/1740774504cn046xx
4. Simon R. New challenges for 21st century clinical trials. *Clin Trials* (2007) **4**:167–9. doi:10.1177/1740774507076800
5. Simon R, Maitournam A. Evaluating the efficiency of targeted designs for randomized clinical trials. *Clin Cancer Res* (2005) **10**:6759–63. doi:10.1158/1078-0432.CCR-04-0496
6. Simon R, Maitournam A. Evaluating the efficiency of targeted designs for randomized clinical trials: supplement and correction. *Clin Cancer Res* (2006) **12**:3229. doi:10.1158/1078-0432.CCR-12-10-COR
7. Maitournam A, Simon R. On the efficiency of targeted clinical trials. *Stat Med* (2005) **24**:329–39. doi:10.1002/sim.1975
8. Hoering A, LeBlanc M, Crowley J. Randomized phase III clinical trial designs for targeted agents. *Clin Cancer Res* (2008) **14**:4358–67. doi:10.1158/1078-0432.CCR-08-0288
9. Mandrekar SJ, Sargent DJ. Clinical trial designs for predictive biomarker validation: theoretical considerations and practical challenges. *J Clin Oncol* (2009) **27**:4027–34. doi:10.1200/JCO.2009.22.3701
10. Simon R, Polley E. Clinical trials for precision oncology using next generation sequencing. *Per Med* (2013) **10**:485–95. doi:10.2217/pme.13.36
11. Simon R. Using genomics in clinical trial design. *Clin Cancer Res* (2008) **14**:5984–93. doi:10.1158/1078-0432.CCR-07-4531
12. Freidlin B, Sun Z, Gray R, Korn EL. Phase III clinical trials that integrate treatment and biomarker evaluation. *J Clin Oncol* (2013) **31**:3158–61. doi:10.1200/JCO.2012.48.3826
13. Simon R, Wang SJ. Use of genomic signatures in therapeutics development. *Pharmacogenomcs J* (2006) **6**:1667–1173. doi:10.1038/sj.tpj.6500349
14. Wang SJ, O'Neill RT, Hung HM. Approaches to evaluation of treatment effect in randomized clinical trials with genomic subset. *Pharm Stat* (2007) **6**:227–44. doi:10.1002/pst.300
15. Freidlin B, McShane LM, Korn EL. Randomized clinical trials with biomarkers: design issues. *J Natl Cancer Inst* (2010) **102**:152–60. doi:10.1093/jnci/djp477
16. Mandrekar SJ, Sargent DJ. Predictive biomarker validation in practice: lessons from real trials. *Clin Trials* (2010) **7**:567–73. doi:10.1177/1740774510368574
17. Freidlin B, McShane LM, Polley MY, Korn EL. Randomized phase II trial designs with biomarkers. *J Clin Oncol* (2012) **28**:3304–9. doi:10.1200/JCO.2012.43.3946
18. Karuri SW, Simon R. A two-stage Bayesian design for co-development of new drugs and companion diagnostics. *Stat Med* (2012) **31**:901–14. doi:10.1002/sim.4462
19. Jiang W, Freidlin B, Simon R. Biomarker adaptive threshold design: a procedure for evaluating treatment with possible biomarker-defined subset effect. *J Natl Cancer Inst* (2007) **99**:1036–43. doi:10.1093/jnci/djm022
20. Simon N, Simon R. Adaptive enrichment designs in clinical trials. *Biostatistics* (2013) **14**:613–25. doi:10.1093/biostatistics/kxt010
21. Wang SJ, Hung HM, O'Neill RT. Adaptive patient enrichment designs in therapeutic trials. *Biom J* (2009) **51**:358–74. doi:10.1002/bimj.200900003
22. Follman D. Adaptively changing subgroup proportions in clinical trials. *Stat Sin* (1997) **7**:1085–102.
23. Rosenblum M, Van der Laan MJ. Optimizing randomized trial designs to distinguish which subpopulations benefit from treatment. *Biometrika* (2011) **98**:845–60. doi:10.1093/biomet/asr055
24. Freidlin B, Simon R. Adaptive signature design: an adaptive clinical trial design for generating and prospectively testing a gene expression signature for sensitive patients. *Clin Cancer Res* (2005) **11**:7872–8. doi:10.1158/1078-0432.CCR-05-0605
25. Wang SJ, Hung HM, O'Neill RT. Impacts on type I error rate with inappropriate use of learn and confirm in confirmatory adaptive design trials. *Biom J* (2010) **52**:798–810. doi:10.1002/bimj.200900207
26. Sher HI, Nasso NF, Rubin E, Simon R. Adaptive clinical trials for simultaneous testing of matched diagnostics and therapeutics. *Clin Cancer Res* (2011) **17**:6634–40. doi:10.1158/1078-0432.CCR-11-1105
27. Matsui S, Simon R, Qu P, Shaughnessy JD, Barlogie B, Crowley J. Developing and validating continuous genomic signatures in randomized clinical trials for predictive medicine. *Clin Cancer Res* (2012) **18**:6065–73. doi:10.1158/1078-0432.CCR-12-1206
28. Gu X, Yin G, Lee JJ. Bayesian two-step lasso strategy for biomarker selection in personalized medicine development for time to event endpoints. *Contemp Clin Trials* (2013) **36**:642–50. doi:10.1016/j.cct.2013.09.009
29. Freidlin B, Jiang W, Simon R. The cross-validated adaptive signature design for predictive analysis of clinical trials. *Clin Cancer Res* (2010) **16**:691–8. doi:10.1158/1078-0432.CCR-09-1357

6

Drug-diagnostics co-development in oncology: Part 2

Jan Trøst Jørgensen*

Dx-Rx Institute, Fredensborg, Denmark
**Correspondence: jan.trost@dx-rx.dk*

Edited and reviewed by:
Olivier Feron, Catholic University of Louvain, Belgium

Keywords: drug-diagnostic co-development, oncology, companion diagnostics, IHC, FISH, NGS, personalized medicine, precision medicine

The idea of combining drugs and diagnostics in oncology is not new. When the selective estrogen-receptor modulator tamoxifen was developed in the 1970s for the treatment of breast cancer, data on estrogen-receptor status were correlated with the treatment outcome. Based on a phase II study performed in patients with advanced breast cancer, published in 1976, the investigators concluded: "a high degree of correlation between response and positive estrogen-receptor assay suggests the value of the diagnostic test as a means to select patients for tamoxifen treatment" (1). Despite the fact that this conclusion was drawn nearly 40 years ago, the adaptation of the drug-diagnostic co-development model has been relatively slow and it is only within the last decade that it has gained widespread acceptance. The parallel development of the monoclonal antibody trastuzumab (Herceptin®, Roche/Genentech) and the companion diagnostics (CDx) assay for HER2 protein overexpression (HercepTest™, Dako) in the 1990s seems to have served as an inspiration to the pharma and biotech companies (2, 3), and the number of drug-diagnostic co-development projects within oncology has increased rapidly within the last decade.

Genomic sequencing has shown that marked heterogeneity exists in cancer, both between and within patients, which mean that "standard" treatments seldom work for everyone (4). The taxonomy of classifying the cancer diseases, according to their sites of origin and histology, also seems to be far from optimal when it comes to the treatment decision. The philosophy of "one-disease-one-target-one drug" is history and the improvement in cancer pharmacotherapy must come from an increased understanding of the underlying molecular mechanisms in the individual patient. These mechanisms are of a complex nature and we are far from a complete understanding. However, what we do understand is that drugs work at the molecular level, and it is here that we must seek the solution to a more rational drug development process and the subsequent treatment of the patients in the clinic (5). Molecular diagnostic testing has provided us with an increased understanding of the cancer biology, which has recently enabled the development of molecular-based targeted therapies such as vemurafenib (Zelboraf®, Roche/Genentech) for melanoma patients harboring a *BRAF* V600E mutation (6), and crizotinib (Xalkori®, Pfizer) and ceritinib (Zykadia®, Novartis), for non-small cell lung cancer (NSCLC) patients with *EML4–ALK* translocation (7, 8). For the latter two compounds, crizotinib and ceritinib, the development time has been remarkably short, which would never have happened without an in-depth molecular understanding of the disease biology and the mechanism of action of the drugs.

The present research topic of *Frontiers in Oncology* aims to provide an update on the wide-ranging area of drug-diagnostic co-development, biomarker research, and CDx. The research topic covers both basic scientific aspects as well as the clinical and regulatory challenges through a number of Review, Original Research, and Clinical Case Study articles. In the review by Olsen and Jørgensen, an introduction to the subject is given and here both the drug-diagnostic co-development model as well as the clinical and regulatory challenges related to CDx development is discussed (9).

The first CDx to obtain approval by the US Food and Drug Administration (FDA) was the assay for HER2 overexpression (HercepTest™, Dako) based on immunohistochemistry (IHC). IHC is a frequently applied method for protein expression analysis in tumor tissue, and despite the current great focus on gene-based assays, especially next-generation sequencing (NGS), this method is still recognized as an important supplement to analysis of different type of gene aberrations. Likewise, there seems to be cancer-related changes in the proteins that are not directly reflected in the changes in RNA and DNA. Gremel et al. review the currently applied CDx tests based on IHC but points also toward the future with regard to mutation-specific antibodies, *in situ* proximity legation assays, and alternative protein binders such as aptamers (10).

Several articles in this research topic touch upon NGS in relation to CDx, but Pant et al. provide the most comprehensive review (11). In this review, the authors exhaustively discuss the different platforms, sequencing technologies, bioinformatics, data reporting, regulatory aspects as well as the potential use of the technology in relation to drug-diagnostic co-development. There is very little doubt that, in the future, NGS will play a prominent role in the development of molecular-based targeted cancer drugs, however, there is still a number of technical, clinical, and regulatory challenges that needs to be overcome.

The review article by Nicolaides et al. suggests a different approach to drug-diagnostic co-development (12). Here, they discuss the use of co-developing diagnostic-targeting vectors to identify patients whose malignant tissue can specifically take up a targeted anti-cancer drug vector prior to treatment. Using this system, the patients can be predetermined in real-time as to whether or not their tumors can specifically take up a drug-linked diagnostic vector, thus inferring the uptake of a similar vector linked to an anti-cancer agent. According to the authors, this approach offers complementary opportunities to the rapid development of broad tumor-specific agents for use in personalized cancer medicine.

Biomarkers may not only serve as an important tool in relation to development of new molecular-based targeted cancer drugs through the drug-diagnostic co-development model but also for repurposing of existing chemotherapeutic anti-cancer drug. The review article by Stenvang et al. describes a strategy of biomarker-guided repurposing of chemotherapeutic drugs for cancer therapy with a specific focus on the topoisomerase I inhibitors and the use of Top1 as a potential predictive biomarker (13).

The recognition of heterogeneity of cancer diseases has called for a rethinking of the clinical trial designs used to demonstrate safety and efficacy of new targeted anti-cancer drugs. The efficacy of these drugs depends on a specific molecular aberration of the tumor that the drug-diagnostics co-development model tries to encounter. In the review by Simon, different clinical trial designs for the parallel development of drugs and diagnostics are discussed both with respect to the use of a single biomarker as well as a genome-wide discovery of a predictive classifier (14).

The development of crizotinib for treatment NSCLC patients with *ALK* rearrangement is definitively a landmark in relation to drug-diagnostic co-development in oncology. This *ALK* rearrangement was discovered in 2007 and already in 2011 crizotinib obtained US FDA approval together with the FISH assay for detection of this specific rearrangement (Vysis *ALK* Break Apart FISH Probe Kit, Abbott Molecular). In the Review/Opinion by Ou et al., the authors discuss the issue of whether the requirements by the US FDA for the simultaneous co-develop of a CDx will delay the approval of receptor tyrosine kinase (RTK) inhibitors for RTK-rearranged NSCLC (15).

Despite great progress in the treatment of cancer achieved with the use of molecular targeted therapy resistance seems to develop to virtually all of the drugs at some point in time. One way to suppress or delay development of resistance might be through the use of combination therapy. In the review article by Goltsov et al., a rational approach to a systematic development of combination therapies is suggested (16). Based on a joint systems analysis of cellular signaling network response and its sensitivity to drug action and oncogenic mutations, they describe an *in silico* method to analyze the targets of drug combinations.

Resistance is also the issue in the research article by Nielsen et al. where the authors look into the link between miR-21 expression and/or cellular localization and resistance to trastuzumab in HER2 positive patients with breast cancer (17). Tumors from 16 HER2 positive patients who underwent adjuvant treatment with trastuzumab were analyzed. Eight of these patients were considered resistant to the treatment. The result of this small study did not show a link between elevated miR-21 expression and resistance to adjuvant treatment with trastuzumab. However, more studies will be needed in order to prove or eliminate the role of miR-21.

In a clinical case study article by Russell et al., tumor profiling for two patients has been described (18). Both patients had advanced-stage cancer and failed standard treatment. The article describes how tumor profiling was used together with a systematic literature review (Caris Molecular Intelligence™) that was used to identify potential beneficial treatments for the patients resulting in disease remission in both cases.

The use of molecular diagnostics has given us new insight into the cancer disease biology, which has enabled development of new anti-cancer drugs with much more specific and well-defined mechanisms of action. When this knowledge is translated into the drug-diagnostic co-development model, remarkable results can be achieved. Crizotinib is one such example, and a similar or even more remarkable example is the recent development of ceritinib, another ALK inhibitor for NSCLC patients with *ALK* rearrangement. In the spring of 2014, ceritinib obtained an accelerated FDA approval based on efficacy data from only 163 metastatic NSCLC patients enrolled in a phase I single-arm, open-label clinical trial (19). Such a result is only achievable with the use of a CDx that enables pre-selection of the patients who are likely responders to the drug, which as for ceritinib resulted in a response rate above 50% even in a phase 1 trial. Despite the challenges that anti-cancer drug development faces, especially the development of resistance to the molecular targeted drugs, the drug-diagnostic co-development model has shown to be an invaluable tool in oncology, which definitively point to the future.

REFERENCES

1. Lerner HJ, Band PR, Israel L, Leung BS. Phase II study of tamoxifen: report of 74 patients with stage IV breast cancer. *Cancer Treat Rep* (1976) **60**:1431–5.
2. Slamon DJ, Leyland-Jones B, Shak S, Fuchs H, Paton V, Bajamonde A, et al. Use of chemotherapy plus a monoclonal antibody against HER2 for metastatic breast cancer that overexpresses HER2. *N Engl J Med* (2001) **344**:783–92. doi:10.1056/NEJM200103153441101
3. Jørgensen JT, Winther H. The development of the HercepTest – from bench to bedside. In: Jørgensen JT, Winther H, editors. *Molecular Diagnostics – The Key Driver of Personalized Cancer Medicine*. Singapore: Pan Stanford Publishing (2010). p. 43–60.
4. Gerlinger M, Rowan AJ, Horswell S, Larkin J, Endesfelder D, Gronroos E, et al. Intratumor heterogeneity and branched evolution revealed by multiregion sequencing. *N Engl J Med* (2012) **366**:883–92. doi:10.1056/NEJMoa1113205
5. Jørgensen JT. A changing drug development process in the era of personalized medicine. *Drug Discov Today* (2011) **16**:891–7. doi:10.1016/j.drudis.2011.09.010
6. Chapman PB, Hauschild A, Robert C, Haanen JB, Ascierto P, Larkin J, et al. Improved survival with vemurafenib in melanoma with BRAF V600E mutation. *N Engl J Med* (2011) **364**:2507–16. doi:10.1056/NEJMoa1103782
7. Kwak EL, Bang YJ, Camidge DR, Shaw AT, Solomon B, Maki RG, et al. Anaplastic lymphoma kinase inhibition in non-small-cell lung cancer. *N Engl J Med* (2010) **363**:1693–703. doi:10.1056/NEJMoa1006448
8. Shaw AT, Kim DW, Mehra R, Tan DS, Felip E, Chow LQ, et al. Ceritinib in ALK-rearranged non-small-cell lung cancer. *N Engl J Med* (2014) **370**:1189–97. doi:10.1056/NEJMoa1311107
9. Olsen D, Jørgensen JT. Companion diagnostics for targeted cancer drugs – clinical and regulatory aspects. *Front Oncol* (2014) **4**:105. doi:10.3389/fonc.2014.00105
10. Gremel G, Grannas K, Sutton LA, Pontén F, Zieba A. In situ protein detection for companion diagnostics. *Front Oncol* (2013) **3**:271. doi:10.3389/fonc.2013.00271
11. Pant S, Weiner R, Marton MJ. Navigating the rapids: the development of regulated next-generation sequencing-based clinical trial assays and companion diagnostics. *Front Oncol* (2014) **4**:78. doi:10.3389/fonc.2014.00078
12. Nicolaides NC, O'Shannessy DJ, Albone E, Grasso L. Co-development of diagnostic vectors to support targeted therapies and theranostics: essential tools in personalized cancer therapy. *Front Oncol* (2014) **4**:141. doi:10.3389/fonc.2014.00141
13. Stenvang J, Kümler I, Nygård SB, Smith DH, Nielsen D, Brünner N, et al. Biomarker-guided repurposing of chemotherapeutic drugs for cancer therapy: a novel strategy in drug development. *Front Oncol* (2013) **3**:313. doi:10.3389/fonc.2013.00313
14. Simon R. Drug-diagnostics co-development in oncology. *Front Oncol* (2013) **3**:315. doi:10.3389/fonc.2013.00315
15. Ou S-HI, Soo RA, Kubo A, Kawaguchi T, Ahn M-J. Will the requirement by the US FDA to simultaneously co-develop companion diagnostics (CDx) delay the approval of receptor tyrosine kinase inhibitors for RTK-rearranged

(ROS1-, RET-, AXL-, PDGFR-α-, NTRK1-) non-small cell lung cancer globally? *Front Oncol* (2014) **4**:58. doi:10.3389/fonc.2014.00058
16. Goltsov A, Langdon SP, Goltsov G, Harrison DJ, Bown J. Customizing the therapeutic response of signaling networks to promote antitumor responses by drug combinations. *Front Oncol* (2014) **4**:13. doi:10.3389/fonc.2014.00013
17. Nielsen BS, Balslev E, Poulsen TS, Nielsen D, Møller T, Mortensen CE, et al. miR-21 expression in cancer cells may not predict resistance to adjuvant trastuzumab in primary breast cancer. *Front Oncol* (2014) **4**:207. doi:10.3389/fonc.2014.00207
18. Russell K, Shunyakov L, Dicke KA, Maney T, Voss A. A practical approach to aid physician interpretation of clinically actionable predictive biomarker results in a multi-platform tumor profiling service. *Front Pharmacol* (2014) **5**:76. doi:10.3389/fphar.2014.00076
19. U S Food and Drug Administration. *Ceritinib.* (2014). Available from: http://www.fda.gov/drugs/informationondrugs/approveddrugs/ucm395386.htm

7

Companion diagnostics for targeted cancer drugs – clinical and regulatory aspects

Dana Olsen*[1] *and Jan Trøst Jørgensen*[2]

[1] Regulatory Affairs, Dako Denmark A/S, an Agilent Technologies Company, Glostrup, Denmark
[2] Dx-Rx Institute, Fredensborg, Denmark

Edited by:
Brian Gabrielli, The University of Queensland, Australia

Reviewed by:
Michelle M. Hill, The University of Queensland, Australia
Hu Liu, Anhui Medical University, China

****Correspondence:***
Jan Trøst Jørgensen, Dx-Rx Institute, Baunevaenget 76, Nodebo, Fredensborg DK-3480, Denmark
e-mail: jan.trost@dx-rx.dk

Companion diagnostics (CDx) holds the promise of improving the predictability of the oncology drug development process and become an important tool for the oncologist in relation to the choice of treatment for the individual patient. A number of drug–diagnostic co-development programs have already been completed successfully, and in the clinic, the use of several targeted cancer drugs is now guided by a CDx. This central role of the CDx assays has attracted the attention of the regulators, and especially the US Food and Drug Administration has been at the forefront in relation to developing regulatory strategies for CDx and the drug–diagnostic co-development project. For an increasing number of cancer patients the treatment selection will depend on the result generated by a CDx assay, and consequently this type of assay has become critical for the care and safety of the patients. In order to secure that the CDx assays have a high degree of analytical and clinical validity, they must undergo an extensive non-clinical and clinical testing before release for routine patient management. This review will give a brief introduction to some of the scientific and medical challenges related to the CDx development with specific emphasis on the regulatory requirements in different regions of the world.

Keywords: companion diagnostics, *in vitro* diagnostics, drug–diagnostic co-development, regulatory requirements, personalized medicine, precision medicine, oncology

INTRODUCTION

The understanding of the molecular mechanisms of cancer has increased considerably within the last 10–20 years, which has resulted in the development of a number of new targeted drugs. A large proportion of these drugs has been developed using the drug–diagnostic co-development model where the diagnostic test and the drug are developed in parallel (1, 2). The use of this model requires a thorough understanding of the underlying molecular pathology and the drug mechanisms of action, in order to link a certain molecular characteristic to the treatment outcome. The first attempt to use the drug–diagnostic co-development model was made when trastuzumab (Herceptin®, Roche/Genentech) and a immunohistochemistry (IHC) assay were developed for HER2 positive advanced breast cancer (3, 4). Since the approval of trastuzumab and the IHC assay for HER2 overexpression (HercepTest™, Dako) in 1998 by the US Food and Drug Administration (FDA), a number of new targeted cancer drugs guided by a diagnostic assay, a companion diagnostic (CDx) test, has been approved and introduced in the clinic to the benefit of the patients (5). The importance of incorporating a CDx in a drug research project has recently been emphasized by the fact that approximately two-thirds of the breakthrough therapy designations granted by the FDA include a diagnostic assay (6).

The main purpose of developing a CDx assay in most oncology drug research programs is to have a test that can predict whether a patient is likely to benefit from the drug in question. Hence, for many targeted cancer drugs the CDx assays will take up a central role as a kind of "decisive" stratification factor, both during development and subsequently after approval when the drug is used in the clinic. The assay will then become a kind of "gatekeeper" in relation to the treatment decision (2). However, if a CDx assay measures a specific biomarker or combination of biomarkers and it turns out that it is not sufficiently correlated with the clinical state, which could be overexpression of a specific protein or genetic mutations, it will not provide meaningful results. Such an erroneous test result could lead to either a false positive or false negative result, which potentially may cause risk and harm to the patient. For example, a false positive result could lead to treatment with a drug where the biological condition for a positive outcome is missing, and consequently the patient is put at risk due to potential toxic side effects from an ineffective treatment. Similarly, a false negative test result could withhold or delay a potentially beneficial treatment and thereby also bringing the patient at risk (7). In oncology, an early and correct diagnosis and intervention are two elements of key importance in the treatment of cancer patients. In case of a wrong treatment decision, the disease may become disseminated with no or very low chances of cure (2).

The central role of CDx assays in relation to both drug development and the clinical use after approval has caught the attention of the regulatory authorities. Especially the FDA has been at the forefront in relation to developing regulatory strategies for drug–diagnostic co-development and personalized medicine. As described above, it is important to avoid false positive and false negative test results and the analytical and clinical validity of any CDx assay must be sufficiently documented before it can be approved for routine use in the clinic (1, 7). In this article some of the scientific and medical challenges related to the CDx development are discussed with specific emphasis on the regulatory requirements.

COMPANION DIAGNOSTICS – TERMINOLOGY AND DEFINITIONS

With regards to the terminology and definitions of a diagnostic assay that is developed in parallel to a targeted drug and used to guide the treatment decision, there seems to be lack of consensus. Different names are used in the literature, such as pharmacodiagnostics, theranostics, pharmacogenomic biomarkers, and companion diagnostics. Within the last few years, the name companion diagnostics has been used more and more frequently and this is also the term that has been adapted by the FDA and now also the European Union (EU), however, theranostics is still used quite frequently especially in the academic literature (2). In 2011, the FDA issued a draft guidance on *In vitro Companion Diagnostics Devices* where a CDx was defined (8). According to this definition a CDx assay is an *in vitro* diagnostic device that provides information that is essential for the safe and effective use of a corresponding therapeutic product. Further, the FDA specifies three areas where a CDx assay is essential: (1) to identify patients who are most likely to benefit from a particular therapeutic product; (2) to identify patients likely to be at increased risk of serious adverse reactions as a result of treatment with a particular therapeutic product; and (3) to monitor response to treatment for the purpose of adjusting treatment (e.g., schedule, dose, discontinuation) to achieve improved safety or effectiveness. So according to the FDA, a CDx assay can be used both to predict outcome (efficacy and safety) and to monitor the response.

The definition that has been proposed by the EU is somewhat narrower and is more or less limited to item 1 in the FDA definition. According to the proposed regulation on *in vitro* diagnostic medical devices from 2012, a CDx is a device specifically intended to select patients with a previously diagnosed condition or predisposition as eligible for a targeted therapy (9). With no doubt the predictive or selective characteristics of a CDx assay has so far attracted the most attention. The use of a CDx assay facilitates the design of clinical trials with a smaller number of subjects, which has a positive effect on the resources and time spent on clinical development (2). A definition that focuses on the predictive or selective characteristics of the CDx assay and makes a link to "personalized medicine" is: "A pre-treatment test performed in order to determine whether or not a patient is likely to respond to a given therapy. This type of test is classified as a predictive or selective test and is a prerequisite for implementation of personalized and stratified medicine" (10).

DRUG–DIAGNOSTIC CO-DEVELOPMENT

In the drug–diagnostic co-development model there is interdependency of drug and diagnostics. The CDx assay is developed in parallel to the drug, as illustrated in **Figure 1**. The success of such a co-development project depends very much on the strength of the biomarker hypothesis, which is often deduced during the early research and preclinical phases of the drug development. As previously mentioned, it requires a thorough molecular understanding of both the pathology and drug mechanisms of action to come up with a solid hypothesis. It might not only be one hypothesis which is tested through prototype assays but several hypotheses. These prototype assays are subsequently used during the clinical phases I and II in order to give an idea of the predictive potential.

If one or more of these hypotheses appears promising the assay will then undergo analytical validation. However, before the analytical validation of the CDx assay can be finalized, the cut-off value must be established, which is usually done based on outcome data from phase I/II clinical trials. During the analytical validation, it must be demonstrated that the assay accurately and reliably measures the biomarker that has been selected earlier on in the development process. In relation to this validation, a number of both internal and external studies must be performed. For the external analytical validation a multi-site study is performed to document reproducibility using the final version of the CDx assay across several laboratories. Before using the CDx assay for patient selection and treatment stratification in a clinical phase III trial,

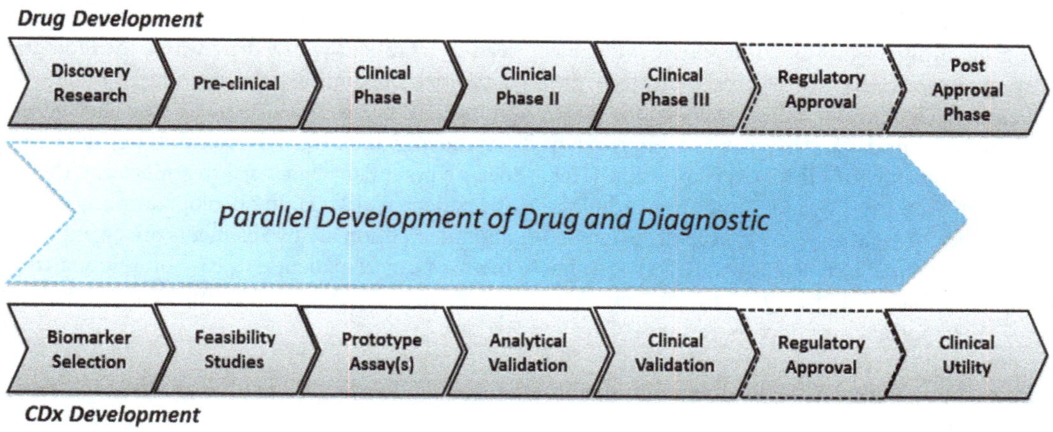

FIGURE 1 | The drug–diagnostic co-development model. The upper parts illustrate the drug development process and the lower parts the parallel CDx development process with an aligned regulatory co-approval at the end of phase III.

Table 1 | Overview of the main clinical trial designs that have been proposed for the parallel development of drugs and diagnostics. The last column in the table lists the diagnostic metrics that can be calculated based on the given clinical trial design. CDx+, test positive patients; CDx−, test negative patients; PPV, positive predictive value; NPV, negative predictive value.

Clinical trial design	Description	Diagnostic metrics
All-comers*	All patients meeting the study eligibility criteria are enrolled in the trial independent of the CDx test results	Sensitivity, specificity, PPV, and NPV
Enrichment	Only patients who are CDx+ and meet the study eligibility criteria are enrolled in the trial	PPV
Stratified	Both CDx+ and CDx− patients meeting the study eligibility criteria are enrolled in the trial and subsequently randomized	Sensitivity, specificity, PPV, and NPV

**Low prevalence of CDx+ patients requires a large sample size.*

it is strongly recommended that the assay is analytically validated (1, 7). Due to challenges with respect to the alignment and timing of the development of the drug and the CDx assay, it is sometimes tempting to start the clinical trial with a prototype assay and then replace it with the validated version later on during the trial. However, such a strategy is not recommendable as it makes it difficult to interpret the clinical trial results due to the fact that the patients have been selected using two different versions of the assay (7). If different versions of an assay have been used during clinical validation a subsequent bridging study will be needed, which is both resource demanding and time consuming. A "golden rule" with regards to the final clinical validation of a CDx is to use only one version of the assay, which is the analytically validated version, and only one testing laboratory in order to reduce possible site to site variation.

In the drug–diagnostic co-development model, phase III is not only used to demonstrate safety and efficacy of the drug, but also to clinically validate the CDx assay. Here, it must be demonstrated that the CDx assay has an ability to predict the treatment outcome in the individual patients (7). A CDx assay will only be useful if it provides information that can discriminate between patients who are likely responders and non-responders, and in this respect the clinical diagnostic accuracy of the assay is important, thus data on the clinical sensitivity, specificity, positive predictive value (PPV), and negative predictive value (NPV) for the CDx assay are important diagnostic metrics to consider. Several trial designs for clinical drug–diagnostic co-development have been proposed, however, not all of them make it possible to calculate the described diagnostic metrics. **Table 1** provides a brief overview of the main clinical trial designs that have been proposed for the parallel development of drug and diagnostic, however, in this article only the enrichment design will be discussed, as it is the design that so far has been used most frequently in relation to drug–diagnostic co-development. Furthermore, a relatively large number of review articles and draft guidance document have been published within the last few years describing these trial designs in more details (1, 2, 11–14).

The enrichment trial design is often used if there is clear evidence of a strong relationship between a positive CDx status and the treatment outcome with the targeted drug (e.g., from previous phase I/II studies) (1, 2). With this design, all the patients are tested by means of a CDx assay, but only the CDx positive patients are enrolled in the study and subsequently randomized to either the new targeted drug or to the standard treatment, as shown in **Figure 2**. The advantage of this design is that it generally requires a smaller number of patients to be randomized compared with the all-comers design, due to the fact that only patients who have a CDx positive status are enrolled in the trial, thus making the study population more homogeneous. However, this design allows only the PPV to be calculated and not sensitivity, specificity, and NPV, which is a limitation of this a trial design (1, 2). The enrichment design was also the one used when trastuzumab went through final phase III testing in women with advanced breast cancer in the 1990s (3). Further, looking at the drug–diagnostic combinations that have obtained FDA approval, the enrichment design is the most frequently used to demonstrate safety and efficacy of the drug and to clinically validate the corresponding CDx assay. Recent examples of targeted cancer drugs that have used this trial designs are vemurafenib (Zelboraf™, Roche/Genentech), crizotinib (Xalkori®, Pfizer), pertuzumab (Perjeta®, Roche/Genentech), ado-trastuzumab emtansine (Kadcyla®, Roche/Genentech), dabrafenib (Tafinlar®, GSK), and trametinib (Mekinist™, GSK). A list of the CDx assays and their corresponding therapeutic product that have been approved by the FDA can be found at the webpage of Center for Devices and Radiological Health (CDRH) (5).

How effective is the use of a CDx in the drug development process? This question was partly answered in an analysis made to estimate the risk of clinical trial failure during non-small cell lung cancer (NSCLC) drug development in the period between 1998 and 2012 (15). The data material was retrieved from different available public sources and 676 clinical trials with 199 unique drug compounds meeting the inclusion criteria of the analysis. The data showed that the success of clinical phase III was the biggest obstacle for drug approval with an overall success rate of only 28%. A small improvement in the success rate was found for the receptor targeted therapies tested in phase III. However, the absolutely highest success rate was observed when the drug was biomarker-guided showing a success rate of 62%, as seen in **Figure 3**. So, the conclusion from this analysis indicates that the use of a CDx assay during phase III drug development improves the success rate considerably. The data from this analysis also seem to confirm the effectiveness of the enrichment design described earlier in this paragraph.

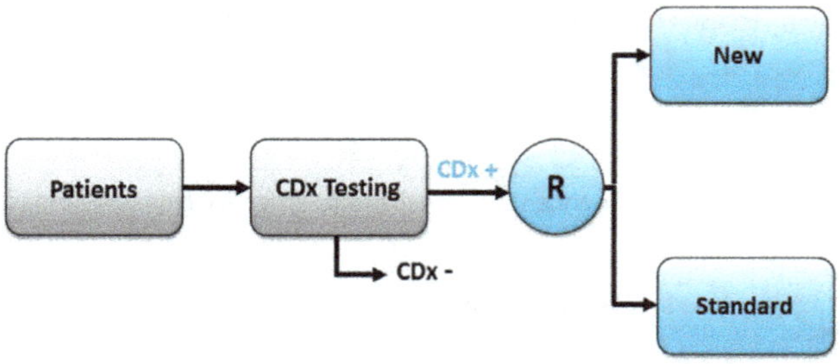

FIGURE 2 | The enrichment clinical trial design. With this design only patients who have a positive CDx assay result are enrolled in the trial and randomized (R) to either the new targeted treatment (New) or standard treatment (Standard). CDx+, indicates test positive patients; CDx−, indicates test negative patients.

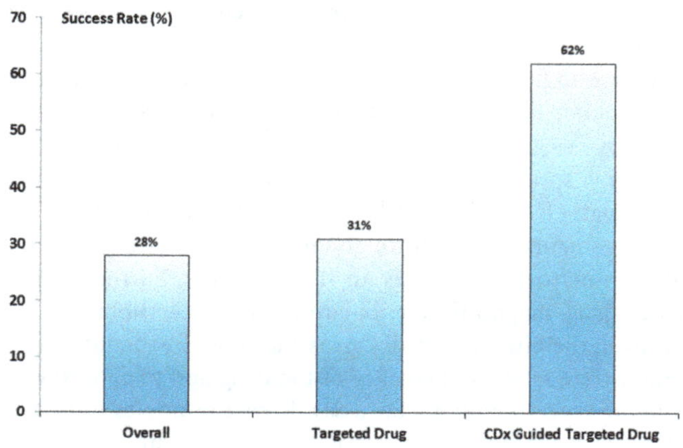

FIGURE 3 | Success rate for NSCLC drugs in phase III clinical trials. Based on the analysis of 676 clinical trials a success rate of 28% was found for all types of drugs, however, if the drug was either a receptor target drug or guided by a CDx assay the success rate increased to 31 and 62%, respectively (15).

COMPANION DIAGNOSTICS AND REGULATORY REQUIREMENTS

Recent developments in the field of personalized medicine and drug–diagnostic co-development have been most challenging, not only for the regulatory professionals but also for regulatory authorities. While drug companies and CDx manufacturers found new grounds in collaboration to jointly bring their products to patients, some regulatory authorities have been too slow to adapt to the changing regulatory landscape caused by the CDx development. A few highlights of the regulatory process for CDx in the major markets are presented and discussed below.

FDA SETTING THE STANDARD FOR REGULATORY PATHWAY OF COMPANION DIAGNOSTICS

In April 2005, the FDA published the Drug–Diagnostic Co-Development Concept Paper. This document labeled by the FDA "Draft Preliminary Concept Paper – Not for Implementation" has become a landmark for the formalization of the drug–diagnostic co-development strategy (1). Even though the pharma and diagnostic companies have seldom found the co-development model for parallel development of drug and diagnostic feasible, it provided grounds for alternative development strategies and for obtaining FDA feedback prior to initiating non-clinical or clinical testing, or prior to intended submission of a marketing application. Since 2005, the FDA has taken the lead and set the standard for the CDx regulatory pathway. This standard also provided inspiration to other authorities and regulatory professionals worldwide. The FDA further strengthened its leading position in defining the regulatory landscape for CDx by creating a personalized medicine group within the Office of *In vitro* Diagnostics and Radiological Health (OIR), formerly, Office of *In vitro* Diagnostics (OIVD) in 2009. This group has contributed to a considerable number of guidance documents related to CDx. Furthermore, FDA is providing transparency of the approval process by including web availability of Safety and Effectiveness Summary documents for the approved CDx.

While waiting for an update of the 2005 concept paper, a draft of the *In vitro* Companion Diagnostic Devices guidance was published in July 2011 (8). This guidance document is not a replacement of the 2005 concept paper, but rather an operational guide for *In vitro* Diagnostics (IVD) of the pharma and biotech industries indicating possible regulatory pathways as well as labeling and regulatory requirements for CDx devices and therapeutic products (5).

Attention should be paid to an important section of the guidance covering the investigational use of CDx. Before the "companion diagnostics era," many of the investigational IVD devices were either exempted from Investigational Device Exemption (IDE) regulations or classified as non-significant risk devices subject to abbreviated IDE requirements. In the case of clinical trials, where companion diagnostics are used to make a medical decision – such as treatment assignment, an IVD is considered a serious risk device requiring IDE approval by the FDA. Typically, a pharma or a biotech company is the sponsor of a drug–diagnostic clinical trial conducted under the Investigational New Drug (IND) regulations. However, it is important that an IDE for the diagnostic is either included in the IND or submitted and approved separately. According to the guidance document, FDA accepts that the IDE information is included in the IND. However, as the IDE format is not compatible with an IND, in some cases, the FDA has expressed that a separate IDE is preferred (16). Hopefully, this will be further clarified in the final version of the guidance, which is expected by October 2014 (17). The content of an IDE is well-defined in the regulations and further specified on the FDA website and in several guidance documents (18). In the case of a combined drug–diagnostic clinical trial, the IDE must, in addition to information on the CDx assay, also include information provided by the drug sponsor, such as the clinical trial protocol, investigational sites, Investigational Review Board (IRB) information, and informed consent material for patients. Thus, in relation to collaboration between a drug company and a diagnostic company, it is important that roles, responsibilities, and timelines are clearly defined between the parties.

In the 2011 guidance document, the FDA declares that "the FDA review of the test/therapeutic product pair will be carried out collaboratively among relevant FDA offices." Truly, FDA offices responsible for each of the products are not only collaborating in the review process but are also announcing approvals of both the drug and CDx concurrently.

Another important guidance, not only for CDx, is the Medical Devices: the Pre-Submission Program and Meetings with FDA Staff published in draft in July 2012. Final version of the guidance was published in February 2014 (19). In this document, the Pre-IDE program was renamed to a Pre-Submission (Pre-Sub) program (19). Since 1995, the Pre-IDE, now Pre-Sub, program, has allowed industry to obtain FDA feedback prior to any kind of device submission and thus providing opportunities for the industry to discuss a drug–diagnostic co-development strategy at any development or testing stage. Even though there is no user fee for a Pre-Sub, the process has become more formalized since authorization of the Medical Device User Fee and Modernization Act (MDUFMA) in 2012 (20). In the new guidance, the FDA provides recommendations to the contents of the Pre-Sub and also clarifies the administrative procedures of the program. The Pre-Sub is a formal, written request for feedback from the FDA regarding analytical or clinical study protocols or a proposed regulatory pathway. A Pre-Sub may also be an appropriate way to acquaint the FDA with a novel technology or design. A Pre-Sub interaction with the FDA is a particularly useful way to discuss testing strategies which are not the ideal co-development scenarios, and where an analytically validated assay is not available at an early stage of the clinical drug development. The benefits of Pre-Subs may include time and cost reduction of research or clinical studies, better understanding of FDA expectations and trends, especially in the area where no guidance documents are available, and, most importantly, may result in a better and more complete marketing application and greater chance of a successful approval. In order to improve the understanding of IVD related issues, it is recommended that the drug sponsor participates in the Pre-Sub process initiated by the diagnostic company. If relevant, CDRH will request Center for Drug Evaluation and Research (CDER) attendance in the process. According to the FDA statistics, the inter-center consultations have increased from 39 in 2010 to 106 in 2012 (16), which is a likely consequence of the increased number of drug–diagnostic co-development projects mainly within oncology.

The controls required by the FDA prior to marketing of a device in the US depend on the classification of the device. Medical devices, including IVDs, are risk-classified as class I, II, or III. The majority of companion diagnostic IVDs are high risk class III devices. This review will not go into details of the regulatory requirements for each product class, but only give a very brief summary. For class I devices, general controls, like establishment registration and device listing, apply; for class II devices, general controls and a premarket clearance [510(k)] is needed; and class III devices require the most stringent approval for medical devices by the FDA, a Premarket Approval Application (PMA) (21).

Briefly, a PMA application may be either traditional or modular. There is no difference in the contents of a traditional or a modular PMA but there is a difference in the way the PMA is submitted for FDA review. In a traditional PMA, all information required by the regulations is submitted at the same time, while for a modular PMA the information is submitted in modules. Thus, analytical performance (non-clinical studies) and manufacturing information may be submitted and reviewed by the FDA while a clinical trial is ongoing. When the clinical trial is completed, the data will then be submitted to the FDA. At this point of time, the other modules have been through FDA review. This approach may allow for a shorter approval process and a better alignment with the drug approval.

A modification in an intended use for a PMA-approved CDx, such as adding a new indication or a new targeted drug, is a complex process which, depending on the type of modification, may require massive analytical and/or clinical data. The FDA is very responsive to Pre-Subs for device modifications and provides feedback to proposed regulatory pathways and studies supporting regulatory submission for the change in the intended use of the specific CDx.

EUROPE TIGHTENS UP THE IVD LEGISLATION

The IVD Directive 98/79/EC regulates *in vitro* diagnostic medical devices in the EU, EU candidate countries, and associated countries (22). The current EU regulatory framework for IVD devices demonstrates how unnoticed CDx IVD devices were at the end of the nineties when the IVD Directive was proposed and subsequently entered into force in 2003. There is no specific mention of CDx in the definition of an IVD, and the classification system of the directive does not consider CDx at all. Also, the IVD Directive list-based classification system has shown its limitations, as only a limited number of IVD devices are considered medium or high risk devices (so-called Annex II devices). All remaining IVDs, including CDx assays, are classified as low risk devices. Adding a new device to the Annex II list has proved to be a cumbersome process. It has taken 4 years to add a variant Creutzfeldt–Jakob disease assay to List A of Annex II, which the United Kingdom requested in 2007, and the decision from the EU Commission came only in 2011 (23).

Briefly, IVD devices placed in the EU market require a CE-mark to indicate conformity with the IVD Directive. For the high risk products listed in Annex II, the involvement of a Notified Body (NB) is required to assess conformity to the IVD Directive before placing the device in the European market. An NB is an organization accredited by a member state to assess the manufacturer's conformity to the essential requirements of the directive.

Currently, any CDx assay entering the EU market is classified as low risk device based on a conformity assessment and CE-marking by the manufacturer, the so-called self-certification procedure. This results in incomprehensible differences in the regulatory pathway to the market between the USA (PMA approval) and the EU (self-certification).

However, there are major changes under way in EU IVD medical device legislation, which will impact CDx assays entering the market. The IVD Directive will be replaced by a Regulation on IVD (9). A regulation is the most powerful, single regulatory framework, which is applicable in a uniform manner at the same time for all EU member states, which leaves no room for divergent transpositions.

A draft of the new IVD Regulation (IVDR) has already been proposed, and obviously, we will be facing a very different regulatory landscape in the EU in the years to come (9). In the classification system proposed in the IVDR, IVDs will be assigned to four classification groups A, B, C, and D, depending on device risk, with class A being the lowest risk class. The four-class system resembles what we already know from the Canadian and Australian regulations, and is similar, but not equal, to what has been proposed by a Global Harmonization Task Force (24). CDx assays will be Class C devices and will require a complex regulatory pathway including a requirement for a Design Examination Certification by an NB. The review by the NB may possibly also be linked to a consultation with the European Medicines Agency (EMA) or, alternatively, compliance to a Common Technical Specifications (CTS) will be required. The CTS for new devices will be drafted as part of the review process. No matter which of the proposed pathways (EMA consultation or CTS) becomes final, the time to the market for a CDx assay will be extended essentially. It is assumed that the proposed IVDR will pass through the Council and Parliament in 2014, and the Regulation will then enter into force in 2017, after a 3-year implementation period.

JAPAN EXPECTED TO MIRROR FDA REVIEW AND APPROVAL PROCESS

In Japan CDx assays are classified as high risk devices (class III), however, the regulatory approval process has until now been disconnected from the approval of the related therapeutic products. In October 2011, the Japan Association of Clinical Reagent Industries (JACRI) addressed the Ministry of Health, Labour and Welfare (MHLW) and the Pharmaceuticals and Medical Devices Agency (PMDA) with a proposal for a regulatory pathway for companion diagnostics (25). At the end of December 2013, the final guidance for CDx and related drugs was announced in the PMDA Notification. The guidance includes a CDx device definition, guidance for application for CDx and therapeutic products, clinical studies of therapeutic products as well as a review system by PMDA. In the original proposal presented to the MHLW/PMDA, JACRI has taken into consideration the FDA draft guidance on *In vitro* Companion Diagnostic Devices that was issued in July 2011 (8). Thus, the final PMDA guidance stresses that application for both a CDx and its corresponding therapeutic product should be submitted and reviewed at the same time under PMDA. Furthermore, it is recommended that drug and diagnostic sponsors seek early consultation with the authorities on the regulatory pathway for CDx, similar to the FDA Pre-Sub program. It is expected that publication of the guidance will improve the review process for companion diagnostics IVDs in Japan and make it more transparent. There is no English version of the guidance available at the moment on the PMDA website (26).

CHINA REGULATORY PATHWAY IS A CHALLENGE

Requirements for registration of IVD devices in China exceed requirements in any of the other countries and regions described above. Here, CDx assays are as in the US and Japan, classified as high risk devices (class III products). So far, there have been no guidance documents issued for CDx assays, but the registration process follows the requirements for class III products and requires extensive documentation and supporting testing data to be submitted to the China Food and Drug Administration. Specific for a class III IVD device in China, there is a requirement for local testing of at least 1000 patient specimens divided among three geographically distinct hospitals. This testing must be performed using three consecutive lots of the device and further detailed lot records, including specific requirements for stability testing and analytical performance testing must be provided. In addition, a number of legal documents are required to be submitted such as legal qualification of the manufacturer and authorization letters for authorized representatives.

CONCLUSION AND FUTURE CONSIDERATIONS

Companion diagnostics holds the promise of improving the predictability of the oncology drug development process and become an important tool for the oncologist in relation to the choice of treatment for the individual patient. A number of drug–diagnostic co-development projects have already been completed successfully, and in the clinic, the use of several targeted cancer drugs are now guided by a CDx. For these drugs the management of the patient partly depends on the result generated by the CDx assay, and consequently this type of assay has become critical for the patient care. In order to avoid "false positive" and "false negative" test results, it must be documented for any CDx assay that it has a high degree of analytical and clinical validity (7). To some extent this is comparable to the safety and efficacy documentation that needs to be generated in order to achieve a marketing authorization for a new drug (27).

The central role of the CDx assays in relation to the current and future pharmacotherapy has attracted the attention of the regulators, especially the US FDA. In the US, CDx assays are in most cases classified as class III, high risk devices, for which the most stringent requirement for safety and effectiveness documentation apply, including submission of a PMA. Knowing the critical role of a CDx assay in relation to patient management this seems only reasonable that a number of other countries including Australia, Canada, China, and Japan have followed suit with regards to stringent requirements. However, for the EU, it has taken some time to realize the critical importance of CDx assays in relation to patient care and safety, and only recently the discussions about a more up to date regulation for IVD medical devices including CDx assay has started. Despite the coming new legislation in the EU not seeming to have the same formalized co-development and co-approval process as in the US, it will most likely increase the patient safety.

Many of the biological characteristics important for a specific drug to be effective, such as mutations, gene rearrangements, gene amplifications, and protein overexpression are typically not present in one cancer type alone, but are often found across several cancer diseases. *HER2* amplification and protein overexpression are such examples, where these characteristics are found in breast and gastric cancer as well as others cancers. Further, it has also been shown that an HER2 targeted drug like trastuzumab is effective in both breast and gastric cancer (3, 28). This and other examples have shown what matters most in relation to determining the response to a specific drug is the molecular pathways driving the growth of the cancer and not from where in the body the tumor originates. Based on this knowledge, we will probably see drug–diagnostic combination being developed for several cancer diseases simultaneously in the future, which will be both scientifically and medically challenging. How the drug regulatory system, such as the FDA, will handle this challenge will also be interesting to see, as both drugs and CDxs have been approved for one cancer disease at a time up to now.

Most of the CDx guided targeted cancer drugs that have been introduced within the last few years have shown significantly high response rates and prolonged progression free survival in specific selected groups of patients. Previously, for many of the treated patients no treatment has been available for their specific disease, and CDx guided drugs definitively represent a real progress within oncology. However, for all these drugs, resistance will develop at some point in time resulting in disease progression. For this reason it is unlikely that "monotherapy" with a targeted cancer drug based on identification of a single biomarker will achieve long-lasting remission, and we will probably need to move away from the "one biomarker one drug" model toward a more multimodal approach (29). This new model will need to integrate multiple biomarkers and multiple targeted cancer drugs and should be based on a simultaneous use of several drugs in order to block more signal pathways, thus to prevent resistance to develop. When it comes to CDx assays, this will make a call on specifically designed multiplex assays most likely based on technologies such as gene expression arrays or next generation sequencing (NGS) (30). Despite the very recent decision by the FDA to grant marketing authorization for the Illumina instrument platform for screening and diagnosis of cystic fibrosis, there still seems to be a number of challenges that must be overcome before we see NGS as CDx for targeted cancer drugs (31, 32). However, the advantages of this type of technology are that they will enable researchers and healthcare professionals to get a broader look at the cancer patients' genetic makeup and probably help them designing more effective treatment modalities. Several CDx possibilities seem to be available to improve the treatment of the cancer patients, however, the development of assays will face a challenging time both with respect to medical/scientific as well as regulatory aspects.

REFERENCES

1. US Food and Drug Administration. *Drug-Diagnostic Co-Development Concept Paper.* Food and Drug Administration (2005). Available from: http://www.fda.gov/downloads/Drugs/ScienceResearch/ResearchAreas/Pharmacogenetics/UCM116689.pdf
2. Jørgensen JT. Companion diagnostics in oncology – current status and future aspects. *Oncology* (2013) **85**:59–68. doi:10.1159/000353454
3. Slamon DJ, Leyland-Jones B, Shak S, Fuchs H, Paton V, Bajamonde A, et al. Use of chemotherapy plus a monoclonal antibody against HER2 for metastatic breast cancer that overexpresses HER2. *N Engl J Med* (2001) **344**:783–92. doi:10.1056/NEJM200103153441101
4. Jørgensen JT, Winther H. The development of the HercepTest – from bench to bedside. In: Jørgensen JT, Winther H, editors. *Molecular Diagnostics – The Key Driver of Personalized Cancer Medicine.* Singapore: Pan Stanford Publishing (2010). p. 43–60.
5. US Food and Drug Administration. *Companion Diagnostic Devices: In vitro and Imaging Tools* (2013). Available from: http://www.fda.gov/MedicalDevices/ProductsandMedicalProcedures/InVitroDiagnostics/ucm301431.htm
6. Varond AJ. *Trends in Personalized Medicine.* Regulatory Focus (2013). Available from: http://www.raps.org/focus-online/news/news-article-view/article/4244/trends-in-personalized-medicine.aspx
7. US Food and Drug Administration. *Paving the Way for Personalized Medicine: FDA's Role in a New Era of Medical Product Development* (2013). Available from: http://www.fda.gov/downloads/ScienceResearch/SpecialTopics/PersonalizedMedicine/UCM372421.pdf
8. US Food and Drug Administration. *Draft Guidance for Industry and Food and Drug Administration Staff – In vitro Companion Diagnostic Devices* (2011). Available from: http://www.fda.gov/MedicalDevices/deviceregulationandguidance/guidancedocuments/default.htm
9. *Proposal for a Regulation of the European Parliament and of the Council on In vitro Diagnostic Medical Devices* (2012). Available from: http://eur-lex.europa.eu/LexUriServ/LexUriServ.do?uri=COM:2012:0541:FIN:EN:PDF
10. Jørgensen JT. Companion diagnostics and the drug-diagnostic co-development model. *Drug Dev Res* (2012) **73**:390–7. doi:10.1002/ddr.21029
11. Simon R. Clinical trial designs for evaluating the medical utility of prognostic and predictive biomarkers in oncology. *Per Med* (2010) **7**:33–47. doi:10.2217/pme.09.49
12. Winther H, Jørgensen JT. Drug-diagnostic co-development in cancer. *Pharm Med* (2010) **24**:363–75. doi:10.1007/BF03256837
13. Fridlyand J, Simon RM, Walrath JC, Roach N, Buller R, Schenkein DP, et al. Considerations for the successful co-development of targeted cancer therapies and companion diagnostics. *Nat Rev Drug Discov* (2013) **12**:743–55. doi:10.1038/nrd4101
14. US Food and Drug Administration. *Guidance for Industry: Enrichment Strategies for Clinical Trials to Support Approval of Human Drugs and Biological Products* (2012). Available from: http://www.fda.gov/downloads/Drugs/GuidanceComplianceRegulatoryInformation/Guidances/UCM332181.pdf
15. Falconi A, Lopes G, Parker JL. Clinical trial risk reduction in non-small cell lung cancer though the use of biomarkers and receptor-targeted therapies. *J Clin Oncol* (2013) **31**:8040. doi:10.1097/JTO.0000000000000075
16. Mansfield E. Personalized medicine: then, now, and future. *Presentation at the AMDM Meeting.* Bethesda, MD (2013).
17. US Food and Drug Administration. *CDRH Fiscal Year 2014 (FY 2014) Proposed Guidance Development* (2014). Available from: http://www.fda.gov/MedicalDevices/DeviceRegulationandGuidance/Overview/MDUFAIII/ucm321367.htm
18. US Food and Drug Administration. *21 Code of Federal Regulations, Part 812* (2013). Available from: http://www.accessdata.fda.gov/scripts/cdrh/cfdocs/cfcfr/CFRSearch.cfm?CFRPart=812
19. US Food and Drug Administration. *Requests for Feedback on Medical Device Submissions: The Pre-Submission Program and Meetings with Food and Drug Administration Staff* (2014). Available from: http://www.fda.gov/downloads/medicaldevices/deviceregulationandguidance/guidancedocuments/ucm311176.pdf
20. US Food and Drug Administration. *Medical Device User Fee Amendments 2012 (MDUFA III)* (2013). Available from: http://www.fda.gov/MedicalDevices/DeviceRegulationandGuidance/Overview/MDUFAIII/default.htm
21. US Food and Drug Administration. *21 Code of Federal Regulations, Part 814* (2013). Available from: http://www.accessdata.fda.gov/scripts/cdrh/cfdocs/cfcfr/CFRSearch.cfm?CFRPart=814
22. *Directive 98/79/EC of the European Parliament and of the Council of 27 October 1998 on In vitro Diagnostic Medical Devices.* Available from: http://eur-lex.europa.eu/LexUriServ/LexUriServ.do?uri=OJ:L:1998:331:0001:0037:EN:PDF
23. *European Commission – Enterprise and Industry* (2013). Available from: http://ec.europa.eu/enterprise/index_en.htm
24. Global Harmonization Task Force. *Principles of In vitro Diagnostic (IVD) Medical Devices Classification, GHTH/SG1/N045:2008* (2008). Available from: http://www.imdrf.org/index.asp
25. *Proposal on Maintaining Infrastructure of Companion Diagnostic Agents to Promote Personalized Medicine.* Japan Association of Clinical Reagents Industries (JACRI) (2011). Available from: http://www.jacr.or.jp/english/news.html
26. PMDA. *Pharmaceuticals and Medical Devices Agency, Japan* (2014). Available from: http://www.pmda.go.jp/english/index.html
27. Hayes DF, Allen J, Compton C, Gustavsen G, Leonard DG, McCormack R, et al. Breaking a vicious cycle. *Sci Transl Med* (2013) **5**:196cm6. doi:10.1126/scitranslmed.3005950
28. Bang YJ, Van Cutsem E, Feyereislova A, Chung HC, Shen L, Sawaki A, et al. Trastuzumab in combination with chemotherapy versus chemotherapy alone for treatment of HER2-positive advanced gastric or gastro-oesophageal junction cancer (ToGA): a phase 3, open-label, randomised controlled trial. *Lancet* (2010) **376**:687–97. doi:10.1016/S0140-6736(10)61121-X
29. Weinstein IB, Joe A. Oncogene addiction. *Cancer Res* (2008) **68**:3077–80. doi:10.1158/0008-5472.CAN-07-3293

30. Jørgensen JT. A changing landscape for companion diagnostics. *Expert Rev Mol Diagn* (2013) **13**:667–9. doi:10.1586/14737159.2013.834799
31. US Food and Drug Administration. *FDA Allows Marketing of Four "Next Generation" Gene Sequencing Devices* (2013). Available from: http://www.fda.gov/newsevents/newsroom/pressannouncements/ucm375742.htm
32. Collins FS, Hamburg MA. First FDA authorization for next-generation sequencer. *N Engl J Med* (2013) **369**:2369–71. doi:10.1056/NEJMp1314561

Multidrug resistance in fungi: regulation of transporter-encoding gene expression

Sanjoy Paul and W. Scott Moye-Rowley*

Department of Molecular Physiology and Biophysics, Carver College of Medicine, University of Iowa, Iowa City, IA, USA

Edited by:
Isabel Sá-Correia, Instituto Superior Técnico, Portugal

Reviewed by:
Miguel Cacho Teixeira, Technical University of Lisbon, Portugal
Frederic Devaux, Universite Pierre et Marie Curie, France

***Correspondence:**
W. Scott Moye-Rowley, Department of Molecular Physiology and Biophysics, Carver College of Medicine, University of Iowa, 6-530 Bowen Science Building, Iowa City, IA 52242, USA
e-mail: scott-moye-rowley@uiowa.edu

A critical risk to the continued success of antifungal chemotherapy is the acquisition of resistance; a risk exacerbated by the few classes of effective antifungal drugs. Predictably, as the use of these drugs increases in the clinic, more resistant organisms can be isolated from patients. A particularly problematic form of drug resistance that routinely emerges in the major fungal pathogens is known as multidrug resistance. Multidrug resistance refers to the simultaneous acquisition of tolerance to a range of drugs via a limited or even single genetic change. This review will focus on recent progress in understanding pathways of multidrug resistance in fungi including those of most medical relevance. Analyses of multidrug resistance in *Saccharomyces cerevisiae* have provided the most detailed outline of multidrug resistance in a eukaryotic microorganism. Multidrug resistant isolates of *S. cerevisiae* typically result from changes in the activity of a pair of related transcription factors that in turn elicit overproduction of several target genes. Chief among these is the ATP-binding cassette (ABC)-encoding gene PDR5. Interestingly, in the medically important *Candida* species, very similar pathways are involved in acquisition of multidrug resistance. In both *C. albicans* and *C. glabrata*, changes in the activity of transcriptional activator proteins elicits overproduction of a protein closely related to *S. cerevisiae* Pdr5 called Cdr1. The major filamentous fungal pathogen, *Aspergillus fumigatus*, was previously thought to acquire resistance to azole compounds (the principal antifungal drug class) via alterations in the azole drug target-encoding gene *cyp51A*. More recent data indicate that pathways in addition to changes in the *cyp51A* gene are important determinants in *A. fumigatus* azole resistance. We will discuss findings that suggest azole resistance in *A. fumigatus* and *Candida* species may share more mechanistic similarities than previously thought.

Keywords: multidrug resistance, transcription, fungal pathogens, ABC transporters, transcription factors, regulation of gene expression

INTRODUCTION

Scientifically, one of the most attractive features of the fungal microorganisms is their striking biological similarity with mammalian cells. This similarity has led to their extensive use as models for basic properties of eukaryotic cells but also illustrates one of the important challenges in dealing with fungal pathogens. Development of antifungal drugs has been slowed by the close relationship between the fundamental cell biology of a fungus and a typical mammalian cell. Early antifungal drugs like amphotericin B were efficacious in treating fungal infections but suffer from high toxicity to the patient (Moen et al., 2009).

More recently developed drugs like the azoles and echinocandins, exhibit better specificity for pathogens but their very success has led to the selection of fungi that are highly tolerant of these antifungal agents (recently discussed in Brown et al., 2012). Azole drugs are the primary antifungal drug used in the clinic and infections associated with azole resistant fungi have dramatically lowered survival rates compared to those associated with azole susceptible organisms (reviewed in Pfaller, 2012). Resistance to azole drugs emerges by two different routes: direct and indirect mechanisms. Direct changes involve changes in the enzyme that is targeted by azole compounds, lanosterol 14α demethylase (See Kristan and Rizner, 2012 for a recent review). This enzyme is encoded by the *ERG11* gene in *Saccharomyces cerevisiae* with azole resistant alleles found to either change the sequence of the protein and/or alter expression levels of this gene product. While these direct changes can be found in *S. cerevisiae* and pathogenic yeast, a common form of azole resistance arises via indirect means. Most typically, selection for azole resistant yeast elicits isolation of strains that overproduce ATP-binding cassette (ABC) transporter proteins. These ABC transporter proteins act to efflux azole drugs from the cell and prevent accumulation of otherwise toxic levels (recently reviewed in Prasad and Goffeau, 2012).

ABC transporter overproduction is a well-known cause of drug resistance in mammalian cells (See Holohan et al., 2013 for a recent discussion). Cancer patients undergoing chemotherapeutic treatment are often found to eventually develop tumors that are termed multidrug resistant. These *in vivo* selected tumors are refractory to growth inhibition caused by a wide range of different chemotherapeutics, even drugs to which the patient was not previously exposed (Szakacs et al., 2006). Multidrug resistant tumors can be associated with gene amplification events that lead to an increase in copy number of genes encoding ABC transporters with a concomitant elevation in protein level (Ambudkar et al., 2003).

In fungal cells, multidrug resistant cells can easily be selected. These mutant strains do not usually have increased gene dosage but rather possess increased expression of ABC transporter-encoding genes (reviewed in Sanglard et al., 2009; Morschhauser, 2010). Elevated gene expression leads to an increase in the protein level of these membrane transporters with accompanying broad range drug tolerance. In every fungus that has been studied, ABC transporters are able to influence azole resistance making this a key issue in treatment of fungal infections.

Given the importance of the level of ABC transporter gene expression in development of azole resistance, their regulation has been the focus of extensive investigation. These studies have led to the identification of dedicated transcription factors dedicated to coordination of their expression with other genes in fungi. Our most detailed picture of the network of transcriptional regulation and multidrug resistance gene is available for the yeast *Saccharomyces cerevisiae*. This network has served as a starting point for the analysis of similar systems in pathogenic fungi and will be discussed below.

TRANSCRIPTIONAL CIRCUITRY CONTROLLING PLEIOTROPIC DRUG RESISTANCE IN *S. CEREVISIAE*

Zn_2Cys_6 ZINC CLUSTER-CONTAINING FACTORS

The first transcription factor discovered to be a determinant of multidrug resistance in *S. cerevisiae* was appropriately designated Pdr1 (Saunders and Rank, 1982). Early genetic work pointed to the existence of dominant alleles of the *PDR1* gene as conferring resistance to a wide range of different toxic compounds (Rank and Bech-Hansen, 1973; Rank et al., 1975, 1976). This broad range resistance phenotype in *S. cerevisiae* was designated pleiotropic drug resistance (Pdr) and is functionally analogous to the multidrug resistance seen in mammalian cells and other fungi. This early work has been the subject of several reviews (Balzi and Goffeau, 1995; Bauer et al., 1999; Gulshan and Moye-Rowley, 2007) and will only be outlined here.

Isolation of the cloned *PDR1* gene by Balzi et al. (1987) led to rapid advances in understanding of the molecular basis of the Pdr phenotype in *S. cerevisiae*. The DNA sequence of *PDR1* led to two important findings. First, this gene encoded a Zn_2Cys_6 cluster-containing transcription factor similar to the previously described Gal4 (Johnston, 1987). Second, sequence of a dominant, multidrug resistant allele of *PDR1* demonstrated that this hypermorphic or gain-of-function (GOF) behavior of Pdr1 was caused by a single amino acid substitution mutation in the central region of the protein. Many different amino acid substitution mutations were eventually discovered that caused Pdr1 to exhibit elevated, constitutive transcriptional activation of target gene expression (Carvajal et al., 1997).

The discovery that Pdr1 was a transcriptional regulator led to work from multiple laboratories to identify genes that were more directly responsible for the observed multidrug resistance phenotype. The first major class of Pdr1 target genes contained several different loci encoding ABC transporter proteins (Balzi et al., 1994; Bissinger and Kuchler, 1994; Hirata et al., 1994a; Katzmann et al., 1995; Mahe et al., 1996). These proteins were typically found in the plasma membrane and thought to act as broad specificity, drug efflux pumps as previously seen in mammalian tumor cells (Gottesman et al., 1995). The *PDR5* locus was found to possess unique central importance among the ABC transporter-encoding genes as the expression level of this gene is the highest of the drug resistance-related ABC transporters and mutants lacking this gene exhibit profound drug hypersensitivities (Leppert et al., 1990; Decottignies et al., 1994). *PDR5* transcription was strongly elevated in cells containing hyperactive *PDR1* dominant alleles through the binding of the transcriptional regulatory protein to three sites in the promoter region (Katzmann et al., 1996). These sites are referred to as Pleiotropic Drug Response Elements or PDREs and have been found upstream of the majority of Pdr1-regulated genes.

A factor closely related to Pdr1 was discovered during genome sequencing experiments and designated *PDR3* (Delaveau et al., 1994). GOF *PDR3* alleles similar to those described for *PDR1* were isolated and elevated *PDR5* transcription and drug resistance found to occur in these strains (Dexter et al., 1994; Nourani et al., 1997; Simonics et al., 2000). Generally speaking, the phenotypic effects of activated alleles of *PDR1* and *PDR3* are very similar. However, a feature unique to the *PDR3* gene was the presence of two PDREs in its promoter (Delahodde et al., 1995). This autoregulatory input was found to be essential for normal function of *PDR3* and is a key component for the regulated expression of this gene (Delahodde et al., 1995; Zhang and Moye-Rowley, 2001).

Along with Pdr1 and Pdr3, several other zinc cluster-containing transcription factors have been associated with the Pdr phenotype. The first of these, Yrr1, was recovered in a screen for tolerance to a cell cycle inhibitor called reveromycin A (Cui et al., 1998). Later work indicated that Yrr1 was both autoregulated and transcriptionally induced by Pdr1/Pdr3 activity (Zhang et al., 2001). Several laboratories discovered that *YRR1* mutants could be recovered that exhibited high constitutive transcriptional activation as previously discussed for similar alleles in *PDR1* and *PDR3* (Cui et al., 1998; Zhang et al., 2001; Keeven et al., 2002; Le Crom et al., 2002). Two homologs of Yrr1 have also been studied: Yrm1 (Lucau-Danila et al., 2003) and Pdr8 (Hikkel et al., 2003).

NON-TRANSPORTER TARGETS GENES OF PDR1/PDR3

While the first genes identified that were controlled by the Pdr regulon were ABC transporters, more recent data make it clear that many different types of proteins are encoded by Pdr1/Pdr3 target genes (Derisi et al., 2000; Devaux et al., 2001, 2002; Traven et al., 2001). These other classes of proteins include 7 transmembrane domain-containing membrane proteins (Rsb1, Rta1) (Kihara and Igarashi, 2004; Panwar and Moye-Rowley, 2006; Kolaczkowska et al., 2012), enzymes involved in sphingolipid biosynthesis (Hallstrom et al., 2001; Kolaczkowski et al., 2004), phospholipid transfer (Van Den Hazel et al., 1999), and other proteins of poorly characterized function. Given the roles for many of these other proteins in lipid homeostasis it is reasonable to propose that the control of lipids has an important effect on drug resistance. Evidence in support of this notion is accumulating in S. cerevisiae and other fungi (Hallstrom et al., 2001; Kolaczkowski et al., 2004; Prasad et al., 2005). While it is important to recognize that the Pdr response involves more than simply transporter genes, these are the best understood in terms of their role in drug resistance. We will focus on the control of transporter genes in this review.

BASIC REGION-LEUCINE ZIPPER-CONTAINING TRANSCRIPTION FACTORS

One of the earliest transcriptional regulators found to influence Pdr was the basic region-leucine zipper (bZip)-containing factor Yap1. Yap1 was isolated in a high-copy-plasmid suppressor screen as *PDR4*, a gene capable of elevating resistance to cycloheximide and the branched chain amino acid biosynthesis inhibitor sulfometuron methyl (Leppert et al., 1990). Later work demonstrated that *YAP1* and *PDR4* were allelic (Hussain and Lenard, 1991) and that Yap1 did not appear to act via *PDR5* (Dexter et al., 1994). Work from several labs demonstrated that the bZip-containing protein Cad1/Yap2 also elevated drug resistance although this effect could only be seen when this protein was overproduced (Bossier et al., 1993; Wu et al., 1993; Hirata et al., 1994b). Similarly, high dosages of the Yap1 homologs Yap5 and Yap6 also conferred resistance to several different drugs (Fernandes et al., 1997; Furuchi et al., 2001).

While there are clear links between the bZip-containing factors and drug resistance, most of the drug resistance effects shown by this group of transcription factors occur when these proteins are overproduced. Disruption mutations rarely exhibit hypersensitivity suggesting either that extensive redundancy exists between these family members or that the normal role of these factors is not to modulate drug resistance. Yap1 is the best understood of these bZip-containing factors in terms of its regulation (reviewed in Toone et al., 2001; Moye-Rowley, 2003a; Rodrigues-Pousada et al., 2004). Loss of the *YAP1* gene has a profound sensitivity to oxidative stress (Schnell et al., 1992; Kuge and Jones, 1994) but little to no consequence on drug resistance (Leppert et al., 1990; Wu et al., 1993; Alarco et al., 1997). An exception to this rule is provided by drugs such as the agrochemical mancozeb that proceed via an oxidative mechanism in which physiological levels of Yap1 are required for normal resistance (Teixeira et al., 2008). Drugs that act through a mechanisms that does not invoke an oxidative stress response typically are insensitive to the presence of Yap1 expressed at normal gene dosage. Yap1 has been thoroughly documented as an important regulator of major facilitator superfamily (MFS) gene expression in the case of *FLR1* (Alarco et al., 1997) and *ATR1* (Coleman et al., 1997). Activation of expression of these genes is likely to explain many of the effects of this transcription factor on drug resistance although little evidence exists that Yap1-dependent transactivation can be stimulated by the presence of drugs. Extensive documentation exists for activation of Yap1 function upon oxidative stress (Kuge et al., 1997; Coleman et al., 1999; Delaunay et al., 2000, 2002). We will focus our discussion on the Zn_2Cys_6 zinc cluster-containing proteins as the paradigms for drug-induced transcriptional activation in *S. cerevisiae* (and likely other fungi as well).

CONTROL OF TRANSCRIPTIONAL ACTIVATION IN *S. CEREVISIAE* MULTIDRUG RESISTANCE

The identification of alleles of *PDR1* as dominant, GOF mutations suggested the possibility of regulatory modulation of the Pdr1 protein. The determination that Pdr1 and Pdr3 were closely related Zn_2Cys_6 zinc cluster-containing transcription factors also argued that these proteins were most likely to be indirect determinants of multidrug resistance via their regulation of direct effectors of this phenotype (such as *PDR5*). Sequence analysis of a large number of these hyperactive mutant alleles of *PDR1* and *PDR3* demonstrated that this multidrug resistant phenotype was routinely caused by single amino acid substitutions in three main regions of these factors (Dexter et al., 1994; Carvajal et al., 1997; Nourani et al., 1997; Simonics et al., 2000). A model of Pdr1 structure is shown in **Figure 1**. Early analyses of these GOF alleles indicated that target genes were overexpressed in the presence of the mutant forms of the transcription regulators. For example, *PDR5* mRNA levels are increased by roughly 10-fold in the presence of a *PDR1* GOF allele compared to levels driven by the wild-type gene (Meyers et al., 1992). This correlates well with the observed increment in drug resistance.

While the characterization of the GOF mutants supported the view that the factors regulating Pdr were under some type of regulatory control, these alleles represent chronic functional alterations in these transcription factors. Here we will summarize more recent progress in elaboration of mechanisms controlling activity of either wild-type Pdr1 or Pdr3. To date, regulatory inputs to these two closely related proteins are unique to each factor and will be considered separately.

PDR1 REGULATION

The first example of a trans-factor influencing Pdr1 activity came from the identification of the Hsp70 protein Ssz1 (originally Pdr13) as a positive regulator of Pdr1 function when overproduced (Hallstrom et al., 1998). Later work demonstrated that this Hsp70 was primarily associated with the ribosome (Hallstrom and Moye-Rowley, 2000a) and has an important role in folding of nascent polypeptide chains (Gautschi et al., 2001). Recently, these findings have been extended with the determination that the dnaJ protein Zuo1 (partner of the dnaK Ssz1 Michimoto et al., 2000) can also stimulate Pdr1 function, possibly by direct binding to

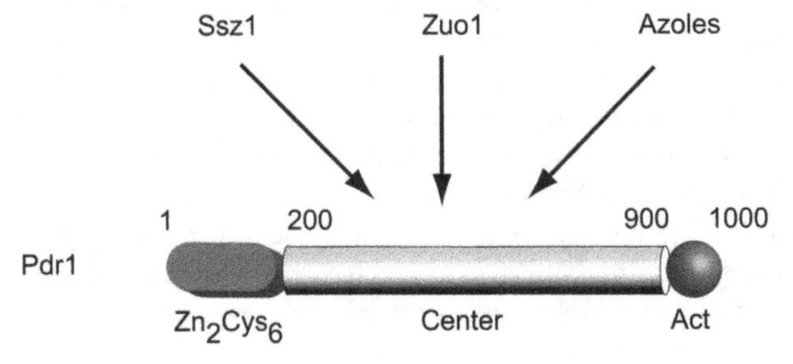

FIGURE 1 | Structure and regulation of *S. cerevisiae* Pdr1. A cartoon of the predicted structure of the *S. cerevisiae* Pdr1 transcription factor is shown. The amino-terminal DNA binding domain containing a Zn_2Cys_6 cluster is located between amino acids 1–200 while the transcriptional activation domain lies at the C-terminus of the protein spanning approximately residues 900–1000. The presumptive regulatory domain that is targeted by several stimulatory signals is referred to as the center domain and lies between residues 200–900. The center domain is thought to be independently regulated by the Hsp70 protein Ssz1, the dnaJ protein Zuo1 and by direct binding to xenobiotics (illustrated here by azole drugs).

this transcription factor (Eisenman and Craig, 2004). Zuo1 contains a short C-terminal region of 13 residues that is necessary and sufficient to induce Pdr1 transcriptional activity (Ducett et al., 2013).

Both Zuo1 and Ssz1 are present at much higher levels than Pdr1 and are thought to have their primary function at the ribosome (Gautschi et al., 2001). Work from the Craig lab has argued that the Zuo1/Ssz1 protein pair can independently activate Pdr1 and are found directly associated with this factor on target promoters (Prunuske et al., 2012). As these findings suggest, the action of Zuo1/Ssz1 in terms of control of Pdr1 activity represents an extra-ribosomal function of these proteins (Eisenman and Craig, 2004). Despite significant effort, the molecular rationale linking activity of these chaperone proteins to Pdr1 remains obscure. An interesting possible tie between Pdr1 and protein folding/degradation came from the finding that the gene encoding the key proteasomal transcriptional regulator Rpn4 is a transcriptional target of Pdr1 (Devaux et al., 2001; Owsianik et al., 2002). Activation of Pdr1 function by Ssz1 can suppress defects in endoplasmic reticulum-associated degradation (Bosis et al., 2010) further strengthening the association of Pdr1 activity with protein homeostasis.

An intriguing model for Pdr1 (and Pdr3) to act as xenobiotic receptor proteins came from studies led by Anders Näär (Thakur et al., 2008). This work provided evidence that the central regions of both these transcription factors could directly bind radioactive fluconazole and that this antifungal drug triggered an increase in Pdr1/3-dependent gene expression. These data support the attractive notion that Pdr1/3 were normally held in a low activity state but could be remodeled in the presence of an appropriate ligand to a more potent transcriptional stimulator.

The simplicity and precedence of this model make it a compelling view for the regulation of Pdr1/3 in physiology. It is still difficult to rationalize why overproduction of either Pdr1 or Pdr3, in the absence of any exogenous drug, can lead to increased gene expression (see for example: Katzmann et al., 1994; Carvajal et al., 1997). If activation of these factors required the presence of a small molecule, then overproduction would not be expected to lead to increase downstream gene expression. In cases where a small molecule is known to be required for activity of a zinc cluster-containing transcription factor, overproduction of the factor leads to downstream repression of gene expression. Examples of this behavior include the heme-dependent activator Hap1 (Zhang et al., 1998) and the leucine biosynthetic activator protein Leu3 (Sze et al., 1993). The genetic behavior of Pdr1/3 seem more easily fit to a situation in which a negative regulatory system is outcompeted when these proteins are overproduced. Further experiments are required to dissect the mechanism of Pdr1/3 control via by small molecules.

PDR3 REGULATION

Although hyperactive alleles of *PDR3* were identified at the inception of the study of the Pdr network in *S. cerevisiae* (Dexter et al., 1994), early analyses of the contribution of Pdr3 to drug resistance suggested that this factor was a less important contributor to transcriptional control than its homolog Pdr1 (Delaveau et al., 1994; Katzmann et al., 1994). Screening a library of random transposon-induced null mutations to identify negative regulators of *PDR5* expression uncovered an array of gene involved in maintaining the mitochondrial genome (Hallstrom and Moye-Rowley, 2000b). Loss of mitochondrial DNA (ρ^0) led to a strong induction of *PDR5* gene expression that was strictly Pdr3-dependent. This was the first example of a situation in yeast in which the level of *PDR5* expression and associated drug resistance rivaled those seen in the presence of a hyperactive allele of either *PDR1* or *PDR3*.

Characterization of the requirements for this mitochondrial signal to trigger Pdr3 induction demonstrated that of the many types of mutations compromising mitochondrial function, only those that also elicited loss of mitochondrial DNA were able to elevate Pdr3 function (Zhang and Moye-Rowley, 2001). The autoregulatory loop of *PDR3* transcription was also essential for the ρ^0 response. However, driving Pdr3 expression from the *PDR1* promoter was still able to produce a ρ^0-dependent induction in drug resistance (Hallstrom and Moye-Rowley, 2000b) arguing that Pdr3 was regulated post-translationally. Together, these findings suggest that a mitochondrial genome-dependent signal leads to a release of Pdr3 from some negative regulatory system. This in turn allows Pdr3 to engage with its own promoter and positively autoregulate transcription. Pdr3 regulation is diagrammed in **Figure 2**.

Further genetic analyses identified several other factors that are required for the normal mitochondrial control of Pdr3. A protein of unknown function called Lge1 was identified as a participant in ρ^0-induced gene expression (Zhang et al., 2005). Lge1 is involved in ubiquitination of histone H2B (Hwang et al., 2003) but this function seems to be distinct from its role in ρ^0 induction of *PDR5* expression (Zhang et al., 2005). Mutants lacking Lge1 fail to fully induce *PDR5* transcription in ρ^0 cells. Overproduction of an enzyme involved in biosynthesis of phosphatidylethanolamine (PE) was discovered to increase Pdr3-dependent transactivation

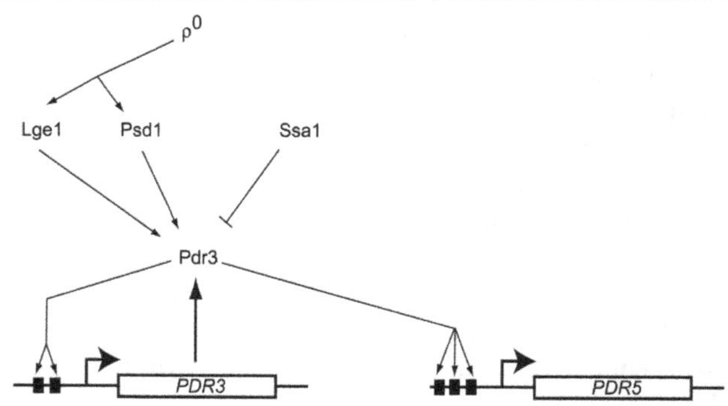

FIGURE 2 | Regulation of *S. cerevisiae* Pdr3. A diagram showing the regulatory inputs modulating Pdr3 function is presented. Loss of mitochondrial DNA (ρ^0) signals move through the PE carboxylase protein Psd1 and via the nuclear factor Lge1. Azole drugs have been demonstrated to directly bind to the center region of Pdr3. The Hsp70 protein Ssa1 associates with and represses activity of Pdr3. The PDR3 gene is under positive autoregulation via the presence of two Pleiotropic Drug Response Elements (PDREs) depicted as solid black boxes. Pdr3 also activates transcription of downstream genes like *PDR5* that confer the multidrug resistance phenotype.

even in ρ^+ cells (Gulshan et al., 2008). This enzyme, called Psd1, is one of two enzymes typically used to produce PE and is located in the inner membrane space of mitochondria (reviewed in Voelker, 1997). Surprisingly, overproduction of a catalytically-inactive form of Psd1 was still capable of inducing *PDR5* expression even though this mutant enzyme could no longer carry out PE biosynthesis (Gulshan et al., 2008). The presence of Psd1 was required for normal ρ^0 signaling to occur consistent with this enzyme having a role in wild-type signal transduction.

Mass spectrometric analysis of purified Pdr3 led to the identification of the Hsp70 protein Ssa1 as a negative regulator of this transcription factor (Shahi et al., 2007). Overproduction of Ssa1 caused a decrease in Pdr3-dependent gene expression and hyperactive mutants exhibited less binding to Ssa1 *in vivo* than wild-type Pdr3. This reduction in Hsp70 association correlated with increased transcriptional activation capability is reminiscent of the regulation of steroid hormone receptors (Pratt and Toft, 1997); however, the presence of other heat shock proteins docked to Pdr3 has not been reported. Interestingly, both Pdr1 and Pdr3 have been reported to be induced by challenge with progesterone, furthering the analogy with a regulatory mechanism resembling steroid hormone receptors (Banerjee et al., 2008).

Further biochemical experiments seeking to identify interacting proteins capable of binding to the KIX domain of the transcriptional Mediator subunit Med15/Gal11 determined that both Pdr1 and Pdr3 interacted with this protein region (Thakur et al., 2008). The Mediator complex is composed of roughly 20 different proteins that act to provide a link between sequence-specific transcriptional regulatory proteins and the RNA polymerase II machinery (see Casamassimi and Napoli, 2007 for a review). Biochemical and genetic experiments have separated the Mediator complex into two different forms referred to as either S-Mediator (or core mediator) containing three and L-Mediator containing four subdomains (Poss et al., 2013). The three subdomains of S-Mediator are called Head, Middle, and Tail with Med15 contributing a component of the Tail complex of proteins (Beve et al., 2005). L-Mediator contains an additional subcomplex consisting of the cyclin-dependent kinase Cdk8 (or Med15/Srb8) and attendant cyclin: cyclinC (Srb11) (reviewed in Conaway and Conaway, 2011). Two other large proteins designated Med12 (Srb8) and Med13 (Srb9) complete the Cdk8 complex.

Interactions between Pdr3 (and Pdr1) and Med15 are crucial for normal levels of downstream gene expression under all conditions (Shahi et al., 2010). However, activation of Pdr3 function in ρ^0 cells still occurs in *med15*Δ cells. Loss of the Med12 protein from the Cdk8 complex completely blocked ρ^0 induction of *PDR5* transcription but had a negligible effect on expression in ρ^+ cells. These findings argue that Med12 is a key target for activated transcription supported by Pdr3, at least in ρ^0 cells. Generally speaking, the Cdk8 complex is thought to serve repressive functions in terms of transcriptional control but more recent data argue that this complex also has positive influences on gene expression as illustrated by the case of Pdr3 activation in ρ^0 cells.

MULTIDRUG RESISTANCE IN *CANDIDA ALBICANS*

The major human fungal pathogen is the yeast *Candida albicans*. This organism, while susceptible to azole drug treatment is readily detected to acquire a multidrug resistance phenotype that includes robust tolerance to this important class of antifungal drug (reviewed in Pfaller, 2012). Next to the current picture of *S. cerevisiae* multidrug resistance, the situation in *C. albicans* is the best understood and has been the focus of authoritative reviews (Cannon et al., 2009; Sanglard et al., 2009; Morschhauser, 2010). Here we will focus our attention on the transcriptional regulatory proteins implicated in clinically relevant resistance phenotypes.

MEMBRANE PROTEINS IMPORTANT IN MULTIDRUG RESISTANCE IN *C. ALBICANS*

The two best characterized genes involved in multidrug resistance in C. albicans are the ABC transporter-encoding *CDR1* gene (Prasad et al., 1995) and the MFS protein-encoding *MDR1* locus (Fling et al., 1991). Both of these resistance determinants are localized to the plasma membrane in *C. albicans* (Manoharlal et al., 2008; Basso et al., 2010; Kapoor et al., 2010). *CDR1* was isolated on the basis of complementation of the drug hypersensitivity of a *pdr5*Δ mutant in *S. cerevisiae*. Loss of *CDR1* led to a pronounced drug sensitive phenotype in *C. albicans*. A closely related ABC transporter-encoding gene, designated *CDR2*, also contributes to drug resistance when overproduced or when *CDR1* is deleted (Sanglard et al., 1997).

MDR1 has been documented to be overexpressed in a number of different clinical isolates (Morschhauser, 2002); however, its loss does not appear to have significant effects on baseline drug resistance. The plasma membrane location of these transporter proteins supports the view that these proteins act as efflux pumps for a range of different drugs (Schuetzer-Muehlbauer et al., 2003; Lettner et al., 2010). Multidrug resistance in *C. albicans* is associated in large part with transcriptional induction of the genes encoding these membrane proteins.

TAC1

The first insight into the molecular basis of transcriptional regulation of multidrug resistance in *C. albicans* came from the identification of the *TAC1* locus. As with *PDR1* and *PDR3* in *S. cerevisiae*, genetic observations drove the discovery of the *TAC1* gene. Analyses of azole tolerant *C. albicans* isolates led to the discovery of loss of heterozygosity/aneuploidy around the mating type loci (MTL) gene cluster (Rustad et al., 2002). Using this observation as a starting point, Sanglard and colleagues took a candidate gene approach by disrupting several different Zn_2Cys_6 zinc cluster-encoding genes in this chromosomal region (Coste et al., 2004). Loss of one of these genes, designated *TAC1* (Transcriptional Activator of Cdr genes), resulted in a strain displaying enhanced azole susceptibility and depressed expression of the *CDR1* ABC transporter-encoding gene.

Along with a requirement for *TAC1* to confer normal wild-type expression of *CDR1* and drug resistance, evidence was obtained that two different changes in the *TAC1* gene influenced its function. First, a number of different substitution and even small deletion mutations strongly enhanced the function of Tac1 (Coste et al., 2007). Secondly, chromosomal rearrangements of chromosome 5 were detected that led to loss of heterozygosity and changes in the dosages of the linked *ERG11* and *TAC1* genes. These structural changes in chromosome 5 were found to lead to the amplification and likely overexpression of *ERG11* and *TAC1* (Coste et al., 2007; Selmecki et al., 2008). These findings are consistent with a model in which Tac1 can be activated either by changes in its primary sequence or simply by overproducing the wild-type factor. Consistent with the notion that increased expression of Tac1 leads to increased function comes from data that the *TAC1* gene is positively autoregulated (Liu et al., 2007; Znaidi et al., 2007).

Although we do not yet know the nature of the signals that control Tac1, the currently available data suggest that its regulation may resemble that of Pdr3 in *S. cerevisiae*. Both of these factors can be activated by mutations along their respective primary sequence and the genes encoding these regulators are positively autoregulated.

Mrr1

A second zinc cluster-containing transcription factor that is an important contributor to drug resistance was identified in cells that were already known to overproduce *MDR1* (Morschhauser et al., 2007). Transcriptional profiling experiments demonstrated that fluconazole resistant isolates shared a common overproduced transcript encoding a zinc cluster-containing transcription factor. This regulatory protein was designated Mrr1 (multidrug resistance regulator). The presence of Mrr1 is required for the observed overproduction of *MDR1* in fluconazole resistant strains. While the *MDR1* promoter contains binding sites for other positive regulators, loss of Mrr1 is sufficient to abrogate the overproduction that occurs in drug resistant isolates. This argues that Mrr1 is the key transcriptional regulator during development of drug resistance involving *MDR1* overproduction (Dunkel et al., 2008). Importantly, azole resistant clinical isolates have been described that overproduce *MDR1* and are dependent upon the presence of this MFS protein for this drug resistance (White, 1997; Wirsching et al., 2000).

Genetic activation of Mrr1 shows similar behavior to other zinc cluster-containing transcription factors in which single amino acid substitutions lead to dramatic induction of Mrr1 transcriptional activity (Dunkel et al., 2008). Detailed analyses of the functional subdomains within Mrr1 indicate that the regulation of this factor is likely to be complex with separable inhibitory and activation domains (Schubert et al., 2011b). Chromatin immunoprecipitation experiments also indicated that Mrr1 is likely to control its own expression (Schubert et al., 2011a) as mentioned above for Tac1. Both these *C. albicans* factors appear to share common overall features with ScPdr3 that is also autoregulated and can be genetically activated by a range of different mutations (reviewed in Moye-Rowley, 2003b).

Along with their important effects on multidrug resistance and critically azole tolerance, these transcription factors have been examined for their influence on virulence. Systematic introduction of GOF forms of *TAC1* and *MRR1* indicated a fitness cost in a gastrointestinal colonization model caused by either mutant gene individually that was exacerbated with their combination (Sasse et al., 2012). These authors suggested an interesting potential rationale for the common observation that clinical isolates of azole resistant *C. albicans* contain either *TAC1* or *MRR1* mutations but not both. Although the double *TAC1 MRR1* strains were robustly azole tolerant, the fitness cost could be so great as to exclude this genetic combination *in vivo*. More recent data suggests that certain combinations of azole resistance mechanisms, including simultaneous presence of mutations in *TAC1* and *MRR1*, may be tolerated (Morio et al., 2013).

A different infection model was used to investigate similar mutations in these same transcription factor genes (tail vein injection) (Lohberger et al., 2014). Using this bloodstream infection model, no significant fitness defect was found consistent with the interpretation that, at least under certain conditions, GOF forms of these transcription factors could be well-tolerated *in vivo*.

OTHER TRANSCRIPTION FACTORS INVOLVED IN DRUG RESISTANCE

The intensive investigation of drug resistance in *C. albicans* has led to identification of a range of different transcriptional regulatory proteins that participate at some level in drug resistance including Ndt80 and Mcm1 among others. These factors in general have not been associated with clinically-relevant drug resistance and seem to play roles as expression modifiers of target genes involved in azole resistance (Mogavero et al., 2011; Sasse et al., 2011).

Two other transcription factors have been linked to certainly azole resistance if not multidrug resistance in *C. albicans*. The Upc2 transcriptional regulator is a positive modulator of sterol biosynthesis and mutations in this factor lead to pronounced azole resistance (Flowers et al., 2012). The effects of Upc2 on drug resistance occur via its role as a key regulator of sterol biosynthesis making this factor unlikely to serve as a true multidrug resistance determinant. *CAP1* encodes the *C. albicans* ScYap1 homolog but does not appear to participate in drug resistance when expressed at normal levels. (Alarco et al., 1997; Alarco and Raymond, 1999). Cap1 clearly regulates *MDR1* (Rognon et al., 2006) but this may have more to do with a role for Mdr1 in the oxidative stress response than drug resistance.

MULTIDRUG RESISTANCE IN *C. GLABRATA*

Candida glabrata is the second most common cause of bloodstream and mucosal candidiasis (10–30%) in the United States, with a high mortality rate (38–53%) (Richter et al., 2005; Pfaller and Diekema, 2007). *C. glabrata* is intrinsically resistant to fluconazole, a common azole drug that targets the fungal specific ergosterol biosynthetic pathway, with resistance known to further increase during drug therapy (8–27% of isolates demonstrating a fluconazole MIC $\geq 64\,\mu g\ ml^{-1}$) (Ostrosky-Zeichner et al., 2003; Pfaller et al., 2004). As for other fungi, *C. glabrata* azole resistance can be the result of an alteration of the target enzyme by either overexpression or mutations in its encoding gene, *ERG11*, that reduces the efficacy of the drug (Henry et al., 2000).

Another frequent basis for multiazole tolerance phenotype is enhanced drug efflux mediated by the activation of expression of ABC transporters like *CgCdr1*, *CgCdr2* (*Pdh1*), and *CgSnq2* (Sanglard et al., 1995, 1997; Miyazaki et al., 1998; Redding et al., 2003; Bennett et al., 2004; Vermitsky and Edlind, 2004; Sanguinetti et al., 2005; Torelli et al., 2008). CgCdr1 seems to be the chief ABC transporter that is constitutively upregulated in most of the drug resistant clinical isolates, either by itself, or as a combination with *CgCdr2* (*Pdh1*) and/or *CgSnq2*. Deletion of *CgCdr1* leads to increased intracellular azole accumulation and hypersensitivity to different azoles, both in clinical isolates as well as lab strains. The ABC transporters mentioned above are regulated by a Zn_2Cys_6 zinc cluster-containing transcription factor encoded by *CgPDR1*. It is now well established that *CgPDR1* exhibits GOF mutations in most of the drug resistant clinical isolates of *C. glabrata* leading to upregulation of the transcription factor, which is responsible for high expression of the target genes that encode drug efflux pumps mediating multidrug resistance. It has been demonstrated that some of these *CgPDR1* GOF mutations also lead to hypervirulence in a mouse model for systemic candidiasis (Ferrari et al., 2009). Interestingly, further work from this same group found that CgPdr1 regulated ABC transporter CgCdr1 and a mitochondrial protein, Pup1, is at least partially responsible for this gain of virulence (Ferrari et al., 2011b).

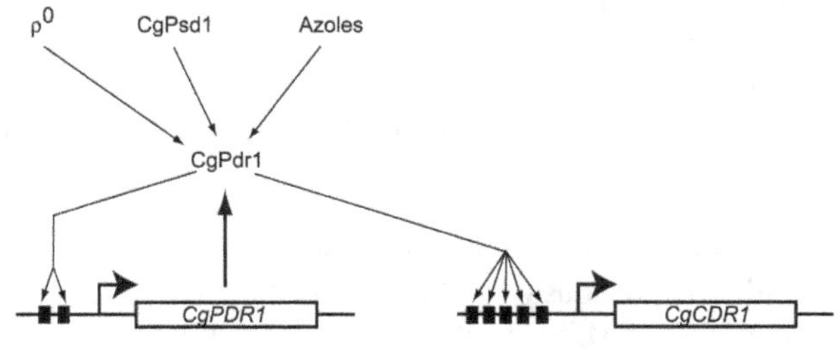

FIGURE 3 | Regulation of multidrug resistance gene expression in *Candida glabrata*. A model reflecting the currently identified players controlling CgPdr1 activity and multidrug resistance gene expression is shown. The solid black boxes indicate the PDREs in the promoters of *CgPDR1* and *CgCDR1*. To date, only signals that positively regulate CgPdr1 have been identified. Note the similarities with ScPdr3 regulation.

CgPdr1

Consistent with the fact that *C. glabrata* is phylogenetically closer to *S. cerevisiae* than *C. albicans*, the multidrug resistance pathways in *S. cerevisiae* and *C. glabrata* share more extensive similarities than with the cognate *C. albicans* system. The molecular players involved in drug resistance, ρ^0-induced PDR pathway activation, and the fact that the pivotal control of multidrug resistance in *C. glabrata* is at the transcriptional level are all shared with *S. cerevisiae*. However, there are interesting differences as well. Unlike *S. cerevisiae*, *C. glabrata* ABC transporters involved in multidrug resistance is regulated by the single transcription factor CgPdr1. CgPdr1 seems to be a blend of transcription factors ScPdr1 and ScPdr3 that modulate drug resistance in *S. cerevisiae*. Though CgPdr1 shares greater identity with ScPdr1 in terms of protein sequence, the *C. glabrata* transcription factor has binding elements in its own promoter contributing to its autoregulation, just as in the case of ScPdr3. Also like ScPdr3, CgPdr1 responds to Pdr pathway activation in ρ^0 cells that lack mitochondrial DNA, as well as when the mitochondrial enzyme phosphatidylserine decarboxylase (ScPsd1) is overproduced (Paul et al., 2011). The role played by the Mediator component Gal11 in regulation of CgPdr1 is also interestingly different in *C. glabrata* when compared to its cognate role in *S. cerevisiae*. There are 2 *GAL11* paralogs (*CgGAL11A* and *CgGAL11B*) in *C. glabrata*, of which only *CgGAL11A* seems to be important for CgPdr1 induced drug resistance (Thakur et al., 2008). The requirement for CgGal11A is however seen only in ρ^+ and not in ρ^0 cells, unlike in *S. cerevisiae* (Paul et al., 2011). Moreover, CgGal11A is required for induction of drug resistance upon azole challenge in ρ^+ cells (**Figure 3**). This phenomenon of xenobiotic/drug-induced efflux pump activation, while not consistently seen in *S. cerevisiae*, is similar to that observed in *C. albicans* (Liu et al., 2005).

C. glabrata respiratory deficient mutants (ρ^0) that have been generated *in vitro* by either ethidium bromide or azole treatment (where ρ^0 cells occur at high frequency), exhibit a growth defect phenotype and reduced virulence (Brun et al., 2005). However, these same cells also possess robust drug resistance that is primarily based on activation of the transcription factor CgPdr1 and upregulation of its target gene CgCdr1 (Vermitsky and Edlind, 2004; Tsai et al., 2006). Interestingly, such mutants have, albeit rarely, been recovered from patients undergoing fluconazole treatment, suggesting that this mechanism of drug resistance may be clinically relevant (Bouchara et al., 2000). Recently, it was reported that an azole resistant *C. glabrata* ρ^0 isolate from the clinic (containing a wild-type *CgPDR1* gene) exhibited higher virulence and *in vivo* fitness in a murine infection model than its azole-susceptible and respiration-competent parental strain (Ferrari et al., 2011a).

Intrinsic low susceptibility and high frequency of resistance to widely used azole antifungals have led to greater use of other drugs, particularly amphotericin B and echinocandins in treatment of candidemias involving *C. glabrata* (Sanguinetti et al., 2005). Echinocandins such as caspofungin and micafungin are lipopeptide inhibitors of β-1,3-glucan synthase and interfere with fungal specific cell wall synthesis. This class of antifungals is active against most *Candida* species, including *C. glabrata* (Ostrosky-Zeichner et al., 2003; Pfaller et al., 2008) and has been used as first-line therapy against *C. glabrata* infections (Pappas et al., 2009). Echinocandin resistance in *C. glabrata* is rare by comparison to azole tolerance but increasing in frequency in response to increasing clinical use (Pfaller et al., 2012). Echinocandin resistance maps to genes encoding components of the β-1,3-glucan synthase (recently discussed in Alexander et al., 2013) and as such is considered outside the typical multidrug resistance determinants in this organism.

To overcome the intrinsic and high frequency acquisition of azole resistance in *C. glabrata*, alternative therapies have also been employed. As mentioned above, echinocandins are effective antifungal agents against *C. glabrata* but resistance to these drugs is on the rise. Combined therapies have also been explored but unexpected complications have arisen in some cases (Alves et al., 2012). An oral drug that represents an alternative to azoles is 5-flurocytosine (5-FC), although there are concerns regarding resistance and toxicity associated with high doses used to negate resistance. Surprisingly, 5-FC/azole combinations have been reported to have an antagonistic effect in *C. glabrata* (Te Dorsthorst et al., 2002; Alves et al., 2012). This antagonistic effect seems to be mediated through the Pdr pathway as it was found that this phenomenon was abrogated in *Cgpdr1*Δ and *Cgcdr1*Δ strains (Steier et al., 2013). 5-FC exposure resulted in 6-fold induction of CgCdr1 that was CgPdr1-dependent even though 5-FC is not a CgCdr1 substrate. Interestingly, 5-FC exposure induced high frequency formation of petite (ρ^0) mutants that upregulate CgPdr1-dependent CgCdr1 activation. Though the molecular mechanism contributing to this antagonistic effect is not clearly understood, it seems that the mitochondrial retrograde signal that activate CgPdr1 is the likely basis for this phenomenon in *C. glabrata.*

OTHER PATHWAYS OF MULTIDRUG RESISTANCE

As mentioned previously for *C. albicans, C. glabrata* also contains a number of MFS-encoding genes. While function of these membrane transporter proteins remains to be characterized, a *C. glabrata* homolog of ScFlr1 has been investigated for its potential role as a multidrug resistance determinant (Chen et al., 2007). The *C. glabrata* homolog was designated *CgFLR1* and as in both *C. albicans* and *S. cerevisiae,* disruption mutations lacking this gene did have drug phenotypes but were unaffected in terms of fluconazole susceptibility. *CgFLR1* is regulated by the *C. glabrata* homolog of ScYap1 (CgAP1) but this regulation does not appear to be involved in normal azole tolerance. More recent experiments have demonstrated that additional MFS proteins contributed to multidrug resistance including CgTPO3 and CgQDR2 (Costa et al., 2013, 2014).

MULTIDRUG RESISTANCE IN *ASPERGILLUS FUMIGATUS*

Significant increases in immunocompromised population over the past few decades have resulted in a concomitant increase in invasive aspergillosis, with *Aspergillus fumigatus* being the most common causative agent (Denning et al., 2013a,b). Invasive aspergillosis is associated with a high rate of morbidity and mortality (as high as 50%) in these patients (Nivoix et al., 2008). However, there are limited effective antifungal drugs available to treat invasive apergillosis (see Pound et al., 2011 for a review). Though amphotericin B has been used with some success, it has been associated with high nephrotoxicity. Echinocandins such as caspofungin have been effective only as a topical agent and has been at best fungistatic. The only oral and the most widespread treatment against invasive aspergillosis has been triazole drugs, particularly itraconazole and voriconazole. However, continuous use of triazoles has led to the development of resistance against different azole drugs used for therapy, with clinical instances of such drug resistance increasing significantly in the last decade.

A prevalent mechanism that is associated with multiazole resistance against *A. fumigatus* has been alterations in the levels of the target enzyme, 14α-sterol demethylase, encoded by *cyp51A* gene (that also happens to have a paralog in *A. fumigatus,* namely *cyp51B*). The L98H mutation in the *cyp51A* gene linked with a 34bp tandem repeat sequence in its promoter has been associated with a large number of multi-azole resistant *A. fumigatus* clinical isolates (Snelders et al., 2008). This mutation was first reported in the Netherlands (where use of azoles as fungicides in agriculture is common), and was later reported from different parts of the world, indicating the spread of this mutation (Lockhart et al., 2011; Camps et al., 2012a; Chowdhary et al., 2012). Other mutational hotspots in *cyp51A* associated with drug resistant isolates have also been identified, though they have been less common and widespread (Recently reviewed in Lelievre et al., 2013).

Since 2008, a large proportion of multi-azole resistant *A. fumigatus* clinical isolates have been shown to be non-*cyp51A* dependent, implicating the role of other drug resistance mechanisms. A comprehensive study involving 64 azole resistant *A. fumigatus* strains done in the United Kingdom revealed that 43% of the cases had no *cyp51A* mutations associated with them (Bueid et al., 2010). Subsequent studies have identified that non-*cyp51A* based drug resistance is on the rise, with more than 50% of the cases involving alternate mechanisms (Camps et al., 2012b; Escribano et al., 2013). Analysis of these non-*cyp51A* based drug resistance isolates have revealed overexpression of ABC transporters in many of these cases, particularly that of cdr1B (abcB) (Fraczek et al., 2013).

Overexpression of efflux pumps is a common and well documented mechanism involved in the drug resistance of pathogenic yeasts such as *C. albicans* and *C. glabrata* as discussed above. They involve two types: the ABC class and the MFS class. The genes encoding these transporters [around 50 ABC (Kovalchuk and Driessen, 2010) and nearly 300 MFS class] are highly redundant in *A. fumigatus,* and some of them have been implicated in multi-azole resistance in *A. fumigatus* in recent years (Slaven et al., 2002; Nascimento et al., 2003; Ferreira et al., 2005). Among the transporters so far characterized in drug resistant clinical isolates of *A. fumigatus, cdr1B* (*abcB*) levels has been found to be most consistently and prominently overexpressed, with *cdr1B* mRNA transcript levels induced between 5–30 fold in these strains. Deletion of *cdr1B* also resulted in a 4-fold increase in susceptibility to itraconazole in both drug susceptible and resistant strains (Fraczek et al., 2013). In an independent study, the *abcB* gene was disrupted in three different *A. fumigatus* genetic backgrounds, resulting in susceptibility to different azoles tested: voriconazole, itraconazole as well as ketoconazole (Paul et al., 2013). Deletion of *abcA,* another ABCG class transporter like *abcB,* also resulted in drug sensitivity, at least in two different *A. fumigatus* genetic backgrounds, although to a lesser extent. Interestingly, overexpression of abcA led to an enhanced tolerance to azole drugs. This study also demonstrated that both *abcA* and *abcB* promoters are induced in the presence of drugs, just like in the case of *CgCDR1.* The action of efflux pumps (AfuMDR4) has also been implicated in fungal resistance within the biofilm, especially in CF patients (Rajendran et al., 2011).

As of yet, we know very little of the identity of transcriptional regulatory proteins involved in control of multidrug resistance in *A. fumigatus.* Analysis of a truncated Afyap1 (*A. fumigatus* homolog of ScYap1) determined that this mutant protein led to antifungal drug resistance (as found for truncated ScYap1-based drug resistance in yeasts), along with conferring tolerance to oxidative stress. However, multiple copies of full-length Afyap1 exhibited voriconazole susceptibility comparable with that of a wild-type *A. fumigatus* strain (Qiao et al., 2010). Together, these data suggest that Afyap1, like the bZip cognate proteins in yeast, exerts effects on antifungal drug resistance only upon mutational activation.

PROSPECTUS

The limited repertoire of antifungal drugs makes developing new modalities an important and pressing need. However, a goal of crucial importance to the enterprise of antifungal therapies in particular and drug-based therapies in general is to understand mechanisms of drug resistance. Multidrug resistance is an especially serious issue as a small number (often one) of genetic changes can lead to loss of susceptibility to multiple drugs simultaneously. In terms of antifungal multidrug resistance, our most developed picture applies to the yeast *Saccharomyces cerevisiae*, due in large part to the facile genetics of this organism. In recent years, important progress has been made in the two major pathogenic *Candida* species, *C. albicans* and *C. glabrata*. While there are significant similarities between the *Candida* species and *S. cerevisiae*, important differences have been described. The increasing development and application of genetic technologies in the *Candida* species will expedite direct study of the resistance mechanisms in these organisms. This is crucial to ensure continued utility of existing and future antifungal drugs.

While we have a fairly extensive catalogue of genes that are likely participants in the process of multidrug resistance, our understanding of how these genes are regulated is still very incomplete. In some cases, the identities of the transcription factors that control the multidrug resistance genes are well-established; yet a detailed picture of how the activity of these factors is regulated is not available. This will be an important future goal as interference with regulation of multidrug resistance gene expression has promise as a potential avenue to prevent development of this phenotype.

Improvements in medical care in regards to longer term survival in the face of immunosuppression has led to a greater chronic reliance on antimicrobial chemotherapy. *Candida* bloodstream infections are now the 4th most common form of nosocomial infection seen (Lewis, 2009). The occurrence of aspergillosis is also on the rise and outcomes associated with azole tolerant forms of this filamental fungal pathogen are dramatically worsened compared to azole susceptible fungi (Van Der Linden et al., 2011). Continued progress in the molecular understanding of antifungal drug resistance is an crucial step toward ensuring the sustainability of antifungal drug therapy and confidently expecting to treat these microbial pathogens in the future.

ACKNOWLEDGMENTS

Our work on multidrug resistance has been supported by NIH grants GM49825 and AI92331.

REFERENCES

Alarco, A. M., Balan, I., Talibi, D., Mainville, N., and Raymond, M. (1997). AP-1-mediated multidrug resistance in *Saccharomyces cerevisiae* requires *FLR1* encoding a transporter of the major facilitator superfamily. *J. Biol. Chem.* 272, 19304–19313. doi: 10.1074/jbc.272.31.19304

Alarco, A. M., and Raymond, M. (1999). The bZip transcription factor Cap1p is involved in multidrug resistance and oxidative stress response in *Candida albicans*. *J. Bacteriol.* 181, 700–708.

Alexander, B. D., Johnson, M. D., Pfeiffer, C. D., Jimenez-Ortigosa, C., Catania, J., Booker, R., et al. (2013). Increasing echinocandin resistance in *Candida glabrata*: clinical failure correlates with presence of FKS mutations and elevated minimum inhibitory concentrations. *Clin. Infect. Dis.* 56, 1724–1732. doi: 10.1093/cid/cit136

Alves, I. A., Bandeira, L. A., Mario, D. A., Denardi, L. B., Neves, L. V., Santurio, J. M., et al. (2012). Effects of antifungal agents alone and in combination against *Candida glabrata* strains susceptible or resistant to fluconazole. *Mycopathologia* 174, 215–221. doi: 10.1007/s11046-012-9538-7

Ambudkar, S. V., Kimchi-Sarfaty, C., Sauna, Z. E., and Gottesman, M. M. (2003). P-glycoprotein: from genomics to mechanism. *Oncogene* 22, 7468–7485. doi: 10.1038/sj.onc.1206948

Balzi, E., Chen, W., Ulaszewski, S., Capieaux, E., and Goffeau, A. (1987). The multidrug resistance gene *PDR1* from *Saccharomyces cerevisiae*. *J. Biol. Chem.* 262, 16871–16879.

Balzi, E., and Goffeau, A. (1995). Yeast multidrug resistance: the *PDR* network. *J. Bioenerget. Biomem.* 27, 71–76. doi: 10.1007/BF02110333

Balzi, E., Wang, M., Leterme, S., Van Dyck, L., and Goffeau, A. (1994). *PDR5*: a novel yeast multidrug resistance transporter controlled by the transcription regulator *PDR1*. *J. Biol. Chem.* 269, 2206–2214.

Banerjee, D., Lelandais, G., Shukla, S., Mukhopadhyay, G., Jacq, C., Devaux, F., et al. (2008). Responses of pathogenic and nonpathogenic yeast species to steroids reveal the functioning and evolution of multidrug resistance transcriptional networks. *Eukaryot. Cell* 7, 68–77. doi: 10.1128/EC.00256-07

Basso, L. R. Jr., Gast, C. E., Mao, Y., and Wong, B. (2010). Fluconazole transport into *Candida albicans* secretory vesicles by the membrane proteins Cdr1p, Cdr2p, and Mdr1p. *Eukaryot. Cell* 9, 960–970. doi: 10.1128/EC.00355-09

Bauer, B. E., Wolfger, H., and Kuchler, K. (1999). Inventory and function of yeast ABC proteins: about sex, stress, pleiotropic drug and heavy metal resistance. *Biochim. Biophys. Acta.* 1461, 217–236. doi: 10.1016/S0005-2736(99)00160-1

Bennett, J. E., Izumikawa, K., and Marr, K. A. (2004). Mechanism of increased fluconazole resistance in *Candida glabrata* during prophylaxis. *Antimicrob. Agents Chemother.* 48, 1773–1777. doi: 10.1128/AAC.48.5.1773-1777.2004

Beve, J., Hu, G. Z., Myers, L. C., Balciunas, D., Werngren, O., Hultenby, K., et al. (2005). The structural and functional role of Med5 in the yeast Mediator tail module. *J. Biol. Chem.* 280, 41366–41372. doi: 10.1074/jbc.M511181200

Bissinger, P. H., and Kuchler, K. (1994). Molecular cloning and expression of the *S. cerevisiae STS1* gene product. *J. Biol. Chem.* 269, 4180–4186.

Bosis, E., Salomon, D., Ohayon, O., Sivan, G., Bar-Nun, S., and Rabinovich, E. (2010). Ssz1 restores endoplasmic reticulum-associated protein degradation in cells expressing defective cdc48-ufd1-npl4 complex by upregulating cdc48. *Genetics* 184, 695–706. doi: 10.1534/genetics.109.111419

Bossier, P., Fernandes, L., Rocha, D., and Rodrigues-Pousada, C. (1993). Overexpression of YAP2, coding for a new yAP protein, and YAP1 in S. cerevisiae alleviates growth inhibition caused by 1,10-phenanthroline. *J. Biol. Chem.* 268, 23640–23645.

Bouchara, J. P., Zouhair, R., Le Boudouil, S., Renier, G., Filmon, R., Chabasse, D., et al. (2000). *In-vivo* selection of an azole-resistant petite mutant of *Candida glabrata*. *J. Med. Microbiol.* 49, 977–984.

Brown, G. D., Denning, D. W., and Levitz, S. M. (2012). Tackling human fungal infections. *Science* 336, 647. doi: 10.1126/science.1222236

Brun, S., Dalle, F., Saulnier, P., Renier, G., Bonnin, A., Chabasse, D., et al. (2005). Biological consequences of petite mutations in *Candida glabrata*. *J. Antimicrob. Chemother.* 56, 307–314. doi: 10.1093/jac/dki200

Bueid, A., Howard, S. J., Moore, C. B., Richardson, M. D., Harrison, E., Bowyer, P., et al. (2010). Azole antifungal resistance in *Aspergillus fumigatus*: 2008 and 2009. *J. Antimicrob. Chemother.* 65, 2116–2118. doi: 10.1093/jac/dkq279

Camps, S. M., Rijs, A. J., Klaassen, C. H., Meis, J. F., O'Gorman, C. M., Dyer, P. S., et al. (2012a). Molecular epidemiology of *Aspergillus fumigatus* isolates harboring the TR34/L98H azole resistance mechanism. *J. Clin. Microbiol.* 50, 2674–2680. doi: 10.1128/JCM.00335-12

Camps, S. M., Van Der Linden, J. W., Li, Y., Kuijper, E. J., Van Dissel, J. T., Verweij, P. E., et al. (2012b). Rapid induction of multiple resistance mechanisms in *Aspergillus fumigatus* during azole therapy: a case study and review of the literature. *Antimicrob. Agents Chemother.* 56, 10–16. doi: 10.1128/AAC.05088-11

Cannon, R. D., Lamping, E., Holmes, A. R., Niimi, K., Baret, P. V., Keniya, M. V., et al. (2009). Efflux-mediated antifungal drug resistance. *Clin. Microbiol. Rev.* 22, 291–321, doi: 10.1128/CMR.00051-08

Carvajal, E., Van Den Hazel, H. B., Cybularz-Kolaczkowska, A., Balzi, E., and Goffeau, A. (1997). Molecular and phenotypic characterization of yeast *PDR1* mutants that show hyperactive transcription of various ABC multidrug transporter genes. *Mol. Gen. Genet.* 256, 406–415. doi: 10.1007/s004380050584

Casamassimi, A., and Napoli, C. (2007). Mediator complexes and eukaryotic transcription regulation: an overview. *Biochemie.* 89, 1439–1446. doi: 10.1016/j.biochi.2007.08.002

Chen, K. H., Miyazaki, T., Tsai, H. F., and Bennett, J. E. (2007). The bZip transcription factor Cgap1p is involved in multidrug resistance and required for activation of multidrug transporter gene CgFLR1 in *Candida glabrata*. *Gene* 386, 63–72. doi: 10.1016/j.gene.2006.08.010

Chowdhary, A., Kathuria, S., Xu, J., Sharma, C., Sundar, G., Singh, P. K., et al. (2012). Clonal expansion and emergence of environmental multiple-triazole-resistant *Aspergillus fumigatus* strains carrying the TR(3)(4)/L98H mutations in the cyp51A gene in India. *PLoS ONE* 7:e52871. doi: 10.1371/journal.pone.0052871

Coleman, S. T., Epping, E. A., Steggerda, S. M., and Moye-Rowley, W. S. (1999). Yap1p activates gene transcription in an oxidant-specific fashion. *Mol. Cell. Biol.* 19, 8302–8313.

Coleman, S. T., Tseng, E., and Moye-Rowley, W. S. (1997). *Saccharomyces cerevisiae* basic region-leucine zipper protein regulatory networks converge at the *ATR1* structural gene. *J. Biol. Chem.* 272, 23224–23230. doi: 10.1074/jbc.272.37.23224

Conaway, R. C., and Conaway, J. W. (2011). Function and regulation of the Mediator complex. *Curr. Opin. Genet. Dev.* 21, 225–230. doi: 10.1016/j.gde.2011.01.013

Costa, C., Nunes, J., Henriques, A., Mira, N. P., Nakayama, H., Chibana, H., et al. (2014). *Candida glabrata* drug:H+ antiporter CgTpo3 (ORF CAGL0I10384g): role in azole drug resistance and polyamine homeostasis. *J. Antimicrob. Chemother.* doi: 10.1093/jac/dku044

Costa, C., Pires, C., Cabrito, T. R., Renaudin, A., Ohno, M., Chibana, H., et al. (2013). *Candida glabrata* drug:H+ antiporter CgQdr2 confers imidazole drug resistance, being activated by transcription factor CgPdr1. *Antimicrob. Agents Chemother.* 57, 3159–3167. doi: 10.1128/AAC.00811-12

Coste, A., Selmecki, A., Forche, A., Diogo, D., Bougnoux, M. E., D'Enfert, C., et al. (2007). Genotypic evolution of azole resistance mechanisms in sequential *Candida albicans* isolates. *Eukaryot. Cell* 6, 1889–1904. doi: 10.1128/EC.00 151-07

Coste, A. T., Karababa, M., Ischer, F., Bille, J., and Sanglard, D. (2004). TAC1, transcriptional activator of CDR genes, is a new transcription factor involved in the regulation of *Candida albicans* ABC transporters CDR1 and CDR2. *Eukaryot. Cell* 3, 1639–1652. doi: 10.1128/EC.3.6.1639-1652.2004

Cui, Z., Shiraki, T., Hirata, D., and Miyakawa, T. (1998). Yeast gene *YRR1*, which is required for resistance to 4-nitroquinoline-N-oxide, mediates transcriptional activation of the multidrug resistance transporter gene *SNQ2*. *Mol. Microbiol.* 29, 1307–1315. doi: 10.1046/j.1365-2958.1998.01027.x

Decottignies, A., Kolaczkowski, M., Balzi, E., and Goffeau, A. (1994). Solubilization and charcterization of the overexpressed PDR5 multidrug resistance nucleotide triphophatase of yeast. *J. Biol. Chem.* 269, 12797–12803.

Delahodde, A., Delaveau, T., and Jacq, C. (1995). Positive autoregulation of the yeast transcription factor Pdr3p, involved in the control of the drug resistance phenomenon. *Mol. Cell. Biol.* 15, 4043–4051.

Delaunay, A., Isnard, A. D., and Toledano, M. B. (2000). H2O2 sensing through oxidation of the Yap1 transcription factor. *EMBO J.* 19, 5157–5166. doi: 10.1093/emboj/19.19.5157

Delaunay, A., Pflieger, D., Barrault, M. B., Vinh, J., and Toledano, M. B. (2002). A thiol peroxidase is an H2O2 receptor and redox-transducer in gene activation. *Cell* 111, 471–481. doi: 10.1016/S0092-8674(02)01048-6

Delaveau, T., Delahodde, A., Carvajal, E., Subik, J., and Jacq, C. (1994). *PDR3*, a new yeast regulatory gene, is homologous to *PDR1* and controls the multidrug resistance phenomenon. *Mol. Gen. Genet.* 244, 501–511. doi: 10.1007/BF00583901

Denning, D. W., Pleuvry, A., and Cole, D. C. (2013a). Global burden of allergic bronchopulmonary aspergillosis with asthma and its complication chronic pulmonary aspergillosis in adults. *Med. Mycol.* 51, 361–370. doi: 10.3109/13693786.2012.738312

Denning, D. W., Pleuvry, A., and Cole, D. C. (2013b). Global burden of chronic pulmonary aspergillosis complicating sarcoidosis. *Eur. Respir. J.* 41, 621–626. doi: 10.1183/09031936.00226911

Derisi, J., Van Den Hazel, B., Marc, P., Balzi, E., Brown, P., Jacq, C., et al. (2000). Genome microarray analysis of transcriptional activation in multidrug resistance yeast mutants. *FEBS Lett.* 470, 156–160. doi: 10.1016/S0014-5793(00)01294-1

Devaux, F., Carvajal, E., Moye-Rowley, S., and Jacq, C. (2002). Genome-wide studies on the nuclear *PDR3*-controlled response to mitochondrial dysfunction in yeast. *FEBS Lett.* 515, 25–28. doi: 10.1016/S0014-5793(02)02387-6

Devaux, F., Marc, P., Bouchoux, C., Delaveau, T., Hikkel, I., Potier, M. C., et al. (2001). An artificial transcription activator mimics the genome-wide properties of the yeast Pdr1 transcription factor. *EMBO Rep.* 2, 493–498. doi: 10.1093/embo-reports/kve114

Dexter, D., Moye-Rowley, W. S., Wu, A.-L., and Golin, J. (1994). Mutations in the yeast *PDR3*, *PDR4*, *PDR7* and *PDR9* pleiotropic drug resistance loci affect the transcript level of an ATP binding cassette transporter encoding gene, *PDR5*. *Genetics* 136, 505–515.

Ducett, J. K., Peterson, F. C., Hoover, L. A., Prunuske, A. J., Volkman, B. F., and Craig, E. A. (2013). Unfolding of the C-terminal domain of the J-protein Zuo1 releases autoinhibition and activates Pdr1-dependent transcription. *J. Mol. Biol.* 425, 19–31. doi: 10.1016/j.jmb.2012.09.020

Dunkel, N., Blass, J., Rogers, P. D., and Morschhauser, J. (2008). Mutations in the multi-drug resistance regulator MRR1, followed by loss of heterozygosity, are the main cause of MDR1 overexpression in fluconazole-resistant *Candida albicans* strains. *Mol. Microbiol.* 69, 827–840. doi: 10.1111/j.1365-2958.2008.06309.x

Eisenman, H. C., and Craig, E. A. (2004). Activation of pleiotropic drug resistance by the J-protein and Hsp70-related proteins, Zuo1 and Ssz1. *Mol. Microbiol.* 53, 335–344. doi: 10.1111/j.1365-2958.2004.04134.x

Escribano, P., Pelaez, T., Munoz, P., Bouza, E., and Guinea, J. (2013). Is azole resistance in *Aspergillus fumigatus* a problem in Spain? *Antimicrob. Agents Chemother.* 57, 2815–2820. doi: 10.1128/AAC.02487-12

Fernandes, L., Rorigues-Pousada, C., and Struhl, K. (1997). Yap, a novel family of eight bZIP proteins in *Saccharomyces cerevisiae* with distinct biological functions. *Mol. Cell. Biol.* 17, 6982–6993.

Ferrari, S., Ischer, F., Calabrese, D., Posteraro, B., Sanguinetti, M., Fadda, G., et al. (2009). Gain of function mutations in CgPDR1 of *Candida glabrata* not only mediate antifungal resistance but also enhance virulence. *PLoS Pathog.* 5:e1000268. doi: 10.1371/journal.ppat.1000268

Ferrari, S., Sanguinetti, M., De Bernardis, F., Torelli, R., Posteraro, B., Vandeputte, P., et al. (2011a). Loss of mitochondrial functions associated with azole resistance in *Candida glabrata* results in enhanced virulence in mice. *Antimicrob. Agents Chemother.* 55, 1852–1860. doi: 10.1128/AAC.01271-10

Ferrari, S., Sanguinetti, M., Torelli, R., Posteraro, B., and Sanglard, D. (2011b). Contribution of CgPDR1-regulated genes in enhanced virulence of azole-resistant *Candida glabrata*. *PLoS ONE* 6:e17589. doi: 10.1371/journal.pone.0017589

Ferreira, M. E., Colombo, A. L., Paulsen, I., Ren, Q., Wortman, J., Huang, J., et al. (2005). The ergosterol biosynthesis pathway, transporter genes, and azole resistance in *Aspergillus fumigatus*. *Med. Mycol.* 43(Suppl. 1), S313–S319. doi: 10.1080/13693780400029114

Fling, M. E., Kopf, J., Tamarkin, A., Gorman, J. A., Smith, H. A., and Koltin, Y. (1991). Analysis of a *Candida albicans* gene that encodes a novel mechanism for resistance to benomyl and methotrexate. *Mol. Gen. Genet.* 227, 318–329. doi: 10.1007/BF00259685

Flowers, S. A., Barker, K. S., Berkow, E. L., Toner, G., Chadwick, S. G., Gygax, S. E., et al. (2012). Gain-of-function mutations in UPC2 are a frequent cause of ERG11 upregulation in azole-resistant clinical isolates of *Candida albicans*. *Eukaryot. Cell* 11, 1289–1299. doi: 10.1128/EC.00215-12

Fraczek, M. G., Bromley, M., Buied, A., Moore, C. B., Rajendran, R., Rautemaa, R., et al. (2013). The cdr1B efflux transporter is associated with non-cyp51a-mediated itraconazole resistance in *Aspergillus fumigatus*. *J. Antimicrob. Chemother.* doi: 10.1093/jac/dkt075

Furuchi, T., Ishikawa, H., Miura, N., Ishizuka, M., Kajiya, K., Kuge, S., et al. (2001). Two nuclear proteins, Cin5 and Ydr259c, confer resistance to cisplatin in *Saccharomyces cerevisiae*. *Mol. Pharmacol.* 59, 470–474.

Gautschi, M., Lilie, H., Funfschilling, U., Mun, A., Ross, S., Lithgow, T., et al. (2001). RAC, a stable ribosome-associated complex in yeast formed by the DNaK-DnaJ homologs Ssz1p and zuotin. *Proc. Natl. Acad. Sci. U.S.A.* 98, 3762–3767. doi: 10.1073/pnas.071057198

Gottesman, M. M., Hrycyna, C. A., Schoenlein, P. V., Germann, U. A., and Pastan, I. (1995). Genetic analysis of the multidrug transporter. *Annu. Rev. Genet.* 29, 607–649. doi: 10.1146/annurev.ge.29.120195.003135

Gulshan, K., and Moye-Rowley, W. S. (2007). Multidrug resistance in fungi. *Eukaryot. Cell* 6, 1933–1942. doi: 10.1128/EC.00254-07

Gulshan, K., Schmidt, J., Shahi, P., and Moye-Rowley, W. S. (2008). Evidence for the bifunctional nature of mitochondrial phosphatidylserine decarboxylase: role in Pdr3-dependent retrograde regulation of PDR5 expression. *Mol. Cell. Biol.* 28, 5851–5864. doi: 10.1128/MCB.00405-08

Hallstrom, T. C., Katzmann, D. J., Torres, R. J., Sharp, W. J., and Moye-Rowley, W. S. (1998). Regulation of transcription factor Pdr1p function by a Hsp70 protein in *Saccharomyces cerevisiae*. *Mol. Cell. Biol.* 18, 1147–1155.

Hallstrom, T. C., Lambert, L., Schorling, S., Balzi, E., Goffeau, A., and Moye-Rowley, W. S. (2001). Coordinate control of sphingolipid biosynthesis and multidrug resistance in *Saccharomyces cerevisiae. J. Biol. Chem.* 276, 23674–23680. doi: 10.1074/jbc.M101568200

Hallstrom, T. C., and Moye-Rowley, W. S. (2000a). Hyperactive forms of the Pdr1p transcription factor fail to respond to positive regulation by the Hsp70 protein Pdr13p. *Mol. Microbiol.* 36, 402–413. doi: 10.1046/j.1365-2958.2000.01858.x

Hallstrom, T. C., and Moye-Rowley, W. S. (2000b). Multiple signals from dysfunctional mitochondria activate the pleiotropic drug resistance pathway in *Saccharomyces cerevisae. J. Biol. Chem.* 275, 37347–37356. doi: 10.1074/jbc.M007338200

Henry, K. W., Nickels, J. T., and Edlind, T. D. (2000). Upregulation of ERG genes in Candida species by azoles and other sterol biosynthesis inhibitors. *Antimicrob. Agents Chemother.* 44, 2693–2700. doi: 10.1128/AAC.44.10.2693-2700.2000

Hikkel, I., Lucau-Danila, A., Delaveau, T., Marc, P., Devaux, F., and Jacq, C. (2003). A general strategy to uncover transcription factor properties identifies a new regulator of drug resistance in yeast. *J. Biol. Chem.* 278, 11427–11432. doi: 10.1074/jbc.M208549200

Hirata, D., Yano, K., Miyahara, K., and Miyakawa, T. (1994a). *Saccharomyces cerevisiae YDR1*, which encodes a member of the ATP-binding cassette (ABC) superfamily, is required for multidrug resistance. *Curr. Genet.* 26, 285–294. doi: 10.1007/BF00310491

Hirata, D., Yano, K., and Miyakawa, T. (1994b). Stress-induced transcriptional activation mediated by *YAP1* and *YAP2* genes that encode the Jun family of transcriptional activators in *Saccharomyces cerevisiae. Mol. Gen. Genet.* 242, 250–256. doi: 10.1007/BF00280413

Holohan, C., Van Schaeybroeck, S., Longley, D. B., and Johnston, P. G. (2013). Cancer drug resistance: an evolving paradigm. *Nat. Rev. Cancer* 13, 714–726. doi: 10.1038/nrc3599

Hussain, M., and Lenard, J. (1991). Characterization of PDR4, a *Saccharomyces cerevisiae* gene that confers pleiotropic drug resistance in high-copy number. *Gene* 101, 149–152. doi: 10.1016/0378-1119(91)90238-7

Hwang, W. W., Venkatasubrahmanyam, S., Ianculescu, A. G., Tong, A., Boone, C., and Madhani, H. D. (2003). A conserved RING finger protein required for histone H2B monoubiquitination and cell size control. *Mol. Cell* 11, 261–266. doi: 10.1016/S1097-2765(02)00826-2

Johnston, M. (1987). A model fungal gene regulatory mechanism: the *GAL* genes of *Saccharomyces cerevisiae. Microbiol. Rev.* 51, 458–476.

Kapoor, K., Rehan, M., Lynn, A. M., and Prasad, R. (2010). Employing information theoretic measures and mutagenesis to identify residues critical for drug-proton antiport function in Mdr1p of *Candida albicans. PLoS ONE* 5:e11041. doi: 10.1371/journal.pone.0011041

Katzmann, D. J., Burnett, P. E., Golin, J., Mahe, Y., and Moye-Rowley, W. S. (1994). Transcriptional control of the yeast *PDR5* gene by the *PDR3* gene product. *Mol. Cell. Biol.* 14, 4653–4661.

Katzmann, D. J., Hallstrom, T. C., Mahe, Y., and Moye-Rowley, W. S. (1996). Multiple Pdr1p/Pdr3p binding sites are essential for normal expression of the ATP binding cassette transporter protein-encoding gene *PDR5. J. Biol. Chem.* 271, 23049–23054. doi: 10.1074/jbc.271.38.23049

Katzmann, D. J., Hallstrom, T. C., Voet, M., Wysock, W., Golin, J., Volckaert, G., et al. (1995). Expression of an ATP-binding cassette transporter encoding gene (*YOR1*) is required for oligomycin resistance in *Saccharomyces cerevisiae. Mol. Cell. Biol.* 15, 6875–6883.

Keeven, J., Ko, D., Shallom, J., Uccellini, B., and Golin, J. (2002). PDR2 gain-of-function mutations eliminate the need for Pdr1 and require the UBP6 product for resistance to translational inhibitors. *Curr. Genet.* 41, 11–19. doi: 10.1007/s00294-002-0274-2

Kihara, A., and Igarashi, Y. (2004). Cross talk between sphingolipids and glycerophospholipids in the establishment of plasma membrane asymmetry. *Mol. Biol. Cell* 15, 4949–4959. doi: 10.1091/mbc.E04-06-0458

Kolaczkowska, A., Manente, M., Kolaczkowski, M., Laba, J., Ghislain, M., and Wawrzycka, D. (2012). The regulatory inputs controlling pleiotropic drug resistance and hypoxic response in yeast converge at the promoter of the aminocholesterol resistance gene RTA1. *FEMS Yeast Res.* 12, 279–292. doi: 10.1111/j.1567-1364.2011.00768.x

Kolaczkowski, M., Kolaczkowska, A., Gaigg, B., Schneiter, R., and Moye-Rowley, W. S. (2004). Differential regulation of ceramide synthase components LAC1 and LAG1 in *Saccharomyces cerevisiae. Eukaryot. Cell* 3, 880–892. doi: 10.1128/EC.3.4.880-892.2004

Kovalchuk, A., and Driessen, A. J. (2010). Phylogenetic analysis of fungal ABC transporters. *BMC Genomics* 11:177. doi: 10.1186/1471-2164-11-177

Kristan, K., and Rizner, T. L. (2012). Steroid-transforming enzymes in fungi. *J. Steroid Biochem. Mol. Biol.* 129, 79–91. doi: 10.1016/j.jsbmb.2011.08.012

Kuge, S., and Jones, N. (1994). *YAP1*-dependent activation of *TRX2* is essential for the response of *S. cerevisiae to oxidative stress by hydroperoxides. EMBO J.* 13, 655–664.

Kuge, S., Jones, N., and Nomoto, A. (1997). Regulation of yAP-1 nuclear localization in response to oxidative stress. *EMBO J.* 16, 1710–1720. doi: 10.1093/emboj/16.7.1710

Le Crom, S., Devaux, F., Marc, P., Zhang, X., Moye-Rowley, W. S., and Jacq, C. (2002). New insights into the pleiotropic drug resistance network from genome-wide characterization of the YRR1 transcription factor regulation system. *Mol. Cell. Biol.* 22, 2642–2649. doi: 10.1128/MCB.22.8.2642-2649.2002

Lelievre, L., Groh, M., Angebault, C., Maherault, A. C., Didier, E., and Bougnoux, M. E. (2013). Azole resistant *Aspergillus fumigatus*: an emerging problem. *Med. Mal. Infect.* 43, 139–145. doi: 10.1016/j.medmal.2013.02.010

Leppert, G., Mcdevitt, R., Falco, S. C., Van Dyk, T. K., Ficke, M. B., and Golin, J. (1990). Cloning by gene amplification of two loci conferring multiple drug resistance in Saccharomyces. *Genetics* 125, 13–20.

Lettner, T., Zeidler, U., Gimona, M., Hauser, M., Breitenbach, M., and Bito, A. (2010). *Candida albicans* AGE3, the ortholog of the S. cerevisiae ARF-GAP-encoding gene GCS1, is required for hyphal growth and drug resistance. *PLoS ONE* 5:e11993. doi: 10.1371/journal.pone.0011993

Lewis, R. E. (2009). Overview of the changing epidemiology of candidemia. *Curr. Med. Res. Opin.* 25, 1732–1740. doi: 10.1185/03007990902990817

Liu, T. T., Lee, R. E., Barker, K. S., Lee, R. E., Wei, L., Homayouni, R., et al. (2005). Genome-wide expression profiling of the response to azole, polyene, echinocandin, and pyrimidine antifungal agents in *Candida albicans. Antimicrob. Agents Chemother.* 49, 2226–2236. doi: 10.1128/AAC.49.6.2226-2236.2005

Liu, T. T., Znaidi, S., Barker, K. S., Xu, L., Homayouni, R., Saidane, S., et al. (2007). Genome-wide expression and location analyses of the *Candida albicans* Tac1p regulon. *Eukaryot. Cell* 6, 2122–2138. doi: 10.1128/EC.00327-07

Lockhart, S. R., Frade, J. P., Etienne, K. A., Pfaller, M. A., Diekema, D. J., and Balajee, S. A. (2011). Azole resistance in *Aspergillus fumigatus* isolates from the ARTEMIS global surveillance study is primarily due to the TR/L98H mutation in the cyp51A gene. *Antimicrob. Agents Chemother.* 55, 4465–4468. doi: 10.1128/AAC.00185-11

Lohberger, A., Coste, A. T., and Sanglard, D. (2014). Distinct roles of *Candida albicans* drug resistance transcription factors TAC1, MRR1, and UPC2 in virulence. *Eukaryot. Cell* 13, 127–142. doi: 10.1128/EC.00245-13

Lucau-Danila, A., Delaveau, T., Lelandais, G., Devaux, F., and Jacq, C. (2003). Competitive promoter occupancy by two yeast paralogous transcription factors controlling the multidrug resistance phenomenon. *J. Biol. Chem.* 278, 52641–52650. doi: 10.1074/jbc.M309580200

Mahe, Y., Parle-Mcdermott, A., Nourani, A., Delahodde, A., Lamprecht, A., and Kuchler, K. (1996). The ATP-binding cassette multidrug transporter Snq2 of *Saccharomyces cerevisiae*: a novel target for the transcription factors Pdr1 and Pdr3. *Mol. Microbiol.* 20, 109–117. doi: 10.1111/j.1365-2958.1996.tb02493.x

Manoharlal, R., Gaur, N. A., Panwar, S. L., Morschhauser, J., and Prasad, R. (2008). Transcriptional activation and increased mRNA stability contribute to overexpression of CDR1 in azole-resistant *Candida albicans. Antimicrob. Agents Chemother.* 52, 1481–1492. doi: 10.1128/AAC.01106-07

Meyers, S., Schauer, W., Balzi, E., Wagner, M., Goffeau, A., and Golin, J. (1992). Interaction of the yeast pleiotropic drug resistance genes PDR1 and PDR5. *Curr. Genet.* 21, 431–436. doi: 10.1007/BF00351651

Michimoto, T., Aoki, T., Toh-E, A., and Kikuchi, Y. (2000). Yeast Pdr13p and Zuo1p molecular chaperones are new functional Hsp70 and Hsp40 partners. *Gene* 257, 131–137. doi: 10.1016/S0378-1119(00)00381-4

Miyazaki, H., Miyazaki, Y., Geber, A., Parkinson, T., Hitchcock, C., Falconer, D. J., et al. (1998). Fluconazole resistance associated with drug efflux and increased transcription of a drug transporter gene, *PDH1*, in *Candida glabrata. Antimicrob. Agents Chemother.* 42, 1695–1701.

Moen, M. D., Lyseng-Williamson, K. A., and Scott, L. J. (2009). Liposomal amphotericin B: a review of its use as empirical therapy in febrile neutropenia and in the treatment of invasive fungal infections. *Drugs* 69, 361–392. doi: 10.2165/00003495-200969030-00010

Mogavero, S., Tavanti, A., Senesi, S., Rogers, P. D., and Morschhauser, J. (2011). Differential requirement of the transcription factor Mcm1 for activation of the *Candida albicans* multidrug efflux pump MDR1 by its regulators Mrr1 and Cap1. *Antimicrob. Agents Chemother.* 55, 2061–2066. doi: 10.1128/AAC.01467-10

Morio, F., Pagniez, F., Besse, M., Gay-Andrieu, F., Miegeville, M., and Le Pape, P. (2013). Deciphering azole resistance mechanisms with a focus on transcription factor-encoding genes TAC1, MRR1 and UPC2 in a set of fluconazole-resistant clinical isolates of *Candida albicans. Int. J. Antimicrob. Agents* 42, 410–415. doi: 10.1016/j.ijantimicag.2013.07.013

Morschhauser, J. (2002). The genetic basis of fluconazole resistance development in *Candida albicans. Biochim. Biophys. Acta* 1587, 240–248. doi: 10.1016/S0925-4439(02)00087-X

Morschhauser, J. (2010). Regulation of multidrug resistance in pathogenic fungi. *Fungal Genet. Biol.* 47, 94–106. doi: 10.1016/j.fgb.2009.08.002

Morschhauser, J., Barker, K. S., Liu, T. T., Blab-Warmuth, J., Homayouni, R., and Rogers, P. D. (2007). The transcription factor Mrr1p controls expression of the MDR1 efflux pump and mediates multidrug resistance in *Candida albicans. PLoS Pathog.* 3:e164. doi: 10.1371/journal.ppat.0030164

Moye-Rowley, W. S. (2003a). Regulation of the transcriptional response to oxidative stress in fungi: similarities and differences. *Eukaryot. Cell* 2, 381–389. doi: 10.1128/EC.2.3.381-389.2003

Moye-Rowley, W. S. (2003b). Transcriptional control of multidrug resistance in the yeast Saccharomyces. *Prog. Nucleic Acids Res. Mol. Biol.* 73, 251–279. doi: 10.1016/S0079-6603(03)01008-0

Nascimento, A. M., Goldman, G. H., Park, S., Marras, S. A., Delmas, G., Oza, U., et al. (2003). Multiple resistance mechanisms among *Aspergillus fumigatus* mutants with high-level resistance to itraconazole. *Antimicrob. Agents Chemother.* 47, 1719–1726. doi: 10.1128/AAC.47.5.1719-1726.2003

Nivoix, Y., Velten, M., Letscher-Bru, V., Moghaddam, A., Natarajan-Ame, S., Fohrer, C., et al. (2008). Factors associated with overall and attributable mortality in invasive aspergillosis. *Clin. Infect. Dis.* 47, 1176–1184. doi: 10.1086/592255

Nourani, A., Papajova, D., Delahodde, A., Jacq, C., and Subik, J. (1997). Clustered amino acid substitutions in the yeast transcription regulator Pdr3p increase pleiotropic drug resistance and identify a new central regulatory domain. *Mol. Gen. Genet.* 256, 397–405. doi: 10.1007/s004380050583

Ostrosky-Zeichner, L., Rex, J., Pappas, P., Hamill, R. J., Larsen, R. A., Horowitz, H. W., et al. (2003). Antifungal susceptibility survey of 2,000 bloodstream Candida *Antimicrob Agents Chemother* 47, 3149–3154. doi: 10.1128/AAC.47.10.3149-3154.2003

Owsianik, G., Balzi, E., and Ghislain, M. (2002). Control of 26S proteasome expression by transcription factors regulating multidrug resistance in *Saccharomyces cerevisiae. Mol. Microbiol.* 43, 1295–1308. doi: 10.1046/j.1365-2958.2002.02823.x

Panwar, S. L., and Moye-Rowley, W. S. (2006). Long chain base tolerance in *Saccharomyces cerevisiae* is induced by retrograde signals from the mitochondria. *J. Biol. Chem.* 281, 6376–6384. doi: 10.1074/jbc.M512115200

Pappas, P. G., Kauffman, C. A., Andes, D., Benjamin, D. K. Jr., Calandra, T. F., Edwards, J. E., et al. (2009). Clinical practice guidelines for the management of candidiasis: 2009 update by the Infectious Diseases Society of America. *Clin. Infect. Dis.* 48, 503–535. doi: 10.1086/596757

Paul, S., Diekema, D., and Moye-Rowley, W. S. (2013). Contributions of *Aspergillus fumigatus* ATP-binding cassette transporter proteins to drug resistance and virulence. *Eukaryot. Cell* 12, 1619–1628. doi: 10.1128/EC.00171-13

Paul, S., Schmidt, J. A., and Moye-Rowley, W. S. (2011). Regulation of the CgPdr1 transcription factor from the pathogen *Candida glabrata. Eukaryot. Cell* 10, 187–197. doi: 10.1128/EC.00277-10

Pfaller, M. A. (2012). Antifungal drug resistance: mechanisms, epidemiology, and consequences for treatment. *Am. J. Med.* 125, S3–S13. doi: 10.1016/j.amjmed.2011.11.001

Pfaller, M. A., Boyken, L., Hollis, R. J., Kroeger, J., Messer, S. A., Tendolkar, S., et al. (2008). *In vitro* susceptibility of invasive isolates of Candida spp. to anidulafungin, caspofungin, and micafungin: six years of global surveillance. *J. Clin. Microbiol.* 46, 150–156. doi: 10.1128/JCM.01901-07

Pfaller, M. A., Castanheira, M., Lockhart, S. R., Ahlquist, A. M., Messer, S. A., and Jones, R. N. (2012). Frequency of decreased susceptibility and resistance to echinocandins among fluconazole-resistant bloodstream isolates of *Candida glabrata. J. Clin. Microbiol.* 50, 1199–1203. doi: 10.1128/JCM.06112-11

Pfaller, M. A., and Diekema, D. J. (2007). Epidemiology of invasive candidiasis: a persistent public health problem. *Clin. Microbiol. Rev.* 20, 133–163. doi: 10.1128/CMR.00029-06

Pfaller, M. A., Messer, S. A., Boyken, L., Hollis, R. J., Rice, C., Tendolkar, S., et al. (2004). *In vitro* activities of voriconazole, posaconazole, and fluconazole against 4,169 clinical isolates of Candida spp. and Cryptococcus neoformans collected during 2001 and 2002 in the ARTEMIS global antifungal surveillance program. *Diagn. Microbiol. Infect. Dis.* 48, 201–205. doi: 10.1016/j.diagmicrobio.2003.09.008

Poss, Z. C., Ebmeier, C. C., and Taatjes, D. J. (2013). The Mediator complex and transcription regulation. *Crit. Rev. Biochem. Mol. Biol.* 48, 575–608. doi: 10.3109/10409238.2013.840259

Pound, M. W., Townsend, M. L., Dimondi, V., Wilson, D., and Drew, R. H. (2011). Overview of treatment options for invasive fungal infections. *Med. Mycol.* 49, 561–580. doi: 10.3109/13693786.2011.560197

Prasad, R., Dewergifosse, P., Goffeau, A., and Balzi, E. (1995). Molecular cloning and characterization of a novel gene of *Candida albicans, CDR1,* conferring multiple resistance to drugs and antifungals. *Curr. Genet.* 27, 320–329. doi: 10.1007/BF00352101

Prasad, R., and Goffeau, A. (2012). Yeast ATP-Binding cassette transporters conferring multidrug resistance. *Annu. Rev. Microbiol.* 39–63. doi: 10.1146/annurev-micro-092611-150111

Prasad, T., Saini, P., Gaur, N. A., Vishwakarma, R. A., Khan, L. A., Haq, Q. M., et al. (2005). Functional analysis of CaIPT1, a sphingolipid biosynthetic gene involved in multidrug resistance and morphogenesis of *Candida albicans. Antimicrob. Agents Chemother.* 49, 3442–3452. doi: 10.1128/AAC.49.8.3442-3452.2005

Pratt, W. B., and Toft, D. O. (1997). Steroid receptor interactions with heat shock protein and immunophilin chaperones. *Endocr. Rev.* 18, 306–360.

Prunuske, A. J., Waltner, J. K., Kuhn, P., Gu, B., and Craig, E. A. (2012). Role for the molecular chaperones Zuo1 and Ssz1 in quorum sensing via activation of the transcription factor Pdr1. *Proc. Natl. Acad. Sci. U.S.A.* 109, 472–477. doi: 10.1073/pnas.1119184109

Qiao, J., Liu, W., and Li, R. (2010). Truncated Afyap1 attenuates antifungal susceptibility of *Aspergillus fumigatus* to voriconazole and confers adaptation of the fungus to oxidative stress. *Mycopathologia* 170, 155–160. doi: 10.1007/s11046-010-9309-2

Rajendran, R., Mowat, E., Mcculloch, E., Lappin, D. F., Jones, B., Lang, S., et al. (2011). Azole resistance of *Aspergillus fumigatus* biofilms is partly associated with efflux pump activity. *Antimicrob. Agents Chemother.* 55, 2092–2097. doi: 10.1128/AAC.01189-10

Rank, G. H., and Bech-Hansen, N. T. (1973). Single nuclear gene inherited cross resistance and collateral sensitivity to 17 inhibitors of mitochondrial function in *Saccharomyces cerevisiae. Mol. Gen. Genet.* 126, 93–102. doi: 10.1007/BF00330986

Rank, G. H., Gerlach, J. H., and Robertson, A. J. (1976). Some physiological alterations associated with pleiotropic cross resistance and collateral sensitivity in *Saccharomyces cerevisiae. Mole. Gen. Genet.* 144, 281–288. doi: 10.1007/BF00341726

Rank, G. H., Robertson, A. J., and Phillips, K. L. (1975). Modification and inheritance of pleiotropic cross resistance and collateral sensitivity in *Saccharomcyes cerevisiae. Genetics* 80, 783–793.

Redding, S. W., Kirkpatrick, W. R., Saville, S., Coco, B. J., White, W., Fothergill, A., et al. (2003). Multiple patterns of resistance to fluconazole in *Candida glabrata* isolates from a patient with oropharyngeal candidiasis receiving head and neck radiation. *J. Clin. Microbiol.* 41, 619–622. doi: 10.1128/JCM.41.2.619-622.2003

Richter, S. S., Galask, R. P., Messer, S. A., Hollis, R. J., Diekema, D. J., and Pfaller, M. A. (2005). Antifungal susceptibilities of Candida species causing vulvovaginitis and epidemiology of recurrent cases. *J. Clin. Microbiol.* 43, 2155–2162. doi: 10.1128/JCM.43.5.2155-2162.2005

Rodrigues-Pousada, C. A., Nevitt, T., Menezes, R., Azevedo, D., Pereira, J., and Amaral, C. (2004). Yeast activator proteins and stress response: an overview. *FEBS Lett.* 567, 80–85. doi: 10.1016/j.febslet.2004.03.119

Rognon, B., Kozovska, Z., Coste, A. T., Pardini, G., and Sanglard, D. (2006). Identification of promoter elements responsible for the regulation of MDR1 from *Candida albicans,* a major facilitator transporter involved in azole resistance. *Microbiology* 152, 3701–3722. doi: 10.1099/mic.0.29277-0

Rustad, T. R., Stevens, D. A., Pfaller, M. A., and White, T. C. (2002). Homozygosity at the *Candida albicans* MTL locus associated with azole resistance. *Microbiology* 148, 1061–1072.

Sanglard, D., Coste, A., and Ferrari, S. (2009). Antifungal drug resistance mechanisms in fungal pathogens from the perspective of transcriptional gene regulation. *FEMS Yeast Res.* 9, 1029–1050. doi: 10.1111/j.1567-1364.2009.00578.x

Sanglard, D., Ischer, F., Monod, M., and Bille, J. (1997). Cloning of *Candida albicans* genes conferring resistance to azole antifungal agents: characterization of *CDR2*, a new multidrug ABC transporter gene. *Microbiology* 143, 405–416. doi: 10.1099/00221287-143-2-405

Sanglard, D., Kuchler, K., Ischer, F., Pagani, J. L., Monod, M., and Bille, J. (1995). Mechanisms of resistance to azole antifungal agents in *Candida albicans* isolates from AIDS patients involve specific multidrug transporters. *Antimicrob. Agents Chemotherap.* 40, 2378–2386. doi: 10.1128/AAC.39.11.2378

Sanguinetti, M., Posteraro, B., Fiori, B., Ranno, S., Torelli, R., and Fadda, G. (2005). Mechanisms of azole resistance in clinical isolates of *Candida glabrata* collected during a hospital survey of antifungal resistance. *Antimicrob. Agents Chemother.* 49, 668–679. doi: 10.1128/AAC.49.2.668-679.2005

Sasse, C., Dunkel, N., Schafer, T., Schneider, S., Dierolf, F., Ohlsen, K., et al. (2012). The stepwise acquisition of fluconazole resistance mutations causes a gradual loss of fitness in *Candida albicans. Mol. Microbiol.* 86, 539–556. doi: 10.1111/j.1365-2958.2012.08210.x

Sasse, C., Schillig, R., Dierolf, F., Weyler, M., Schneider, S., Mogavero, S., et al. (2011). The transcription factor Ndt80 does not contribute to Mrr1-, Tac1-, and Upc2-mediated fluconazole resistance in *Candida albicans. PLoS ONE* 6:e25623. doi: 10.1371/journal.pone.0025623

Saunders, G. W., and Rank, G. H. (1982). Allelism of pleiotropic drug resistance in *S. cerevisiae. Can. J. Genet. Cytol.* 24, 493–502.

Schnell, N., Krems, B., and Entian, K.-D. (1992). The PAR1 (YAP1/SNQ3) gene of *Saccharomyces cerevisiae*, a c-jun homolog, is involved in oxygen metabolism. *Curr. Genet.* 21, 269–273. doi: 10.1007/BF00351681

Schubert, S., Barker, K. S., Znaidi, S., Schneider, S., Dierolf, F., Dunkel, N., et al. (2011a). Regulation of efflux pump expression and drug resistance by the transcription factors Mrr1, Upc2, and Cap1 in *Candida albicans. Antimicrob. Agents Chemother.* 55, 2212–2223. doi: 10.1128/AAC.01343-10

Schubert, S., Popp, C., Rogers, P. D., and Morschhauser, J. (2011b). Functional dissection of a *Candida albicans* zinc cluster transcription factor, the multidrug resistance regulator Mrr1. *Eukaryot. Cell* 10, 1110–1121. doi: 10.1128/EC.05100-11

Schuetzer-Muehlbauer, M., Willinger, B., Krapf, G., Enzinger, S., Presterl, E., and Kuchler, K. (2003). The *Candida albicans* Cdr2p ATP-binding cassette (ABC) transporter confers resistance to caspofungin. *Mol. Microbiol.* 48, 225–235. doi: 10.1046/j.1365-2958.2003.03430.x

Selmecki, A., Gerami-Nejad, M., Paulson, C., Forche, A., and Berman, J. (2008). An isochromosome confers drug resistance *in vivo* by amplification of two genes, ERG11 and TAC1. *Mol. Microbiol.* 68, 624–641. doi: 10.1111/j.1365-2958.2008.06176.x

Shahi, P., Gulshan, K., and Moye-Rowley, W. S. (2007). Negative transcriptional regulation of multidrug resistance gene expression by an Hsp70 protein. *J. Biol. Chem.* 282, 26822–26831. doi: 10.1074/jbc.M704772200

Shahi, P., Gulshan, K., Naar, A. M., and Moye-Rowley, W. S. (2010). Differential roles of transcriptional mediator subunits in regulation of multidrug resistance gene expression in *Saccharomyces cerevisiae. Mol. Biol. Cell* 21, 2469–2482. doi: 10.1091/mbc.E09-10-0899

Simonics, T., Kozovska, Z., Michalkova-Papajova, D., Delahodde, A., Jacq, C., and Subik, J. (2000). Isolation and molecular characterization of the carboxy-terminal *pdr3* mutants in *Saccharomyces cerevisiae. Curr. Genet.* 38, 248–255. doi: 10.1007/s002940000164

Slaven, J. W., Anderson, M. J., Sanglard, D., Dixon, G. K., Bille, J., Roberts, I. S., et al. (2002). Increased expression of a novel *Aspergillus fumigatus* ABC transporter gene, atrF, in the presence of itraconazole in an itraconazole resistant clinical isolate. *Fungal Genet. Biol.* 36, 199–206. doi: 10.1016/S1087-1845(02)00016-6

Snelders, E., Van Der Lee, H. A., Kuijpers, J., Rijs, A. J., Varga, J., Samson, R. A., et al. (2008). Emergence of azole resistance in *Aspergillus fumigatus* and spread of a single resistance mechanism. *PLoS Med.* 5:e219. doi: 10.1371/journal.pmed.0050219

Steier, Z., Vermitsky, J. P., Toner, G., Gygax, S. E., Edlind, T., and Katiyar, S. (2013). Flucytosine antagonism of azole activity versus *Candida glabrata*: role of transcription factor Pdr1 and multidrug transporter Cdr1. *Antimicrob. Agents Chemother.* 57, 5543–5547. doi: 10.1128/AAC.02394-12

Szakacs, G., Paterson, J. K., Ludwig, J. A., Booth-Genthe, C., and Gottesman, M. M. (2006). Targeting multidrug resistance in cancer. *Nat. Rev. Drug Discov.* 5, 219–234. doi: 10.1038/nrd1984

Sze, J. Y., Remboutsika, E., and Kohlhaw, G. B. (1993). Transcriptional regulator Leu3 of *Saccharomyces cerevisiae*: separation of activator and repressor functions. *Mol. Cell. Biol.* 13, 5702–5709.

Te Dorsthorst, D. T., Verweij, P. E., Meletiadis, J., Bergervoet, M., Punt, N. C., Meis, J. F., et al. (2002). *In vitro* interaction of flucytosine combined with amphotericin B or fluconazole against thirty-five yeast isolates determined by both the fractional inhibitory concentration index and the response surface approach. *Antimicrob. Agents Chemother.* 46, 2982–2989. doi: 10.1128/AAC.46.9.2982-2989.2002

Teixeira, M. C., Dias, P. J., Simoes, T., and Sa-Correia, I. (2008). Yeast adaptation to mancozeb involves the up-regulation of FLR1 under the coordinate control of Yap1, Rpn4, Pdr3, and Yrr1. *Biochem. Biophys. Res. Commun.* 367, 249–255. doi: 10.1016/j.bbrc.2007.12.056

Thakur, J. K., Arthanari, H., Yang, F., Pan, S.-J., Fan, X., Breger, J., et al. (2008). A nuclear receptor-like pathway regulating multidrug resistance in fungi. *Nature* 452, 604–609. doi: 10.1038/nature06836

Toone, W. M., Morgan, B. A., and Jones, N. (2001). Redox control of AP-1-like factors in yeast and beyond. *Oncogene* 20, 2336–2346. doi: 10.1038/sj.onc.1204384

Torelli, R., Posteraro, B., Ferrari, S., La Sorda, M., Fadda, G., Sanglard, D., et al. (2008). The ATP-binding cassette transporter-encoding gene CgSNQ2 is contributing to the CgPDR1-dependent azole resistance of *Candida glabrata. Mol. Microbiol.* 68, 186–201. doi: 10.1111/j.1365-2958.2008.06143.x

Traven, A., Wong, J. M., Xu, D., Sopta, M., and Ingles, C. J. (2001). Interorganellar communication. Altered nuclear gene expression profiles in a yeast mitochondrial DNA mutant. *J. Biol. Chem.* 276, 4020–4027. doi: 10.1074/jbc.M006807200

Tsai, H. F., Krol, A. A., Sarti, K. E., and Bennett, J. E. (2006). *Candida glabrata* PDR1, a transcriptional regulator of a pleiotropic drug resistance network, mediates azole resistance in clinical isolates and petite mutants. *Antimicrob. Agents Chemother.* 50, 1384–1392. doi: 10.1128/AAC.50.4.1384-1392.2006

Van Den Hazel, H. B., Pichler, H., Do Valle Matta, M. A., Leitner, E., Goffeau, A., and Daum, G. (1999). *PDR16* and *PDR17*, two homologous genes of *Saccharomyces cerevisiae*, affect lipid biosynthesis and resistance to multiple drugs. *J. Biol. Chem.* 274, 1934–1941. doi: 10.1074/jbc.274.4.1934

Van Der Linden, J. W., Snelders, E., Kampinga, G. A., Rijnders, B. J., Mattsson, E., Debets-Ossenkopp, Y. J., et al. (2011). Clinical implications of azole resistance in *Aspergillus fumigatus*, The Netherlands, 2007-2009. *Emerging Infect. Dis.* 17, 1846–1854. doi: 10.3201/eid1710.110226

Vermitsky, J. P., and Edlind, T. D. (2004). Azole resistance in *Candida glabrata*: coordinate upregulation of multidrug transporters and evidence for a Pdr1-like transcription factor. *Antimicrob. Agents Chemother.* 48, 3773–3781. doi: 10.1128/AAC.48.10.3773-3781.2004

Voelker, D. R. (1997). Phosphatidylserine decarboxylase. *Biochim. Biophys. Acta* 1348, 236–244. doi: 10.1016/S0005-2760(97)00101-X

White, T. C. (1997). Increased mRNA levels of *ERG16*, *CDR* and *MDR1* correlate with increases in azole resistance in *Candida albicans* isolates from a patient infected with human immunodeficiency virus. *Antimicrob. Agents Chemother.* 41, 1482–1487.

Wirsching, S., Michel, S., and Morschhauser, J. (2000). Targeted gene disruption in *Candida albicans* wild-type strains: the role of the MDR1 gene in fluconazole resistance of clinical *Candida albicans* isolates. *Mol. Microbiol.* 36, 856–865. doi: 10.1046/j.1365-2958.2000.01899.x

Wu, A., Wemmie, J. A., Edgington, N. P., Goebl, M., Guevara, J. L., and Moye-Rowley, W. S. (1993). Yeast bZIP proteins mediate pleiotropic drug and metal resistance. *J. Biol. Chem.* 268, 18850–18858.

Zhang, L., Hach, A., and Wang, C. (1998). Molecular mechanism governing heme signaling in yeast: a higher-order complex mediates heme regulation of the transcriptional activator HAP1. *Mol. Cell. Biol.* 18, 3819–3828.

Zhang, X., Cui, Z., Miyakawa, T., and Moye-Rowley, W. S. (2001). Cross-talk between transcriptional regulators of multidrug resistance in *Saccharomyces cerevisiae. J. Biol. Chem.* 276, 8812–8819. doi: 10.1074/jbc.M010686200

Zhang, X., Kolaczkowska, A., Devaux, F., Panwar, S. L., Hallstrom, T. C., Jacq, C., et al. (2005). Transcriptional regulation by Lge1p requires a function independent of its role in histone H2B ubiquitination. *J. Biol. Chem.* 280, 2759–2770. doi: 10.1074/jbc.M408333200

Zhang, X., and Moye-Rowley, W. S. (2001). *Saccharomyces cerevisiae* multidrug resistance gene expression inversely correlates with the status of the Fo component of the mitochondrial ATPase. *J. Biol. Chem.* 276, 47844–47852. doi: 10.1074/jbc.M106285200

Znaidi, S., De Deken, X., Weber, S., Rigby, T., Nantel, A., and Raymond, M. (2007). The zinc cluster transcription factor Tac1p regulates PDR16 expression in *Candida albicans*. *Mol. Microbiol.* 66, 440–452. doi: 10.1111/j.1365-2958.2007.05931.x

9

Complex interplay between the P-glycoprotein multidrug efflux pump and the membrane: its role in modulating protein function

Frances Jane Sharom*

Department of Molecular and Cellular Biology, University of Guelph, Guelph, ON, Canada

Edited by:
Stefania Nobili, University of Florence, Italy

Reviewed by:
Marc Poirot, Institut National de la Santé et de la Recherche Médicale, France
Saibal Dey, Uniformed Services University of the Health Sciences, USA

****Correspondence:***
Frances Jane Sharom, Department of Molecular and Cellular Biology, University of Guelph, Guelph, ON N1G 2W1, Canada
e-mail: fsharom@uoguelph.ca

Multidrug resistance in cancer is linked to expression of the P-glycoprotein multidrug transporter (Pgp, ABCB1), which exports many structurally diverse compounds from cells. Substrates first partition into the bilayer and then interact with a large flexible binding pocket within the transporter's transmembrane regions. Pgp has been described as a hydrophobic vacuum cleaner or an outwardly directed drug/lipid flippase. Recent X-ray crystal structures have shed some light on the nature of the drug-binding pocket and suggested routes by which substrates can enter it from the membrane. Detergents have profound effects on Pgp function, and several appear to be substrates. Biochemical and biophysical studies *in vitro*, some using purified reconstituted protein, have explored the effects of the membrane environment. They have demonstrated that Pgp is involved in a complex relationship with its lipid environment, which modulates the behavior of its substrates, as well as various functions of the protein, including ATP hydrolysis, drug binding, and drug transport. Membrane lipid composition and fluidity, phospholipid headgroup and acyl chain length all influence Pgp function. Recent studies focusing on thermodynamics and kinetics have revealed some important principles governing Pgp–lipid and substrate–lipid interactions, and how these affect drug-binding and transport. In some cells, Pgp is associated with cholesterol-rich microdomains, which may modulate its functions. The relationship between Pgp and cholesterol remains an open question; however, it clearly affects several aspects of its function in addition to substrate–membrane partitioning. The action of Pgp modulators appears to depend on their membrane permeability, and membrane fluidizers and surfactants reverse drug resistance, likely via an indirect mechanism. A detailed understanding of how the membrane affects Pgp substrates and Pgp's catalytic cycle may lead to new strategies to combat clinical drug resistance.

Keywords: P-glycoprotein (ABCB1), phospholipids, detergents, cholesterol, ATP hydrolysis, membrane partitioning, membrane transport, drug binding

INTRODUCTION

Many human cancers, including breast, kidney, and colon carcinomas, leukemias, multiple myeloma, and several pediatric cancers, develop multidrug resistance (MDR), which is a major obstacle to chemotherapeutic treatment (1, 2). MDR tumors are cross-resistant to a broad spectrum of structurally unrelated cytotoxic drugs, including the *Vinca* alkaloids (vinblastine, vincristine), anthracyclines (doxorubicin, daunorubicin), and taxanes. Physiologically, a complex network of ATP-binding cassette (ABC) proteins is involved in drug detoxification and protection of tissues from xenobiotics, including administered therapeutic drugs. Three of these ATP-driven drug efflux pumps are widely expressed in tumors, and have been linked to drug resistance; P-glycoprotein (Pgp; ABCB1), ABCG2 and ABCC1 (MRP1) (3, 4). Pgp and MRP1 exist as large single polypeptides, whereas ABCG2 is a "half-transporter" that functions as a homodimer. Together, these three proteins are able to carry out efflux of a wide range of anti-cancer drugs that are in common use clinically. The ability to inhibit the action of these drug efflux pumps has the potential to greatly improve the outcome of chemotherapy treatment, and the development of strategies to achieve this has been ongoing for many years.

Since Pgp was the first ABC drug efflux pump to be identified (5), and has been intensively studied for more than 35 years, it is the one we know most about. Hundreds of Pgp substrates have been identified over the years, including many clinically used drugs, chemotherapeutic agents, natural products, linear and cyclic peptides, amphiphiles, and fluorescent dyes (3, 4). The protein displays basal ATPase activity, which is often (but not always) stimulated by substrates, and it hydrolyzes ATP to power active transport, generating a drug concentration gradient across the membrane (6). Pgp and other ABC transporters are believed to operate by an alternating access model. The first step in transport involves binding of drug to the inward-facing conformation from the cytosolic side of the membrane. This is followed by a switch to the outward-facing conformation, which reorients the binding site to the extracellular side, resulting in drug release. ATP hydrolysis provides the energy for the switch between these two conformations. Despite recent progress in determining the high resolution structure of Pgp, there are still many gaps in our understanding of how the protein functions at the molecular level.

It was evident some time ago that the host membrane plays a central role in Pgp-mediated MDR (7, 8), and the complexity of this relationship has become more apparent as our knowledge of the protein has advanced. First, the membrane has a profound effect on Pgp's lipophilic substrates, affecting both their lipid partitioning and transbilayer movement. Second, many aspects of Pgp structure (such as its stability and conformation) and function (including ATP binding, ATP hydrolysis, drug binding, and drug transport) are especially sensitive to the properties and composition of the surrounding membrane. It is important to understand how Pgp function is modulated by membrane properties, since this may influence transporter activity in tumors. Indeed, MDR was successfully reversed *in vitro* simply by altering the biophysical characteristics of the membrane (9). Changing membrane properties may thus be a useful approach for clinical reversal of MDR. The importance of the membrane in drug efflux also suggests additional approaches for development of new anti-cancer drugs and modulators with increased clinical effectiveness; for example, chemical modification of existing compounds may alter their interactions with the membrane, and their ability to access Pgp. If such strategies are to be successful, it is clearly important to have a detailed understanding of how the properties of the lipid environment affect all aspects of the Pgp catalytic cycle.

This review focuses on the complexity of the interactions of Pgp and its substrates with their membrane environment, the effect of these interactions on many different aspects of Pgp function, and how understanding them can help shed light on the molecular details of drug transport. Our current knowledge of Pgp has been gleaned from both *in vitro* and cellular studies of the transporter. The majority of these studies have been carried out with either rodent Pgp (Chinese hamster and mouse) or the human protein. The latter is clearly the clinically important homolog, but (as discussed further below) high resolution structures are currently available only for the mouse and *Caenorhabditis elegans* proteins. The rodent Pgps are highly active, relatively stable, and have proved extremely useful for *in vitro* studies of the structure and mechanism of action of the purified protein. The human protein, on the other hand, appears to be relatively unstable and is more difficult to express and purify [e.g., Ref. (10)]. The rodent Pgps are very closely related to the human homolog (e.g., 87% sequence identity and 93% sequence similarity between Chinese hamster and human Pgp), and only small differences in substrate specificity have been observed in cell-based transport assays. Recent work using purified hamster Pgp in a liposomal assay system to quantify drug interactions reported that results correlated very well with clinically relevant data on disposition of Pgp transport substrates in human subjects (11). Rodent Pgps thus remain very important models for understanding the function of the human protein.

PGP IN HUMAN CANCER: ITS ROLE AND POTENTIAL MODULATION

P-glycoprotein expression is widespread in clinical cancer. The U.S. National Cancer Institute uses a panel of 60 tumor cell lines to identify and evaluate new anti-cancer agents. Expression of Pgp was detected in 39 of these cell lines, including renal and colon carcinomas, melanomas, and central nervous system tumors (12). Expression of Pgp was also highly correlated with resistance of these cell lines to anti-cancer drugs. Pgp has also been found in many human tumors (13, 14), with levels often increasing substantially after one or more rounds of chemotherapy, especially in acute myelogenous leukemia and lymphomas. Even very low levels of Pgp that are difficult to detect in tumor tissue significantly affect the sensitivity of cells to drugs. Although multiple mechanisms are undoubtedly responsible for drug resistance *in vivo* (15), Pgp is the single most important cause of MDR, representing an attractive target for intervention. Pgp expression has been linked to reduced responses to chemotherapy and poor clinical outcome for breast cancer, sarcomas, hematological malignancies such as leukemias, and pediatric cancers [reviewed in Refs. (1, 16)]. An important goal in cancer therapy has been the development of compounds that can effectively inhibit Pgp-mediated MDR. Such modulators (also known as chemosensitizers) have been identified based on their ability to reverse drug resistance in MDR cells *in vitro*. Pgp modulators commonly used in biochemical studies include verapamil and cyclosporin A. Since MDR is probably the single greatest barrier to successful chemotherapy, the ability to circumvent Pgp-mediated drug resistance could lead to improved treatment outcomes.

Three different strategies for defeating Pgp have been described (1); "engage" (co-administration of anti-cancer drugs and modulators), "evade" (the use of anti-cancer drugs that are poor Pgp substrates), and "exploit" (specific targeting of the Pgp molecule). Many clinical trials have been carried out to evaluate the hypothesis that co-administration of modulators would improve the effectiveness of chemotherapy drugs, thus leading to increased efficacy in patients [reviewed in Ref. (16)]. Early promising results obtained for pediatric cancers using cyclosporin A (17) generated optimism that this approach might be useful in tumors where Pgp expression is the primary cause of MDR. However, success in adult cancers has been elusive, in part because of poor clinical trial design and patient selection, and also because first and second generation modulators showed toxicity, sub-optimal effectiveness, and serious pharmacokinetic drug interactions (16, 18, 19). Since then, much more potent and less toxic third generation modulators have been developed to target Pgp specifically, such as LY336979 (zosuquidar) and XR9576 (tariquidar). However, they, too, failed to improve patient outcome in clinical trials [see Ref. (16)]. Several non-toxic plant natural products have also been proposed as MDR modulators, including curcumin (20), polyphenols (21), and flavonoids (22), however, these have not yet been tested in clinical trials. Given the disappointing outcome of the modulator strategy to date, it is not clear whether this line of attack will be successful. Designing novel approaches to specifically target Pgp in MDR will require detailed knowledge of the various steps in the catalytic cycle.

VACUUM CLEANER AND FLIPPASE MODELS FOR PGP FUNCTION

PGP AS A HYDROPHOBIC VACUUM CLEANER

The compounds that Pgp transports are typically lipophilic, so they accumulate within the lipid bilayer. Pgp substrates are also generally amphipathic molecules, and rather than distributing uniformly in the hydrophobic core of the lipid bilayer, they align themselves in the interfacial region. NMR studies have shown that they tend to concentrate between the lipid headgroup and the first few carbon atoms of the lipid acyl chains (23). Early work strongly suggested that Pgp effluxes drugs directly from the membrane, rather than the aqueous phase (6). Acetoxymethyl ester derivatives of various fluorescent calcium and pH indicators entering intact cells from the extracellular side are intercepted and extruded without entering the cytosol (24). A Förster resonance energy transfer (FRET) study in which the transporter was photolabeled with the lipophilic probe iodonaphthalene-1-azide showed that the substrate doxorubicin was present within the membrane close to Pgp (25). This suggested that Pgp may interact with its substrates within the membrane and subsequently efflux them to the extracellular medium. These observations and others led to the proposal by Higgins and Gottesman that the transporter was a hydrophobic "vacuum cleaner" (**Figure 1**) responsible for removal of potentially harmful lipophilic compounds from the membrane (26). Later work showed that the rate of Hoechst 33342 efflux by Pgp was directly proportional to the membrane concentration of the fluorescent dye, but inversely proportional to its aqueous concentration, supporting the idea that transport takes place from the bilayer interior (27). In addition, studies employing a deletion mutant of Pgp showed that the transmembrane (TM) domains of the transporter were sufficient to bind drug substrates (28). The vacuum cleaner model is now widely accepted, and was a key concept in our understanding of the relationship between Pgp and its membrane environment.

Transport studies using reconstituted Pgp, plasma membrane vesicles, and intact MDR cells showed that several fluorescent substrates (Hoechst 33342, LDS-751, and a rhodamine derivative)

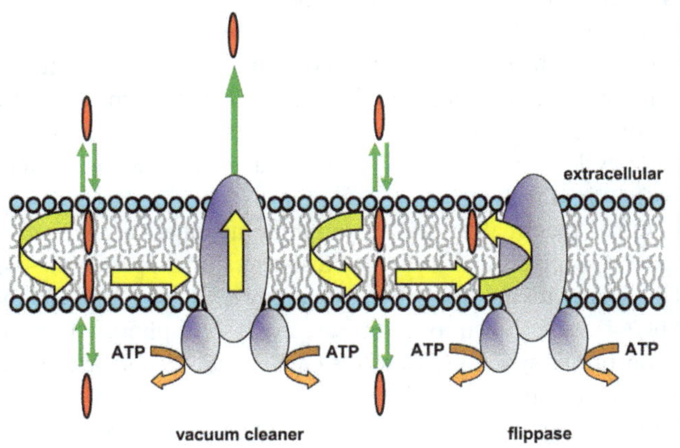

FIGURE 1 | Hydrophobic vacuum cleaner and flippase models of Pgp function. In the vacuum cleaner model, drugs partition into the membrane, spontaneously translocate to the cytoplasmic leaflet, and gain access to the Pgp substrate-binding pocket from within the bilayer interior. They are subsequently effluxed into the extracellular aqueous phase. In the flippase model, drugs partition into the membrane, spontaneously translocate to the inner leaflet, interact with the Pgp substrate-binding pocket, and are then flipped to the outer membrane leaflet. The drug concentration will be higher in the outer leaflet compared to the inner leaflet, and a concentration gradient is generated when drugs rapidly partition from the two membrane leaflets into the aqueous phase on either side of the membrane.

were extracted from the cytoplasmic membrane leaflet (29–31). FRET studies designed to pinpoint the location of the binding sites for Hoechst 33342 and LDS-751 also showed that they were situated within the TM regions of Pgp, in the cytoplasmic leaflet of the membrane (32, 33). The recent X-ray crystal structures of Pgp from mouse (34) and *C. elegans* (35) have allowed a closer view of the potential routes that substrate molecules may follow from the bilayer inner leaflet into the binding pocket of the protein (see below).

PGP AS A DRUG AND LIPID FLIPPASE

P-glycoprotein may be envisaged as expelling its substrates directly into the extracellular medium, which would have an energy cost for lipophilic species. The protein has also been proposed to operate as a drug translocase or flippase (**Figure 1**), moving its substrates from the inner to the outer leaflet of the membrane (26). This mechanism requires that drug molecules have a specific localization within each bilayer leaflet, rather than being randomly distributed in the hydrophobic core. An NMR study of Pgp substrates and modulators confirmed that this is the case, and showed that these molecules align with the phospholipid acyl chains (23). After reaching the outer leaflet, substrates would then either passively diffuse into the extracellular aqueous phase (a very fast process), or move back to the inner leaflet by spontaneous flip–flop. In order to maintain a substrate concentration gradient across the membrane, the rate of passive transbilayer flip–flop of substrate would need to be slower than the rate of Pgp-mediated flipping, so that its concentration remains higher in the outer leaflet. Indeed, the rate of drug movement between leaflets is variable, and can be quite slow, with half-times ranging from minutes to hours depending on the structure of the compound (36, 37). The flippase model involves delivery of drug to the outer leaflet, followed by rapid partitioning into the extracellular medium, while in the vacuum cleaner model, drug is delivered to the extracellular medium, followed by rapid partitioning into the outer leaflet. Since the same equilibrium state is reached in each case, it is not currently possible to distinguish experimentally between these two models, and they are not mutually exclusive. Energetic considerations suggest that release of a dehydrated lipophilic substrate into the outer membrane leaflet would be energetically more favorable than transfer into the aqueous phase followed by hydration, but it is possible that both of these locations are accessible to the substrate-binding pocket of Pgp during the transport process.

There is substantial evidence supporting the flippase model for Pgp function. Indeed, the protein is able to act as an outwardly directed flippase for several fluorescent phospholipid and glycosphingolipid molecules in both intact cells and reconstituted proteoliposomes. Cells overexpressing native or recombinant Pgp showed altered distribution of fluorescent phosphatidylcholine (PC), phosphatidylethanolamine (PE), and sphingomyelin (SM), accumulated lower amounts of both short- and long-chain fluorescent phospholipid derivatives, and displayed increased outward transport of these analogs, which decreased after treatment with Pgp modulators (38–42). These observations strongly suggested that the lipids were Pgp substrates. Sharom and co-workers showed directly that purified Pgp reconstituted into proteoliposomes can act as a broad-specificity, outwardly directed flippase for a variety of both short-chain and long-chain nitrobenzo-2-oxa-1,3-diazole (NBD)-labeled phospholipids (43). Phospholipids with the fluorescent NBD group on both the acyl chain and the headgroup were translocated. Simple glycosphingolipids, such as glucosyl- and galactosylceramide were also flipped by reconstituted Pgp, as was lactosylceramide, although at a greatly reduced rate (44). Species with headgroups larger than two sugar residues are unlikely to be substrates. Like drug transport, phospholipid and glycolipid flippase activity required ATP hydrolysis, and was inhibited by the phosphate analog, *ortho*-vanadate. Flippase activity was inhibited in a concentration-dependent manner by known Pgp substrates, and inhibitory potency was highly correlated with their Pgp binding affinity, suggesting that drugs and membrane lipids follow the same route through the transporter. Taken together, these observations suggest that Pgp-mediated drug efflux probably takes place by a flippase-like mechanism.

INTERACTION OF LIPIDS AND LIPID-LIKE MOLECULES WITH PGP

Eckford and Sharom (45) used several functional screens to identify a number of lipid-based molecules that interact directly with Pgp with high affinity (**Figure 2**). These compounds resulted in inhibition of ATPase activity, competition for transport of two drugs, and competition for translocation of NBD–PC (16:0, 6:0), suggesting that they are substrates for Pgp. Included in these lipid species are platelet-activating factors (PAFs), ether–phospholipid signaling molecules that are probably endogenous substrates for the transporter (46, 47). Pgp is also able to bind and transport hexadecylphosphocholine (also known as miltefosine), an anti-cancer drug structurally related to PC (48). Other anti-cancer agents such as the alkyl phospholipids, edelfosine, and ilmofosine, and the related compounds, D-20133 and D-21266, also interact with the transporter, leading to resistance (45, 48). In support of these results, yeast cells expressing Pgp were previously reported to be resistant to the cytotoxicity of edelfosine (49). Pgp–lipid interactions thus have important consequences for cancer treatment using these lipid-based drugs.

Metabolic labeling of Pgp, followed by purification and organic solvent extraction, was used to isolate and identify the membrane lipids closely associated with Pgp (50). These proved to be enriched in PE and to a lesser extent phosphatidylserine (PS), but contained little PC or SM, despite the fact that these choline phospholipids are major components of the plasma membrane from which the transporter was solubilized. Thus Pgp associates preferentially with certain phospholipids; in this respect, it is interesting that PE and PS are enriched in the inner leaflet of the plasma membrane, whereas PC and SM are found primarily in the outer leaflet.

A recent mass spectrometry (MS) study (51) examined lipid interactions with Pgp using purified mouse protein in micelles of the detergent *n*-dodecyl-β-D-maltoside (DDM). Gas phase Pgp ions were released and retained only one to two detergent molecules, possibly in the binding pocket. MS could detect simultaneous binding of lipids, drugs, and nucleotides. Estimates of apparent K_d values, which were in the micromolar range, indicated that negatively charged lipids bind to Pgp more favorably than zwitterionic lipids, and both steric effects and headgroup charge modulated binding. Binding of the cyclic peptide, cyclosporin A, was observed to promote subsequent lipid binding. Interestingly, cardiolipin, a bulky anionic mitochondrial lipid, was also able to bind to Pgp. It was suggested that lipid molecules could interact with the transporter inside the large binding cavity and also at the interface between the protein and the lipid bilayer. This novel approach shows promise in the direct study of drug and lipid interactions with Pgp.

PHYSIOLOGICAL ROLE OF PGP–LIPID FLIPPASE ACTIVITY

The physiological significance of Pgp's lipid flippase activity is still the subject of speculation. The protein may be the primary means of exporting PAFs *in vivo*, by translocating them from the cytoplasmic to the extracellular membrane leaflet, from which they can diffuse into the aqueous external environment. Other probable endogenous Pgp substrates include steroid hormones such as aldosterone (52) and β-estradiol-17β-D-glucuronide (53). Indeed, the transporter is known to interact with several steroids (54, 55), and a role in transporting these hormones could explain Pgp expression in the adrenal gland. Pgp may also play a physiological role in the biosynthesis of complex glycosphingolipids in the Golgi by translocating glucosylceramide from the cytoplasmic to the luminal membrane leaflet. The protein most closely related to Pgp, ABCB4 (78% sequence similarity), acts primarily as a PC-specific flippase in the liver, exporting phospholipid into the bile (56, 57), although it can also transport some drugs at a low rate (58). Thus Pgp and ABCB4 may function in a similar manner.

It seems unlikely that the primary role of Pgp *in vivo* is that of a lipid flippase, because the rate of flipping is relatively low (43, 44), and Pgp could not rescue a knockout of ABCB4, even when both proteins were expressed in the liver canalicular membrane (59). However, differing expression levels of each protein could confound this observation. Another consideration is the existence of the plasma membrane aminophospholipid translocase, ATP8a1, which is a member of the P4-ATPase family. This protein normally translocates PE and PS to the inner leaflet, thus maintaining bilayer asymmetry (60). If Pgp moves these endogenous lipids from the inner to the outer leaflet at a significant rate, it would counteract the action of the translocase, resulting in a futile cycle of phospholipid flip–flop accompanied by wasteful hydrolysis of ATP.

Other mammalian ABC superfamily members are known to operate as physiological lipid transporters or flippases (61–63). Three proteins in the ABCA subfamily (ABCA1, ABCA7, and ABCA4) were shown to translocate fluorescent phospholipids in reconstituted systems (64). ABCA1 and ABCA7 transported lipids from the cytoplasmic to the extracellular leaflet, whereas ABCA4 is the only known eukaryotic ABC protein to move substrate in the opposite direction.

PGP STRUCTURE

Like other ABC proteins, Pgp comprises two homologous halves, each consisting of six TM segments, and two nucleotide-binding (NB) domains on the cytosolic side where ATP binds and is hydrolyzed (**Figure 3A**) (65, 66). The NB domains of ABC proteins contain three highly conserved sequences; the Walker A and B motifs (found in many ATP-binding proteins) and the C (or ABC signature) motif that is unique to this superfamily (67). It is now clear that nucleotide binding to ABC transporters is

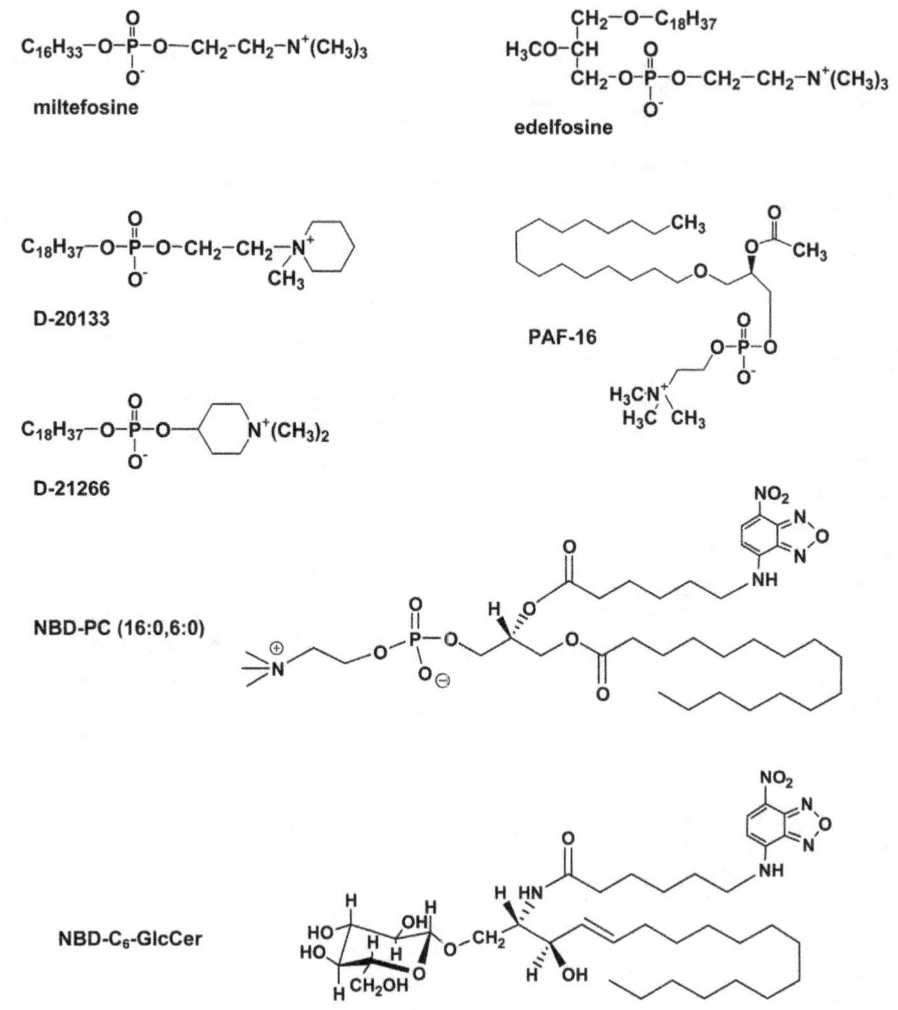

FIGURE 2 | Structures of some lipid-based Pgp substrates.

driven by dimerization of the NB domains (66, 68), which is essential for ATP-driven transport. The X-ray crystal structures of several isolated NB subunits of bacterial ABC proteins showed an interdigitated head-to-tail arrangement, a so-called sandwich dimer. Two ATP molecules are bound at the interface of the sandwich dimer, each interacting with the Walker A and B motifs of one NB domain and the C motif of the partner domain. These stable symmetric dimers are only observed when the NB domains are in an inactive state, either by mutation of an amino acid residue essential for catalysis, or in the absence of Mg^{2+} (69, 70). Thus, they probably do not represent a true catalytic intermediate.

Early electron microscopy (EM) studies provided the first glimpses of Pgp's three-dimensional structure [reviewed in Ref. (71)]. A medium-resolution EM structure of Chinese hamster Pgp at 8-Å resolution was obtained by cryo-electron crystallography of two-dimensional crystals (72). The protein contained bound nucleotide (AMP-PNP), and showed an asymmetric conformation. Other EM studies showed that the two NB domains of Pgp are closely apposed, leading to a closed conformation that was attributed to a sandwich dimer (73, 74).

In the past few years, important advances have been made in understanding the nature of the Pgp-drug-binding pocket [e.g., Ref. (32, 33, 75, 76)]. Mutagenesis studies suggested that the pocket was located at the interface between the two TM halves (77), and this was later confirmed by photoaffinity labeling in conjunction with MS (78, 79). The first X-ray crystal structures of mouse Pgp in an inward-facing conformation appeared in 2009 (34). The structures were determined in the absence of nucleotide, with and without bound cyclic peptide substrates, which are located in a drug-binding pocket within the TM regions of the protein. This large flexible cavity is made up of two bundles of six helices, each composed of portions from both the N- and C-terminal halves (**Figure 3B**). This phenomenon, known as domain swapping, has also been reported for other ABC exporters. The pocket is accessible from the cytoplasmic leaflet of the membrane, as expected. The drug-binding region is partially lined with aromatic and hydrophobic residues, which are proposed to bind substrates via

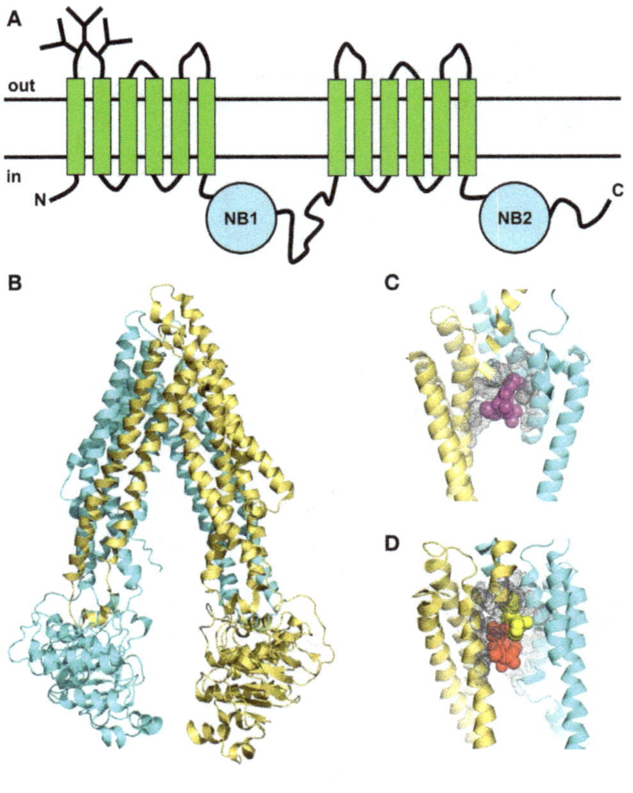

FIGURE 3 | Topology and X-ray crystal structures of Pgp. (A) The membrane topology shows two homologous halves, each with six TM segments and a NB domain on the cytoplasmic side, which binds and hydrolyzes ATP. **(B)** X-ray crystal structure of mouse Pgp (34) shows an inward-facing conformation in the absence of nucleotide (PDB 3G61). **(C,D)** The drug-binding pocket of mouse Pgp as seen in the X-ray crystal structure. **(C)** Close-up view (4.4 Å resolution) of one molecule of the cyclic peptide modulator QZ59-RRR (magenta, space-filling format) occupying the middle site inside the drug-binding pocket, with the volumes of nearby side-chains shown in gray (PDB 3G60). **(D)** Close-up view of two molecules of the cyclic peptide modulator QZ59-SSS occupying the upper and lower sites (yellow and red, respectively, space-filling format) inside the drug-binding pocket, with the volumes of nearby side-chains shown in gray (PDB 3G61).

hydrophobic and van der Waals interactions. Different stereoisomers of the same cyclic peptide substrate are held in different sub-sites by a unique set of interactions, and two molecules of the same substrate can fit into the pocket simultaneously, via different sets of interactions (**Figures 3C,D**). The presence of overlapping sub-sites inside the binding pocket helps to explain the extraordinary range of chemical structures that interact with Pgp. Although the mouse structures are not of very high resolution, they provided some useful information that will help to guide future studies. However, they have not settled any of the outstanding controversies in the field, such as the extent of the separation and movement of the NB domains during the catalytic cycle. Some new mouse Pgp structures show wider separations of the two NB domains (80). One structure shows a complex with a nanobody inhibitor, which appears to inhibit ATP hydrolysis by binding to an epitope on the N-terminal NB domain, thus preventing dimerization of the two domains.

A higher resolution structure (3.4 Δ) of *C. elegans* Pgp in an inward-facing conformation, without bound substrate or nucleotide, appeared in 2012 (35). It shows a portal leading from the cytoplasmic side of the bilayer to the central cavity where substrates are presumed to bind. This structure is compatible with decades of biochemical analysis on the human protein, and helps to explain perplexing functional data on the Phe335Ala mutant. Homology models of human Pgp derived from the *C. elegans* and mouse Pgp structures differ significantly in their orientation of TM helices 3–5, and recent work suggests that the *C. elegans* model is most likely correct (81).

Recent simulation studies of mouse Pgp in a model membrane showed a wide range of NB domain separations, underscoring the apparent high flexibility of the inward-facing protein conformation (82). Of great interest is the observation that the acyl chain of a membrane lipid slid into the cleft between TM helix 4 and TM helix 6, and remained there for the duration of the 50-ns simulation. The tip of the penetrating chain, which was more than 10 carbon atoms long, made contact with several amino acid residues lining the substrate-binding pocket that are known to be involved in drug binding. It is possible that the binding pocket of Pgp may be occupied by endogenous membrane phospholipids in the absence of drug substrates, in line with the idea that it also functions as a low activity lipid flippase. Occupation of the binding pocket by lipids might also explain the high basal ATPase activity observed for Pgp from mouse and Chinese hamster. If these lipids bind with relatively low affinity, they may be displaced by high affinity drug substrates, which would thus be transported preferentially.

To date, only inward-facing conformations of Pgp have been obtained using crystallographic studies, and there is still no nucleotide-bound structure available. Until these two "missing links" are obtained, it will be difficult to make progress on understanding the structural changes that take place during the catalytic and transport cycles. The difficulty in crystallizing Pgp in the outward-facing or nucleotide-bound forms might arise from either the high dynamic flexibility or low stability of these conformations.

MODEL SYSTEMS FOR STUDYING THE INTERPLAY BETWEEN PGP AND LIPIDS

The vacuum cleaner and flippase models predict that Pgp will be very sensitive to its membrane microenvironment. Because of the complexities of intact cells, they have limited usefulness in exploring the relationship between transporter function and membrane properties. Plasma membrane fluidity can be altered by growing cells in medium containing saturated fatty acids, which alters the endogenous lipid composition of cellular membranes. Membrane properties can also be changed by adding exogenous amphiphiles, or membrane rigidifying or fluidizing agents [e.g., Ref. (9)]. Experimental observables are typically restricted to indirect measures of Pgp function, such as total cellular drug uptake, or cell survival in the presence of drug.

Simpler model systems have provided unique opportunities to explore the structure and function of Pgp. Mammalian MDR cell lines selected with cytotoxic drugs can express very high levels of Pgp [up to 30% of the total plasma membrane protein

(83)], and have been popular choices as the starting material for model systems. Sealed inside-out plasma membrane vesicles have been used for studies of ATP-driven drug transport [see Ref. (6)], and also as a source of purified active protein for biochemical and spectroscopic characterization. These studies have typically relied on the use of exogenous agents to alter membrane fluidity. For example, the ability of Pgp in canalicular membrane vesicles to transport daunorubicin and vinblastine was reduced two- to four-fold by benzyl alcohol, a known membrane fluidizer (84).

Several research groups have reported successful purification of Chinese hamster, mouse, and human Pgp from drug-selected MDR cell lines, or cells expressing recombinant protein [reviewed in Ref. (6)]. The use of solubilizing detergents is clearly essential in the extraction and purification of Pgp from native cell membranes. The choice of detergent is a critical step, and is typically governed in the first instance by the necessity of maintaining various functions of the protein, including ATP binding, ATP hydrolysis, drug binding, and drug transport. A second consideration is the compatibility of the chosen detergent with reconstitution, if this is a desired goal (85). Detergents with very low critical micelle concentrations (CMCs), such as Triton X-100, are usually very difficult to remove by dialysis, gel filtration chromatography, or dilution, and are not a good choice for reconstitution. The mild detergents 3-[3-(cholamidopropyl) dimethyl amino]-1-propanesulfonate (CHAPS) and octyl-β-D-glucoside (OG) have relatively high CMC values, and have been used successfully for purification and functional reconstitution of both Chinese hamster and human Pgp from mammalian cells (86–89).

Purified Pgp of mouse or Chinese hamster origin typically displays high levels of both basal and drug-stimulated ATPase activity (2–3 μmol/min/mg), and can carry out ATP-dependent active transport of drugs and hydrophobic peptides after reconstitution [summarized in Ref. (90)]. However, the basal rate of ATP hydrolysis of purified human Pgp is much lower than that of the rodent proteins, and it appears to require the presence of both drug substrates and lipids for activity. The rodent and human proteins are highly homologous, and the underlying reason for this difference in behavior is not clear. Human Pgp was recently reconstituted into lipid nanodiscs composed of *Escherichia coli* lipids, where it retained robust levels of both basal and drug-stimulated ATPase activity (91). Surface plasmon resonance was used to probe conformational changes in Pgp associated with progression through the ATP hydrolysis cycle. This novel nanodisc platform may prove useful in the further study of human Pgp.

Many of the purified Pgp preparations described in the literature employ the addition of exogenous lipids to maintain its function. Very few research groups have isolated Pgp in the absence of added exogenous lipids (50, 92). This approach allowed the development of experimental protocols to reconstitute Pgp into proteoliposomes of defined phospholipids, either synthetic or natural mixtures (92–94). Using these model systems has permitted detailed investigation of how Pgp function is modulated by membrane properties, leading to unique insights into transporter behavior. Further details of these studies are provided below.

DETERGENT INTERACTIONS AND EFFECTS ON PGP FUNCTION

The interaction of Pgp with detergents has been examined from two different aspects. First, the effectiveness of different detergents in solubilization and functional reconstitution of Pgp has been studied by several groups. Coupled with this has been the investigation of how exposure to various detergents stabilizes or destabilizes the protein. Second, the role of detergents as specific Pgp substrates and modulators has been explored, with a view to probing the nature of their interactions with the drug-binding pocket.

Sharom and co-workers established a protocol for partial purification of Chinese hamster Pgp with high levels of ATPase activity using the zwitterionic detergent CHAPS (95), in the absence of any exogenously added lipids. This allowed subsequent exploration of the effects of various detergents on the protein's activity and stability (96). Only the high CMC detergents, CHAPS and OG, were able to preserve ATPase activity at higher concentrations (4 mM for OG, 10 mM for CHAPS), whereas Triton X-100, digitonin and SDS resulted in complete loss of activity at 100 μM levels. The ability of CHAPS to preserve Pgp ATPase activity, while other detergents caused loss of activity was later confirmed by Orlowski et al. (97). They noted that drug stimulation of ATPase activity was restored after dilution of detergent to a concentration below its CMC. Even after almost complete removal of CHAPS from purified Pgp by dialysis, 80–90% of the ATPase activity remained (96), suggesting that the protein still retained a substantial annual lipid layer around it, which provided protection from denaturation. Later work used metabolic labeling to show that highly purified Pgp in CHAPS solution retained 53–56 tightly bound phospholipids per protein molecule (50). This amount may be sufficient to surround the TM domains of the protein, thus assisting in maintaining its native conformation and function.

The non-ionic detergents DDM and zwittergent 3–12 were reported to inactivate Chinese hamster Pgp function at low concentrations, below their CMCs, while OG inhibited activity in the millimolar range (98). In all cases, loss of ATPase activity and reduced drug-binding activity were prevented by the addition of 0.2% w/w of a crude lipid mixture. It was suggested that these detergents disrupted the lipid–protein interface, which is essential for Pgp to maintain its functional conformation. Similarly, the non-ionic *n*-alkyl-β-D-maltosides and *n*-ethyleneglycol monododecyl ethers were reported to reduce Pgp ATPase activity at concentrations well below their CMC values (99).

Naito and Tsuruo carried out the purification of human Pgp from MDR K562 cells using a panel of 12 detergents, and assessed its function following reconstitution into proteoliposomes (100). They reported that only cholate, glycocholate, and taurocholate were able to extract the protein and maintain its activity. However, the measured ATPase and transport activities were extremely low, likely as a result of protein denaturation during immunoaffinity elution. The overall conclusion from all of these studies is that the sensitivity of Pgp to inactivation by detergents depends on the lipids present in its immediate environment.

P-glycoprotein was reported to be dimeric or multimeric in the plasma membrane of some MDR cells (101–103), however, the minimal functional unit of the protein appears to be a monomer (104). Poruchynsky and Ling reported that detergent extracts from hamster and human MDR cell lines contained Pgp in an oligomerized form (105). CHAPS resulted in a high proportion of oligomerized Pgp, whereas only monomers were found after SDS treatment, suggesting that the nature of the detergent is important in either the formation or preservation of oligomers. Both Pgp monomers and oligomers appeared functional, in that they bound photoactive nucleotide and drug analogs. However, other studies have failed to find any evidence of Pgp dimerization using both biochemical and genetic approaches (106). The existence and functional role, if any, of oligomeric forms of Pgp is, therefore, still not clear.

Doige and Sharom first noted that Triton X-100 stimulated Pgp ATPase activity at low concentrations and inhibited it at higher concentrations, suggesting that it interacted specifically with the transporter (96). Triton X-100 was also observed to inhibit photoaffinity labeling of Pgp by the substrate ^{3}H-azidopine at low concentrations (107, 108). It was later confirmed to be a high affinity substrate for Pgp ($K_d = \sim 0.4\ \mu M$) using fluorescence quenching of purified protein (109). Several cationic amphiphiles, including the detergents benzalkonium chloride, methylbenzethonium chloride, cetylpyridinium chloride, and dodecyltrimethylammonium chloride, also appear to be Pgp substrates (107, 108). Both drug-selected MDR cells and Pgp transfectants showed cross-resistance to these compounds, which was effectively sensitized by the modulator verapamil. The synthetic surfactant, nonylphenol ethoxylate, which is a common component of various household detergents, was identified as a constituent of human urine, and *in vitro* studies confirmed that it is also a Pgp substrate (110). These findings indicate that the compound is excreted into the urine *in vivo* by kidney Pgp, in keeping with the proposed physiological role of the transporter in elimination of potentially toxic compounds.

Seelig's group further pursued the idea that detergents may be Pgp substrates using the non-ionic species Triton X-100, $C_{12}EO_8$ (dodecyloctaglycol), and Tween 80 (polysorbate-80) (111). The bell-shaped curves obtained for the effect of these detergents on Pgp ATPase activity suggested that they behaved like substrates, and interacted directly with Pgp with high affinity (K_d values $\sim 1\ \mu M$). Thermodynamic measurements showed that the ethoxyl groups of these detergents formed H-bonds with donor amino acid residues in the TM regions of Pgp, and their binding affinity increased with the number of these groups. Further investigation used a large series of polyoxyethylene alkylether detergents with varying numbers of methylene and ethoxyl residues (C_mEO_n), to systematically dissect the role of hydrophobic and H-bonding in binding of these compounds (112). Thermodynamic parameters indicated that detergent binding to the Pgp substrate cavity is driven exclusively by H-bonding or weak electrostatic forces, and not by hydrophobic interactions. Binding to Pgp is only achieved if the detergent has at least two hydrogen bond acceptor units within its chemical structure, supporting earlier work that used a large number of structurally diverse substrates (113). It is energetically unfavorable for the non-polar moiety of the detergent (the methylene chain) to enter the substrate-binding pocket, and it likely remains in contact with the hydrophobic lipid bilayer, where it may assist in flipping of the molecule to the other leaflet (112). This concept appears counter-intuitive, since the existence of hydrophobic and aromatic interactions between bound substrates and the surrounding cavity was suggested based on the X-ray crystal structures of mouse Pgp (34), and many QSAR studies have also stressed the importance of non-polar groups in binding to the transporter. However, the primary role of these groups may actually be to promote partitioning of the substrate into the bilayer, where it can then gain access to the protein's binding cavity.

Some detergents were reported to produce unexpectedly large down-modulation of Pgp ATPase activity, which was not a result of membrane disordering (114). The ratio of the free energy of detergent partitioning into the membrane (from K_{lip}) and the free energy of detergent binding to Pgp from within the membrane (from K_{dlip}) appeared to control the rate of ATP hydrolysis induced by the detergent, and probably the rate of its transport. Deviations from an optimal ratio of these free energies led to reduced rates of ATP hydrolysis and, by extension, transport. It was suggested that similar principles apply to drugs that are Pgp substrates and modulators.

PERTURBATION OF LIPID BILAYERS BY PGP

Early work on drug-selected MDR cell lines indicated that overexpression of Pgp led to secondary changes in the properties of their plasma membrane [summarized in Refs. (107, 115)]. It seemed likely that insertion of this large hydrophobic protein perturbs the physiochemical properties of the membrane, especially in cell lines where Pgp may represent as much as 20–30% of the total plasma membrane protein (83, 92). Loe and Sharom used the fluorescent probe merocyanine 540 to examine the local microenvironment in the plasma membrane of various CHO cell lines expressing Pgp (107). This negatively charged dye localizes in the outer leaflet of the plasma membrane, and the extent of its partitioning into membranes depending on the lipid packing density. Increasing levels of cellular drug resistance led to a progressive shift in the mean cell fluorescence to lower levels, indicating that the molecular packing of lipids in the outer leaflet of MDR cells increases with higher levels of Pgp expression.

The availability of purified Pgp led to further studies in reconstituted systems. Differential scanning calorimetry was first carried out by Romsicki and Sharom, using the synthetic phospholipid dimyristoyl-PC (DMPC) as the host lipid (116). Inclusion of increasing mole ratios of Pgp led to a decrease in the melting temperature of the bilayer, T_m. The cooperativity of the lipid melting transition was greatly reduced, and the transition enthalpy, ΔH, decreased linearly as the Pgp content increased to a lipid:protein ratio of 16:1 (w/w). Pgp was found to perturb a large number of bilayer phospholipids, preventing 375–485 of them from participating in the phase transition. As the Pgp content of the bilayers increased, the transition enthalpy was observed to increase again, an effect likely arising from either aggregation/oligomerization of the transporter, or a change in its mode of interaction with the bilayer. Oleinikov et al. explored the perturbing effects of Pgp in its native environment by forming monolayers from membrane fractions derived from a series of MDR cell lines in which the

Pgp content varied from 0 to 32% (w/w) (117). Compression of the Langmuir–Blodgett monolayers showed that 11 and 24% Pgp decreased monolayer stability without altering the surface area, while 32% Pgp increased both the stability and the surface area. Raman spectroscopy indicated that the presence of 32% Pgp reduced the lipid transition temperature by 7°C, and the number of perturbed lipids per protein was estimated at 400–500 (117), thus confirming the results seen in reconstituted systems (116).

Callaghan and co-workers reported that incorporation of Pgp into bilayers of PC–PE altered their overall fluidity, increased their permeability to polar compounds, and modified the packing organization of fluorescent lipid probes (115). The presence of the transporter also increased the flip–flop rate of short-chain phospholipids between bilayer leaflets, but this did not require ATP hydrolysis, so it likely takes place by an indirect mechanism.

Similar types of perturbing effects have previously been noted when other large hydrophobic proteins are inserted into lipid bilayers [e.g., Refs. (118, 119)]. Effects specific to Pgp may arise from its oligomerization behavior, and the ability of the transporter to interact with, and translocate, membrane lipids.

MODULATION OF PGP FUNCTIONS BY THE MEMBRANE

The availability of purified Pgp, both in detergent solution and reconstituted proteoliposomes, coupled with the development of biochemical and spectroscopic techniques for assessing many aspects of Pgp function, have greatly increased our understanding of the ways in which the lipid environment can modulate the transporter. The catalytic cycle of Pgp involves several steps, including nucleotide binding, drug binding from within the membrane, nucleotide hydrolysis, and drug translocation. Each of these steps may be subject to the influence of the surrounding membrane. In recent years, greater emphasis has been placed on the importance of measuring thermodynamic and kinetic constants for the various steps, since these provide a sound basis for construction of a detailed, experimentally testable model of the catalytic cycle.

DRUG-MEMBRANE PARTITIONING

P-glycoprotein substrates are typically lipid-soluble and amphipathic, and it is now clear that their binding to the protein takes place in two steps: partitioning into the lipid bilayer, followed by interaction with the substrate-binding pocket located within the TM domains. The presence of a drug within the membrane inner leaflet is thus a primary determinant of its recognition by the transporter. Amphipathic molecules are not randomly distributed in the bilayer, but orient themselves in an anisotropic manner at the lipid–water interface, parallel to the long axis of the membrane phospholipids (23, 120, 121). Their polar moieties interact with water and phospholipid headgroups, and (depending on the compound) their hydrophobic moieties may enter the non-polar core of the bilayer. Modeling studies suggest that a specific molecular conformation may also be required for partitioning of, for example, verapamil into the bilayer (120).

Since substrates gain access to Pgp from within the membrane, the lipid–water partition coefficient, K_{lip}, is an important molecular property affecting their interactions with the transporter. Lipid bilayers are multilayered, amphipathic structures (essentially highly ordered liquid crystals), and cannot be readily mimicked by isotropic systems such as octanol or olive oil. Experimental measurement of K_{lip} values using lipid bilayers is thus important for a quantitative understanding of the contribution of substrate partitioning to interaction with Pgp. K_{lip} values for Pgp substrates, whose structures are extremely diverse, range from 50 to 10^5 (111, 112, 114, 122–126). The high lipid–water partition coefficients of a series of polyoxyethylene alkylether detergents resulted in their concentration in a palmitoyloleoyl-PC (POPC) bilayer (112). Calorimetric measurements indicated that lipid partitioning was an entropy-driven hydrophobic event, driven by release of water molecules from the detergent when it entered the bilayer.

The passive diffusion and spontaneous flip–flop of small molecules across membranes decline exponentially with an increase in lateral packing density (127), which in turn depends on lipid composition and temperature. Native plasma membranes with high lateral packing density, such as these found in endothelial cells of the blood brain barrier, may thus make it easier for Pgp to establish a drug concentration gradient. Phospholipid bilayers exist in a rigid gel phase below the phase transition (melting) temperature, T_m, and a fluid liquid-crystalline phase above this temperature. These two phases are characterized by different packing densities, diffusion rates, fluidity, and lipid conformations. In an effort to understand the effects of membrane biophysical properties on partitioning of Pgp substrates, Clay and Sharom measured K_{lip} for three structurally unrelated Pgp substrates (LDS-751, H33342, and MK-571) in DMPC and palmitoylmyristoyl-PC (PMPC) bilayers over a temperature range that spanned T_m (122). Membrane partitioning of all three drugs was greatly favored in the fluid liquid-crystalline phase relative to the more rigid gel phase. The volume of the lipid bilayer increases by 4% when it melts (128), so drugs can fit more easily into the additional space present in the membrane in the liquid-crystalline phase, resulting in higher partitioning. The membrane partitioning of these three substrates was greatly affected by small changes in acyl chain length and lipid phase state, implying that such changes in membrane properties can readily modify Pgp's ability to bind drugs within the bilayer and transport them to the aqueous phase. Lipid rafts are small cholesterol- and glycosphingolipid-rich microdomains which display altered lipid composition, including acyl chain length, and also exist in a phase with reduced fluidity (the liquid-ordered phase, l_o), compared to the bulk membrane. Pgp appears to be located within rafts in some cell types (see below), and may move in and out of them in a dynamic fashion, thus potentially changing its access to drug substrates within the bilayer.

ATP BINDING AND HYDROLYSIS

Although the NB domains of Pgp are envisaged as being located in the cytoplasmic compartment, they appear to be almost completely dependent on the presence of membrane lipids for their catalytic activity. Early work showed that a Pgp-β-galactosidase fusion protein required phospholipids for ATPase activity (129). Detergent delipidation of Pgp results in complete loss of ATPase activity, which is readily and rapidly reversible by addition of lipids (96, 98, 130), suggesting that the loss of activity does not involve denaturation of the protein.

The ability of bulk exogenous phospholipids to protect Pgp catalytic activity from thermal inactivation was tested by Sharom and co-workers, using partially purified Chinese hamster Pgp in CHAPS solution (96). Asolectin, a mixture of soybean phospholipids, provided complete protection of the ATPase activity at 0.25 mg/mL, whereas various PC species did not. PS was also able to maintain the ATPase activity, and various PE species, either alone or mixed with PC, actually stimulated activity. Restoration of ATPase activity following detergent delipidation with Triton X-100 and deoxycholate required a different set of phospholipids, likely reflecting the intimately associated annular lipids that Pgp prefers (96). In general, short, unsaturated fluid lipids were better able to restore activity than longer, saturated species. The ATPase activity of purified Chinese hamster Pgp in CHAPS solution was altered by incubation with various phospholipids, some of which stimulated activity, while others caused inhibition (50). The best stimulatory lipid, dipalmitoyl-PE, was a mixed activator, increasing V_{max} and decreasing the K_M for ATP. Exogenous lipids are probably able to exchange into the annular lipid region of Pgp in the presence of small amounts of detergent, thus modulating protein function. Mixed activation is a common observation with Pgp-drug substrates. The ability of phospholipids to modulate ATP hydrolysis could also be because they are actually transport substrates, as discussed previously in the context of the documented flippase activity of the transporter.

Urbatsch and Senior solubilized Chinese hamster Pgp using OG and attempted to purify it in the absence of exogenous lipids (86). This resulted in completely inactive protein that could not be restored by reconstitution. When Pgp was purified in the presence of three natural lipid mixtures, activity was maintained, and they were able to reconstitute it into proteoliposomes of these lipids (86). They noted different effects on the level of ATPase activity and its stimulation by drugs, depending on the host lipid. The level of drug stimulation, which may reflect coupling between drug binding and ATP hydrolysis, was also reported by other groups to be increased after reconstitution of Pgp (87, 131), as was high affinity drug binding (98).

To explore the effects of lipid melting on catalytic activity, purified Pgp was reconstituted into synthetic phospholipid bilayers with a defined melting temperature, composed of DMPC ($T_m = {\sim}23$(C) and PMPC ($T_m = {\sim}28$(C) (132). Both ATP binding and ATP hydrolysis were found to be modulated by the phase state of the membrane. The kinetic parameters and activation energy for ATP hydrolysis, as well as K_d for ATP binding, were significantly different above and below the bilayer melting temperature, and there was a sharp discontinuity at T_m. The binding affinity for ATP was higher in the fluid liquid-crystalline phase, whereas the K_M for ATP hydrolysis was lower in the rigid gel phase. No changes in these parameters were observed at the same temperatures with Pgp in detergent solution. Thus, the conformation and/or folding of the NB domains may be affected by the fluidity and/or packing density of the membrane, which in turn affects nucleotide binding and hydrolysis. The opposite effects observed for K_d and K_M are not contradictory, since these parameters can only be considered equivalent for a simple Michaelis–Menten reaction scheme, and the catalytic cycle for Pgp is likely much more complex, with multiple steps.

Using drug-induced modulation of ATPase activity as a surrogate measure of drug binding, Seelig and co-workers were able to estimate the thermodynamic parameters for ATP hydrolysis (133). They showed that although the membrane lateral packing density only modulates the overall ATPase activity by up to two-fold, it substantially affected the thermodynamics of the transporter, which operated in an enthalpy-driven manner at low packing densities, but was driven by entropy at high densities. Partitioning of highly lipophilic Pgp substrates into the bilayer, and their accumulation to high concentrations (see above), may increase the fluidity and reduce the lateral packing density of the membrane. However, this appears to have only small effects on the thermodynamics of ATPase activity (133).

A FRET study showed that the NB domains of Pgp lie close to the membrane surface (134). In addition, when expressed in *E. coli*, the C-terminal NB domain was associated with the membrane fraction, indicating that it might interact preferentially with lipid surfaces (135). Taken together, this suggests that Pgp's NB domains may be in physical contact with the membrane surface, much like peripheral proteins, explaining why membrane fluidity and packing density affect their function. The lipid requirement for catalytic activity may be interpreted in two ways. Either the lipids are needed for stabilization of the TM regions which in turn stabilize the NB domains, or the NB domains interact with the membrane directly and require phospholipids for their catalytic function and, possibly, their structural integrity.

Rodent and human Pgp appear to differ in terms of their stability and lipid requirements for activity. The human protein typically displays very low basal ATPase activity compared to the Chinese hamster protein, but shows much higher levels of drug-stimulated activity. Reconstitution into lipid is often necessary for observation of any ATPase activity at all [for example, see Ref. (136)]. The drug-stimulated activity of human Pgp also appears to be highly dependent on the presence of cholesterol (137). Kodan et al. carried out a systematic study of factors promoting the stability of human Pgp expressed in insect cells (10). They noted a remarkable stabilizing effect of cholesteryl hemisuccinate (CHS) on the stability of the protein's ATPase activity after DDM solubilization; only 50% of the activity remained after 1 h at 25°C in the absence of CHS, whereas 50% activity was still present after 30 days at 4°C in the presence of 0.02% CHS. CHS has been noted to stabilize other human membrane proteins after DDM solubilization (138).

DRUG BINDING

Measurement of equilibrium drug binding to Pgp in plasma membrane vesicles from MDR cells has been carried out using radiolabeled substrates and modulators (139). This approach is technically difficult because the hydrophobic compounds give rise to high levels of non-specific background association with the membrane. Fluorescence spectroscopic methods using purified Pgp in detergent solution and reconstituted proteoliposomes have allowed quantitative estimates of K_d for binding of many substrates and modulators, without the need to separate free and Pgp-bound drugs [reviewed in Refs. (140, 141)]. The affinity of Pgp for binding a large group of compounds with diverse structures covers a range of ${\sim}10^4$, from 37 nM to160 μM.

Because of the difficulty of directly assessing drug binding, several groups have used drug or modulator stimulation of Pgp ATPase activity as a surrogate measure. Changing patterns of substrate-induced ATPase stimulation in the presence of different lipids suggests that either drug binding itself, or the coupling between drug binding and ATP hydrolysis, is altered by the membrane environment. Following Pgp purification and reconstitution into three natural lipid mixtures, Urbatsch and Senior noted different effects on the level of stimulation of ATPase activity by three substrates and one modulator, depending on the host lipid (86). Other groups also reported that after reconstitution of Pgp the level of drug stimulation of ATP hydrolysis (87, 131), and the affinity of drug binding (98) were increased.

For a substrate to interact with Pgp, two distinct steps must take place. The drug must first partition from the aqueous phase into the bilayer, and then it must enter the binding pocket of the transporter. Seelig and co-workers proposed that Pgp functions optimally when the free energies for these two processes fall in a narrow range (114). The first step is defined by the lipid–water partition coefficient for the drug, K_{lip}, and the second step is defined by the dissociation constant for binding of the drug to Pgp within the membrane, K_{dlip} (see **Figure 4**). The apparent binding affinity of Pgp for drugs measured from the aqueous phase, K_{d}, is related to K_{dlip} by:

$$K_{\mathrm{dlip}} = \frac{K_d}{\left(\frac{V_{\mathrm{lip}}}{V} + \frac{1}{K_{\mathrm{lip}}}\right)}$$

where V is the total volume of the system, and V_{lip} is the volume of lipid (122). Thus experimental measurement of K_{lip} and K_{d} can provide an estimate of the "true" affinity of Pgp for binding drugs from within the lipid bilayer.

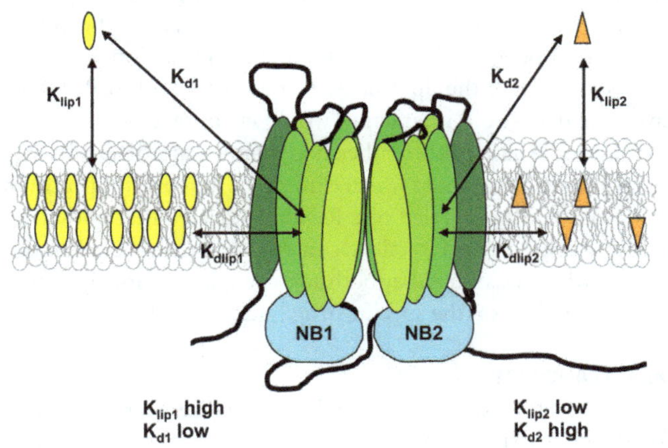

FIGURE 4 | Substrate–membrane relationships and their role in drug binding to Pgp. Pgp substrates partition into the lipid bilayer from the aqueous phase in accordance with their lipid–water partition coefficients (K_{lip}). The drug on the left of the figure has a high K_{lip} value and thus reaches a high concentration in the lipid phase, whereas the drug on the right of the figure has a low K_{lip} value, and therefore has a much lower membrane concentration. K_{lip} values measured for Pgp substrates are typically in the range 300–20,000. The apparent binding affinity (K_{d}) is determined using aqueous drug concentrations, and depends on both drug partitioning into the lipid phase and drug binding to the transporter from within the membrane. The intrinsic affinity of Pgp for binding substrate from the lipid bilayer (K_{dlip}) can be estimated from the values of K_{lip} and K_{d}, and is relatively low, in the range 0.5–70 mM.

For reconstituted Pgp in three different lipid systems, a high-fluidity lipid (egg PC) gave a large increase in binding affinity (determined by fluorescence quenching) compared to a low-fluidity lipid (dipalmitoyl-PC; DPPC) for vinblastine and verapamil (6- to 15-fold reduction in K_{d} value), while daunorubicin showed a much smaller change (two-fold reduction) (124). K_{d} was also correlated with the value of K_{lip} for vinblastine and verapamil. The highest apparent binding affinity was observed for substrates that had the greatest partitioning into lipid, in other words, the highest concentration in the bilayer (**Figure 4**). This suggests that the bilayer drug concentration is a major determinant of binding affinity, in agreement with the vacuum cleaner model. Pgp may thus have a relatively low "true" affinity for binding within the bilayer (i.e., K_{dlip} is high), but the membrane highly concentrates its substrates. A large fraction of the free energy of drug binding to the protein from the aqueous phase was shown to be provided by the free energy of drug–lipid partitioning, on the order of 75% (122, 126). In concert with changes in binding affinity, different host lipids also produced an altered ATPase stimulation profile for verapamil. Higher drug-binding affinity led to higher levels of stimulation of activity, whereas the concentration of verapamil required for half-maximal stimulation remained unchanged (124).

The extent of partitioning of substrates into the membrane is thus important for their interaction with Pgp, because it essentially controls the effective concentration presented to the transporter. For example, the apparent binding affinity of *C. elegans* Pgp for paclitaxel and actinomycin D was increased 100- and 4,000-fold, respectively, when the protein was in a membrane environment compared to detergent solution (35). Seelig and co-workers were the first to address this idea directly, using the drug concentration required for half-maximal ATPase stimulation as an indirect measure of its binding affinity (142). By calculating the free energy of drug binding from the aqueous phase to Pgp in the membrane, and combining this with drug–lipid partitioning data, they were able to estimate the affinity of Pgp for binding three drugs from the lipid phase. K_{dlip} values were in the range 0.5–4 mM for three substrates (142), providing the first evidence that Pgp binds its substrates from the membrane with low affinity. Recent work by Clay and Sharom using reconstituted Pgp in DMPC and PMPC bilayers directly measured the K_{d} for binding to Pgp from the aqueous phase, and also the lipid–water partition coefficient for three structurally unrelated substrates (122). Estimated K_{dlip} values were high, in the range 9–70 mM, confirming that Pgp has an intrinsically weak interaction with substrates within the lipid bilayer.

Defined reconstituted systems provide a powerful tool to define the effect of bilayer physicochemical properties on drug binding. Romsicki and Sharom first made the interesting (and paradoxical) observation that the binding affinity for vinblastine, verapamil and daunorubicin was higher in gel phase DMPC bilayers, despite the fact that drug partitioning is substantially lower for gel phase lipid (124). More recent work using Pgp reconstituted into DMPC and PMPC bilayers showed that this relationship held true for the substrates H33342, LDS-751, and MK-571 (122); both K_{d} and K_{dlip} values are lower (i.e., binding affinity is higher) in rigid gel phase bilayers. Van't Hoff plots of binding parameters over a wide temperature range showed different values of the binding free energy above and below the lipid phase transition. Since substrates must leave the lipid bilayer when they bind to Pgp, a less favorable drug–lipid interaction would encourage binding to the transporter. Analysis of the thermodynamic parameters for Pgp-drug binding in a manner which eliminated the contribution of the lipid was therefore carried out. Results indicated that both drug–lipid and drug–Pgp interactions contributed to the overall binding affinity, which was altered by both acyl chain length and lipid phase state, depending on the specific drug under consideration.

DRUG TRANSPORT

Early work showed that small molecule fluidizers and surfactants could reduce Pgp transport function in plasma membrane vesicles and intact MDR cells, leading to increased accumulation of drugs and reversal of drug resistance (9, 84, 143–145). Transport inhibition does not appear to involve direct interaction between these agents and Pgp, and is probably linked to increases in membrane fluidity or permeability (146, 147).

A transport study using Pgp reconstituted into bilayers of the synthetic phospholipid DMPC found that ATP-driven transport of [^{3}H]colchicine into reconstituted proteoliposomes determined by rapid filtration was more than two-fold higher at the T_m of 24°C than in the fluid liquid-crystalline phase at 32°C (8). Using Pgp in bilayers of DMPC and PMPC, the effect of bilayer phase state on the kinetics of ATP-driven transport was explored further (148). The initial rate of transport of the high affinity substrate tetramethylrosamine (TMR, a rhodamine derivative) was measured using a continuous real-time fluorescence assay over a time-scale of less than 1 min. Results showed that drug transport was modulated by the fluidity of the host membrane, with biphasic temperature dependence. The transport rate was high in rigid gel phase lipid, reached a maximum at the melting temperature of the bilayer, and then declined in fluid liquid-crystalline phase lipid. This behavior is unusual, as many membrane transport proteins show low or non-existent transport activity in rigid gel phase lipid, compared with activity in the fluid liquid-crystalline phase. Rigid gel phase lipid is poorly compressible, and it is thought that rate-limiting protein conformational changes are hindered in such an environment. It is possible that Pgp does not have a conformational barrier of this nature.

The rate of transport by Pgp likely depends directly on the drug concentration within the bilayer, and this, in turn, is controlled by the level of membrane partitioning of the substrate. Thus, the rate of drug transport may depend directly on the lipid–water partition coefficient, K_{lip}. Rogers and Davis reported that partitioning of various *p*-alkylphenols into DMPC bilayers also showed biphasic temperature dependence (149). The value of K_{lip} showed a maximum at T_m, declined substantially at temperatures higher than T_m, and remained constant, or declined slightly at temperatures lower than T_m, a pattern very similar to that seen for TMR transport by Pgp in bilayers of DMPC and PMPC (148). The temperature dependence of drug transport by Pgp may thus reflect the temperature dependence of K_{lip} for the substrate.

A recent study examined the effect of bilayer properties on Pgp-mediated transport of H33342 and LDS-751 in DMPC and PMPC bilayers, using real-time fluorescence measurements (122). Membrane partitioning data were also collected for these substrates, which allowed Pgp transport turnover numbers to be obtained in a reconstituted system for the first time. For both drugs, there is a clear discontinuity in transport rates above and below T_m, however, in contrast to the previous studies using TMR, higher transport rates were observed in the liquid-crystalline phase relative to the gel phase. Different temperature dependence of partitioning of the three substrates into gel and liquid-crystalline lipid bilayers may be responsible for this difference in behavior. LDS-751 and H33342 displayed the opposite behavior to TMR; their lipid–water partition coefficients increased with temperature in liquid-crystalline phase bilayers.

Overall, these studies clearly indicate that the membrane phase state is an important factor affecting Pgp's ability to transport drugs. One proposed strategy for reducing the transport activity of Pgp, thus reversing MDR, involves modifying the fluidity of the lipid environment (144). Since the effect of lipid fluidity on drug transport appears to vary depending on the specific substrate being transported, such an approach may not be feasible.

INTERACTIONS OF PGP WITH STEROLS

Cholesterol is a major component of mammalian plasma membranes, making up about 50% of the lipid content on a mole basis, and there have been many observations linking this sterol to Pgp function. Early work in intact cells suggesting the involvement of Pgp in cholesterol esterification was plagued by contradictions and confusion [reviewed in Ref. (123)] resulting from the use of Pgp modulators that later turned out to also inhibit cholesterol metabolism. Drug-selected MDR cells typically show changes in lipid composition, including cholesterol content, which may incidentally affect Pgp function. A study using cell lines where Pgp was inducible concluded that expression of the protein does not play a major role in cholesterol homeostasis (150), and that effects previously noted in drug-selected cells expressing Pgp might result from changes in other pathways that accompany selection. However, a possible physiological role for Pgp in intracellular cholesterol trafficking has been suggested (151). Using Pgp-deficient fibroblasts, replication of *Toxoplasma gondii* was shown to be critically dependent on Pgp, which played a role in the transport of host-derived cholesterol to the intracellular parasite.

Many studies investigating the role of cholesterol in Pgp function in intact cells and native membrane vesicles made use of methyl-β-cyclodextrin (MβCD), a cholesterol-extracting agent, to alter the amount of cholesterol in the plasma membrane (152–155). Essentially, all the cholesterol can be removed from membranes by this compound at a sufficiently high concentration, and inclusion complexes of MβCD with cholesterol can also be used to achieve controlled cholesterol repletion. However, MβCD was shown to directly inhibit the catalytic activity of Pgp, independent of its ability to extract cholesterol from membranes (123), calling into question the conclusions of studies that used this reagent.

Many groups have reported that the presence of cholesterol affects the catalytic activity of Pgp and its stimulation by substrates and modulators. When mouse Pgp was partially purified by hydroxyapatite FPLC using SDS, reconstitution into bilayers without cholesterol was reported to result in four- to five-fold reduced ATPase activity relative to bilayers where 20–40% cholesterol was incorporated (156). In addition, no stimulation of the activity by verapamil was observed unless cholesterol was included in the bilayer. Further studies showed that the lipids α-tocopherol and DPPC could also enhance verapamil stimulation, although they had no effect on basal ATPase activity (157). However, the ATPase activity of this Pgp preparation was very low, and it is possible that it was either partially denatured or not properly folded because of the somewhat harsh solubilization conditions, which likely strip away endogenous lipids. Callaghan and co-workers reported that the basal ATPase activity of partially purified hamster Pgp in PC–PE liposomes was increased ~two-fold on incorporation of 0–30% cholesterol (115). The fold-stimulation of ATPase activity induced by verapamil was reduced at higher cholesterol levels, although the absolute level of activity increased. Eckford and Sharom found that cholesterol had only a modest overall effect on catalytic activity. Purified Chinese hamster Pgp reconstituted into DMPC bilayers showed a small increase in basal ATPase activity, but a decrease in the level of verapamil-stimulated activity, with increasing cholesterol content from 0 to 30% (123). Cholesterol at high concentrations was able to partially restore the activity of delipidated Pgp, but less effectively than either PC or a PC-cholesterol mixture. Using purified reconstituted human Pgp, Kimura et al. reported that increasing cholesterol in the bilayer from 0 to 20% increased basal ATPase activity and modulated drug-stimulated activity (137).

However, cholesterol is not strictly required for Pgp function. Pgp purified using CHAPS is fully active (ATPase activity and drug transport) in proteoliposomes composed of synthetic phospholipids in the absence of added cholesterol [for example, see Refs. (122, 123, 132, 148)]. Perhaps this is because CHAPS-purified Pgp appears to retain an annular phospholipid layer around it (50). Alternatively, the sterol-like structure of CHAPS may interact with Pgp in a favorable manner, mimicking cholesterol. However, CHAPS does not stimulate Pgp ATPase activity like other detergents that are known to be substrates (96). It seems likely that the effects of cholesterol on both basal and drug-stimulated ATPase activity will differ depending on the specific detergent used to solubilize the protein, the extent to which endogenous lipids have been removed, and the lipid mixture used for reconstitution.

Cholesterol is well known to alter membrane packing, order, and fluidity. Such changes in the local environment may directly modulate the ability of Pgp to bind and hydrolyze ATP, and to transport drugs. Physicochemical changes in the membrane induced by cholesterol may also affect the concentration of drugs in the bilayer by changing their lipid–water partition coefficients. The inclusion of 30% cholesterol in DMPC proteoliposomes reduced Pgp's binding affinity for ATP by ~2.5-fold (123). This is in agreement with a previous report that ATP-binding affinity decreased in bilayers with lower fluidity (132). Photoaffinity labeling of Pgp by the substrate [^{3}H]azidopine was altered by yeast sterols, and cholesterol, suggesting that these lipids affected drug binding (158, 159). Later studies using fluorescence quenching to quantify drug interactions with purified reconstituted Pgp found that inclusion of cholesterol in the bilayer alters binding affinity (123, 124). The effects were dependent on the specific substrate used, with some drugs (e.g., vinblastine) showing a 10-fold increase in K_d value as cholesterol levels increased from 0 to 30%, while others (e.g., daunorubicin) showed essentially no change (123). These complex effects of cholesterol are different for individual drugs, and may be related to drug–lipid partitioning. Eckford and Sharom found that cholesterol had a large effect on drug partitioning into lipid bilayers, reducing the K_{lip} value by two- to nine-fold for several common Pgp substrates, with the exception of Hoechst 33342, which displayed a ~two-fold increase in K_{lip} (123). These differences may arise from the specific localization within the bilayer of drugs and cholesterol, which will modify the properties of different regions of the membrane selectively.

A water-soluble cholesterol analog, polyoxyethylcholesteryl sebacate, competed with daunorubicin for binding to Pgp (160), and cholesterol co-eluted with purified Pgp in detergent (137), however, it is still not clear whether these interactions are specific. Using the kinetics of drug-stimulated ATPase activity as a surrogate measure for drug-binding affinity, Kimura et al. reported that the presence of cholesterol in reconstituted proteoliposomes increased Pgp's binding affinity for small molecular mass drugs (<500 Da), but not for larger drugs (800–900 Da) (137). They proposed that cholesterol may occupy the substrate-binding pocket simultaneously with smaller drug molecules, filling the empty space and thus promoting their binding (161). However, when drug binding to reconstituted Pgp was measured directly using fluorescence quenching, no relationship between drug size and the effect of cholesterol on binding affinity was found (123). A large drug (vinblastine) showed a large reduction in binding affinity at high bilayer cholesterol, whereas a small drug (daunorubicin) showed little change in affinity.

The effect of cholesterol on the ability of Pgp to flip fluorescent NBD–PC and transport three different substrates were explored in reconstituted proteoliposomes (123). A modest decrease in flippase activity was noted at 20–30% cholesterol, and the ability of vinblastine to compete for flippase activity was enhanced. Inclusion of cholesterol in the bilayer showed biphasic effects on the initial rate of transport of TMR and Hoechst 33342. Net transport into proteoliposomes is a balance between inward active pumping of substrate by Pgp and passive outward efflux through the bilayer. These results were explained by cholesterol altering the membrane permeability and partitioning of substrates, which affect transport indirectly (123).

Whether Pgp is directly involved in outward movement of cholesterol across the plasma membrane has been the subject of debate. The effect of Pgp on the transbilayer distribution of cholesterol in native membrane vesicles was monitored using cholesterol oxidation by cholesterol oxidase. (152). It was concluded that Pgp was responsible for ATP-dependent transport of cholesterol from the cytoplasmic to the extracellular leaflet of the membrane. However, the estimated rate of spontaneous cholesterol movement between membrane leaflets was very slow, with a half-time of ~10 min. This contradicts other reports of very fast intrinsic flip–flop [reviewed in Ref. (162)], which suggest that cholesterol does not require a transport protein to move between bilayer leaflets. Eckford and Sharom confirmed rapid flip–flop of two cholesterol analogs in native membrane vesicles and proteoliposomes, faster than the time-resolution of the cholesterol oxidase assay, and also failed to show Pgp-mediated flip–flop of cholesterol (123). Since Pgp mediates ATP-dependent translocation of SM (44), which has a high affinity for cholesterol (163), it may indirectly influence cholesterol distribution in membranes. It is unlikely that Pgp is directly involved in moving cholesterol between membrane leaflets.

LIPID RAFTS AND PGP

The cholesterol content of the plasma membrane is highly regulated and relatively invariant. However, some domains are selectively enriched in cholesterol, namely lipid rafts and caveolae, which are characterized by the presence of higher lipid order, lower density, and detergent resistance (164). In intact cells, dynamic movement of Pgp into and out of these more ordered, cholesterol-rich domains could potentially regulate its functions. Pgp has been proposed to localize in low density raft microdomains and caveolae in some cell and tissue types [for a detailed list, see Ref. (165)]. However, in one MDR cell line, Pgp was present in intermediate density Brij-96 domains that were biochemically and physically distinct from both classical low density lipid rafts and caveolae (166), and in another case, Pgp was found not to be associated with lipid rafts at all (167). Thus, any proposed role for these domains in functional modulation of Pgp must necessarily be cell type-specific. Typically, treatments that break up lipid rafts (e.g., MβCD) result in loss of Pgp from raft domains, and a decrease in its function [for example, see Ref. (168)]. However, interpretation of these results is complicated by the fact that MβCD has secondary effects besides cholesterol sequestration; it can extract other membrane components such as phospholipids (169), and it is also known to inhibit Pgp catalytic function directly (123). One other source of variation in assessing the association of Pgp with these domains is the methodology used to isolate lipid rafts. Several different detergents have been commonly used for their extraction from intact cells, including Triton X-100, Brij-96, and Lubrol, and detergent-free approaches using carbonate have also been employed [see Ref. (165)]. It has been suggested that lipid rafts domains are concentric layered structures, with different sensitivities to detergent extraction at their periphery compared to the central core (170). This may explain why Pgp is typically strongly associated with Lubrol- or Brij-96-based rafts, but less so with Triton X-100 rafts (171).

Perhaps not surprisingly, Callaghan and co-workers showed that Pgp was fully functional after reconstitution into liquid-ordered (l_o phase) membranes rich in sphingolipids and cholesterol, i.e., with a typical "lipid raft" composition (172). The main difference noted between Pgp behavior in raft-like proteoliposomes and in those composed of PC alone was that drugs were able to stimulate or inhibit ATPase activity at lower concentrations. This is compatible with reports that Pgp binds its substrates more tightly in less fluid lipid bilayers (122, 124).

DETERGENTS AND MEMBRANE FLUIDIZERS AS PGP MODULATORS

Lipophilic compounds cross lipid bilayers by a three-step process involving partitioning into the interfacial region, diffusion through the hydrophobic core, and desorption from the opposite side of the membrane. Since many compounds, including Pgp substrates, are localized in specific regions of a lipid bilayer, the second step may be thought of as flip–flop (173), and is the slowest, rate-limiting step for movement of amphiphilic species across membranes. For example, doxorubicin flip–flop across lipid bilayers occurs with a half-time of ~1 min (174). The ability of substrates and modulators to interact with Pgp may depend on their ability to flip–flop between membrane leaflets. For example, some positively charged drugs and peptide modulators cannot interact with Pgp in intact cells if supplied on the extracellular side, probably because they have a very low rate of flip–flop to the inner leaflet (175). However, they can interact with Pgp in membrane vesicles, where the cytoplasmic leaflet is accessible. In support of this idea, substrate concentrations were found to be significantly lower in the cytosolic leaflet of intact cells expressing Pgp than in the cytosolic leaflet of inside-out membrane vesicles (176).

P-glycoprotein may handle classical modulators in exactly the same way as drugs, i.e., they are transported with hydrolysis of ATP (37, 177). The difference in the behavior of modulators and drugs may be related to their rate of flip–flop across the membrane (37). Pgp substrates were found to cross lipid bilayers relatively slowly (half-time for rhodamine 123 of ~3 min), while the transbilayer diffusion rates of several modulators were extremely fast. Pgp moves drugs and modulators (those that are transported) to the outer membrane leaflet, or they re-enter it after being moved to the extracellular medium. The rate of flip–flop to the inner leaflet is proposed to be slow for substrates, so that Pgp can keep pace, establish a drug concentration gradient across the membrane, and ultimately cause drug resistance. The long residence time of substrates in the inner leaflet also allows more opportunity for interaction with Pgp (174). For modulators, the rate of transbilayer flip–flop is so rapid that Pgp cannot keep pace or establish a concentration gradient, and MDR cells are not resistant to them. Work by Seelig and co-workers confirmed these ideas (176). Pgp in intact cells was found to transport substrates at a rate proportional to that of ATP hydrolysis, however, it could only prevent substrates from entering the cytosol if their rate of diffusion across the lipid bilayer was slow, in a range similar to that of Pgp-mediated efflux. This model suggests that for a modulator to be effective, it should bind to Pgp with high affinity and also have a high transbilayer diffusion rate (36, 177). If a compound modifies membrane properties to increase the rate of transbilayer movement of a drug sufficiently, it may be able to circumvent resistance without interacting specifically with Pgp. Thus, a second class of Pgp modulators may exist, consisting of agents such as surfactants and membrane fluidizers. In fact, several compounds that fall into this category are already known to reverse MDR (e.g., Pluronic block copolymers, Cremophor EL, Solutol HS15, Tween 80) (143, 178). Surfactants are ubiquitous in cleaning products, and are also present as additives in food and cosmetics. Since they are typically of very low toxicity, they may represent a useful class of Pgp modulators.

Evidence for the idea that Pgp-mediated MDR can be modulated by acceleration of passive drug permeation across the plasma membrane is contradictory. Tween 80 and Cremophor EL inhibited Pgp function in cell monolayers, increasing the apical-to-basolateral permeability and decreasing the basolateral-to-apical permeability of the substrate rhodamine 123 (179). These effects were related to the ability of the surfactants to increase membrane fluidity, in contrast with OG, which did not either modulate membrane fluidity or affect Pgp transport. However, polyoxyethylene surfactants that reversed MDR actually decreased lipid fluidity in plasma membrane vesicles from MDR cells, as assessed using several fluorescent probes (147), whereas surfactants that did not reverse MDR did not influence membrane fluidity. Low concentrations of Pluronic 61 were found to greatly increase the rates of phospholipid flip–flop and transbilayer movement of doxorubicin in lipid bilayers (180). Anesthetics (benzyl alcohol, chloroform, and diethylether) and non-ionic detergents (Tween-20, Nonidet P-40, and Triton X-100), increase membrane fluidity and the rate of transbilayer drug flip–flop (144). These compounds also abolish Pgp ATPase activity and drug binding, possibly by increasing membrane fluidity. Recent work in intact cells reported different results from experiments using liposomes and plasma membrane vesicles (146). Anesthetics were found to modulate MDR by accelerating transbilayer drug movement, whereas Pluronic P85, Tween-20, Triton X-100, and Cremophor EL had no effect on drug movement, and modulated MDR by inhibiting Pgp-mediated efflux. No correlation was found between the ability of surfactants to accelerate drug movement and their membrane fluidizing effects (146). Thus the molecular mechanism by which surfactants and membrane fluidizers inhibit the action of Pgp is still very much an open question.

CONCLUSION AND FUTURE PROSPECTS

P-glycoprotein is an unusual transporter, and various aspects of its function appear to be modulated by the lipid environment in novel and complex ways. Its mode of action as a hydrophobic vacuum cleaner and lipid/drug flippase make it especially sensitive to the properties of the surrounding lipid bilayer. Membrane composition, fluidity, and phase state all appear to be important parameters affecting Pgp stability, ATP binding, ATP hydrolysis, drug binding, and drug transport. Substrate interactions with the lipid bilayer play a critical role in the overall process of drug binding to Pgp, and are also modulated by the physicochemical properties of the membrane. It has been proposed that changing the properties of the host membrane may be a useful approach for clinical modulation of MDR. Clearly, an enhanced understanding of how all aspects of the Pgp catalytic cycle are affected by the local lipid microenvironment is essential if this strategy is to be successful. For example, the relationship between membrane partitioning and the binding affinity of Pgp substrates suggests one way to reduce or circumvent drug resistance. If a chemotherapeutic drug can be chemically modified to reduce its lipid–water partition coefficient, the ability of Pgp to transport it might be reduced. This would allow the drug to reach its intracellular targets, and thus increase its clinical effectiveness. Recent work on Pgp-membrane interactions has advanced to the point where it is now possible to measure thermodynamic and kinetic constants for the various steps of the catalytic cycle in model systems. Although the relationship between Pgp and its membrane environment is likely to be much more complex in living cells, this approach may provide a rational basis for novel strategies to overcome Pgp-mediated MDR in human tumors. It may also lead to a better understanding of the molecular mechanism of this enigmatic transporter.

ACKNOWLEDGMENTS

Original work in the author's laboratory reviewed in this article was supported by an operating grant from the Canadian Cancer Society (Grant 700248).

REFERENCES

1. Szakacs G, Paterson JK, Ludwig JA, Booth-Genthe C, Gottesman MM. Targeting multidrug resistance in cancer. *Nat Rev Drug Discov* (2006) **5**:219–34. doi:10.1038/nrd1984
2. Ambudkar SV, Dey S, Hrycyna CA, Ramachandra M, Pastan I, Gottesman MM. Biochemical, cellular, and pharmacological aspects of the multidrug transporter. *Annu Rev Pharmacol Toxicol* (1999) **39**:361–98. doi:10.1146/annurev.pharmtox.39.1.361
3. Sharom FJ. ABC multidrug transporters: structure, function and role in chemoresistance. *Pharmacogenomics* (2008) **9**:105–27. doi:10.2217/14622416.9.1.105
4. Eckford PD, Sharom FJ. ABC efflux pump-based resistance to chemotherapy drugs. *Chem Rev* (2009) **109**:2989–3011. doi:10.1021/cr9000226
5. Juliano RL, Ling V. A surface glycoprotein modulating drug permeability in Chinese hamster ovary cell mutants. *Biochim Biophys Acta* (1976) **455**:152–62. doi:10.1016/0005-2736(76)90160-7
6. Sharom FJ. The P-glycoprotein efflux pump: how does it transport drugs? *J Membr Biol* (1997) **160**:161–75. doi:10.1007/s002329900305
7. Ferté J. Analysis of the tangled relationships between P-glycoprotein-mediated multidrug resistance and the lipid phase of the cell membrane. *Eur J Biochem* (2000) **267**:277–94. doi:10.1046/j.1432-1327.2000.01046.x
8. Sharom FJ. The P-glycoprotein multidrug transporter: interactions with membrane lipids, and their modulation of activity. *Biochem Soc Trans* (1997) **25**:1088–96.
9. Callaghan R, Stafford A, Epand RM. Increased accumulation of drugs in a multidrug resistant cell line by alteration of membrane biophysical properties. *Biochim Biophys Acta* (1993) **1175**:277–82. doi:10.1016/0167-4889(93)90217-D
10. Kodan A, Shibata H, Matsumoto T, Terakado K, Sakiyama K, Matsuo M, et al. Improved expression and purification of human multidrug resistance protein MDR1 from baculovirus-infected insect cells. *Protein Expr Purif* (2009) **66**:7–14. doi:10.1016/j.pep.2009.02.010
11. Melchior DL, Sharom FJ, Evers R, Wright GE, Chu JW, Wright SE, et al. Determining P-glycoprotein-drug interactions: evaluation of reconstituted P-glycoprotein in a liposomal system and LLC-MDR1 polarized cell monolayers. *J Pharmacol Toxicol Methods* (2012) **65**:64–74. doi:10.1016/j.vascn.2012.02.002
12. Alvarez M, Paull K, Monks A, Hose C, Lee JS, Weinstein J, et al. Generation of a drug resistance profile by quantitation of mdr-1/P-glycoprotein in the cell lines of the National Cancer Institute Anticancer Drug Screen. *J Clin Invest* (1995) **95**:2205–14. doi:10.1172/JCI117910
13. Noonan KE, Beck C, Holzmayer TA, Chin JE, Wunder JS, Andrulis IL, et al. Quantitative analysis of MDR1 (multidrug resistance) gene expression in human tumors by polymerase chain reaction. *Proc Natl Acad Sci U S A* (1990) **87**:7160–4. doi:10.1073/pnas.87.18.7160
14. Lum BL, Gosland MP, Kaubisch S, Sikic BI. Molecular targets in oncology: implications of the multidrug resistance gene. *Pharmacotherapy* (1993) **13**:88–109.
15. Mattern J. Drug resistance in cancer: a multifactorial problem. *Anticancer Res* (2003) **23**:1769–72.
16. Tamaki A, Ierano C, Szakacs G, Robey RW, Bates SE. The controversial role of ABC transporters in clinical oncology. *Essays Biochem* (2011) **50**:209–32. doi:10.1042/bse0500209
17. Chan HS, DeBoer G, Thiessen JJ, Budning A, Kingston JE, O'Brien JM, et al. Combining cyclosporin with chemotherapy controls intraocular retinoblastoma without requiring radiation. *Clin Cancer Res* (1996) **2**:1499–508.
18. Leonard GD, Fojo T, Bates SE. The role of ABC transporters in clinical practice. *Oncologist* (2003) **8**:411–24. doi:10.1634/theoncologist.8-5-411
19. Robey RW, Massey PR, Amiri-Kordestani L, Bates SE. ABC transporters: unvalidated therapeutic targets in cancer and the CNS. *Anticancer Agents Med Chem* (2010) **10**:625–33. doi:10.2174/187152010794473957
20. Limtrakul P, Chearwae W, Shukla S, Phisalphong C, Ambudkar SV. Modulation of function of three ABC drug transporters, P-glycoprotein (ABCB1), mitoxantrone resistance protein (ABCG2) and multidrug resistance protein 1

(ABCC1) by tetrahydrocurcumin, a major metabolite of curcumin. *Mol Cell Biochem* (2007) **296**:85–95. doi:10.1007/s11010-006-9302-8

21. Michalak K, Wesolowska O. Polyphenols counteract tumor cell chemoresistance conferred by multidrug resistance proteins. *Anticancer Agents Med Chem* (2012) **12**:880–90. doi:10.2174/187152012802650011
22. Di Pietro A, Conseil G, Perez-Victoria JM, Dayan G, Baubichon-Cortay H, Trompier D, et al. Modulation by flavonoids of cell multidrug resistance mediated by P-glycoprotein and related ABC transporters. *Cell Mol Life Sci* (2002) **59**:307–22. doi:10.1007/s00018-002-8424-8
23. Siarheyeva A, Lopez JJ, Glaubitz C. Localization of multidrug transporter substrates within model membranes. *Biochemistry* (2006) **45**:6203–11. doi:10.1021/bi0524870
24. Homolya L, Hollo Z, Germann UA, Pastan I, Gottesman MM, Sarkadi B. Fluorescent cellular indicators are extruded by the multidrug resistance protein. *J Biol Chem* (1993) **268**:21493–6.
25. Raviv Y, Pollard HB, Bruggemann EP, Pastan I, Gottesman MM. Photosensitized labeling of a functional multidrug transporter in living drug-resistant tumor cells. *J Biol Chem* (1990) **265**:3975–80.
26. Higgins CF, Gottesman MM. Is the multidrug transporter a flippase? *Trends Biochem Sci* (1992) **17**:18–21. doi:10.1016/0968-0004(92)90419-A
27. Shapiro AB, Corder AB, Ling V. P-glycoprotein-mediated Hoechst 33342 transport out of the lipid bilayer. *Eur J Biochem* (1997) **250**:115–21. doi:10.1111/j.1432-1033.1997.00115.x
28. Loo TW, Clarke DM. The transmembrane domains of the human multidrug resistance P-glycoprotein are sufficient to mediate drug binding and trafficking to the cell surface. *J Biol Chem* (1999) **274**:24759–65. doi:10.1074/jbc.274.35.24759
29. Shapiro AB, Ling V. Extraction of Hoechst 33342 from the cytoplasmic leaflet of the plasma membrane by P-glycoprotein. *Eur J Biochem* (1997) **250**:122–9. doi:10.1111/j.1432-1033.1997.00122.x
30. Shapiro AB, Ling V. Transport of LDS-751 from the cytoplasmic leaflet of the plasma membrane by the rhodamine-123-selective site of P-glycoprotein. *Eur J Biochem* (1998) **254**:181–8. doi:10.1046/j.1432-1327.1998.2540181.x
31. Katzir H, Yeheskely-Hayon D, Regev R, Eytan GD. Role of the plasma membrane leaflets in drug uptake and multidrug resistance. *FEBS J* (2010) **277**:1234–44. doi:10.1111/j.1742-4658.2009.07555.x
32. Qu Q, Sharom FJ. Proximity of bound Hoechst 33342 to the ATPase catalytic sites places the drug binding site of P-glycoprotein within the cytoplasmic membrane leaflet. *Biochemistry* (2002) **41**:4744–52. doi:10.1021/bi0120897
33. Lugo MR, Sharom FJ. Interaction of LDS-751 with P-glycoprotein and mapping of the location of the R drug binding site. *Biochemistry* (2005) **44**:643–55. doi:10.1021/bi0511179
34. Aller SG, Yu J, Ward A, Weng Y, Chittaboina S, Zhuo R, et al. Structure of P-glycoprotein reveals a molecular basis for poly-specific drug binding. *Science* (2009) **323**:1718–22. doi:10.1126/science.1168750
35. Jin MS, Oldham ML, Zhang Q, Chen J. Crystal structure of the multidrug transporter P-glycoprotein from *Caenorhabditis elegans*. *Nature* (2012) **490**:566–9. doi:10.1038/nature11448
36. Eytan GD. Mechanism of multidrug resistance in relation to passive membrane permeation. *Biomed Pharmacother* (2005) **59**:90–7. doi:10.1016/j.biopha.2005.01.003
37. Eytan GD, Regev R, Oren G, Assaraf YG. The role of passive transbilayer drug movement in multidrug resistance and its modulation. *J Biol Chem* (1996) **271**:12897–902. doi:10.1074/jbc.271.22.12897
38. Abulrob AG, Gumbleton M. Transport of phosphatidylcholine in MDR3-negative epithelial cell lines via drug-induced MDR1 P-glycoprotein. *Biochem Biophys Res Commun* (1999) **262**:121–6. doi:10.1006/bbrc.1999.1120
39. Bosch I, Dunussi-Joannopoulos K, Wu RL, Furlong ST, Croop J. Phosphatidylcholine and phosphatidylethanolamine behave as substrates of the human MDR1 P-glycoprotein. *Biochemistry* (1997) **36**:5685–94. doi:10.1021/bi962728r
40. van Helvoort A, Smith AJ, Sprong H, Fritzsche I, Schinkel AH, Borst P, et al. MDR1 P-glycoprotein is a lipid translocase of broad specificity, while MDR3 P-glycoprotein specifically translocates phosphatidylcholine. *Cell* (1996) **87**:507–17. doi:10.1016/S0092-8674(00)81370-7
41. van Helvoort A, Giudici ML, Thielemans M, van Meer G. Transport of sphingomyelin to the cell surface is inhibited by brefeldin A and in mitosis, where C_6-NBD-sphingomyelin is translocated across the plasma membrane by a multidrug transporter activity. *J Cell Sci* (1997) **110**:75–83.
42. Pohl A, Lage H, Muller P, Pomorski T, Herrmann A. Transport of phosphatidylserine via MDR1 (multidrug resistance 1) P-glycoprotein in a human gastric carcinoma cell line. *Biochem J* (2002) **365**:259–68. doi:10.1042/BJ20011880
43. Romsicki Y, Sharom FJ. Phospholipid flippase activity of the reconstituted P-glycoprotein multidrug transporter. *Biochemistry* (2001) **40**:6937–47. doi:10.1021/bi0024456
44. Eckford PD, Sharom FJ. The reconstituted P-glycoprotein multidrug transporter is a flippase for glucosylceramide and other simple glycosphingolipids. *Biochem J* (2005) **389**:517–26. doi:10.1042/BJ20050047
45. Eckford PD, Sharom FJ. P-glycoprotein (ABCB1) interacts directly with lipid-based anti-cancer drugs and platelet-activating factors. *Biochem Cell Biol* (2006) **84**:1022–33. doi:10.1139/o06-196
46. Raggers RJ, Vogels I, van Meer G. Multidrug-resistance P-glycoprotein (MDR1) secretes platelet-activating factor. *Biochem J* (2001) **357**:859–65. doi:10.1042/0264-6021:3570859
47. Ernest S, Bello-Reuss E. Secretion of platelet-activating factor is mediated by MDR1 P-glycoprotein in cultured human mesangial cells. *J Am Soc Nephrol* (1999) **10**:2306–13.
48. Rybczynska M, Liu R, Lu P, Sharom FJ, Steinfels E, Pietro AD, et al. MDR1 causes resistance to the antitumour drug miltefosine. *Br J Cancer* (2001) **84**:1405–11. doi:10.1054/bjoc.2001.1776
49. Ruetz S, Brault M, Dalton W, Gros P. Functional interactions between synthetic alkyl phospholipids and the ABC transporters P-glycoprotein, Ste-6, MRP, and Pgh 1. *Biochemistry* (1997) **36**:8180–8.
50. Sharom FJ, Yu X, Chu JW, Doige CA. Characterization of the ATPase activity of P-glycoprotein from multidrug-resistant Chinese hamster ovary cells. *Biochem J* (1995) **308**:381–90.
51. Marcoux J, Wang SC, Politis A, Reading E, Ma J, Biggin PC, et al. Mass spectrometry reveals synergistic effects of nucleotides, lipids, and drugs binding to a multidrug resistance efflux pump. *Proc Natl Acad Sci U S A* (2013) **110**:9704–9. doi:10.1073/pnas.1303888110
52. Bello-Reuss E, Ernest S, Holland OB, Hellmich MR. Role of multidrug resistance P-glycoprotein in the secretion of aldosterone by human adrenal NCI-H295 cells. *Am J Physiol Cell Physiol* (2000) **278**:C1256–65.
53. Liu Y, Huang L, Hoffman T, Gosland M, Vore M. MDR1 substrates/modulators protect against β-estradiol-17β-D-glucuronide cholestasis in rat liver. *Cancer Res* (1996) **56**:4992–7.
54. Orlowski S, Mir LM, Belehradek J Jr, Garrigos M. Effects of steroids and verapamil on P-glycoprotein ATPase activity: progesterone, desoxycorticosterone, corticosterone and verapamil are mutually non-exclusive modulators. *Biochem J* (1996) **317**(Pt 2):515–22.
55. Rao US, Fine RL, Scarborough GA. Antiestrogens and steroid hormones: substrates of the human P-glycoprotein. *Biochem Pharmacol* (1994) **48**:287–92. doi:10.1016/0006-2952(94)90099-X
56. Ruetz S, Gros P. Phosphatidylcholine translocase: a physiological role for the *mdr2* gene. *Cell* (1994) **77**:1071–81. doi:10.1016/0092-8674(94)90446-4
57. Smith AJ, Timmermans-Hereijgers JL, Roelofsen B, Wirtz KW, van Blitterswijk WJ, Smit JJ, et al. The human MDR3 P-glycoprotein promotes translocation of phosphatidylcholine through the plasma membrane of fibroblasts from transgenic mice. *FEBS Lett* (1994) **354**:263–6. doi:10.1016/0014-5793(94)01135-4
58. Smith AJ, van Helvoort A, van Meer G, Szabo K, Welker E, Szakacs G, et al. MDR3 P-glycoprotein, a phosphatidylcholine translocase, transports several cytotoxic drugs and directly interacts with drugs as judged by interference with nucleotide trapping. *J Biol Chem* (2000) **275**:23530–9. doi:10.1074/jbc.M909002199
59. Frijters CMG, Tuijn CJ, Ottenhoff R, Zegers BN, Groen AK, Elferink RPJO. The role of different P-glycoproteins in hepatobiliary secretion of fluorescently labeled short-chain phospholipids. *J Lipid Res* (1999) **40**:1950–7.
60. Sharom FJ. Flipping and flopping – lipids on the move. *IUBMB Life* (2011) **63**:736–46. doi:10.1002/iub.515
61. Quazi F, Molday RS. Lipid transport by mammalian ABC proteins. *Essays Biochem* (2011) **50**:265–90. doi:10.1042/bse0500265
62. Borst P, Zelcer N, van Helvoort A. ABC transporters in lipid transport. *Biochim Biophys Acta* (2000) **1486**:128–44. doi:10.1016/S1388-1981(00)00053-6

63. van Meer G, Halter D, Sprong H, Somerharju P, Egmond MR. ABC lipid transporters: extruders, flippases, or flopless activators? *FEBS Lett* (2006) **580**:1171–7. doi:10.1016/j.febslet.2005.12.019
64. Quazi F, Molday RS. Differential phospholipid substrates and directional transport by ATP binding cassette proteins ABCA1, ABCA7, and ABCA4 and disease-causing mutants. *J Biol Chem* (2013) **288**:34414–26. doi:10.1074/jbc.M113.508812
65. Sharom FJ. The P-glycoprotein multidrug transporter. *Essays Biochem* (2011) **50**:161–78. doi:10.1042/bse0500161
66. Zolnerciks JK, Andress EJ, Nicolaou M, Linton KJ. Structure of ABC transporters. *Essays Biochem* (2011) **50**:43–61. doi:10.1042/bse0500043
67. Holland IB, Blight MA. ABC-ATPases, adaptable energy generators fuelling transmembrane movement of a variety of molecules in organisms from bacteria to humans. *J Mol Biol* (1999) **293**:381–99. doi:10.1006/jmbi.1999.2993
68. Jones PM, George AM. Subunit interactions in ABC transporters: towards a functional architecture. *FEMS Microbiol Lett* (1999) **179**:187–202. doi:10.1111/j.1574-6968.1999.tb08727.x
69. Jones PM, George AM. Mechanism of the ABC transporter ATPase domains: catalytic models and the biochemical and biophysical record. *Crit Rev Biochem Mol Biol* (2013) **48**:39–50. doi:10.3109/10409238.2012.735644
70. George AM, Jones PM. Perspectives on the structure-function of ABC transporters: the Switch and Constant Contact models. *Prog Biophys Mol Biol* (2012) **109**:95–107. doi:10.1016/j.pbiomolbio.2012.06.003
71. Sharom FJ, Liu R, Romsicki Y. Spectroscopic and biophysical approaches for studying the structure and function of the P-glycoprotein multidrug transporter. *Biochem Cell Biol* (1998) **76**:695–708. doi:10.1139/o98-075
72. Rosenberg MF, Callaghan R, Modok S, Higgins CF, Ford RC. Three-dimensional structure of P-glycoprotein: the transmembrane regions adopt an asymmetric configuration in the nucleotide-bound state. *J Biol Chem* (2005) **280**:2857–62. doi:10.1074/jbc.M410296200
73. Lee JY, Urbatsch IL, Senior AE, Wilkens S. Projection structure of P-glycoprotein by electron microscopy. Evidence for a closed conformation of the nucleotide binding domains. *J Biol Chem* (2002) **277**:40125–31. doi:10.1074/jbc.M206871200
74. Lee JY, Urbatsch IL, Senior AE, Wilkens S. Nucleotide-induced structural changes in P-glycoprotein observed by electron microscopy. *J Biol Chem* (2008) **283**:5769–79. doi:10.1074/jbc.M707028200
75. Lugo MR, Sharom FJ. Interaction of LDS-751 and rhodamine 123 with P-glycoprotein: evidence for simultaneous binding of both drugs. *Biochemistry* (2005) **44**:14020–9. doi:10.1021/bi0511179
76. Lugo MR, Sharom FJ. Interaction of LDS-751 with the drug-binding site of P-glycoprotein: a Trp fluorescence steady-state and lifetime study. *Arch Biochem Biophys* (2009) **492**:17–28. doi:10.1016/j.abb.2009.10.002
77. Loo TW, Clarke DM. Mutational analysis of ABC proteins. *Arch Biochem Biophys* (2008) **476**:51–64. doi:10.1016/j.abb.2008.02.025
78. Pleban K, Kopp S, Csaszar E, Peer M, Hrebicek T, Rizzi A, et al. P-glycoprotein substrate binding domains are located at the transmembrane domain/transmembrane domain interfaces: a combined photoaffinity labeling-protein homology modeling approach. *Mol Pharmacol* (2005) **67**:365–74. doi:10.1124/mol.104.006973
79. Parveen Z, Stockner T, Bentele C, Pferschy S, Kraupp M, Freissmuth M, et al. Molecular dissection of dual pseudosymmetric solute translocation pathways in human P-glycoprotein. *Mol Pharmacol* (2011) **79**:443–52. doi:10.1124/mol.110.067611
80. Ward AB, Szewczyk P, Grimard V, Lee CW, Martinez L, Doshi R, et al. Structures of P-glycoprotein reveal its conformational flexibility and an epitope on the nucleotide-binding domain. *Proc Natl Acad Sci U S A* (2013) **110**:13386–91. doi:10.1073/pnas.1309275110
81. Loo TW, Clarke DM. Drug rescue distinguishes between different structural models of human P-glycoprotein. *Biochemistry* (2013) **52**:7167–9. doi:10.1021/bi401269m
82. Wen PC, Verhalen B, Wilkens S, Mchaourab HS, Tajkhorshid E. On the origin of large flexibility of P-glycoprotein in the inward-facing state. *J Biol Chem* (2013) **288**:19211–20. doi:10.1074/jbc.M113.450114
83. al-Shawi MK, Senior AE. Characterization of the adenosine triphosphatase activity of Chinese hamster P-glycoprotein. *J Biol Chem* (1993) **268**:4197–206.
84. Sinicrope FA, Dudeja PK, Bissonnette BM, Safa AR, Brasitus TA. Modulation of P-glycoprotein-mediated drug transport by alterations in lipid fluidity of rat liver canalicular membrane vesicles. *J Biol Chem* (1992) **267**:24995–5002.
85. Sharom FJ, Eckford PD. Reconstitution of membrane transporters. *Methods Mol Biol* (2003) **227**:129–54.
86. Urbatsch IL, Senior AE. Effects of lipids on ATPase activity of purified Chinese hamster P-glycoprotein. *Arch Biochem Biophys* (1995) **316**:135–40. doi:10.1006/abbi.1995.1020
87. Sharom FJ, Yu X, Doige CA. Functional reconstitution of drug transport and ATPase activity in proteoliposomes containing partially purified P-glycoprotein. *J Biol Chem* (1993) **268**:24197–202.
88. Shapiro AB, Ling V. Reconstitution of drug transport by purified P-glycoprotein. *J Biol Chem* (1995) **270**:16167–75. doi:10.1074/jbc.270.27.16167
89. Ambudkar SV. Purification and reconstitution of functional human P-glycoprotein. *J Bioenerg Biomembr* (1995) **27**:23–9. doi:10.1007/BF02110327
90. Sharom FJ. Multidrug resistance protein: P-glycoprotein. In: You G, Morris ME, editors. *Drug Transporters: Molecular Characterization and Role in Drug Disposition.* Hoboken, NJ: John Wiley & Sons (2007). p. 223–62.
91. Ritchie TK, Kwon H, Atkins WM. Conformational analysis of human ATP-binding cassette transporter ABCB1 in lipid nanodiscs and inhibition by the antibodies MRK16 and UIC2. *J Biol Chem* (2011) **286**:39489–96. doi:10.1074/jbc.M111.284554
92. Dong M, Penin F, Baggetto LG. Efficient purification and reconstitution of P-glycoprotein for functional and structural studies. *J Biol Chem* (1996) **271**:28875–83. doi:10.1074/jbc.271.46.28875
93. Sharom FJ, Liu R, Vinepal B. Fluorescence studies of drug binding and translocation by membrane transporters. In: Yan Q, editor. *Methods in Molecular Biology: Membrane Transporters in Drug Discovery and Development.* Totowa, NJ: Springer Science+Business Media (2009). p. 133–48.
94. Sharom FJ. Characterization and functional reconstitution of the multidrug transporter. *J Bioenerg Biomembr* (1995) **27**:15–22. doi:10.1007/BF02110326
95. Doige CA, Yu X, Sharom FJ. ATPase activity of partially purified P-glycoprotein from multidrug-resistant Chinese hamster ovary cells. *Biochim Biophys Acta* (1992) **1109**:149–60. doi:10.1016/0005-2736(92)90079-2
96. Doige CA, Yu X, Sharom FJ. The effects of lipids and detergents on ATPase-active P-glycoprotein. *Biochim Biophys Acta* (1993) **1146**:65–72. doi:10.1016/0005-2736(93)90339-2
97. Orlowski S, Selosse MA, Boudon C, Micoud C, Mir LM, Belehradek J Jr, et al. Effects of detergents on P-glycoprotein ATPase activity: differences in perturbations of basal and verapamil-dependent activities. *Cancer Biochem Biophys* (1998) **16**:85–110.
98. Callaghan R, Berridge G, Ferry DR, Higgins CF. The functional purification of P-glycoprotein is dependent on maintenance of a lipid-protein interface. *Biochim Biophys Acta* (1997) **1328**:109–24. doi:10.1016/S0005-2736(97)00079-5
99. Beck A, Aanismaa P, Li-Blatter X, Dawson R, Locher K, Seelig A. Sav1866 from *Staphylococcus aureus* and P-glycoprotein: similarities and differences in ATPase activity assessed with detergents as allocrites. *Biochemistry* (2013) **52**:3297–309. doi:10.1021/bi400203d
100. Naito M, Tsuruo T. Reconstitution of purified P-glycoprotein into liposomes. *J Cancer Res Clin Oncol* (1995) **121**:582–6. doi:10.1007/BF01197774
101. Naito M, Tsuruo T. Functionally active homodimer of P-glycoprotein in multidrug-resistant tumor cells. *Biochem Biophys Res Commun* (1992) **185**:284–90. doi:10.1016/S0006-291X(05)80988-X
102. Boscoboinik D, Debanne MT, Stafford AR, Jung CY, Gupta RS, Epand RM. Dimerization of the P-glycoprotein in membranes. *Biochim Biophys Acta* (1990) **1027**:225–8. doi:10.1016/0005-2736(90)90311-B
103. Sehested M, Simpson D, Skovsgaard T, Buhl-Jensen P. Freeze-fracture study of plasma membranes in wild type and daunorubicin-resistant Ehrlich ascites tumor and P388 leukemia cells. *Virchows Arch B Cell Pathol Incl Mol Pathol* (1989) **56**:327–35. doi:10.1007/BF02890034
104. Loo TW, Clarke DM. The minimum functional unit of human P-glycoprotein appears to be a monomer. *J Biol Chem* (1996) **271**:27488–92. doi:10.1074/jbc.271.44.27488

105. Poruchynsky MS, Ling V. Detection of oligomeric and monomeric forms of P-glycoprotein in multidrug resistant cells. *Biochemistry* (1994) **33**:4163–74. doi:10.1021/bi00196a023
106. Taylor JC, Horvath AR, Higgins CF, Begley GS. The multidrug resistance P-glycoprotein. Oligomeric state and intramolecular interactions. *J Biol Chem* (2001) **276**:36075–8. doi:10.1074/jbc.C100345200
107. Loe DW, Sharom FJ. Interaction of multidrug-resistant Chinese hamster ovary cells with amphiphiles. *Br J Cancer* (1993) **68**:342–51. doi:10.1038/bjc.1993.338
108. Zordan-Nudo T, Ling V, Liu Z, Georges E. Effects of nonionic detergents on P-glycoprotein drug binding and reversal of multidrug resistance. *Cancer Res* (1993) **53**:5994–6000.
109. Sharom FJ, Liu R, Romsicki Y, Lu P. Insights into the structure and substrate interactions of the P-glycoprotein multidrug transporter from spectroscopic studies. *Biochim Biophys Acta* (1999) **1461**:327–45. doi:10.1016/S0005-2736(99)00166-2
110. Charuk JH, Grey AA, Reithmeier RA. Identification of the synthetic surfactant nonylphenol ethoxylate: a P-glycoprotein substrate in human urine. *Am J Physiol* (1998) **274**:F1127–39.
111. Li-Blatter X, Nervi P, Seelig A. Detergents as intrinsic P-glycoprotein substrates and inhibitors. *Biochim Biophys Acta* (2009) **1788**:2335–44. doi:10.1016/j.bbamem.2009.07.010
112. Li-Blatter X, Seelig A. Exploring the P-glycoprotein binding cavity with polyoxyethylene alkyl ethers. *Biophys J* (2010) **99**:3589–98. doi:10.1016/j.bpj.2010.10.033
113. Seelig A. A general pattern for substrate recognition by P-glycoprotein. *Eur J Biochem* (1998) **251**:252–61. doi:10.1046/j.1432-1327.1998.2510252.x
114. Li-Blatter X, Beck A, Seelig A. P-Glycoprotein-ATPase modulation: the molecular mechanisms. *Biophys J* (2012) **102**:1383–93. doi:10.1016/j.bpj.2012.02.018
115. Rothnie A, Theron D, Soceneantu L, Martin C, Traikia M, Berridge G, et al. The importance of cholesterol in maintenance of P-glycoprotein activity and its membrane perturbing influence. *Eur Biophys J* (2001) **30**:430–42. doi:10.1007/s002490100156
116. Romsicki Y, Sharom FJ. Interaction of P-glycoprotein with defined phospholipid bilayers: a differential scanning calorimetric study. *Biochemistry* (1997) **36**:9807–15. doi:10.1021/bi963120l
117. Oleinikov VA, Fleury F, Ianoul A, Zaitsev S, Nabiev I. P-glycoprotein effect on the properties of its natural lipid environment probed by Raman spectroscopy and Langmuir-Blodgett technique. *FEBS Lett* (2006) **580**:4953–8. doi:10.1016/j.febslet.2006.07.069
118. Lentz BR, Clubb KW, Barrow DA, Meissner G. Ordered and disordered phospholipid domains coexist in membranes containing the calcium pump protein of sarcoplasmic reticulum. *Proc Natl Acad Sci U S A* (1983) **80**:2917–21. doi:10.1073/pnas.80.10.2917
119. Chicken CA, Sharom FJ. Lipid-protein interactions of the human erythrocyte concanavalin A receptor in phospholipid bilayers. *Biochim Biophys Acta* (1984) **774**:110–8. doi:10.1016/0005-2736(84)90281-5
120. Gerebtzoff G, Seelig A. In silico prediction of blood-brain barrier permeation using the calculated molecular cross-sectional area as main parameter. *J Chem Inf Model* (2006) **46**:2638–50. doi:10.1021/ci0600814
121. Omote H, al-Shawi MK. Interaction of transported drugs with the lipid bilayer and P-glycoprotein through a solvation exchange mechanism. *Biophys J* (2006) **90**:4046–59. doi:10.1529/biophysj.105.077743
122. Clay AT, Sharom FJ. Lipid bilayer properties control membrane partitioning, binding, and transport of P-glycoprotein substrates. *Biochemistry* (2013) **52**:343–54. doi:10.1021/bi301532c
123. Eckford PD, Sharom FJ. Interaction of the P-glycoprotein multidrug efflux pump with cholesterol: effects on ATPase activity, drug binding and transport. *Biochemistry* (2008) **47**:13686–98. doi:10.1021/bi801409r
124. Romsicki Y, Sharom FJ. The membrane lipid environment modulates drug interactions with the P-glycoprotein multidrug transporter. *Biochemistry* (1999) **38**:6887–96. doi:10.1021/bi990064q
125. Seelig A, Landwojtowicz E. Structure-activity relationship of P-glycoprotein substrates and modifiers. *Eur J Pharm Sci* (2000) **12**:31–40. doi:10.1016/S0928-0987(00)00177-9
126. Gatlik-Landwojtowicz E, Aanismaa P, Seelig A. Quantification and characterization of P-glycoprotein-substrate interactions. *Biochemistry* (2006) **45**:3020–32. doi:10.1021/bi051380+
127. Aanismaa P, Seelig A. P-Glycoprotein kinetics measured in plasma membrane vesicles and living cells. *Biochemistry* (2007) **46**:3394–404. doi:10.1021/bi0619526
128. Heimburg T. Mechanical aspects of membrane thermodynamics. Estimation of the mechanical properties of lipid membranes close to the chain melting transition from calorimetry. *Biochim Biophys Acta* (1998) **1415**:147–62. doi:10.1016/S0005-2736(98)00189-8
129. Shimabuku AM, Nishimoto T, Ueda K, Komano T. P-glycoprotein. ATP hydrolysis by the N-terminal nucleotide-binding domain. *J Biol Chem* (1992) **267**:4308–11.
130. Lerner-Marmarosh N, Gimi K, Urbatsch IL, Gros P, Senior AE. Large scale purification of detergent-soluble P-glycoprotein from *Pichia pastoris* cells and characterization of nucleotide binding properties of wild-type, Walker A, and Walker B mutant proteins. *J Biol Chem* (1999) **274**:34711–8. doi:10.1074/jbc.274.49.34711
131. Ambudkar SV, Lelong IH, Zhang J, Cardarelli CO, Gottesman MM, Pastan I. Partial purification and reconstitution of the human multidrug-resistance pump: characterization of the drug-stimulatable ATP hydrolysis. *Proc Natl Acad Sci U S A* (1992) **89**:8472–6. doi:10.1073/pnas.89.18.8472
132. Romsicki Y, Sharom FJ. The ATPase and ATP-binding functions of P-glycoprotein-modulation by interaction with defined phospholipids. *Eur J Biochem* (1998) **256**:170–8. doi:10.1046/j.1432-1327.1998.2560170.x
133. Aanismaa P, Gatlik-Landwojtowicz E, Seelig A. P-glycoprotein senses its substrates and the lateral membrane packing density: consequences for the catalytic cycle. *Biochemistry* (2008) **47**:10197–207. doi:10.1021/bi800209h
134. Liu R, Sharom FJ. Proximity of the nucleotide binding domains of the P-glycoprotein multidrug transporter to the membrane surface: a resonance energy transfer study. *Biochemistry* (1998) **37**:6503–12. doi:10.1021/bi973031o
135. Sharma S, Rose DR. Cloning, overexpression, purification, and characterization of the carboxyl-terminal nucleotide binding domain of P-glycoprotein. *J Biol Chem* (1995) **270**:14085–93. doi:10.1074/jbc.270.23.14085
136. Loo TW, Clarke DM. Rapid purification of human P-glycoprotein mutants expressed transiently in HEK 293 cells by nickel-chelate chromatography and characterization of their drug-stimulated ATPase activities. *J Biol Chem* (1995) **270**:21449–52. doi:10.1074/jbc.270.37.21449
137. Kimura Y, Kioka N, Kato H, Matsuo M, Ueda K. Modulation of drug-stimulated ATPase activity of human MDR1/P-glycoprotein by cholesterol. *Biochem J* (2007) **401**:597–605. doi:10.1042/BJ20060632
138. Weiss HM, Grisshammer R. Purification and characterization of the human adenosine A(2a) receptor functionally expressed in *Escherichia coli*. *Eur J Biochem* (2002) **269**:82–92. doi:10.1046/j.0014-2956.2002.02618.x
139. Martin C, Berridge G, Higgins CF, Mistry P, Charlton P, Callaghan R. Communication between multiple drug binding sites on P-glycoprotein. *Mol Pharmacol* (2000) **58**:624–32. doi:10.1124/mol.58.3.624
140. Sharom FJ, Liu R, Qu Q, Romsicki Y. Exploring the structure and function of the P-glycoprotein multidrug transporter using fluorescence spectroscopic tools. *Semin Cell Dev Biol* (2001) **12**:257–65. doi:10.1006/scdb.2000.0251
141. Sharom FJ. Shedding light on drug transport: structure and function of the P-glycoprotein multidrug transporter (ABCB1). *Biochem Cell Biol* (2006) **84**:979–92. doi:10.1139/o06-199
142. Meier M, Blatter XL, Seelig A, Seelig J. Interaction of verapamil with lipid membranes and P-glycoprotein: connecting thermodynamics and membrane structure with functional activity. *Biophys J* (2006) **91**:2943–55. doi:10.1529/biophysj.106.089581
143. Woodcock DM, Linsenmeyer ME, Chojnowski G, Kriegler AB, Nink V, Webster LK, et al. Reversal of multidrug resistance by surfactants. *Br J Cancer* (1992) **66**:62–8. doi:10.1038/bjc.1992.217
144. Regev R, Assaraf YG, Eytan GD. Membrane fluidization by ether, other anesthetics, and certain agents abolishes P-glycoprotein ATPase activity and modulates efflux from multidrug-resistant cells. *Eur J Biochem* (1999) **259**:18–24. doi:10.1046/j.1432-1327.1999.00037.x
145. Coon JS, Knudson W, Clodfelter K, Lu B, Weinstein RS. Solutol HS 15, nontoxic polyoxyethylene esters of 12-hydroxystearic acid, reverses multidrug resistance. *Cancer Res* (1991) **51**:897–902.
146. Regev R, Katzir H, Yeheskely-Hayon D, Eytan GD. Modulation of P-glycoprotein-mediated multidrug resistance by acceleration of passive drug permeation across the plasma membrane. *FEBS J* (2007) **274**:6204–14. doi:10.1111/j.1742-4658.2007.06140.x

147. Dudeja PK, Anderson KM, Harris JS, Buckingham L, Coon JS. Reversal of multidrug resistance phenotype by surfactants: relationship to membrane lipid fluidity. *Arch Biochem Biophys* (1995) **319**:309–15.
148. Lu P, Liu R, Sharom FJ. Drug transport by reconstituted P-glycoprotein in proteoliposomes. Effect of substrates and modulators, and dependence on bilayer phase state. *Eur J Biochem* (2001) **268**:1687–97. doi:10.1046/j.1432-1327.2001.02041.x
149. Rogers JA, Davis SS. Functional group contributions to the partitioning of phenols between liposomes and water. *Biochim Biophys Acta* (1980) **598**:392–404. doi:10.1016/0005-2736(80)90017-6
150. Le Goff W, Settle M, Greene DJ, Morton RE, Smith JD. Reevaluation of the role of the multidrug-resistant P-glycoprotein in cellular cholesterol homeostasis. *J Lipid Res* (2006) **47**:51–8. doi:10.1194/jlr.M500255-JLR200
151. Bottova I, Hehl AB, Stefanic S, Fabrias G, Casas J, Schraner E, et al. Host cell P-glycoprotein is essential for cholesterol uptake and replication of *Toxoplasma gondii*. *J Biol Chem* (2009) **284**:17438–48. doi:10.1074/jbc.M809420200
152. Garrigues A, Escargueil AE, Orlowski S. The multidrug transporter, P-glycoprotein, actively mediates cholesterol redistribution in the cell membrane. *Proc Natl Acad Sci U S A* (2002) **99**:10347–52. doi:10.1073/pnas.162366399
153. Gayet L, Dayan G, Barakat S, Labialle S, Michaud M, Cogne S, et al. Control of P-glycoprotein activity by membrane cholesterol amounts and their relation to multidrug resistance in human CEM leukemia cells. *Biochemistry* (2005) **44**:4499–509. doi:10.1021/bi048669w
154. Mayer dos Santos S, Weber CC, Franke C, Muller WE, Eckert GP. Cholesterol: coupling between membrane microenvironment and ABC transporter activity. *Biochem Biophys Res Commun* (2007) **354**:216–21. doi:10.1016/j.bbrc.2006.12.202
155. Arima H, Yunomae K, Morikawa T, Hirayama F, Uekama K. Contribution of cholesterol and phospholipids to inhibitory effect of dimethyl-β-cyclodextrin on efflux function of P-glycoprotein and multidrug resistance-associated protein 2 in vinblastine-resistant Caco-2 cell monolayers. *Pharm Res* (2004) **21**:625–34. doi:10.1023/B:PHAM.0000022409.27896.d4
156. Bucher K, Belli S, Wunderli-Allenspach H, Kramer SD. P-glycoprotein in proteoliposomes with low residual detergent: the effects of cholesterol. *Pharm Res* (2007) **24**:1993–2004. doi:10.1007/s11095-007-9326-0
157. Belli S, Elsener PM, Wunderli-Allenspach H, Kramer SD. Cholesterol-mediated activation of P-glycoprotein: distinct effects on basal and drug-induced ATPase activities. *J Pharm Sci* (2009) **98**:1905–18. doi:10.1002/jps.21558
158. Saeki T, Shimabuku AM, Azuma Y, Shibano Y, Komano T, Ueda K. Expression of human P-glycoprotein in yeast cells-effects of membrane component sterols on the activity of P-glycoprotein. *Agric Biol Chem* (1991) **55**:1859–65. doi:10.1271/bbb1961.55.1859
159. Saeki T, Shimabuku AM, Ueda K, Komano T. Specific drug binding by purified lipid-reconstituted P-glycoprotein: dependence on the lipid composition. *Biochim Biophys Acta* (1992) **1107**:105–10. doi:10.1016/0005-2736(92)90334-I
160. Wang EJ, Casciano CN, Clement RP, Johnson WW. Cholesterol interaction with the daunorubicin binding site of P-glycoprotein. *Biochem Biophys Res Commun* (2000) **276**:909–16. doi:10.1006/bbrc.2000.3554
161. Kimura Y, Morita SY, Matsuo M, Ueda K. Mechanism of multidrug recognition by MDR1/ABCB1. *Cancer Sci* (2007) **98**:1303–10. doi:10.1111/j.1349-7006.2007.00538.x
162. Hamilton JA. Fast flip-flop of cholesterol and fatty acids in membranes: implications for membrane transport proteins. *Curr Opin Lipidol* (2003) **14**:263–71. doi:10.1097/00041433-200306000-00006
163. Leventis R, Silvius JR. Use of cyclodextrins to monitor transbilayer movement and differential lipid affinities of cholesterol. *Biophys J* (2001) **81**:2257–67. doi:10.1016/S0006-3495(01)75873-0
164. Brown DA, London E. Functions of lipid rafts in biological membranes. *Annu Rev Cell Dev Biol* (1998) **14**:111–36. doi:10.1146/annurev.cellbio.14.1.111
165. Orlowski S, Martin S, Escargueil A. P-glycoprotein and 'lipid rafts': some ambiguous mutual relationships (floating on them, building them or meeting them by chance?). *Cell Mol Life Sci* (2006) **63**:1038–59. doi:10.1007/s00018-005-5554-9
166. Radeva G, Perabo J, Sharom FJ. P-Glycoprotein is localized in intermediate-density membrane microdomains distinct from classical lipid rafts and caveolar domains. *FEBS J* (2005) **272**:4924–37. doi:10.1111/j.1742-4658.2005.04905.x
167. Reungpatthanaphong P, Marbeuf-Gueye C, Le Moyec L, Salerno M, Garnier-Suillerot A. Decrease of P-glycoprotein activity in K562/ADR cells by MβCD and filipin and lack of effect induced by cholesterol oxidase indicate that this transporter is not located in rafts. *J Bioenerg Biomembr* (2004) **36**:533–43.
168. Kamau SW, Kramer SD, Gunthert M, Wunderli-Allenspach H. Effect of the modulation of the membrane lipid composition on the localization and function of P-glycoprotein in MDR1-MDCK cells. *In vitro Cell Dev Biol Anim* (2005) **41**:207–16. doi:10.1290/0502016.1
169. Anderson TG, Tan A, Ganz P, Seelig J. Calorimetric measurement of phospholipid interaction with methyl-β-cyclodextrin. *Biochemistry* (2004) **43**:2251–61. doi:10.1021/bi0358869
170. Klappe K, Hummel I, Hoekstra D, Kok JW. Lipid dependence of ABC transporter localization and function. *Chem Phys Lipids* (2009) **161**:57–64. doi:10.1016/j.chemphyslip.2009.07.004
171. Hinrichs JW, Klappe K, Van Riezen M, Kok JW. Drug resistance-associated changes in sphingolipids and ABC transporters occur in different regions of membrane domains. *J Lipid Res* (2005) **46**:2367–76. doi:10.1194/jlr.M500070-JLR200
172. Modok S, Heyward C, Callaghan R. P-glycoprotein retains function when reconstituted into a sphingolipid- and cholesterol-rich environment. *J Lipid Res* (2004) **45**:1910–8. doi:10.1194/jlr.M400220-JLR200
173. Kramer SD, Lombardi D, Primorac A, Thomae AV, Wunderli-Allenspach H. Lipid-bilayer permeation of drug-like compounds. *Chem Biodivers* (2009) **6**:1900–16. doi:10.1002/cbdv.200900122
174. Regev R, Eytan GD. Flip-flop of doxorubicin across erythrocyte and lipid membranes. *Biochem Pharmacol* (1997) **54**:1151–8. doi:10.1016/S0006-2952(97)00326-2
175. Sharom FJ, Lu P, Liu R, Yu X. Linear and cyclic peptides as substrates and modulators of P-glycoprotein: peptide binding and effects on drug transport and accumulation. *Biochem J* (1998) **333**:621–30.
176. Nervi P, Li-Blatter X, Aanismaa P, Seelig A. P-glycoprotein substrate transport assessed by comparing cellular and vesicular ATPase activity. *Biochim Biophys Acta* (2010) **1798**:515–25. doi:10.1016/j.bbamem.2009.11.022
177. Eytan GD, Kuchel PW. Mechanism of action of P-glycoprotein in relation to passive membrane permeation. *Int Rev Cytol* (1999) **190**:175–250. doi:10.1016/S0074-7696(08)62148-8
178. Kabanov AV, Batrakova EV, Alakhov VY. Pluronic block copolymers for overcoming drug resistance in cancer. *Adv Drug Deliv Rev* (2002) **54**:759–79. doi:10.1016/S0169-409X(02)00047-9
179. Rege BD, Kao JP, Polli JE. Effects of nonionic surfactants on membrane transporters in Caco-2 cell monolayers. *Eur J Pharm Sci* (2002) **16**:237–46. doi:10.1016/S0928-0987(02)00055-6
180. Krylova OO, Melik-Nubarov NS, Badun GA, Ksenofontov AL, Menger FM, Yaroslavov AA. Pluronic L61 accelerates flip-flop and transbilayer doxorubicin permeation. *Chemistry* (2003) **9**:3930–6. doi:10.1002/chem.200204621

10

Will the requirement by the US FDA to simultaneously co-develop companion diagnostics (CDx) delay the approval of receptor tyrosine kinase inhibitors for RTK-rearranged (*ROS1-, RET-, AXL-, PDGFR-α-, NTRK1-*) non-small cell lung cancer globally?

Sai-Hong Ignatius Ou[1]*, Ross A. Soo[2], Akihito Kubo[3], Tomoya Kawaguchi[4] and Myung-Ju Ahn[5]

[1] *Chao Family Comprehensive Cancer Center, University of California Irvine School of Medicine, Orange, CA, USA*
[2] *National University Health System and Cancer Science Institute of Singapore, Singapore*
[3] *Aichi Medical University School of Medicine, Nagakute, Japan*
[4] *National Hospital Organization Kinki-Chuo Chest Medical Center, Sakai City, Japan*
[5] *Division of Hematology-Oncology, Department of Medicine, Samsung Medical Center, Sungkyunkwan University School of Medicine, Seoul, South Korea*

Edited by:
Jan Trøst Jørgensen, Dx-Rx Institute, Denmark

Reviewed by:
Brion William Murray, Pfizer Worldwide Research & Development, USA
Amit K. Tiwari, Tuskegee University, USA

****Correspondence:***
Sai-Hong Ignatius Ou, Division of Hematology-Oncology, Department of Medicine, Chao Family Comprehensive Cancer Center, University of California Irvine Medical Center, University of California Irvine School of Medicine, 101 City Drive, Building 56, RT81, Orange, CA 92868-3298, USA
e-mail: ignatius.ou@uci.edu

The discovery of anaplastic lymphoma kinase (*ALK*) rearrangement in non-small cell lung cancer (NSCLC) in 2007 and the approval of crizotinib for the treatment of advanced *ALK*-rearranged NSCLC in 2011 represents a landmark in the development of targeted oncology therapy. The approval of crizotinib was accompanied simultaneously by the approval of the Vysis (Abbott Molecular) break-apart fluorescence *in situ* hybridization (FISH) test as the companion diagnostic (CDx) test to detect *ALK* rearrangement. Pfizer, the manufacturer of crizotinib, sponsored the screening of thousands of patients and the standardization of the *ALK* FISH test as part of the approval process for crizotinib, a first in class ALK inhibitor. Many pharmaceutical companies are now using the Food and Drug Administration (FDA)-approved *ALK* FISH assay to enroll patients onto trials for their own respective ALK inhibitors. In essence they are "piggy-backing" on the FDA-approved *ALK* FISH assay without having to pay for the development of a CDx, nor screening for *ALK*-rearranged NSCLC patients in the protocols because screening for *ALK* rearrangement is now the standard of care in NSCLC after the approval of crizotinib. Since 2007, rearrangement in more receptor tyrosine kinases (RTKs) such as *ROS1, RET, AXL, PDGFR-α, and NTRK1* have been discovered in NSCLC but the incidence of each subtype of RTK-rearranged NSCLC is quite rare. Crizotinib has now demonstrated significant clinical activity in *ROS1*-rearranged NSCLC patients. Whether crizotinib will gain official FDA approval for use in *ROS1*-rearranged NSCLC, on the other hand, remains unclear as there is no test for *ROS1*-rearrangement currently being developed to support US FDA approval as a CDx. This may be due in part to the fact that the full cost associated with the development of a pre-market approved-approved CDx must be borne by the company seeking the first drug approval in a new indication. Given the low incidence of *ROS1*-rearrangement in NSCLC, and the availability of crizotinib in most countries, a more cost-effective way is for crizotinib to gain compendium listing for *ROS1*-rearranged NSCLC in treatment guidelines. However, without a formal indication from the FDA, a drug cannot be marketed for off label use, it is unlikely that payers public or private will routinely pay for molecular testing for *ROS1*-rearrangement in NSCLC let alone reimburse off label use of crizotinib. Similarly, several marketed tyrosine kinase inhibitors (TKIs) in the US (sorafenib, sunitinib, vandetanib, cabozantinib, regorafenib) are potent RET inhibitors *in vitro*. It does not make sense for any one pharmaceutical company to shoulder the full cost of developing a particular CDx for *RET*-rearranged NSCLC where, once approved, it may be used by other pharmaceutical companies to gain addition labeling approval for their own RET inhibitors. Thus, the requirement by the US FDA that a specific CDx have to be co-developed and standardized for each of the molecular subtype of NSCLC as part of the drug approval process, while prudent, may have the un-intended consequence of deterring clinical development of these TKIs in these very rare molecular subsets of NSCLC. While we all march to the drumbeat of precision cancer medicine, the stringent requirement of co-development CDx for each molecular subtype of solid tumor may inadvertently make this goal substantially more difficult to achieve.

Keywords: companion diagnostics, *ALK*-rearranged NSCLC, *ROS1*-rearranged NSCLC, *RET*-rearranged NSCLC, fluorescence *in situ* hybridization, immunohistochemistry, next generation sequencing, reverse transcription-polymerase chain reaction

INTRODUCTION

Achieving personalized medicine is the "holy grail" in oncology. The approval of crizotinib in the US, an anaplastic lymphoma kinase (ALK)/ROS1/MET multi-targeted tyrosine kinase inhibitor (TKI), merely 4 years after the discovery of rearrangement in ALK in non-small cell lung cancer (NSCLC) represented a landmark in oncology drug development and a significant step toward the goal of personalized medicine in oncology (1). The approval of crizotinib was accompanied the simultaneous approval of the Vysis (Abbott Molecular) break-apart fluorescence *in situ* hybridization (FISH) companion diagnostics (CDx) assay by the US Food and Drug Administration (FDA) for the detection of *ALK* rearrangement in NSCLC. The success of crizotinib has shone a bright spotlight on the existence of molecular subsets of NSCLC and other epithelial malignancies that are driven by rearrangement in receptor tyrosine kinases (RTKs) and heralded the era of RTK rearrangement in solid tumor oncology. Since 2007 other RTK-rearrangements in NSCLC have been discovered (**Table 1**). Concurrently, various diagnostic tests besides FISH have been offered by major commercial diagnostic companies in the US to detect the different RTK-rearrangements. Given the rarity of RTK rearrangement in NSCLC and the requirement by US FDA to develop an analytically and clinically validated CDx for approval of TKIs against each RTK-rearranged molecular cohort, challenges abound in persuading many pharmaceutical companies to pursue a simultaneous registration strategy. We will review the lessons learned from the development of crizotinib for *ALK*-rearranged NSCLC where several second generation ALK inhibitors are in now development due to the existence of an FDA-approved CDx, the ongoing challenges in gaining additional FDA approval for crizotinib in the treatment of *ROS1*-rearranged NSCLC due to a lack of an approved CDx for *ROS1*-rearranged NSCLC, the immense challenges in gaining approval for any currently marketed TKI that are also potential RET TKI for the treatment of *RET*-rearranged NSCLC due to again the lack of an FDA-approved CDx for *RET* rearrangement (**Table 2**). Additionally, we will discuss whether the first FDA-approved CDx is the optimal CDx going forward given the inevitability of technology obsolescence coupled with the exponential gain in knowledge in the understanding of these subsets of molecularly defined NSCLC. Finally, we speculate that if the current challenges of co-CDx approval are not overcame how the development of precision cancer medicine may be impeded.

THE DISCOVERY OF RECEPTOR TYROSINE KINASE-REARRANGED (*ALK-*, *ROS1-*, *RET-*, *AXL-*, *PDGFR-α-*, *NTRK1-*) NSCLC

All the RTK-rearrangements identified in NSCLC occur in genes of the human RTK family, which consists of 58 members (11). The discovery of *ALK* rearrangement in NSCLC in 2007 was significant because prior to the discovery it was believed that gene fusions especially involving RTK rearrangement were believed to be rare in epithelial tumors (12). It is abundantly clear that each subtype of RTK-rearranged NSCLC is itself a heterogeneous disease made up many different (and yet to be discovered) fusion partners translocated to the same RTK (**Table 1**). The complexity within each molecular subtype of RTK-rearranged NSCLC have implications on the CDx. Ideally a CDx should be technically simple and/or be easily standardized, cost-effective, but also provide "forward-looking" information such as the exact fusion variant with at the exact breakpoint so that subtle differences among the various fusion variants within each molecular subtype of RTK-rearranged NSCLC can be elucidated.

Rearrangement of *ROS1* in NSCLC was discovered contemporaneously in 2007 by one of the two groups that discovered *ALK* rearrangement (13). *ROS1* shares extensive amino acid sequence homology with ALK in particular within the kinase domain making ROS1 a potential target for ALK inhibitors (14). Prior to 2007, *ROS1*-rearrangement was discovered in glioblastoma multiforme (15) and subsequently has been discovered in other major epithelial tumor types including gastric (16) and colorectal adenocarcinoma (17).

The *RET* (rearranged during transfection) proto-oncogene was first identified in 1985 through transfection of NIH3T3 cells with human lymphoma DNA (18). RET rearrangement has also been well characterized in thyroid cancer (19). Since 2012, multiple groups using various techniques published the rearrangement of RET in NSCLC with four identified fusion partners so far (*KIF5B-CCDC6-*, *NOCA4-*, *TRIM33-*) (2) (**Table 1**).

Rearrangement of the tropomyosin-related kinase gene (TRKA) was first biologically characterized in 1986 in a colorectal carcinoma patient (20), when tropomyosin was found to be fused to an unknown DNA sequence that likely codes for a transmembrane RTK (*TPM3-TRKA*) (20). The normal function of TRKA is the receptor for neurotrophins and is responsible for differentiation into subtypes of sensory neurons. TRKA has been renamed as neurotrophic tyrosine receptor kinase 1 (NTRK1) as it is one of three members of NTRK family (21). In 2013, rearrangement in NTRK1 was reported in NSCLC involving fusion partners with CD74 and MPRIP as fusion partners (*CD74-NTRK1*, *MPRIP-NTRK1*) (4). Screening a panel of NSCLC that are pan-negative for oncogenic driver mutations, they found 3 out of 91 (3.3%) were positive for *NTRK1* rearrangement. Cell-based and xenograft assays using NTRK1 inhibitors in NTRK1 transformed cells led to inhibition of cellular proliferation and tumor shrinkage, respectively, indicated *NTRK1* rearrangement are indeed a driver mutation in NSCLC (4). Of note similar to RET, rearrangement of *NTRK1* has been described in thyroid cancer (*TPM3-NTRK1*, *TPR-NTRK1*, *TFG-NTRK1*) (22).

AXL, termed from the Greek word anexelekto, or uncontrolled, was identified initially as a transforming oncogene in two chronic myelogeneous leukemia (CML) patients in 1991 (23). In 2012, *AXL* was found to be fused to MAP3K12 binding inhibitory protein 1 (MBIP) resulting in *AXL-MBIP* fusion variant by whole genome sequencing (WGS) (3). In the same study, Seo et al. also discovered the platelet derived growth factor receptor-alpha (*PDGFR-α*) was fused to SR-related CTD-associated factor 11 (*SCAF11-PDGFR-α*) in NSCLC (3). Prior to that, rearrangement in *PGDFR-α* was found in myeloid and lymphoid neoplasms with esinophilia where *PDGFR-α* is fused to Flip1-like 1 gene (FIP1L1) (*FIP1L1-PDGFR-α*) (24). Interesting aberrantly activation by phosphorylation of *PDGFR-α* was demonstrated in one cell line (H1703) and several patient samples in 2007 but no rearrangement was discovered (13). In summary, many of the RTK-rearrangements in NSCLC were discovered in other tumors but because of the success of crizotinib

Table 1 | Characteristics of RTK rearrangement in NSCLC.

RTK rearrangement	Year identified	Fusion partners	Estimate prevalence (%)	Methods of initial identification	Select reference
ALK	2007	EML4-, KIF5B-, KCL-, TFG-	~5–8	Tumor DNA transfection, Phospho-kinase activation	Ou et al. (1)
ROS1	2007	CD74-, SDC4-, SLC34A2-,TPM3-, FIG-, KDEL2-, CCDC6-, LRIG3-, ERZ-	~2	Phospho-kinase activation	Gainor and Shaw (2)
RET	2012	KIF5B-, CCDC6-, NOCA4-, TRIM33-	~2	FISH, NGS, WGS	Gainor and Shaw (2)
AXL	2012	MBIP-	NA	WGS	Seo et al. (3)
PDGFR-α	2012	SCAF11-	NA	WGS	Seo et al. (3)
NTRK1	2013	CD74-, MPRIP-	~3[a]	FISH, NGS	Vaishnavi et al. (4)

[a]3.3% in ALK, ROS1, RET negative NSCLC.

the discovery of these RTK-rearrangements in NSCLC has drawn increased attention to these RTKs in all tumor types (25).

ALK INHIBITORS FOR THE TREATMENT OF *ALK*- AND *ROS1*-REARRANGED NSCLC

While crizotinib is the first and only ALK inhibitor approved for the treatment of advanced *ALK*-rearranged NSCLC since August 2011, the majority of patients invariably progress on crizotinib with a median progression-free survival of about 8 months (26). The incorporation of break-apart ALK FISH as the FDA-approved CDx for detection of *ALK* rearrangement through the approval of crizotinib has provided a new standard of care with an established assay to screen for and enroll these *ALK*-rearranged NSCLC patients onto clinical trials of these ALK inhibitors. Pfizer, the manufacturer of crizotinib, engaged a diagnostic company to support both the development and technical validation of the *ALK* FISH CDx. In this case, Abbott Molecular sponsored the *ALK* FISH screening test and the validity of the CDx and the regulatory approval of the CDx as well as all screening of patients, to support the drug approval but Pfizer paid for everything Abbott Molecular. In retrospect, Pfizer essentially paved the way for competitors to more easily develop follow-on ALK inhibitors by establishing the clinical validity of a CDx test and screening for *ALK*-rearranged NSCLC patients. This realization, we believe has important implications on how the CDx for the other unique RTK-rearranged NSCLC may be developed by pharmaceutical companies.

Crizotinib has also shown significant clinical activity in *ROS1*-rearranged NSCLC due to the homology between the kinase domain (27). As part of the original phase I crizotinib trial (PROFILE1001, NCT00585195), the assay for the trial to detect *ROS1*-rearrangement is a locally developed laboratory-based test and no formal CDx is being developed for FDA approval in conjunction with the trial. In order for Pfizer to gain formal FDA approval for crizotinib in *ROS1*-rearranged NSCLC, Pfizer may have to sponsor another large scale trial and more importantly pay for the screening and analytical and clinical validation of a *ROS1* CDx (likely be FISH again) so that a CDx can be submitted simultaneously for FDA approval in support for the clinical activity of crizotinib in *ROS1*-rearranged NSCLC. However, once a CDx for *ROS1*-rearrangement is approved by the US FDA, other pharmaceutical companies can take advantage of the existence of an FDA-approved ROS1 CDx to develop their own ROS1 inhibitors similarly to the situations for current ALK inhibitors in clinical development. Given the low incidence of *ROS1*-rearranged NSCLC (~2%), Pfizer or other pharmaceutical companies is unlikely to make this investment given crizotinib is already available in many countries. Furthermore, although many Clinical Laboratory Improvement Amendments (CLIA)-certified commercial diagnostic companies in the US are offering *ROS1*-rearrangement testing [either by break-apart FISH, reverse transcription-polymerase chain reaction (RT-PCR), or even next generation sequencing (NGS)], without an official indication from the US FDA, screening for *ROS1*-rearrangement among community oncologists in the US will not be a common practice. Without an official FDA indication of crizotinib for *ROS1*-rearranged NSCLC, even with the endorsement of the National Comprehensive Cancer Centers Network (NCCN) guidelines, insurance companies may not pay for crizotinib for the few *ROS1*-positive NSCLC patients, even if their oncologists prescribe it. Furthermore, without an FDA indication for *ROS1*-rearranged NSCLC, the research of *ROS1*-rearrangement in other major epithelial tumor types such as colon (17) and gastric cancer (16), the cost of co-developing a companion diagnostics for *ROS1*-rearrangement will dissuade a lot of pharmaceutical companies to pursue a registration strategy in any *ROS1*-rearranged tumors even if they have potent ROS1 inhibitors in the pipeline.

WILL A RET INHIBITOR EVER BE FORMALLY APPROVED BY THE US FDA FOR *RET*-REARRANGED NSCLC AND WHAT IS THE IMPLICATION IF THE ANSWER IS NO?

We ask this question because the clinical reality of *RET*-rearranged NSCLC is even more relevant in illustrating the central theme of this perspective. There are currently at least six marketed TKIs (regorafenib, cabozantinib, ponatinib, sunitinib, sorafenib, vandetanib) in the US that are also potent *in vitro* RET inhibitors (**Table 2**). Under the current US FDA regulations, manufacturers of any one of the above marketed TKIs who wants to gain an additional approval for treatment of *RET*-rearranged NSCLC will have

Table 2 | List of potential RET inhibitors potentially for the treatment of RET-rearranged NSCLC.

Compound	Trade name	Manufacturer	*In vitro* kinase IC_{50} (nM) against RET	*In vitro* cellular kinase IC_{50} (nM) against RET	*In vitro* IC50 (nm) against RET V804 mutant	Other targets	Approved indications in the US	In clinical trial for RET-rearranged NSCLC	CDx used to detect *RET* rearrangement in NSCLC trials
Regorafenib (5)	Stivarga	Bayer	1.5	~10	NR	VEGFR1-3, KIT, RAF-1, BRAF, BRAFV600E, PDGFR-β	Treatment refractory colorectal adenocarcinoma	No	N/A
Ponatinib (6)	Iclusig	ARIAD	7	0.7–11	12	Bcr-abl, FGFR1-4,	TKI resistance CML or Ph + ALL	Yes[a] NCT01813734	FISH, NGS
Cabozantinib (7)	Cometriq	Exelixis	5.2	27–85	>5000	VEGFR2, c-MET	Medullary thyroid cancer	Yes NCT01639508	FISH, NGS
Lenvatinib (E7080) (8)	N/A	Eisai	1.5	48 (CCDC6-RET)	NR	VEGFR1-3, FGFR1-3, PDGFR, c-kit	N/A	Yes NCT01877083	NGS
Sunitinib (6)	Sutent	Pfizer	30	40–164	55	PDGFR, VEGFRs, c-kit, FLT-3	RCC, GIST, unresectable/ metastatic PNET	Yes NCT01829217	FISH, NGS
Sorefenib (9)	Nexaavar	Bayer	47	~20–50	55	Raf, PDGFR, VEGFR2, VEGFR3, c-kit,	HCC, RCC,	No	N/A
Vandetanib (10)	Caprelsa	AstraZeneca	100	NR	NR	VEGFR, EGFR	Medullary thyroid cancer	Yes NCT01823068	FISH

[a] *Currently on hold.*

N/A, not applicable; NR, not reported.

PDGFR, platelet derived growth factor receptor; NGS, next generation sequencing; PNET, pancreatic neuroendocrine tumor; VEGFR, vascular endothelial growth factor receptor.

to pay for the screening for thousands of NSCLC patients and the development of a *RET*-rearrangement CDx. Again given the low incidence of *RET*-rearranged of NSCLC (~2%) and the potential crowded market for RET inhibitors, it is unlikely manufacturer of any one of the six potential marketed RET inhibitors will sponsor such as a trial, lest it will allow competitors to piggyback on the CDx to gain approval of their TKIs without shouldering the cost for patient screening and developing an approvable CDx. This is currently, the case as all the clinical trials in these marketed TKIs are investigator-initiated trials with a diverse platforms to screen for *RET* rearrangement (**Table 2**). Indeed, preliminary clinical activity of cabozantinib in three *RET*-rearranged NSCLC patients has been recently published (28). The exception is the manufacturer of lenvatinib (E7080) (Eisai Company, Ltd.) who is sponsoring a trial of lenvatinib in *RET*-rearranged NSLCL primarily in Asia using NGS as the primary CDx (NCT01829217) (**Table 2**). Without a US FDA-approved RET CDx, not only will potential RET inhibitors not gain US FDA approval to treat *RET*-rearranged NSCLC but other *RET*-rearranged malignancies such as thyroid cancer (19) or chronic myelomonocytic leukemia (CMML) (29).

Going forward, many small molecular inhibitors are being developed against *AXL* (30) and *NTRK1* (31, 32). Additionally, imatinib has shown excellent clinical activity against myeloid and lymphoid malignancies harboring *FIP1L1-PDGFR-α* rearrangement (33). Thus, achieving the goal of precision cancer medicine hinges on formal approval of these inhibitors to treat these various rare but diverse molecularly defined and driven malignancies and the requirement to co-develop a CDx may be a huge impediment to achieving this goal.

IS THE FIRST APPROVED CDx THE BEST CDx CONSIDERING THE ISSUES OF COST-EFFECTIVENESS, KNOWLEDGE ADVANCEMENT, AND TECHNOLOGY OBSOLESCENCE?

The approval of the Abbott Vysis break-apart FISH assay by the FDA as the CDx for the diagnosis of *ALK*-rearranged NSCLC seemed to have established break-apart FISH as the lead method platform to diagnose RTK rearrangement in NSCLC. However, break-apart FISH is probably "the worst of both worlds" as a CDx platform. There are three major criteria that have to be satisfied for a break-apart FISH to be considered positive: (1) a minimum of 50 cells have to be counted; (2) signals are considered "break-apart" when they are separated by at least two diameter in length OR only the 3′ signal is present; (3) at least 15% of the cells have to contain the break-apart signals. Polysomy is common in *ALK*-rearranged lung cancer tumor (34) thus, identifying all these criteria requires technical expertise and expert interpretation and is labor-intensive and time consuming. Additionally, FISH is prohibitively expensive as a mass screening method for many countries. Finally, FISH will not identify the specific fusion partner to the rearranged RTK gene. As our knowledge about RTK-rearranged NSCLC grows, it is highly likely that different RTK fusion variant will have different clinicopathologic characteristics such as extent of disease, site of metastasis, and differential response to TKIs (35), which required even more tailored treatment in the future. In summary, FISH is neither an inexpensive mass screening CDx nor does it lead to further understanding of the pathogenesis of RTK-rearranged NSCLC.

In contrast, ALK protein is only expressed in tumor tissue due to transcriptional activation from the promoter of the 5′-fusion partner to ALK but not in normal tissue and can be easily detected by immunohistochemistry (IHC). IHC is inexpensive and easily performed by all pathologists. Furthermore, ALK IHC has been demonstrated to show high concordance to ALK FISH (36). Since October 2012, IHC (Ventana automated staining system using D5F3 antibody from Cell Signaling Inc.) has been approved in the European Union (EU) as a CDx to detect *ALK* rearrangement along with break-apart FISH. This automated ALK IHC staining platform has shown extremely high sensitivity and specificity to ALK FISH (37). In September 2013 China approved the same method approved in EU to detect *ALK* rearrangement.

Immunohistochemistry has been used to detect *ROS1*-rearrangement in NSCLC and the sensitivity and specificity of ROS1 IHC is found to be 100 and 92%, respectively (38). Thus, it is likely with further refinement, IHC will likely be widely used to detect *ROS1*-rearrangement. On the other hand, RET is highly expressed in normal tissue and the sensitivity of RET IHC is low and thus, IHC may not be an ideal CDx to diagnose *RET* rearrangement (39). Thus, while IHC is a standard pathology procedure and cheaper than FISH, it is not applicable to all the different RTK-rearrangements depending on the normal expression pattern of the RTK in that particular tumor type. Much remain to be discovered on the expression level of *TRK1*-, *AXL*-, and *PDGFRα*- fusion proteins in NSCLC before we can really assess the utility of IHC in the detecting of these newly discovered molecular subtypes of RTK-rearranged NSCLC.

Reverse transcription-polymerase chain reaction is another commonly utilized research technique to detect RTK rearrangement. RT-PCR is highly specific and can be easily performed in standard diagnostic laboratories. However, most of the RT-PCR studies require large volume of tumor tissue snapped frozen from surgical resection. In daily oncology practice, the vast majority of the NSCLC are diagnosed from fine or core needle biopsy from which the tissue is placed in formalin instead of snap frozen at −80°C. RNA is not easily preserved in formalin-fixed tissues and thus RT-PCR may not be technically feasible in many of the samples. Also given that each unique molecular subtype of RTK-rearranged NSCLC has many different fusion variants; in order to identify all the known fusion variants the PCR has to contain primers to all the fusion partners. Any un-reported/un-discovered fusion partner will be missed by RT-PCR. In the case of *ROS1*-rearrangement, at least nine sets of primers for the nine reported fusion partners have to be present in the RT-PCR. Therefore, although RT-PCR has been commercialized in the US to detect RTK-rearranged NSCLC (40), it is not a widely adopted CDx and unlikely to gain global acceptance.

Next generation sequencing is a broad term that generally describes the massively parallel sequencing approach and employing various detection methods on a panel of genes that are altered in cancer. Many NGS panels of varying number of gene are now being offered commercially. For example, Foundation Medicine Inc., is offering a 236 gene test that can detect mutations, copy number alterations, and 19 gene rearrangements that has been used commercially used to detect new *RET* rearrangement in an investigator-initiated trial (28) or previously undetected *ALK* rearrangement (41).

Advances in the understanding of neoplastic diseases couple with technical advancement in the field of diagnostic tests raise the ongoing issue of technology obsolescence supporting the original FDA-approved test. Technology obsolescence will invariably poses a significant problem with time because one particular technology/diagnostic platform (i.e., FISH) is essentially linked to drug labeling by the FDA. With time that one specific diagnostic platform may turn out to be expensive, highly operator dependent with a steep learning curve, not easily automatable, and provide scant clinical information (e.g., FISH does not provide the fusion partner nor the break-point, which may be important in underlying the clinicopathologic and natural history of that particular RTK rearrangement). The ideal future CDx should be able to pinpoint chromosomal breakpoint and to identify the various fusion partners to a particular RTK rearrangement so that, we can continue to advance our molecular understanding of oncology in order to refine our approach to personalized medicine.

However, to get a different CDx platform approved by the FDA will again incur significant expense not only in standardization and validation of the new CDx but the cost of conducting a clinical trial "reinventing" the original approval process.

SAMPLE SURVEY OF THE APPROVED INDICATIONS FOR CRIZOTINIB OUTSIDE THE US

Crizotinib received conditional approval in the EU in July 2012 for previously treated ALK-positive NSCLC with the recommendation that a validated test for *ALK* rearrangement be used. Similarly crizotinib was approved in Singapore in 2013 for the treatment of locally advanced or metastatic *ALK*-rearranged NSCLC detected by an accurate and validated test. However, no one particular CDx (such as FISH) was specified by the approval in both EU and Singapore. Granted that in EU the approval of medicines and CDx are coordinated by two different agencies (42). Indeed, since October 2012, Vetana ALK IHC has been approved as a CDx for *ALK* rearrangement also. In Korea (2012), Japan (2012), and Australia (2013), crizotinib was approved for treatment of *ALK*-rearranged NSCLC without mention of the detection method. Granted by 2012, there is plentiful data supporting high concordance FISH and IHC (36) or even NGS (41) thus it is not necessary to pigeonhole a drug approval to one particular CDx. However, without the initial US FDA approval of crizotinib and the advance in knowledge over the intervening years it is likely that "relaxed" CDx requirement will not be possible in many countries. Thus, approval of the US FDA remains the gold standard for the drug regulatory agencies and authorities in many countries.

CONCLUDING PERSPECTIVES

Many of the RTKs discussed in this perspective were discovered in 1980s as transformed oncogenes due to elegant basic science research. It has been more than 30 years since then to now where we are at the cusp of realizing precision cancer medicine by successfully translating these discoveries to therapeutic approvals and finally bearing fruit of all the research funding for the benefit of patients. The successful launch of crizotinib has been an inspiring example of this development.

The technologies to screen for these RTKs in all tumors are commercially available; inhibitors to these RTKs are either approved for other indication or in early clinical development. Because of the rarity of these RTK-rearrangements, the cost of sponsoring a registration trial for a particular TKI and simultaneous development of a CDx is prohibitively expensive and clinical progress is being delayed due to reluctance of pharmaceutical companies to pursue such narrow indications in rare disease populations.

One attractive though organizationally challenging solution may be to foster a collaboration of government, pharmaceutical companies, and diagnostic companies pooling resources together to an independent consortium to establish analytical and clinical validity of CDx platforms for detection of RTK-rearrangements and potentially other cancer genes. The US FDA may then approve these CDx platforms such as FISH, IHC, or NGS for each or several RTK-rearrangements and then allowing pharmaceutical companies to sponsor the trials and select any of the CDx platforms to demonstrate clinical benefit. This will alleviate the burden of simultaneously developing a CDx that can then be "piggy-backed" by other pharmaceutical companies developing their own inhibitors. Additionally, this will eliminate potential conflict of interest as some global pharmaceutical companies also own major diagnostic companies (i.e., Ventana Medical Systems by F. Hoffmann-La Roche, Genoptix by Novartis) where one particular diagnostic platform may be favored by one pharmaceutical company due to technological knowhow and/or existing patents.

Short of industry-wide cooperation, regulatory policy may be used to lower regulatory burdens and create a more favorable incentive structure for therapeutic and diagnostics companies pursuing targeted therapy and CDx development. For instance, to reduce CDx costs, certain CDx quality systems and validation requirements may be simplified or deferred to the post-approval period, given appropriate risk determination. And as above, some assays may be approvable based on analytical validation data alone, decoupling diagnostic from therapeutic development decisions and thus streamlining coordination.

The requirement for co-development and co-approval of CDx in order to get TKIs approved against these RTK (*ROS1, RET, NTRK1, AXL, PDGFR-α*) rearrangement lung cancer represents the daunting challenge to successfully translate decades of basic science research into benefit of cancer patients. However, the successful approval of TKIs to treat *ROS1-*, *RET-*, *NTRK1-*, *PDGFR-α*, and *AXL*-rearranged NSCLC is vitally important as it sets the example for approval of TKIs to treat the same RTK-rearranged common epithelial tumors such as colon, gastric, and breast cancers (25). Using NSCLC as a tumor example, we wish this perspective contributed to the ongoing in-depth discussions about how to optimally and expeditiously develop TKIs to receive US FDA approval in the current regulatory environment where co-development and co-approval of a CDx is required for a drug in other TK-driven cancers.

REFERENCES

1. Ou SI, Barlett CH, Mino-Kneudson M, Cui J, Iafrate AJ. Crizotinib for the treatment of *ALK*-rearranged non-small cell lung cancer: a success story to usher in the second decade of molecular targeted therapy in oncology. *Oncologist* (2012) **17**:1351–75. doi:10.1634/theoncologist.2012-0311

2. Gainor JF, Shaw AT. Novel targets in non-small cell lung cancer. *ROS1* and *RET* fusions. *Oncologist* (2013) **18**:865–75. doi:10.1634/theoncologist.2013-0095
3. Seo J, Ju YS, Lee W, Shin J, Lee JK, Bleazard T, et al. The transcriptional landscape and mutational profile of lung adenocarcinoma. *Genome Res* (2012) **22**:2109–19. doi:10.1101/gr.145144.112
4. Vaishnavi A, Capelletti M, Le AT, Kako S, Butaney M, Ercan D, et al. Oncogenic and drug-sensitive *NTRK1* rearrangement in lung cancer. *Nat Med* (2013) **19**:1469–72. doi:10.1038/nm.3352
5. Wilheim SM, Dumas J, Adnane L, Lynch M, Carter CA, Schutz G, et al. Regorafenib (BAY 73-4506): a new oral multikinase inhibitor of angiogenic, stromal and oncogenic receptor tyrosine kinases with potent preclinical antitumor activity. *Int J Cancer* (2011) **129**:245–55. doi:10.1002/ijc.25864
6. Mologni L, Radaelli S, Morandi A, Plaza-Menacho I, Gambacorti-Passerini C. Ponatinib is a potent inhibitor of wild-type and drug-resistant gatekeeper mutant RET kinase. *Mol Cell Endocrinol* (2013) **377**:1–6. doi:10.1016/j.mce.2013.06.025
7. Bentzien F, Zuzow M, Heald N, Gibson A, Shi Y, Goon L, et al. *In vitro* and *in vivo* activity of cabozantinib (XL184), an inhibitor of RET, MET, and VEGFR2, in a model of medullary thyroid cancer. *Thyroid* (2013) **23**:1569–77. doi:10.1089/thy.2013.0137
8. Okamoto K, Kodama K, Takase K, Sugi NH, Yamamoto Y, Iwata M, et al. Antitumor activities of the targeted multi-tyrosine kinase inhibitor lenvatinib (E7080) against RET gene fusion-driven tumor models. *Cancer Lett* (2013) **340**:97–103. doi:10.1016/j.canlet.2013.07.007
9. Carlomagno F, Anaganti S, Guida T, Salvatore G, Troncone G, Wilhelm SM, et al. Bayer 43-9006 inhibition of oncogenic RET mutants. *J Natl Cancer Inst* (2006) **98**:326–34. doi:10.1093/jnci/djj069
10. Carlomagno F, Vitagliano D, Guida T, Clardiello F, Tortora G, Vecchio G, et al. ZD6474, an orally available inhibitor of KDR tyrosine kinase activity, efficiently blocks oncogenic RET kinases. *Cancer Res* (2002) **62**:7284–90.
11. Blume-Jensen P, Hunter T. Oncogenic kinase signalling. *Nature* (2001) **411**:355–65. doi:10.1038/35077225
12. Mitelman F, Johansson B, Mertens F. Fusion genes and rearranged genes as a linear function of chromosome aberrations in cancer. *Nat Genet* (2004) **36**:331–4. doi:10.1038/ng1335
13. Rikova K, Guo A, Zeng Q, Possemato A, Yu J, Haack H, et al. Global survey of phosphotyrosine signaling identifies oncogenic kinases in lung cancer. *Cell* (2007) **131**:1190–203. doi:10.1016/j.cell.2007.11.025
14. Ou SI, Tan J, Yen Y, Soo RA. ROS1 as a 'druggable' receptor tyrosine kinase: lessons learned from inhibiting the ALK pathway. *Expert Rev Anticancer Ther* (2012) **12**:447–56. doi:10.1586/era.12.17
15. Charest A, Lane K, McMahon K, Park J, Preisinger E, Conroy H, et al. Fusion of FIG to the receptor tyrosine kinase ROS in a glioblastoma with an interstitial del(6)(q21q21). *Genes Chromosomes Cancer* (2003) **37**:58–71. doi:10.1002/gcc.10207
16. Lee J, Lee SE, Kang SY, Do I, Lee S, Ha SY, et al. Identification of ROS1 rearrangement in gastric adenocarcinoma. *Cancer* (2013) **119**:1627–35. doi:10.1002/cncr.27967
17. Aisner DL, Nguyen TT, Paskulin DD, Le AT, Haney J, Schulte N, et al. *ROS1* and *ALK* fusions in colorectal cancer, with evidence of intratumoral heterogeneity for molecular drivers. *Mol Cancer Res* (2013) **12**:111–8. doi:10.1158/1541-7786.MCR-13-0479-T
18. Takahashi M, Ritz J, Cooper GM. Activation of a novel human transforming gene, ret, by DNA rearrangement. *Cell* (1985) **42**:581–8. doi:10.1016/0092-8674(85)90115-1
19. Santoro M, Melillo RM, Fusco A. RET/PTC activation in papillary thyroid cancer: European Journal of Endocrinology prize lecture. *Eur J Endocrinol* (2006) **155**:645–53. doi:10.1530/eje.1.02289
20. Martin-Zanca D, Hughes SH, Barbacid M. A human oncogene formed by the fusion of truncated tropomyosin and protein tyrosine kinase sequences. *Nature* (1986) **319**:741–8. doi:10.1038/319743a0
21. Longo FM, Massa SM. Small molecule modulation of neurotrophin receptors: a strategy for the treatment of neurological disease. *Nat Rev Drug Discov* (2013) **12**:507–25. doi:10.1038/nrd4024
22. Greco A, Miranda C, Pierotti MA. Rearrangements of *NTRK1* gene in papillary thyroid carcinoma. *Mol Cell Endocrinol* (2010) **321**:44–9. doi:10.1016/j.mce.2009.10.009
23. O'Bryan JP, Frye RA, Cogswell PC, Neubauer A, Kitch B, Prokop C, et al. axl, a transforming gene isolated from primary human myeloid leukemia cells, encodes a novel receptor tyrosine kinase. *Mol Cell Biol* (1991) **11**:5016–31.
24. Gotlib J, Cools J. Five years since the discovery of *PIP1L1-PDGFRA*: what we have learned about the fusion and other molecularly defined eosinophilias. *Leukemia* (2008) **22**:1999–2010. doi:10.1038/leu.2008.287
25. Shaw AT, Hsu PP, Awad MM, Engelman JA. Tyrosine kinase gene rearrangements in epithelial malignancies. *Nat Rev Cancer* (2013) **11**:772–87. doi:10.1038/nrc3612
26. Shaw AT, Kim DW, Nakagawa K, Seto T, Crinó L, Ahn MJ, et al. Crizotinib versus chemotherapy in advanced ALK-positive lung cancer. *N Engl J Med* (2013) **368**:2385–94. doi:10.1056/NEJMoa1214886
27. Ou SHI, Bang YJ, Camidge DR, Riely GR, Salgia R, Shapiro G, et al. Efficacy and safety of crizotinib in patients with advanced *ROS1*-rearranged non-small cell lung cancer (NSCLC). *J Clin Oncol* (2013) **31**(Suppl.):abstr. 8032.
28. Drilon A, Wang L, Hasanovic A, Suehara Y, Lipson D, Stephens P, et al. Response to cabozantinib in patients with RET fusion-positive lung adenocarcinomas. *Cancer Discov* (2013) **3**:630–5. doi:10.1158/2159-8290.CD-13-0035
29. Ballerini P, Struski S, Cresson C, Prade N, Toujani S, Deswarte C, et al. *RET* fusion genes are associated with chronic myelomonocytic leukemia and enhance monocytic differentiation. *Leukemia* (2012) **26**:2384–9. doi:10.1038/leu.2012.109
30. Verma A, Warner SL, Vankayalapati H, Bearss DJ, Sharma S. Targeting Axl and Mer kinases in cancer. *Mol Cancer Ther* (2011) **10**:1763–73. doi:10.1158/1535-7163.MCT-11-0116
31. Thress K, MacIntyre T, Wang H, Whitston D, Liu ZY, Hoffmann E, et al. Identification and preclinical characterization of AZ-23, a novel, selective, and orally bioavailable inhibitor of the Trk kinase pathway. *Mol Cancer Ther* (2009) **8**:1818–27. doi:10.1158/1535-7163.MCT-09-0036
32. Weiss GJ, Hidalgo M, Borad MJ, Laheru D, Tibes R, Ramanathan RK, et al. Phase I study of the safety, tolerability and pharmacokinetics of PHA-848125AC, a dual tropomyosin receptor kinase A and cyclin-dependent kinase inhibitor, in patients with advanced solid malignancies. *Invest New Drugs* (2012) **30**:2334–43. doi:10.1007/s10637-011-9774-6
33. Baccarani M, Cilloni D, Rondoni M, Ottaviani E, Messa F, Merante S, et al. The efficacy of imatinib mesylate in patients with PIP1L1-PDGFRa-positive hypereosinophilic syndrome. Results of a multicenter prospective study. *Haematologica* (2007) **92**:1173–9. doi:10.3324/haematol.11420
34. Salido M, Pijuan L, Martinez-Aviles L, Galvan AB, Canada I, Rovira A, et al. Increased ALK gene copy number and amplification are frequent in non-small cell lung cancer. *J Thorac Oncol* (2011) **6**:21–7. doi:10.1097/JTO.0b013e3181fb7cd6
35. Heuckmann JM, Balke-Want H, Malchers F, Peifer M, Sos ML, Koker M, et al. Differential protein stability and ALK inhibitor sensitivity of EML4-ALK fusion variants. *Clin Cancer Res* (2012) **18**:4682–90. doi:10.1158/1078-0432.CCR-11-3260
36. Paik JJ, Choe G, Kim H, Choe J, Lee JL, Lee C, et al. Screening of anaplastic lymphoma kinase rearrangement by immunohistochemistry in non-small cell lung cancer. Correlation with fluorescence in situ hybridization. *J Thorac Oncol* (2011) **6**:466–72. doi:10.1097/JTO.0b013e31820b82e8
37. Ying J, Guo L, Qiu T, Shan L, Ling Y, Liu X, et al. Diagnostic value of a novel fully automated immunochemistry assay for detection of *ALK* rearrangement in primary lung adenocarcinoma. *Ann Oncol* (2013) **24**:2589–93. doi:10.1093/annonc/mdt295
38. Sholl LM, Sun H, Butaney M, Zhang C, Lee C, Janne PA, et al. ROS1 immunohistochemistry for detection of *ROS1*-rearranged lung adenocarcinomas. *Am J Surg Pathol* (2013) **37**:1441–9. doi:10.1097/PAS.0b013e3182960fa7
39. Wang R, Hu H, Pan Y, Li Y, Ye T, Li C, et al. RET fusions define a unique molecular and clinicopathologic subtype of non-small-cell lung cancer. *J Clin Oncol* (2012) **30**:4352–9. doi:10.1200/JCO.2012.44.1477
40. Li T, Maus MKH, Desai SJ, Beckett LA, Stephens C, Huang E, et al. Large-scale screening and molecular characterization of EML4-ALK fusion variants in archival non-small-cell lung cancer tumor specimens using quantitative reverse transcription polymerase chain reaction assays. *J Thorac Oncol* (2014) **9**:18–25. doi:10.1097/JTO.0000000000000030
41. Peled N, Palmer G, Hirsch FR, Wynes MW, Ilouze M, Varella-Garcia M, et al. Next-generation sequencing identifies and immunohistochemistry confirms a novel crizotinib-sensitive ALK rearrangement in a patient with metastatic non-small-cell lung cancer. *J Thorac Oncol* (2012) **7**:e14–6. doi:10.1097/JTO.0b013e3182614ab5

11

Nanodrug delivery in reversing multidrug resistance in cancer cells

Sonali Kapse-Mistry[1], Thirumala Govender[2], Rohit Srivastava[3] and Mayur Yergeri[4]*

[1] Department of Pharmaceutics, SVKM's Dr. Bhanuben Nanavati College of Pharmacy, University of Mumbai, Mumbai, India
[2] Discipline of Pharmaceutical Sciences, School of Health Sciences, University of KwaZulu-Natal, Durban, South Africa
[3] Department of Biosciences and Bioengineering, Indian Institute of Technology Bombay, Mumbai, India
[4] Department of Pharmaceutical Chemistry, SVKM's Dr. Bhanuben Nanavati College of Pharmacy, University of Mumbai, Mumbai, India

Edited by:
Alexandre Arcaro, University of Bern, Switzerland

Reviewed by:
Marcel Verheij, The Netherlands Cancer Institute - Antoni van Leeuwenhoek Hospital, Netherlands
Olivier Feron, University of Louvain (UCL), Belgium

****Correspondence:***
Mayur Yergeri, Department of Pharmaceutical Chemistry, SVKM's Dr. Bhanuben Nanavati College of Pharmacy, University of Mumbai, Vile-Parle (West), Mumbai 400 056, India
e-mail: mayuryc@rediffmail.com

Different mechanisms in cancer cells become resistant to one or more chemotherapeutics is known as multidrug resistance (MDR) which hinders chemotherapy efficacy. Potential factors for MDR includes enhanced drug detoxification, decreased drug uptake, increased intracellular nucleophiles levels, enhanced repair of drug induced DNA damage, overexpression of drug transporter such as P-glycoprotein(P-gp), multidrug resistance-associated proteins (MRP1, MRP2), and breast cancer resistance protein (BCRP). Currently nanoassemblies such as polymeric/solid lipid/inorganic/metal nanoparticles, quantum dots, dendrimers, liposomes, micelles has emerged as an innovative, effective, and promising platforms for treatment of drug resistant cancer cells. Nanocarriers have potential to improve drug therapeutic index, ability for multifunctionality, divert ABC-transporter mediated drug efflux mechanism and selective targeting to tumor cells, cancer stem cells, tumor initiating cells, or cancer microenvironment. Selective nanocarrier targeting to tumor overcomes dose-limiting side effects, lack of selectivity, tissue toxicity, limited drug access to tumor tissues, high drug doses, and emergence of multiple drug resistance with conventional or combination chemotherapy. Current review highlights various nanodrug delivery systems to overcome mechanism of MDR by neutralizing, evading, or exploiting the drug efflux pumps and those independent of drug efflux pump mechanism by silencing Bcl-2 and HIF1α gene expressions by siRNA and miRNA, modulating ceramide levels and targeting NF-κB. "Theragnostics" combining a cytotoxic agent, targeting moiety, chemosensitizing agent, and diagnostic imaging aid are highlighted as effective and innovative systems for tumor localization and overcoming MDR. Physical approaches such as combination of drug with thermal/ultrasound/photodynamic therapies to overcome MDR are focused. The review focuses on newer drug delivery systems developed to overcome MDR in cancer cell.

Keywords: tumor microenvironment, drug efflux pumps, multidrug resistance, nanodrug delivery systems, theragnostic

INTRODUCTION

Cancer is a heterogeneous disease and use of multiple drugs simultaneously can result in drug resistance which is either intrinsic or acquired known as multidrug resistance (MDR). MDR renders cancer cells immune to standard treatments with many anticancer agents and is a major challenge in cancer therapy as it needs to address multiple phenotypes including MDR phenotypes. Tumor heterogeneity and tumor cell resistance to anticancer drugs thus remains key formidable challenges for effective targeting of drug delivery systems for successful chemotherapy. Drug resistance toward antineoplastic agents is a result of reduction in the effective concentration of drug in the cell prior to its interaction with the target or due to a combination of processes. The numerous mechanism of drug resistance reported includes (a) over expression of drug efflux pumps such as permeability glycoprotein (P-gp), multidrug resistance associated protein (MRP), and breast cancer resistance protein (BCRP) (b) alterations in lipid metabolism (ceramide pathway) (c) drug elimination by detoxification systems (d) drug test sequestration inside lysosomes and endosomes (e) reduced drug uptake due to altered surface receptors/carriers (f) inactivation of drugs via glutathione-mediated reduction (g) over expression of target enzymes such as up-regulated thymidylate synthase (h) altered drug targets such as topoisomerase II (i) increased DNA repair capacity (j) reduced ability to undergo apoptosis (k) hypoxia up-regulated expression of MDR-linked genes such as ABC transporters, Bcl-2 family genes, glutathione, metallothionein, etc. through activation of transcription factor HIF1 (l) chromosomal abnormalities in cancer cells lead to over-expression of anti-apoptotic genes (m) altered signal transduction pathways in cancer cells governed via integrin receptors, growth factor receptors etc. leads to blockage of apoptosis and expression of MDR-linked genes those involved in DNA repair and drug-efflux pumps (Broxterman et al., 2003).

Drug resistance mechanism of antineoplastic agents (**Table 1**) and mechanism of MDR in tumor cells is shown in **Figure 1**.

MULTIDRUG EFFLUX PUMPS

Drug efflux pumps expressed on human cancer cells majorly contribute to MDR (Sharom, 1997). These efflux pumps belong to ATP-binding cassette (ABC) family and include (a) **P-gp** also known as multidrug resistance protein 1 (MDR1) or cluster of differentiation 243 (CD243) a ATP-binding cassette sub-family B member 1 encoded in human by *ABCB1* gene (b) **Multidrug Resistance Associated Protein 1 (MRP1)** a ATP-binding cassette sub-family C member 1 encoded in human by *ABCC1* gene, **Multidrug Resistance Associated Protein 2 (MRP2)** also called as canalicular multispecific organic anion transporter 1 (cMOAT) a ATP-binding cassette sub-family C member 2 encoded in human by *ABCC2* gene (c) **BCRP** also known as cluster of differentiation (CDw338) a member of white sub-family and ATP-binding cassette G member 2 encoded in human by *ABCG2* gene (Ozben, 2006).

P-GLYCOPROTEIN (P-gp)

P-gp is the first member of ABC super family and is an ATP-powered drug efflux pump membrane transporter (Fardel et al., 1996; Sharom, 1997). Over-expression of P-gp in mammalian and human cancer cells results in MDR. P-gp has two isoforms expressed in human, class I and III isoforms are drug transporters (*MDR1/ABCB1*) while class II isoforms export phosphatidylcholine into bile (*MDR2/3/ABCB4*) (Sharom, 1997). P-gp encoded by MDR1 gene is present in human tissues including liver, kidney, pancreas, small and large intestine while P-gp encoded by MDR2 gene is present at high levels only in liver (Fardel et al., 1996). Carcinoma of colon, kidney, adrenal gland, pancreas, and liver express high P-gp levels while intermediate P-gp levels are expressed in neuroblastomas, soft tissue carcinomas, hematological malignancies including CD34-positive acute myeloid leukemias, etc. with low P-gp levels expressed in malignancies of lung, esophagus, stomach, ovary, breast, melanomas, lymphomas, multiple myelomas, and acute promyelocytic leukemia but may display elevated P-gp levels after chemotherapy due to acquired drug resistance (Velingkar and Dandekar, 2010). P-gp interacts with structurally diverse substrates such as anticancer drugs, HIV protease inhibitors, analgesics, calcium channel blockers, immunosuppressive agents, cardiac glycosides, antihelminthics, antibiotics, H_2-receptor antagonists, steroids, fluorescent dyes, linear and cyclic peptides, ionophores, peptides, lipids, small cytokines such as interleukin-2, intereukin-4, and interferon-γ, MDR chemosensitizers, and many more (Velingkar and Dandekar, 2010).

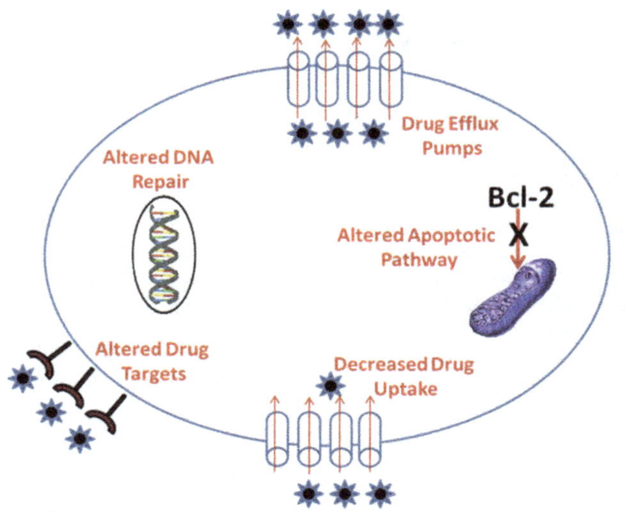

FIGURE 1 | Mechanism of multidrug resistance in tumor cell.

Table 1 | Drug resistance mechanisms of anticancer drugs.

Class	Example	Cytotoxicity mechanism	Molecules in resistance mechanism
Intercalators	Doxorubicin Daunomycin	Topoisomerase II inhibitor, superoxides and free radicals	P-gp, Topoisomerase II, MRP, GST
Alkylators	Cyclophosphamide	DNA alkylation	O^6-alkylguanine-DNA alkyltransferase, Glutathione, Aldehyde dehydrogenase
	Cisplatin	DNA alkylation	Glutathione, Metallothionein, DNA repair enzyme, multispecific organic anion transporter
Antimetabolites	BCNU Methotrexate	DNA alkylation Folic acid antagonist	O^6-alkylguanine-DNA alkyltransferase Amplification of dihydrofolate reductase, MRP, decreased reduced folate carrier expression
Vinca alkaloids	5-Fluorouracil Vinblastine Vincristine	Uracil analog Tubulin Polymerization inhibitor	Amplification of thymidylate synthase P-gp, MRP, Tubulin Mutation
Epidophylotoxins	Etoposide	Topoisomerase II inhibitor	MRP, Glutathione, P-gp, Topoisomerase I
Taxanes	Paclitaxel	Microtubule assembly inhibitor	P-gp, altered α/β Tubulin

FIRST GENERATION INHIBITORS

These are non-selective, less potent with poor, and low binding affinity; requiring high doses to achieve plasma levels to reverse MDR, resulting in unacceptable patient toxicity. They are substrates for P-gp and act as competitive inhibitors thereby requiring high serum concentrations of chemosensitizers to produce adequate intracellular concentrations of cytotoxic drug due to which these inhibitors are unsuccessful in clinical trials (Dantzig et al., 2003). First generation inhibitors include Verapamil, Trifluoperazine, Cyclosporine-A, Quinidine and Reserpine, Vincristine, Yohimbine, Tamoxifen, and Toremifene. Due to unpredictable pharmacokinetic interactions of these substrates in presence of chemotherapy agents several novel chemosensitizers analogs were developed with less toxicity and greater potency.

SECOND GENERATION INHIBITORS

Structural modifications of first generation inhibitors resulted in more potent second generation P-gp modulators with better pharmacological profile, reduced toxicity, and better tolerability. They significantly inhibit metabolism and excretion of cytotoxic agents leading to unacceptable toxicity necessitating chemotherapy dose reductions. Successful treatment of refractory cancers and reversal of MDR in clinical trials have been possible by co-administration of these modulators with chemotherapy agents. Modulators include Dexverapamil, Dexniguldipine, Valspodar (PSC 833), and Biricodar citrate (VX-710).

THIRD GENERATION INHIBITORS

They have high potency and specificity for P-gp transporters over second generation agents. They do not interfere with cytochrome P450 3A4 unaffecting drug pharmacokinetics with no dose alterations in chemotherapy. They include Tariquidar-XR9576, Zosuquidar-LY335979, Laniquidar-R101933, ONT-093 (substituted diarylimidazole), Elacridar-GF120918, OC 144-093, Mitotane (NSC-38721), Annamycin, and R101933 (Ozben, 2006). Most promising Tariquidar (non-transported P-gp inhibitor) which inhibits ATPase by interaction with protein is currently in phase III trials for non-small cell lung cancer but still suspended due to unfavorable toxicity. Clinical trial studies revealed that Tariquidar, LY335979, R101933, and ONT-093 can be administered with therapeutic doses and minimal interference with pharmacokinetics of cytotoxic agents. They have shown promise in clinical trials and continued development of these agents may establish the true therapeutic potential of P-gp mediated MDR reversal.

Tariquidar a third generation inhibitor with no limitations of first and second generation inhibitors, have highest specificity which specifically and potently inhibits P-gp. Inhibition of ATPase activity of P-gp suggests that the modulating effect is derived from inhibition of substrate binding, inhibition of ATP hydrolysis and or both (Fox and Bates, 2007). Clinical trials of third-generation inhibitors (Thomas and Coley, 2003) showed better tolerability of Tariquidar with no significant pharmacokinetic interaction with chemotherapy. This makes Tariquidar an ideal agent for demonstrating P-gp inhibition activity in cancer. Targeted delivery of paclitaxel and tariquidar co-encapsulated in biotin functionalized PLGA nanoparticles revealed significantly higher cytotoxicity *in vitro* and greater tumor growth inhibition *in vivo* in drug-resistant tumor mouse model compared to paclitaxel nanoparticles alone with promising results in clinical trials (Patil et al., 2009b).

TUMOR MICROENVIRONMENT AND MDR

Tumors are core-shell structures with hypoxic core surrounded by tissues and proliferative cells. Tumor microenvironment is made of complex tissues containing extracellular matrix, activated fibroblasts, immune cells, pericytes, adipocytes, epithelial cells, glial cells, vascular and lymphatic endothelial cells, and numerous proteins (van Kempen et al., 2003; Weber and Kuo, 2012). The proliferative cells are highly vascularized, unorganized and discontinuous resulting in enhanced permeability and retention (EPR) effect widely exploited for passive targeting. The major factors contributing to tumor progression and metastasis, enhanced drug resistance, poor prognosis, and response to therapies includes cell mobility, survival potential, capacity to degrade extracellular tissue matrix, and ability to adjust in new tissue environment (Otranto et al., 2012; Singh and Kaur, in press). All solid tumor microenvironment possess the following characteristics (Milane et al., 2011) (**Table 2**) (a) leaky and unorganized tumor vasculature (b) hypoxia region (c) up-regulation of oncogenes (d) DNA repair mechanisms (e) down regulation of tumor suppressors and cell cycle regulation (f) increased growth factor receptors (g) low nutrients. Tumor microenvironment significantly contributes to drug resistance by reducing drug accessibility to tumor cells and reduces the oxygen radicals generated by antitumor drugs (Otranto et al., 2012; Singh and Kaur, in press). Hypoxia and acidity with low nutrient levels remains the two key factors characterizing tumor microenvironment (Schornack and Gillies, 2003; Wouters et al., 2003). Tumor hypoxia is low oxygen regions with partial oxygen pressure (pO_2) levels below 10 mm-Hg where normal tissues range from 24 to 66 mm-Hg (Rofstad, 2000). Hypoxia microenvironment is characterized by low pH (acidic cell environment) and can be associated with activation of proteases that contributes to metastasis, low glucose levels, high interstitial fluid pressure due to leaky vasculature, impaired lymphatic drainage, and high levels of P-gp (Tomida and Tsuruo, 2002). Hypoxia Inducible Factor (HIF) (Harris, 2002) is another mechanism that induces MDR and metastasis by up-regulating target genes by binding to hypoxia-response element (HRE) in

Table 2 | Tumor microenvironment characteristics contributing toward MDR.

Increased levels	Decreased levels
Oncogenes	Tumor suppressors
Growth factors/receptors	Oxidative phosphorylation
Nutrient importers	pH
ABC transporters	Cell cycle regulation
Aerobic glycolysis	Increased apoptosis
Interstitial fluid pressure	
DNA repair	
Detoxification enzymes	

the target. HIF-1 is a transcription factor activated in hypoxia. While tumor acidic pH results in poor tumor perfusion due to abnormal vascularization, hypoxia, and metabolic abnormalities are associated with cell growth and increased capacity for transmembrane pH regulation (Simon et al., 1994). Both pO_2 and pH are important determinants of tumor growth, metabolism, and response to variety of therapies (Fukumura and Jain, 2007). Acidic extracellular pH restricts uptake of weak base drugs such as Adriamycin, Doxorubicin, and Mitoxantrone. Both hypoxia and acidic pH contributes to growth and tumor metastasis (Harris, 2002). Hypoxia upregulates various angiogenic growth factors including Vascular Endothelial Growth Factor (VEGF), Angiopoietin (Ang) 2, Platelet Derived Growth Factor (PDGF), Placenta Growth Factor (PGF), Transforming Growth Factor α (TGFα), Interleukin (IL)-8, and Hepatocyte Growth Factor (HGF) of which Hypoxia Inducible Factor 1α (HIF1α) is considered the master regulator of oxygen homeostasis.

STRATEGIES TO OVERCOME MDR IN CANCER CELLS

MODIFICATION OF CHEMOTHERAPY REGIMENS

Chemotherapy regimen includes "induction regimen" and "maintenance regimen" refers to initial disease treatment and ongoing chemotherapy to reduce chances of cancer recurrence or prevent growth of an existing cancer, respectively. Combination chemotherapy utilizes synergistic effect of multiple antineoplastic drugs acting through different mechanisms, but due to their different dose-limiting adverse effects they are given together in chemotherapy regimens. Chemotherapy regimen needs to balance efficacy and toxicity through proper dosing schedule. Dose-dense regimens have more toxic effects than standard regimen causing treatment delays and toxicity with few survival improvements and early treatment discontinuation. A dose-dense approach is more effective than standard approach, as it hampers formation of blood vessels that feed tumors and tumor shrinkage following treatment promoting tumor dormancy by maintaining tumor size and preventing outgrowth. Chemotherapy regimens are identified by acronyms, identifying the drug combination agents. E.g., (i) Breast cancer: AC (Adriamycin, Cyclophosphamide), CAF (Cyclophosphamide, Adriamycin, Flurouracil), EC (Epirubicin, Cyclophosphamide), FEC (Flurouracil, Epirubicin, Cyclophosphamide); (ii) Colorectal cancer: FL (Fluorouracil, Leucovorin), FOLFOX (Fluorouracil, Leucovorin, Oxaliplatin), FOLFIRI (Fluorouracil, Leucovorin, Irinotecan). Chemotherapy regimen is based on the assumption that the mutations conferring drug resistance will not convey resistance to all the agents in the regimen and high-dose chemotherapy regimens could be given to cancer patients. Such approach assumes that despite resistance to standard doses of anticancer drugs, a dose-response relationship exists for tumors and high doses of chemotherapy might overcome the resistance.

INACTIVATION OF MDR-ASSOCIATED GENES BY TARGETING SPECIFIC mRNA FOR DEGRADATION

Strategies to overcome multi drug resistance by silencing the expression of gene encoding P-gp efflux transporter, i.e., MDR-1 or Survivin through RNA interference (RNAi) or small interfering RNA (siRNA) has been explored. Transient RNAi mediated silencing can be achieved by siRNA or stable RNAi-mediated gene silencing through short hairpin RNA (shRNA) transfection. The siRNAs assembles into endoribonuclease inside the cells containing complexes known as RNA-Induced Silencing Complexes (RISCs) which guides the RISCs to complementary RNA molecules, cleaving and destroying the target RNA. Antisense oligonucleotides and catalytic RNAs have been successful in inhibiting P-gp, MRP, and BCRP expression and sensitized drug-resistant cells (Nadali et al., 2007; Ren et al., 2008). *In vitro* and *in vivo* studies with biotin-functionalized nanoparticles co-encapsulating paclitaxel and P-gp targeted siRNA partially overcame tumor drug resistance (Patil et al., 2010). Two groups, Nieth et al. (2003) and Wu et al. demonstrated that RNAi knock downs the MDR1/P-gp encoding mRNA and reverse the MDR phenotype of cancer cells. They further chemically synthesized siRNA to transiently down regulate MDR1/P-gp mRNA and protein expression. To overcome MDR in cancer, Lage (2009) developed anti-ABC transporter shRNA expression vectors with high potential to overcome MDR through silencing specific ABC transporter transcripts. These studies revealed total knock down of mRNA and protein by inhibition of P-gp and reversal of drug-resistant phenotype. Efficiency of RNAi to overcome MDR *in vivo* were performed by transfecting MDR cancer cells with anti-MDR shRNA expression plasmids. Treatment of these cells grown as xenografts in nude mice with vincristine revealed tumor growth inhibitin by 42% for the shRNA expressing tumors. Tumor growth inhibition by 80-fold was observed in cells transfected with anti-MDR1/P-gp shRNA expressing retroviruses implanted in nude mice (Milane et al., 2011).

MONOCLONAL ANTIBODIES FOR P-gp

Monoclonal antibodies (MAbs) have potential for targeting P-gp and kill MDR tumor cells. Anti-P-gp MAbs such as MRK-16 and MRK-17 along with chemosensitizers reverses P-gp mediated MDR and conjugated MAbs such as bispecific antibody, immunotoxin and radioisotope conjugates enhance anti-tumor activity. Combination of MRK-16 with Cyclosporin-A or PSC-833 reversed Doxorubicin resistance in K562/ADM cells and inhibited tumor growth in athymic mice bearing HCT-15/ADM2-2 xenografts. MRK-16 increased Cyclosporine-A accumulation in MDR cells but not affected intracellular PSC-833 accumulation in MDR cells, instead Cyclosporin-A and PSC-833 increased MRK-16 binding to P-gp revealing a synergistic MDR reversal activity. MAbs with other anti-P-gp MAbs such as UIC2, 4E3, and series of HYB antibodies have potential to inhibit drug transport (Tomida and Tsuruo, 2002).

DEVELOPMENT OF NEW ANTICANCER DRUGS THAT ARE NOT SUBSTRATES OF P-gp

Drug analogs such as Taxane analogs DJ-927 (Phase I), BMS-184476 (Phase I), RPR 109881A (Phase II), Ortataxel (Phase II), Trabectedin-ET-743 (Phase II and III) are not recognized by P-gp transporter and are evaluated in clinical trials for their broad spectrum activity in sensitive and resistant tumor cell lines to overcome MDR (Dong and Mumper, 2010). DJ-927 was more potent and cytotoxic than paclitaxel and docetaxel when compared *in vitro* and *in vivo* in various P-gp expressing tumor cell lines with high intracellular accumulation in P-gp positive cells. The expression of P-gp levels or P-gp modulators did not affect the tumoricidal efficacy of DJ-927. Phase I study of DJ-927 in combination with capecitabine was acceptable with no pharmacokinetic drug interactions in patients with advanced solid tumor malignancies and is recommended for further clinical studies. Preclinical studies showed that BMS-184476 was more potent than paclitaxel against taxane sensitive and resistant tumors. The P-gp over-expressing human colon cancer cell line (HCT-116/MDR) was 62-fold more resistant to paclitaxel and 15-fold resistant to BMS-184476. Also the human ovarian cancer cells with acquired taxane resistance expressed 9-fold resistance to BMS-184467 and 32-fold to paclitaxel. Studies of BMS-184476 against human tumor xenografts with both acquired and primary taxane resistance models revealed superiority of BMS-184476 (Yared and Tkaczuk, 2012).

INHIBITORS OF ABC TRANSPORTERS TO REVERSE MDR

Inhibition of ABC transporters should reverse MDR by increasing intracellular drug concentrations in tumor cells and restore drug sensitivity. These inhibitors transport themselves and then act as competitive antagonists while others are not transported but affect transporter function (Dong and Mumper, 2010). Preclinical trials of first and second generation ABC transport inhibitors were not successful. They failed in clinical trials due to their non-specificity, high concentrations to inhibit activity, undesirable drug interactions due to co-administration of inhibitors and anticancer drugs (e.g., verapamil and doxorubicin), substrates of cytochrome P-450 and increased toxicity of anticancer drugs. Clinical trials of third generation inhibitors with LY335979 (Zosuquidar), GF120918 (Elacridar), R101933 and XR9576 (Tariquidar) are ongoing. Tariquidar in phase I studies revealed high potency in *in vitro* and *in vivo* studies. LY335979 prolonged survival by reducing tumor growth in mice with drug resistant tumors, GF120918 enhanced topotecan bioavailability in mice by sensitizing human MDR sarcoma MES-Dx5 cells. Although phase I and II clinical trials of third generation inhibitors are promising but are limited to unpredictable pharmacokinetic drug interactions, simultaneous involvement of several drug transporters and variability in drug transporter expression levels among individuals restricts restoration of drug sensitivity of such modulators in clinic (Wu et al., 2008).

NANOTECHNOLOGY BASED APPROACHES TO OVERCOME MDR

Nanocarriers to overcome MDR are extensively discussed in section "Nanocarriers as potential drug delivery systems in cancer therapy." Nanocarriers have been developed encapsulating anticancer drugs as P-gp substrates and/or with P-gp substrates.

INHIBITION OF MDR USING PEPTIDES

Synthetic P-gp peptides derived from fragments of extracellular loops of murine P-gp coupled with polyethylene glycol and loaded in Doxorubicin liposomes have shown MDR reversal with 83% increase in survival time of mice inoculated with P388R cells. Antitumor effect of peptide-conjugated Doxorubicin in human erythroleukemic (K562/ADR) resistant cells showed dose-dependent inhibition of cell growth against K562/ADR cells as compared with Doxorubicin alone (Dong and Mumper, 2010).

NANOCARRIERS AS POTENTIAL DRUG DELIVERY SYSTEMS IN CANCER THERAPY

Nanovehicles such as polymeric nanoparticles, solid lipid nanoparticles, magnetic nanoparticles, dendrimers, liposomes, micelles, quantum dots, etc. are extensively explored for cancer diagnosis, treatment, imaging, and as ideal vectors to overcome drug resistance by diverting ABC-transporter mediated drug efflux mechanisms. The major classes of nanocarriers utilized for chemotherapeutic drug delivery are listed in **Table 3** (Ayers and Nasti, 2012).

POLYMERIC NANOPARTICLES

Polymeric nanoparticles have emerged as a versatile nanotechnology platform for controlled, sustained and targeted delivery of anticancer agents including small molecular weight drugs and macromolecules such as genes and proteins (Wang et al., 2009; Sahay et al., 2010; Tang et al., 2010). A significant reduction in tumor size and increased animal survival rate in rat xenograft glioma model with indomethacin loaded nanocapsules was observed by Bernardi et al. (2009). PLGA loaded cystatin nanoparticles and PLGA loaded cytokeratin specific monoclonal antibody nanoparticles neutralized excessive proteolysis preventing metastatic and invasive potential of breast tumor cells (Kos et al., 2009). Paclitaxel loaded PLA immunonanoparticles covalently coupled with humanized monoclonal antibodies (antiHER2) actively targeted tumor cells over expressing HER2 receptors (Cirstoiu-Hapca et al., 2009). Folic acid receptors over-expressed on human cancer cells (Antony, 1996; Wang et al., 2010) are studied in tumor models including mouse M109 carcinoma, KB human epidermal carcinoma cell line and mouse J6456 lymphoma (Alberto et al., 2004). Paclitaxel loaded PLA-PEG-ligand conjugated nanoparticles functionalized with biotin and folic acid enhanced drug accumulation in MCF-7 tumor xenograft model (Patil et al., 2009b). Lee et al. found that folic acid conjugated chitosan nanoparticles showed higher transfection activity than unmodified chitosan nanoparticles (Lee et al., 2006). Wang et al. (2010) observed 35% reduction in tumor growth, inhibition of P-gp and mdr1 gene levels in KB-A-1 cells implanted in Balb/c-nu/nu mice targeted by folic acid conjugated antisense oligodeoxynucleotides-hydroxypropyl-chitosan nanoparticles compared to bare antisense oligodeoxynucleotides to overcome tumor drug resistance. Folate functionalized PLGA nanoparticles loaded with anti-cancer drug nutlin-3a and chemosensitizer Curcumin enhanced therapeutic potential of nutlin-3a by modulating MDR of Y79 retinoblastoma cell through Curcumin and enhanced the anticancer activity of nutlin-3a in drug resistance Y79 cells. Dual drug loaded nanoparticles revealed better therapeutic efficacy with enhanced expression or down regulation of proapoptotic/antiapoptotic proteins and down-regulation of Bcl2 and NF-κB protein. Study demonstrated the role of Curcumin as MDR modulator to enhance the therapeutic potential of nutlin-3a for targeting MDR cancer (Das and Sahoo, 2012).

Silencing P-gp expression by RNAi with reduction-sensitive linear cationic click polymer nanoparticles (RCPNs) loaded with plasmid iMDR1-pDNA for gene delivery revealed higher transfection efficiency and lower cytotoxicity than PEI/DNA

Table 3 | Chemotherapeutic nanodrug delivery systems.

Nanocarriers	Properties	Characteristics
Solid lipid nanoparticle (SLNs)	Release drug in acidic microenvironment of multidrug resistance cells	Delivers anticancer drugs to overcome P-gp mediated multidrug resistance
Polymeric nanoparticles (NPs)	Versatile platform for controlled, sustained, and targeted delivery of anticancer agents including small molecular weight drugs and macromolecules (genes and proteins)	Enhanced drug accumulation, reduction in tumor size/volume, increased animal survival rate in rat models, minimal cytotoxicity in cancer cell lines, high transfection activity, potential to overcome multidrug resistance
Liposomes (LIPO)	Made of lipid bilayers encapsulating both hydrophobic and hydrophilic drugs, stealth liposomes are surface coated with PEG	Long-circulating, prevents non-specific interactions, preferential accumulation in tumor tissues via enhanced permeability, and retention effect to overcome drug resistance
Micelles (MI)	Small size, high payload capacity, greater solubilization potential for hydrophobic drugs, improved stability, long circulation	Selective targeting, P-gp inhibitory action, altered drug internalization, and sub-cellular localization properties
Mesoporous silica nanoparticles (MSNPs)	Inorganic nanocarriers with tunable size and shape, high drug loading due to high pore volume and surface area, multifunctionalization for targeted, and controlled delivery	Enhanced cellular uptake and bioavailability, circumvents unwanted biological interactions, delivers therapeutics at cellular levels for therapeutic, and imaging in cancer
Inorganic nanoparticles (a) Iron oxide magnetic nanoparticles	Unique optical, electrical, magnetic and/or electrochemical properties, inert, stable, ease of functionalization	Circumvents drug resistance associated with over expression of ATP-binding cassette transporters, increased intracellular drug retention, enhanced loss of cell viability
(b) Gold nanoparticles (AuNPs)	Shape and size dependent on electronic characteristics, versatile drug delivery system due to tunable optical properties	Induces cellular DNA damage
(c) Quantum dots (QD)	Semiconductor inorganic fluorescent nanocrystals, small (1–20 nm), and uniform size, high surface to volume ratio, surface conjugation with multiple ligands, biocompatible, fluorescence properties help real time tracks within target cells	Release of toxic compounds (cadmium) and generation of reactive oxygen species can result in long term toxicity

nanoparticles against human breast cancer MCF-7 cells and drug-resistant MCF-7/ADR cells (Gao et al., 2011). Vincristine sulfate loaded nanoassemblies enhanced cytotoxicity by 36.5-fold and cellular accumulation by 12.6-fold in MCF-7 and P-gp over expressing MCF-7/ADR cells compared to vincristine sulfate solution and overcome MDR by clathrin and caveolae mediated endocytosis pathways (Zhang et al., 2011b). Co-delivery of Paclitaxel and survivin shRNA nanoparticles lowered IC_{50} by 360-fold in Paclitaxel resistant lung cancer cells against A549/T cells compared to free Paclitaxel and enhanced efficacy with Paclitaxel induced apoptosis and cell arrest in G2/M phase. Nanoparticles facilitated drug accumulation in tumor cells and down-regulated of survivin shRNA into nuclei of lung cancer cells lowering the apoptosis threshold of drug resistant cells and renders chemotherapeutic agents more effective to overcome MDR (Shen et al., 2012). Docetaxel loaded poly(ε-caprolactone)/Pluronic F68 nanoparticles increased drug uptake and enhanced cytotoxicity in docetaxel-resistance human breast cancer cell line and MCF-7 TAX30 compared to poly caprolactone nanoparticles indicating its potential to overcome MDR (Mei et al., 2009). Lipid/particle assemblies (LNPs) loaded with Doxorubicin in DMAB-modified PLGA nanoparticles coated with DPPC lipid shell significantly increased accumulation and improved nucleus targeting in MCF-7 cells and P-gp over expressing resistant MCF-7/ADR cells relative to free drug and reversed the transporter-mediated drug resistance in human breast cancer. Cytotoxicity (IC_{50}) of Doxorubicin loaded-LNPs was 30-fold lower than free Doxorubicin in MCF-7/ADR, indicating intracellular retention of Doxorubicin and bypassing drug resistance (Li et al., 2012a). Co-delivery of MDR1 siRNA via lipid-modified dextran-based polymeric nanoparticles with Doxorubicin increased intracellular drug concentration in MDR cell nucleus and efficiently suppressed P-gp expression in drug resistant osteosarcoma cell lines ($KHOS_{R2}$ and $U\text{-}2OS_{R2}$) (Susa et al., 2010). Pramanik et al. developed composite nanoparticles of Doxorubicin with Curcumin a potent MDR inhibitor to overcome Doxorubicin resistance in multiple *in-vivo* models such as multiple myeloma, acute leukemia, prostate and ovarian cancers. Composite nanoparticles revealed no cardiac toxicity or bone marrow suppression compared to free Doxorubicin (Pramanik et al., 2012). P-glycoprotein mediated efflux can be effectively circumvented by co-administration of P-gp inhibitor/s and anticancer drug/s in nanoparticles which evades P-gp recognition at cell membrane and delivers drug in the cell cytoplasm or nucleus thereby sustaining delivery of the drug inside the cell. Chavanpatil et al. encapsulated paclitaxel a P-gp substrate and verapamil a P-gp inhibitor in PLGA nanoparticles to circumvent P-gp-mediated drug efflux in MDR tumor cells (Chavanpatil et al., 2006). Doxorubicin loaded aerosol OT (AOT)-alginate nanoparticles enhanced the cellular delivery and therapeutic efficacy of P-gp substrates in P-gp over expressing cells (Chavanpatil et al., 2007). Novel polymer-lipid hybrid nanoparticle loaded with doxorubicin and chemosensitizer (GG918) evaluated in human MDR breast cancer cell line (MDA435/LCC6/MDR1) demonstrated nuclear drug localization and anticancer activity toward MDR cells, while co-administration of the single-agents loaded nanoparticles resulted in high cellular internalization but were ineffective (Wong et al., 2006). Encapsulation of paclitaxel with P-gp modulator tariquidar in poly (D, L-lactide-co-glycolide) nanoparticles functionalized with biotin revealed higher *in-vitro* cytotoxicity and increased intracellular accumulation compared to paclitaxel nanoparticles alone in drug-resistant tumor cells to overcome tumor drug resistance through biotin receptor-mediated endocytosis (Patil et al., 2009a).

SOLID LIPID NANOPARTICLES (SLNS)

In-vitro cytotoxicity in resistant P388/ADR cell line and *in-vivo* studies in P388/ADR leukemia mouse model revealed lowering of IC_{50} value by 9-fold and greater median survival time about 20 days (3.5 mg/kg dose) with Doxorubicin SLN compared to Doxorubicin solution. While comparable cell uptake and IC_{50} values were obtained with both Idarubicin SLN and free Idarubicin in P-gp over expressing P388/ADR and HCT-15 cells mouse tumor models. Study revealed the potential of Doxorubicin SLN in overcoming P-gp-mediated MDR both *in-vitro* in P388/ADR leukemia cells and *in-vivo* in murine leukemia mouse model (Ma et al., 2009). Greater accumulation of Doxorubicin SLN in MCF-7/ADR cells over expressing P-gp with enhanced apoptotic cell death and decreased cell viability compared to plain Doxorubicin revealed the potential of Doxorubicin SLNs to overcome chemoresistance in adriamycin-resistant breast cancer cell line. Decrease in the intensity of 116-kDa PARP band (DNA repair enzyme activated by DNA damage and used as apoptosis biochemical marker) in MCF-7/ADR cells treated with 3 μM either of Doxorubicin or SLN alone or Doxorubicin SLN indicated efficiency of Doxorubicin SLN to cause cell death through induction of apoptosis in Doxorubicin resistant cancer cells. Cellular uptake of Doxorubicin SLN was 17.1-fold and 21.6-fold higher than Doxorubicin alone implying potential of SLNs in diminishing P-gp mediated drug efflux (Kang et al., 2010). SLNs being easily internalized enhanced cellular uptake and cytotoxicity of Doxorubicin and Paclitaxel loaded solid lipid nanospheres in human promyelocytic leukemia cells (HL60) and human breast carcinoma cells (MCF-7) compared to free drug solutions. Paclitaxel solid lipid nanospheres were 100-fold more effective than free Paclitaxel in MCF-7 cells with low sensitivity on HL60 cells. Doxorubicin SLN enhanced cytotoxicity and sensitivity on MCF-7 cells (10-fold) and on HL60 cells (>40-fold) with IC_{50} at 1 ng/ml compared to Doxorubicin solution reducing drug cell resistance. Such increased cytotoxicity of Doxorubicin nanocarriers compared to solution has been earlier reported with polymeric nanoparticles, micelles and liposomes. Enhanced intracellular accumulation and cytotoxicity of Doxorubicin loaded pluronic copolymer micelles have been reported by Kabanov and coworkers. Couvreur reported that Doxorubicin loaded polyalkylcyanoacrylate nanoparticle were more cytotoxic than Doxorubicin solution against P388 leukemia cells overcomed MDR and decreased cell viability against resistant MCF-7 cell-lines (Couvreur and Vauthier, 1991). Paclitaxel SLN enhanced cytotoxicity (100-fold) at concentration >5 ng/ml on HL60 cells and at 1 ng/ml on MCF-7 cells (Miglietta et al., 2000). Polymer-lipid hybrid nanoparticle with Doxorubicin and chemosensitizer (GG918) or their combination revealed high Doxorubicin uptake in human MDR breast cancer cell line (MDA435/LCC6/MDR1) compared to co-administration of two single-agent/s loaded hybrid nanoparticles (Wong et al., 2006). Tween®80 coated Edelfosine lipid nanoparticles revealed antiproliferative effect due to P-gp inhibitory action on C6 glioma cell lines and significantly reduced the tumor growth within 14 days post treatment in nude mice bearing C6 glioma xenograft tumor (Mendoza et al., 2011). Paclitaxel and Doxorubicin SLN exhibited higher cytotoxicity in human breast tumor drug sensitive MCF-7 and drug resistant MCF-7/ADR cells compared to Taxol and Doxorubicin solution. Paclitaxel and Doxorubicin loaded SLN revealed 31.0- and 4.3-fold reversal in drug resistance of MCF-7 cells compared to MCF-7/ADR cells respectively (Miao et al., 2013). Doxorubicin-mitomycin co-loaded stealth polymer-lipid hybrid nanoparticles enhanced efficacy in sensitive and MDR human mammary tumor xenografts with 3-fold increase in life span, 10–20% tumor cure rate, inhibition of tumor angiogenesis with no severe tissue toxicity compared to liposomal Doxorubicin (Prasad et al., 2013). P-glycoprotein efflux at the brain limits entry of Docetaxel for cancer treatment. Folic acid modified solid lipid nanoparticles loaded with docetaxel and ketoconazole (P-gp inhibitor) evaluated in brain endothelial cell lines for cytotoxicity and cell uptake revealed a brain permeation coefficient 44 times higher than that of Taxotere® (Venishetty et al., 2013). Docetaxel loaded hepatoma-targeted SLNs revealed high cellular uptake by hepatoma cells, better biodistribution and enhanced antitumor efficacy due to increased drug accumulation and cytotoxicity in murine model bearing hepatoma and hepatocellular carcinoma cell line BEL7402 compared to Taxotere® or non-targeted SLNs for treatment of advanced and metastatic hepatocellular carcinoma (Xu et al., 2009). A lipophilic paclitaxel derivative (2′-behenoyl-paclitaxel) (C22-PX) conjugated in lipid nanoparticle for metastatic breast cancer improved antitumor efficacy, tumor retention, better tolerability, and higher plasma levels compared to Taxol in a subcutaneous 4T1 mouse mammary carcinoma model (Ma et al., 2013).

LIPOSOMES

Liposomal anthracyclines approved by US FDA for treatment of AIDS-related Kaposi's sarcoma are pegylated liposomal doxorubicin (Doxil®/Caelyx®) and liposomal daunorubicin (DaunoXome®) which preferentially accumulates in tumor tissues via EPR effect to overcome drug resistance or accumulates within extracellular space of tumor stroma and leaks into tumor environment which provides pharmacologic advantage for liposomes over free drug to overcome drug resistance (**Table 4**). Currently liposomes of Paclitaxel, Camptothecins and Vincristine are in clinical development. Liposomal strategies to enhance drug bioavailability and efficacy in drug-resistant cancer include (i) liposomes modified for controlled release (ii) ligand targeted liposomes such as immunoliposomes for intracellular drug delivery in tumor cells.

Liposomes directly interact with P-gp and inhibit P-gp through endocytosis. Liposome co-encapsulating Doxorubicin and Verapamil conjugated with human transferrin (Tf) showed greater cytotoxicity, selective targeting and reversal of P-gp mediated drug resistance in resistant leukemia K562 cells than non-targeted co-loaded liposomes. Doxorubicin liposomes increased cytotoxicity on HL60 cells and Vincristine resistant HL60 cells due to rapid internalization and drug release inside the cells (Gokhale et al., 1996). Robert Lee et al. found that uptake of folate-PEG-liposomal Doxorubicin by KB cells was 45-fold higher than non-targeted liposomal Doxorubicin (Lee and Low, 1995). Liposomes overcome drug resistance due to endothelial P-gp efflux mechanism at blood-brain and blood-tumor barriers in brain tumors where the barriers allows extravasation of long circulating liposomes and circumvent drug resistance with stabilized liposomal Doxorubicin in rat intracranial sarcoma model (Siegal et al., 1995) and rat intracranial 9L gliosarcoma model (Zhou et al., 2002).

MODIFIED LIPOSOMES TO OVERCOME DRUG RESISTANCE

New liposomal systems developed for treatment of drug-resistant cancers are listed in **Tables 5, 6**.

MICELLES

Micelles are efficient drug carriers with potential P-gp inhibitory action, altered drug internalization, subcellular localization and selective targeting. Seven anti-tumor drugs loaded polymeric micelles in clinical trials are Genexol®-PM, NK105, NC-6004, NC-4016, NK012, NK911 and SP1049C (Gong et al., 2012). Micelles overcome drug resistance by combination of mechanisms including EPR effect, active internalization, endosomal-triggered release and drug escape. Folate decorated pH-sensitive Doxorubicin micelles showed high drug concentration in cytosol and nucleus due to triggered release in early endosomes (~pH 6) and high cytotoxicity in Doxorubicin resistant MCF-7 (MCF-7/DOXR) cells due to internalization via folate-receptor mediated endocytosis to overcome P-gp (Lee et al., 2005). Folate functionalized micelles co-encapsulating Paclitaxel and Verapamil in O-carboxymethylated chitosan modified with deoxycholic acid revealed greater cytotoxicity and higher cellular uptake in drug resistance MCF-7 and multi-drug-resistant MCF-7/ADR cells through synergistic effect of folate receptor-mediated endocytosis and Verapamil mediated efflux mechanism to overcome drug resistance in tumor cells (Wang et al., 2011a). Wei et al. revealed that pluronics lowered the IC_{50} in human lung adenocarcinoma cell lines SPC-A1 (8.7 ± 0.4 ng/ml) and A-549 (0.10 ± 0.04 μg/ml) with Paclitaxel-Pluronic P123/F127

Table 5 | Modified liposome approaches to overcome multidrug resistance.

Modified liposomes	Mechanism of action
Anionic liposomes	Anionic lipids (Cardiolipin and Phosphatidylserine) inhibits P-gp by direct interaction with membrane lipids, enhance cellular absorption, and cellular toxicity compared to free drugs
Inhibitory phospholipids	Inhibits P-gp to overcome multidrug resistance
Stimuli responsive liposomes	Modified liposomes which release drug in target tissue upon hyperthermia treatment/temperature change, pH change, or other stimuli
Liposomes in combination with resistance inhibitors	Liposome inhibits P-gp and successfully delivers chemotherapeutic to cancer cells and increase drug therapeutic index
Liposomes encapsulating drug analogs	Liposomes delivers hydrophobic drugs that are not substrates for P-gp or not effluxed by P-gp
Gene therapy approaches	Non-viral delivery of nucleic acid to tumor cells circumvents drug resistance, non-viral delivery of resistance genes to normal tissues gives chemoprotection

Table 4 | Marketed liposomal delivery systems to overcome drug resistance.

Marketed liposomes	Rationale	Mechanism
Pegylated liposomal Doxorubicin (Doxil®/Caelyx®)	Long-circulating liposomes preferentially accumulates in tumor tissue	Increased tumor exposure
Non-pegylated liposomal Doxorubicin (Myocet™)	Liposome leads to altered biodistribution, reduced drug toxicity profiles with new chemotherapeutics combinations to overcome drug resistance	Reduced toxicity profile
Liposomal Daunorubicin (DaunoXome®)	Liposomal encapsulated Doxorubicin is less cardiotoxic than unencapsulated Doxorubicin and can be safely used in concurrent combination with other cardiotoxic chemotherapy drugs such as Trastuzumab Minimal side effects allow substitution with Doxorubicin in same treatment regimen improving safety with no loss of efficacy	

Table 6 | Immunoliposomes and ligands-liposomes to overcome drug resistance.

Liposomes	Mechanism
Immunoliposomes for growth factor receptors	Targeting growth factor receptors with liposomes encapsulating monoclonal antibodies (MAbs) for targeting undergo endocytosis pathways to overcome drug efflux pumps
Immunoliposomes for endothelial receptors	Unlike cancer cells, endothelial cells do not develop multidrug resistance
Immunoliposomes for P-gp	Multidrug resistance is reversed with MAbs against P-gp

mixed polymeric micelles compared to Taxol and free Paclitaxel (Wei et al., 2009). Lu et al. developed dendrimer phthalocyanine-encapsulated polymeric micelle with Doxorubicin and revealed nuclear accumulation of Doxorubicin in doxorubicin-resistant MCF-7 breast cancer cells and xenograft model after photoirradiation with higher antitumor activity compared to photodynamic therapy alone (Lu et al., 2011). Cambón et al., synthesized reverse poly(butylene oxide)-poly(ethylene oxide)-poly(butylene oxide) block copolymers with potential P-gp inhibitory action in MDR cell line. Doxorubicin loaded in these polymeric micelles enhanced cell accumulation and cytotoxicity in MDR ovarian NCIADR-RES cell line over expressing P-gp (Cambón et al., 2013). Methotrexate conjugated mixed micelles of pluronic F127 and P105 suppressed tumor growth in KBv MDR cells compared to physically entraped mixed micelles due to combined effect of tumor chemosensitization by pluronic and passive targeting by micelles (Chen et al., 2013). Vincristine sulfate nanocarriers improved cellular uptake, cytotoxicity in MCF-7 and P-gp over expressing MCF-7/Adr resistant cancer cells by bypass P-gp due to endocytosis mediated by clathrin and caveolae pathways (Zhang et al., 2011b). Chemosensitizing ability of pluronics suppressed Doxorubicin induced MDR in murine lymphocytic leukemia cells (P388) and in BDF1 mice bearing (P388) ascite cancer cells with Doxorubicin-Pluronic P85 micelles (Sharma et al., 2008). Pluronics modulate MDR by intracellular ATP depletion, decreased mitochondrial potential and passive targeting. IC_{50} values of Paclitaxel-Pluronic P123/F127 mixed micelles revealed anti-proliferation activity against lung resistance protein over expressing human lung adenocarcinoma A-549 cells with 3-fold longer mean residence time and 31.8% reduction in tumor volume compared to Taxol after 28 days (Wei et al., 2010). Polyethylene glycol-polycaprolactone or Pluronic P105 micelle down-regulated the mitochondrial membrane potential and reduced ATP level to improve cytotoxicity (4 times), intracellular accumulation and overcome Doxorubicin resistance in human myelogenous leukemia (K562/ADR) cells compared to Doxorubicin solution at 12 ng/mL (Han et al., 2011).

MESOPOROUS SILICA NANOPARTICLES (MSNPS)

Mesoporous silica nanoparticles (**Figure 2**) have high drug loading due to high pore volume and surface area, multifunctionalization for targeted and controlled delivery, enhanced cellular uptake and delivers therapeutics at cellular levels in cancer (Mai and Meng, 2013; Mamaeva et al., 2013). Doxorubicin MSNPs surface conjugated with TAT peptide facilitated intranuclear drug localization in multidrug resistant MCF-7/ADR cancer cells and overcome MDR compared to free Doxorubicin or non-TAT peptide conjugated nanoparticles (Pan et al., 2013). Doxorubicin MSNPs lowered the IC_{50} value 8-fold compared to free Doxorubicin and overcome MDR in Doxorubicin resistant and P-gp over expressing cancer cell line MCF-7/ADR by increased cell proliferation suppression effect (Shen et al., 2011). Chemotherapy efficacy was enhanced bypassing the efflux pump resistance in multidrug-resistance cancer cells by co-delivery of Doxorubicin and siRNAs in MSNPs (Chen et al., 2009a). Rapid internalization of siRNA loaded magnetic MSNPs coated with polyethylenimine and surface modified with fusogenic peptide (KALA) in the tumor cells resulted in knockdown of enhanced green fluorescent protein (EGFP) and VEGF and inhibited tumor growth by suppression of tumor neovascularization (Li et al., 2013b). Doxorubicin-CTAB micelles co-loaded pH responsive MSNPs overcome multi-drug resistance in both drug-resistant MCF-7/ADR cells and drug-sensitive MCF-7 cells due to chemosensitization potential of CTAB arresting the cell cycle and inducing apoptosis (He et al., 2011). Manganese oxide-based MSNPs loaded with Doxorubicin multifunctionalized as theranostics circumvented MDR, restored drugs anti-proliferative effect by endocytosis, P-gp inhibition and ATP depletion in cancer cells (Chen et al., 2012). Anticancer drug loaded magnetic MSNPs were internalized by A549 cells through an energy-dependent clathrin induced endocytosis pathway and inhibited cancer cell growth under magnetic field (Liu et al., 2012; Sekhon, 2012). Exposure of Doxorubicin loaded zinc doped iron oxide nanocrystals in mesoporous silica framework surface-modified with pseudorotaxanes to AC field caused death of (MDA-MB-231) breast cancer cells (Thomas et al., 2010). Hyperthermia stimulated the intracellular GSH level in A549 human lung cancer cells and enhanced anti-cancer efficacy of Doxorubicin MSNPs by inducing cell death and apoptosis (Lee et al., 2011). Lejiao Jia et al. developed Paclitaxel MSNPs and revealed that anti-tumor activity of Paclitaxel in breast cancer cells (MCF-7) was dependent on pore-size and apoptosis increased with increased nanoparticle pore size (Jia et al., 2013). Galactose functionalized Camptothecin MSNPs

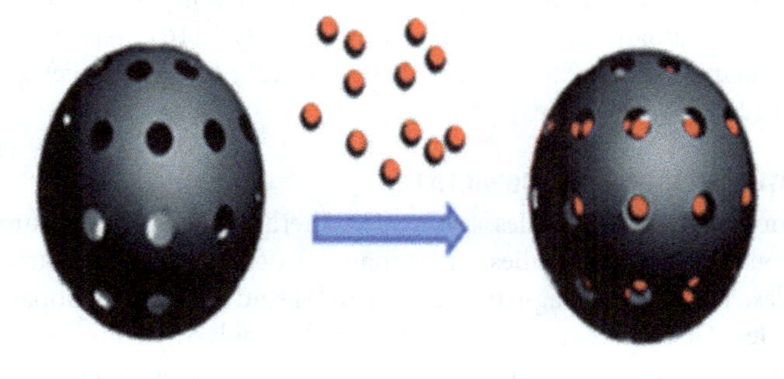

FIGURE 2 | Mesoporous silica nanoparticles (MSNPs).

with photosensitizer (porphyrin) enhanced anti-cancer activity in human cell lines of colorectal (HCT-116), pancreatic (Capan-1) and breast cancer (MDA-MB-231) (Gary-Bobo et al., 2012).

OTHER INORGANIC NANOPARTICLES

Inorganic nanoparticles for cancer therapy include quantum dots, carbon nanotubes, silica nanoparticles, gold nanoparticles, iron oxide magnetic nanoparticles and ceramic nanoparticles. Doxorubicin covalently bounded to polyethylenimine via pH sensitive hydrazone linkage and conjugated to iron oxide nanoparticles functionalized with polyethylene glycol circumvented MDR and reduced cell viability in DOX-resistant cells over-expressed in rat glioma C6 cells compared to free drug (Kievit et al., 2011). Wu Yanan et al. studies reversed the effect of 5-Bromotetrandrine and magnetic iron oxide nanoparticle combining Daunorubicin in xenograft leukemia model and inhibited expression of Bcl-2 protein and up-regulated BAX and CASPASE-3 protein expression in K562/A02 cells xenograft tumor (Yanan et al., 2009). Doxorubicin loaded pH sensitive poly (beta-amino ester) copolymer superparamagnetic iron oxide nanoparticle in drug-resistant C6 glioma cell lines (C6-ADR) revealed 300% higher cellular internalization 24 h post-treatment and reduced IC_{50} by 65% at 72 h post-treatment compared to free Doxorubicin (Fang et al., 2012). Co-administration of Doxorubicin and magnetite nanoparticles in presence of magnetic field showed cytotoxic effects against breast cancer cell lines MDA-MB-468 with greater than 80% cell death in hyperthermia combination than with Doxorubicin alone (Sadeghi-Aliabadi et al., 2013). Similar drug resistance inhibitory effect of magnetite nanoparticles loaded with Doxorubicin and Tetrandrine against K562 leukemia cells have been reported by Wang et al. (2007), Chen et al. (2008). Significant reduction in transcriptions of Mdr-1 and Bcl-2 gene and increased expressions of Bax and caspase-3 in K562-n and K562-n/VCR cells *in-vivo* in nude mice revealed the potential of Daunorubicin magnetic nanoparticles to overcome multi-drug resistance (Chen et al., 2009b). MDR1-siRNA encapsulated magnetic chitosan iron oxide nanoparticle reversed MDR effect on MDR1 gene in BT325 glioblastoma cell line with 70–80% transfection efficiency by reduced expression of MDR1 at mRNA and protein level and decreased IC_{50} values in normal BT325 and transfected cell (Zhao et al., 2013). Lectin functionalized Paclitaxel magnetic nanoparticles lowered the IC_{50} with higher cellular uptake and cytotoxic effect on Bcr-Abl positive K562 cells in chronic myelogenous leukemia (Singh et al., 2011). Cisplatin magnetic nanoparticles enhanced inhibition of A549 cells and cisplatin-resistant A549 cells in MDR lung cancer cells, lowered the levels of MRP1, lung resistance-related protein, Akt and Bad pathways and increased the levels of caspase-3 genes and proteins (Li et al., 2013a). Single drug Tetrandrine loaded magnetic nanoparticles revealed a 100-fold lowering in mdrl mRNA level but no reduction in total P-gp content while magnetic nanoparticles loaded with Adriamycin and Tetrandrine synergistically reversed multidrug resistant in K562/A02 resistant cell lines (Chen et al., 2008). Heparin coated Doxorubicin superparamagnetic iron oxide nanoparticles promoted apoptosis due to regulation of anti-apoptotic genes including caspase-3, bax, bcl-2 and surviving in human ovarian cancer cell lines A2780 (Javid et al., 2011).

Gold nanoparticles (AuNPs) are versatile platform for cancer drug delivery (Kumar and Liang, 2011; Kumar et al., 2013) and have recently entered cancer clinical trials phase I and II (Thakor et al., 2011; Vigderman and Zubarev, 2012). Gu et al. successfully synthesized doxorubicin grafted-PEGylated gold nanoparticles to overcome Doxorubicin resistant in cell lines (Gu et al., 2012). Oxaliplatin grafted on PEGylated AuNPs rapidly distributed in the nucleus and enhanced the chemotherapeutic efficacy (Brown et al., 2010). AuNPs surface conjugated with therapeutic peptide (PMI or p12) and targeted peptide (CRGDK) was rapidly internalized for better efficacy in overcoming breast cancer (Kumar et al., 2012). AuNPs covalently grafted with doxorubicin through thioctic acid-PEG linker inhibited growth of drug resistant breast cancer cells due to high drug concentrations inside cancer cells due to acid sensitive release from endosomes (Wang et al., 2011b). Zhang et al. observed similar effects with gold nanoparticle–DNA–paclitaxel conjugate (Zhang et al., 2011d). Gold nanorods functionalized with gastrin-releasing peptide (Bombesin) showed uptake via GRP receptor-mediated endocytosis with high binding affinity to breast cancer cells (Chanda et al., 2009, 2010). Selenium nanoparticles significantly enhanced the expression of pp38, Bax and cytochrome C in estrogen receptor-α positive cells (MCF-7) but not in estrogen receptor-α-negative cells (MDA-MB-231) and prevented mammary tumor growth by inducing cell death (Vekariya et al., 2012).

Quantum dots are semiconductor inorganic fluorescent nanocrystals with small and uniform sizes (1–20 nm), high surface to volume ratio, surface conjugation with multiple ligands and biocompatibility (Zhang et al., 2008a; Geszke-Moritz and Moritz, 2013). Water-soluble cadmium telluride (CdTe) quantum dots capped with negatively charged 3-mercapitalpropionic acid combined with Daunorubicin as a biomarker for simultaneous cellular imaging and inhibition of MDR for treatment of drug-sensitive leukemia K562 and drug-resistant leukemia K562/A02 cell lines was developed by Yanyan Zhou et al. The study revealed significant drug uptake in target cancer cells and cytotoxicity suppression in both cell lines (Zhou et al., 2010). Further Zhang et al. demonstrated rapid uptake and increased apoptosis rate which activated apoptosis-related caspases protein expression in drug-resistant human hepatoma HepG2/ADM cells with Daunorubicin-3-mercaptopropionic acid-capped Cadmium telluride quantum dots (Zhang et al., 2011a). Paclitaxel-loaded PLGA quantum dots were more cytotoxic than free Paclitaxel in paclitaxel-resistant KB paclitaxel-50 cells than paclitaxel-sensitive KB, however treatment with Verapamil reversed the MDR activity and reduced viability of KB paclitaxel-50 cell (Kuo et al., 2009). Doxorubicin conjugated via pH-sensitive hydrazone bond and aptamer to quantum dots when targeted to mutated MUC1 mucin over expressed in ovarian carcinoma revealed higher cytotoxicity than free drug with preferential accumulation in ovarian tumor and drug release in acidic environment of cancer cells (Savla et al., 2011).

DENDRIMERS

Novel delivery systems comprising of Doxorubicin, dendrimer and vector protein rAFP3D to bind alpha-fetoprotein receptors on tumor cell surface accumulated in the cells by receptor mediated endocytosis and demonstrated high cytotoxicity against human ovarian adenocarcinoma cell lines - Doxorubicin-sensitive SKOV3 cells and Doxorubicin-resistant SKVLB cells revealed low toxicity against human peripheral blood lymphocytes reversing the MDR in Doxorubicin-resistant cells (Yabbarov et al., 2013). The cancer-targeting potential of folate/dextran/galactose ligands anchored on poly(propylene imine) dendrimers evaluated on HeLa and SiHa cell lines indicated an IC_{50} values of 0.05, 0.2, 0.8 and 0.08 µM for folate, dextran, galactose formulations and free paclitaxel respectively on HeLa cells while the IC_{50} values of 0.6, 0.8, 10 and 6 µM with folate, dextran and galactose formulations and free PTX respectively with SiHa cells. The study revealed the targeting potential of ligands in the order folate > dextran > galactose (Kesharwani et al., 2011). Dendrimer phthalocyanine-encapsulated polymeric micelle combined with doxorubicin and mediated by photochemical internalization showed doxorubicin release from endo-lysosomes to nuclei after photoirradiation and nuclear accumulation of doxorubicin, higher antitumor activity than DPc/m-PDT alone in drug-resistant MCF-7 cells and xenograft model (Lu et al., 2011). Biotin, a cell growth promoter is required for rapid proliferation of cancer cells and is overexpressed on cancer cell surface than normal tissue. Bifunctional dendrimer conjugated with biotin a targeting moiety and fluorescein isothiocyanate an imaging moiety exhibited higher cellular uptake by an energy-dependent process in HeLa cells than conjugate without biotin. Conjugation of targeting moieties such as sugar, folic acid, antibody, peptide and epidermal growth factor to dendrimers leads to preferential accumulation of drug in the targeted tissue or cells. Similar biotin-conjugate carriers have been reported to increase uptake of anti-cancer drugs in tumor cells (Yang et al., 2009a). Cytotoxicity of dendrimers-chlorambucil conjugate and inhibition of [3H] thymidine incorporated in DNA on both MDA-MB-231 and MCF-7 breast cancer cells demonstrated that the conjugate had more potent antiproliferative activity and actively inhibited collagen biosynthesis than chlorambucil (Bielawski et al., 2011). Similar cytotoxicity effects have been reported by Khandare et al. for conjugation of paclitaxel to linear PEG polymers and PAMAM dendrimers. PAMAM dendrimer-paclitaxel conjugate showed significantly higher toxicity while linear PEG-paclitaxel conjugate showed more than 25-fold lower toxicity compared to free drug with increased IC_{50} dose (Khandare et al., 2006). Surface modified G3 PAMAM dendrimers with permeation enhancing lauryl chains conjugated with Paclitaxel via glutaric anhydride linker revealed the potential to cross cellular barriers in cell monolayers indicated by increased apparent permeability coefficient and increased cytotoxicity in both human colon adenocarcinoma cell line (Caco-2) and primary cultured porcine brain endothelial cells (PBECs). The interactions of hydrophobic lauryl moieties of L6-G3-glu-pac dendrimer conjugate with plasma membrane revealed 12-fold greater permeability across both cell monolayers than free Paclitaxel (Teow et al., 2013). Dendrimer conjugated with methotrexate a dual-acting molecule showed cytotoxicity due to its potent inhibitory activity against dihydrofolate reductase and binds folic acid receptor, upregulated on cancer cell surface (Li et al., 2012b).

NANOSTRUCTURED LIPID CARRIERS (NLCs)

Mitoxantrone hydrochloride nanostructured lipid-dextran sulfate hybrid carriers enhanced cytotoxicity and invaded cells by clathrin-mediated endocytosis with high drug accumulation in BCRP overexpressing MCF-7/MX cells and overcome MDR compared to solution (Zhang et al., 2012). Oral bioavailability of Etoposide was enhanced 1.8-, 3.0-, and 3.5-fold in NLCs, PEG40-NLCs and DSPE-NLCs respectively compared to suspension. Etoposide DSPE-NLCs and NLCs revealed highest cytotoxicity, lower cellular viability and strong inhibitory effects against human epithelial-like lung carcinoma cells (A549) than etoposide with IC_{50} values of 40.61 ± 6.15 nM, 61.78 ± 7.49 nM, and 210.87 ± 0.76 nM respectively after 24 h (Némati et al., 1996; Zhang et al., 2011c). Oleh Taratula et al. developed dual targeting NLCs loaded with an anticancer drug (Doxorubicin or Paclitaxel) to induce cell death and siRNA to target MRP1 mRNA and BCL2 mRNA to suppress pump and nonpump cellular resistance in lung cancer cells respectively and overcome resistance. Further conjugation of targeting moiety Luteinizing Hormone Releasing Hormone (LHRH peptide) to NLCs enhanced the targeting specificity to cancer cells overexpressing LHRH receptors (Taratula et al., 2013). Folate decorated Paclitaxel and Doxorubicin loaded NLCs designed by Xing-Guo Zhang et al. exhibited high cytotoxicity against human breast cancer (MCF-7) cells and multi-drug resistant (MCF-7/ADR) cells with Paclitaxel NLCs and in MCF-7/ADR cells with Doxorubicin NLCs with MDR reversal potential of 34.3-fold for Paclitaxel NLCs and 6.4-fold for Doxorubicin NLCs. Similar cytotoxicity trend was observed against human ovarian cancer (SKOV3) cells and multi-drug resistant ($SKOV3_{TR}$) cells with reversal power of 31.3 and 2.2-fold for Paclitaxel NLCs and Doxorubicin NLCs respectively compared to Taxol and Doxorubicin solution (Zhang et al., 2008b). Potential of active targeting the low density lipoprotein (LDL) receptors over expressed on cancer cells was utilized by Jaber Emami et al. and developed Paclitaxel loaded cholesterol NLCs which were taken by human colorectal cancer cell line (HT-29) through LDL receptor endocytic pathway and revealed IC_{50} values of 5.24 ± 0.96 ng/mL compared to 8.32 ± 1.35 ng/mL of free Paclitaxel solubilized in Cremophor-EL after 72 h exposure (Emami et al., 2012). Folate decorated Paclitaxel and Doxorubicin NLCs exhibited high cytotoxicity in MCF-7 and MCF-7/ADR cells while Doxorubicin NLCs revealed high cytotoxicity only in MCF-7/ADR cells compared to Taxol and Doxorubicin solution, while Paclitaxel and Doxorubicin NLCs revealed same cytotoxicity trends against human ovarian cancer cells (SKOV3) and their multidrug resistant ($SKOV3_{TR}$) cells. The reversal power of Paclitaxel and Doxorubicin NLCs were 34.3- and 6.4-folds, respectively (Zhang et al., 2008b).

Nanovehicles enhance chemotherapeutics solubility, bioavailability, therapeutic index and overcome dose-limiting toxicity, non-specific biodistribution, non-targeting and emerging drug resistance in cancer therapy. Multifunctional nanocarriers along with distinct size and surface characteristics are able to target tumor cells through active and passive targeting approaches. Nanocarrier's ability to down regulate ABC transporters or carry gene expression modulator/inhibitor enhance drugs intracellular tumor concentrations improving the chemotherapeutic efficacy. Thus nanotechnology is a novel approach for specific delivery of chemotherapeutics with potential to overcome complexity of MDR in tumors treatments.

NANOCARRIERS INHIBITING MDR BASED ON DRUG EFFLUX PUMPS

SILENCING OF DRUG RESISTANCE GENES

RNAi technology has been explored as a therapeutic strategy to overcome MDR by silencing drug efflux transporter genes such as P-gp/MDR1 and MRP1. RNAi mediated silencing through siRNA, through transfection with shRNA (Saad et al., 2008; MacDiarmid et al., 2009; Chen et al., 2010; Patil et al., 2010) and decreased MDR1 expression with antisense oligodeoxynucleotides (Wang et al., 2010) are strategies to overcome P-gp associated MDR using RNAi. Targeting transferrin receptors with PEG coated siRNA nanoparticles silenced target gene M2 ribonucleotide reductase in refractory metastatic melanoma (Davis et al., 2010). Cationic and anionic liposome polycation-DNA nanoparticles loaded with C-Myc siRNA and Doxorubicin suppressed MDR1 gene expression via silencing the transcription level by targeting transcription factors, intercalation of Doxorubicin, topoisomerase II inhibition, transcription inhibition of resistant tumors and tumor regression (Chen et al., 2010). Sigma receptors overexpressed on non-small cell lung cancer, breast tumor and prostate cancer targeted with anisamide decorated nanoparticles reduced tumor growth of C-Myc siRNA, down-regulated MDR1 expression and increased Doxorubicin accumulation in xenograft model of NCI/ADR-RES (OVCAR-8 derived) tumor (Banerjee et al., 2004). Bacterially derived minicells encapsulating siRNA targeting MDR1 gene transcripts with cytotoxic drugs down-regulated P-gp and increased survival of mice bearing human tumor xenografts (MacDiarmid et al., 2009).

INHIBITION OF DRUG RESISTANCE PROTEINS

To overcome MDR, colloidal carries inhibiting drug resistance proteins P-gp includes polymeric nanoparticles (Khdair et al., 2009; Kuo et al., 2009; Patil et al., 2009a; Song et al., 2009), quantum dots (Kuo et al., 2009), liposomes (Wu et al., 2007), nanoemulsions (Ganta and Amiji, 2009) etc. which contains combination of P-gp inhibitors with anticancer drugs such as Paclitaxel, Vincristine, or Doxorubicin. Biotin or folic acid functionalized PLGA nanoparticles encapsulating Tariquidar and Paclitaxel resulted in higher cytotoxicity and inhibited tumor growth in human MDR tumor xenografts compared to Paclitaxel nanoparticles alone (Robey et al., 2008; Patil et al., 2009b). Paclitaxel loaded theragnostic PLGA nanoparticles conjugated to quantum dots were more effective than free Paclitaxel in Paclitaxel-sensitive nasopharyngeal KB carcinoma cells and Paclitaxel-resistant KB PTX-50 while cytotoxicity enhanced in presence of Paclitaxel-loaded nanoparticles with Verapamil (Kuo et al., 2009). Transferrin coated liposomes co-encapsulating Doxorubicin and Verapamil exhibited 5 and 3-fold cytotoxicity in Doxorubicin-resistant human erythroleukemia K562 cells compared to non-targeted liposomes and transferrin targeted liposomes with Doxorubicin alone respectively (Wu et al., 2007).

NANOCARRIERS SUPPRESSING MECHANISM OF DRUG RESISTANCE INDEPENDENT OF EFFLUX TRANSPORTERS

SILENCING OF Bcl-2 AND HIF1α GENE EXPRESSION

Nanotechnology approaches suppressing drug resistance mechanisms independent of drug efflux pumps are silencing of B-cell lymphoma 2 (Bcl-2) (Indran et al., 2011) (**Figure 3**) and hypoxia-inducible factor alpha (HIF1-α) genes. Bcl-2 family proteins are regulators of apoptosis and HIF1-α gene encodes a transcription factor in cellular response to hypoxia (Rapisarda and Melillo, 2009). Two isoforms of Bcl-2, Isoform 1 (1G5M) and Isoform 2 (1G5O/1GJH) exhibit similar fold antiapoptotic activity, however their ability to bind the BAD and BAK proteins suggest differences in antiapoptotic activity of the isoforms. Bcl-2 gene damage is a major cause of cancer and resistance to cancer treatments because over-expression of anti-apoptotic genes and under-expression of pro-apoptotic genes results in lack of cell death. Hypoxia regions present in solid tumors are indicators of malignant progression, metastatic development and chemoresistance. The degree of intra-tumoral hypoxia depends on expression of HIF-1 which is composed of 2 sub-units HIF-1α and HIF-1β and is major factor for cell survival in hypoxic environment (O'Donnell et al., 2006). Matrine (active component of Sophora flavescence dry roots) in human gastric cancer MKN45 tumor cells activates caspase-3, 7 and up-regulates pro-apoptotic molecules Bok, Bak, Bax, Puma, Bim and induces apoptosis via Bcl-2 (Noguchi et al., 2003;

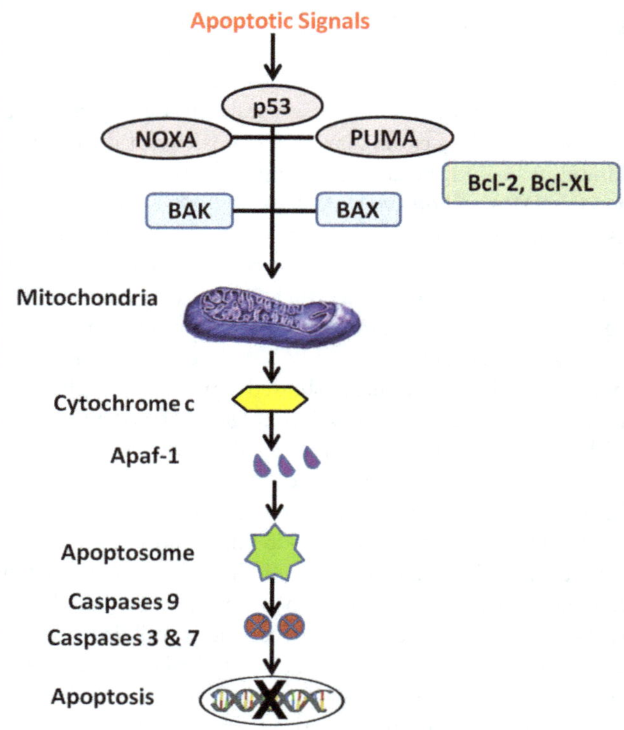

FIGURE 3 | Mitochondrial pathway.

Luo et al., 2007). Cationic cholesterol derivative with hydroxyethylamino head group, cholesteryl-3bcarboxyamidoethylene-*N*-hydroxyethylamine (I) on liposome significantly promoted gene transfection, Bcl-2 antisense phosphorothioate oligonucleotides complexed with cationic liposomes suppressed human cancer cell growth and induced apoptosis in human cervix epithelial carcinoma cell lines HeLa and mouse fibroblast NIH3T3 cells (Okayama et al., 1997). Positively charged chitosan coated PLGA nanoparticles with siRNA increased transfection and blocked the expression of anti-apoptotic Bcl-2 gene with significant cellular uptake and tumor regression (Jagani et al., 2013). Dong-feng Yu et al. developed cationic liposomes to downregulate the expression of Bcl-2 gene with siRNA transfection with enhanced apoptosis and sensitivity of 5-Fluorouracil in gastric adenocarcinoma SGC-7901 cell (Yu et al., 2013). Suppression of Bcl-xL gene through co-delivery of Doxorubicin and small hairpin RNA (shRNA) in polyplexes conjugated with an anti-PSMA aptamer specifically binds the prostate-specific membrane antigen expressed on prostate cancer cell surface. Aptamer polyplexes revealed excellent tumoricidal efficacy and significantly lowered the IC_{50} values by 17-fold compared to mixture of shRNA and Doxorubin (Kim et al., 2010a). Gene silencing capability of siRNA loaded magnetic MSNPs coated with polyethyleneimine effectively knock downed both exogenous enhanced green fluorescent protein (EGFP) gene and endogenous Bcl-2 gene with negligible cytotoxicity and released siRNA in cancer cells (Li et al., 2011). Glycoprotein transferrin (Tf) is a ligand for transferrin receptors (TfR) overexpressed on cancer cells and internalized by receptor-mediated endocytosis. Novel transferrin receptor-targeted liposomes delivered phosphorothioate antisense oligodeoxyribonucleotide (ODN-G3139) in TfR positive K562 leukemia cells and downregulated Bcl-2 protein in K562 cells 2-fold greater than non-targeted liposomes and 10-fold greater than free G3139. Tf-conjugated liposomes with G3139 reduced Bcl-2 transcription by >80%, lowered IC_{50} from 1.8 to 0.18 μM and sensitized K562 cells to Daunorubicin (Chiu et al., 2006).

MODULATION OF CERAMIDE LEVELS

Ceramide lipids are endogenous lipids and potent mediators of cellular responses in cancer including apoptosis, cell growth suppressor, differentiation, cell migration and adhesion. Ceramides are located in cell membranes and mitochondrial outer membrane, releasing pro-apoptotic factors Cytochrome c by forming permeable channels. Few sphingolipids are vital signal transducer and cell regulator in growth suppression and apoptosis. Extracellular agent such as tumor necrosis factor α activates sphingomyelinase and cleaves membrane sphingomyelin to generate cellular ceramide. Ceramide are converted to sphingolipids in presence of P-gp and accelerates cancer cell death by co-administration of P-gp antagonists with short-chain ceramides (C_6-ceramide) (Hannun and Obeid, 1995; Pettus et al., 2002; Boddapati et al., 2008). Exposure to chemotherapy and/or anticancer drugs increase intracellular ceramide levels in cancer cells and is involved in membrane clustering of the death receptor. Most anticancer chemotherapeutics stimulate ceramide accumulation through increased ceramide synthesis or inhibition of ceramide catabolism. Neutralization of ceramide via glycosylation or phosphorylation in malignant cells is linked to MDR. New therapeutic strategies to overcome resistance focus on increasing endogenous ceramide levels by stimulating ceramide synthesis, inhibiting ceramide neutralization, or direct delivery of exogenous ceramide (Barth et al., 2011). Cytotoxicity of C_6-ceramide nanoliposomes with P-gp antagonist (Tamoxifen, Cyclosporine-A, VX-710 (Biricodar), Verapamil) in human CRC cell lines (HCT-15, HT-29, LoVo) revealed synergistic effect of caspase dependent apoptosis, poly ADP ribose polymerase(PARP) cleavage, DNA fragmentation, cell cycle arrest, increased mitochondrial membrane permeability and enhanced protein expression of tumor suppressor p53 (Morad et al., 2013). Shabbits and Mayer (2003) revealed that cytotoxicity and cellular uptake of ceramides are dependent on acyl chain length with the most active C_6-ceramide (IC_{50} value = 3–14 μM) and least active C16-ceramide (IC_{50} value = 100 μM) in MDA435/LCC6 human breast cancer and J774 mouse macrophage cell lines (Shabbits and Mayer, 2003). Cisplatin-Fe_3O_4 magnetic nanoparticles reversed resistance of ovarian carcinoma cell line SKOV3/DDP by 2.2-fold and down-regulated mRNA levels of Bcl-2 and survivin expression with increased cell apoptosis (Jiang et al., 2009). Similarly Daunorubicin-Fe_3O_4 magnetic nanoparticles lowered the transcriptions of Mdr-1 and Bcl-2 gene and increased the transcriptions and expressions of Bax and caspase-3 in K562-n and K562-n/VCR cells in nude mice to overcome MDR (Chen et al., 2009b). Lonidamine and Paclitaxel dual loaded PLGA/PEG/EGFR-peptide targeted nanoparticles at 1 μM paclitaxel/10 μM lonidamine dose revealed <10% cell viability for all hypoxic cell lines and <5% cell viability for all normoxic cell lines overexpressing EGFR in human breast and ovarian cancer cell lines. EGFR-peptide targeted nanoparticles promoted mitochondrial binding of Bcl-2 proteins (Lonidamine) and hyperstabilizing microtubules (Paclitaxel) to overcome MDR (Milane et al., 2011). siRNA cationic polymeric nanoparticles downregulated Bcl-2 mRNA expression levels (<10%) in HepG2, HeLa and MDA-MB-231 cell lines and sensitized HeLa cells to Paclitaxel (Beh et al., 2009). Transferrin targeted protamine lipid nanoparticles of antisense oligonucleotide (G3139) down-regulated Bcl-2 to overcome resistance in K562, MV4-11 and Raji leukemia cell lines and was more effective than non-targeted lipid nanoparticles and frees G3139 and induced caspase-dependent apoptosis (Yang et al., 2009b). Co-administration of Paclitaxel (20 mg/kg) and C_6-ceramide (100 mg/kg) in poly(ethylene oxide)-modified poly(epsilon-caprolactone) nanoparticles revealed > 4.3- and 3-fold increase in tumor growth delay and 3.6- and 3-fold increase in tumor volume doubling time in wild-type SKOV-3 and multidrug resistant (MDR-1 positive) SKOV-3_{TR} models respectively compared to individual agents (Devalapally et al., 2007). Tumor accumulation of Paclitaxel from Paclitaxel-C_6-ceramide poly (beta-amino ester) nanoparticles was high compared to free drug in sensitive MCF-7 and multidrug resistant MCF-7TR (MDR-1 positive) human breast adenocarcinoma (van Vlerken et al., 2008). C_6-ceramide nanoliposomes revealed caspase-dependent apoptosis and diminished survivin protein expression in treatment of human and rat natural killer-large granular lymphocytic leukemia cells (Liu et al., 2010). C_6-ceramide loaded temperature-sensitive linear-dendritic nanoparticle revealed preferential uptake of fluorescein isothiocyanate-labeled linear-dendritic nanoparticles into human MDA-MB-231 breast adenocarcinoma cells with growth inhibition and solid tumor apoptosis with hyperthermia (Stover et al., 2008). Cytotoxicity of cetyltrimethyl ammonium bromide stabilized SLNs loaded MBO-asGCS oligonucleotide with or without C_6-ceramide evaluated in NCI/ADR-RES human ovary cancer cells revealed enhanced uptake of MBO-asGCS oligonucleotide with downregulation of GCS reversing resistance of cells to Doxorubicin (Siddiqui et al., 2010). Docetaxel loaded hyaluronic acid-ceramide nanoparticles enhanced intracellular uptake in CD44-overexpressing cell line (MCF-7) and revealed MDR effect in MCF-7/ADR cells (Cho et al., 2011). Doxorubicin loaded polyethylene glycol conjugated hyaluronic acid-ceramide revealed greater uptake in CD44 receptor expressed in SCC7 cell line (Cho et al., 2012). C_6-ceramide nanoliposomal with Gemcitabine or an inhibitor of glucosylceramide synthase [D-threo-1-phenyl-2-decanoylamino-3-morpholino-1-propanol (PDMP)] in Gemcitabine resistant human pancreatic cancer cell line revealed cytotoxicity and inhibited tumor growth (Jiang et al., 2011). Transferrin modified ceramide liposomes initiated lysosomal membrane permeabilization resulting in leakage of hydrolytic enzymes (cathepsins) into cytoplasm, induced cancer cells apoptosis and revealed antitumor and pro-apoptotic effects in A2780-ovarian carcinoma xenograft mouse model compared to ceramide-free and ceramide-loaded non-modified liposomes (Koshkaryev et al., 2012). Co-administration of Tamoxifen and Paclitaxel in poly (ethylene oxide) modified poly (epsilon-caprolactone) polymeric nanoparticles enhanced antitumor efficacy, lowered IC_{50} of Paclitaxel by 10- and 3-fold in SKOV3 cells and P-gp over-expressing $SKOV3_{TR}$ cells respectively (Devalapally et al., 2008). Polymeric nanoparticles co-encapsulating Paclitaxel and C_6-ceramide enhanced apoptotic signaling and reduced tumor volume 2-fold over standard Paclitaxel monotherapy (van Vlerken et al., 2010). Ceramide-generating properties of 4-HPR (Fenretinide) are being evaluated in phase II study of recurrent ovarian cancer and C_6-ceramide nanoliposomes are being evaluated as neoplastic-selective agent (Chapman et al., 2010).

TARGETING NF-κB

Transcriptional factor nuclear factor-kappa B (NF-κB) plays vital role in cancer development and resistance. Degradation of inhibitor κB after phosphorylation by inhibitor κB kinases activates NF-κB translocating into nucleus and initiating transcription contributing to tumor development, progression, chemoresistance, inflammation, and autoimmune diseases (Zingarelli et al., 2003; Li and Sethi, 2010). NF-κB is involved in multiple cellular processes including stress, cytokine gene expression, free radicals, cellular adhesion, cell cycle activation, apoptosis, and oncogenesis (Baud and Karin, 2009). NF-κB is activated via two distinct signal transduction pathways in cancer, the canonical and non-canonical pathways. NF-κB regulates expression of key proteins such as Bcl-2, Bcl-XL, cellular inhibitors of apoptosis, survivin, TRAF, Cox-2, MMP9, iNOS, and cell cycle regulatory components. Thus, NF-κB is a potential target for cancer therapeutics since inhibitors of NF-κB mediates antitumor responses and enhances tumor sensitivity to anticancer drugs (Luqman and Pezzuto, 2010). Activation of NF-κB affects cancer cell survival while inhibition of NF-κB enhances sensitivity of cancer cells to antineoplastic agents (Schwartz et al., 1999). NF-κB is important in tumorigenic process due to its strong anti-apoptotic functions in cancer cells (Magné et al., 2006). Polyethylene glycol-5000 coated Curcumin PLGA nanoparticles induced apoptosis of leukemic cells, inhibited TNF-induced NF-κB activation and suppressed NF-κB-regulated proteins involved in cell proliferation (cyclin D1), invasion (MMP-9) and angiogenesis (VEGF) (Nair et al., 2010). Micellar aggregates of cross-linked copolymers N-isopropylacrylamide with N-vinyl-2-pyrrolidone and poly(ethyleneglycol) monoacrylate encapsulating Curcumin induced cellular apoptosis, blocked NF-κB activation and down-regulated proinflammatory cytokines (IL-6, IL-8 and TNFα) in human pancreatic cancer cell lines (Bisht et al., 2007). Silica nanoparticles (50–200 μg/mL) generated reactive oxygen species, mitochondrial depolarization and apoptosis in human umbilical vein endothelial cells (HUVECs), activated c-Jun N-terminal kinase (JNK), c-Jun, p53, caspase-3 and NF-κB, increased Bax expression and suppressed Bcl-2 protein while the highest concentration significantly increased the necrotic rate, LDH leakage, expression of CD54 and CD62E and release of TF, IL-6, IL-8 and MCP-1 (Liu and Sun, 2010). Potential of gene therapy for targeting NF-κB has recently been explored as a new strategy in cancer (Tas et al., 2009). Degradation of TSP [Tween 85-s-s-polyethyleneimine (TSP)] a non-viral gene vector for p65 (shRNA) from TSP/p65 shRNA nanoparticles with release of shRNA blocked NF-κB signaling pathway, induced cell apoptosis and down-regulated p65 expression in breast cancer cells (Xiao et al., 2013). Inhibition of NF-κB with pyrrolidine dithiocarbamate (PDTC) an antioxidant and heavy metals chelator suppressed release of IκBα from NF-κB and induced cell death in neuroblastoma cells (Schreck et al., 1992). Doxorubicin and NF-κB inhibitor PDTC entrapped folic acid conjugated chitosan nanoparticles enhanced intracellular targeting of tumor cells via folic acid receptor mediated endocytosis and lowered IC_{50} values compared to free drug to overcome resistance (Fan et al., 2010).

NANOCARRIERS ADDRESSING EFFLUX PUMP DEPENDENT AND INDEPENDENT DRUG RESISTANCE MECHANISMS

Simultaneously delivery of single/multiple anticancer agents in nanocarriers addressing both efflux pump dependent (P-gp) and independent (NF-κB) drug resistance mechanisms enhances cell apoptosis and induce cancer cell death. Paclitaxel and Curcumin (NF-κB and P-gp inhibitor) co-encapsulated in flaxseed oil nanoemulsion enhanced cancer cell sensitivity to Paclitaxel and cytotoxicity in SKOV3 and drug resistant $SKOV3_{TR}$ human ovarian adenocarcinoma cells (Ganta and Amiji, 2009). Doxorubicin and siRNA containing cationic liposomes simultaneously silenced MRP1 and Bcl-2 (Saad et al., 2008). Doxorubicin/Mitomycin/5-Fluorouracil loaded hydroxyapatite nanoparticles acted synergistically with recombinant mutant human tumor necrosis factor-α (rmhTNFα) reduced P-gp levels of mRNA, increased intracellular concentration in human hepatoma xenografts of HepG2/ADM cells and suppressed tumor cell growth by apoptosis (Al-Bataineh et al., 2010; Ronaldson et al., 2010).

PHYSICAL APPROACHES TO OVERCOME MDR

DRUG DELIVERY WITH THERMAL THERAPY

In hyperthermia therapy, cells undergo heat stress (41–46°C) resulting in activation and/or initiation of intracellular and extracellular degradation mechanisms like protein denaturation, protein folding, aggregation and DNA cross linking, changing tumor cell physiology and leading to apoptosis or making cancer cells more sensitive to anti-cancer drugs. Hyperthermia increases blood flow to the tumor cells and enhances delivery of nanocarriers and thus used as an adjunct treatment to increase efficacy of chemotherapy and enhance radiation induced tumor damage. Depending on the degree of temperature, hyperthermia is classified (i) in-thermo ablation; tumor subjected to >46°C (upto 56°C) causes cells to undergo direct tissue necrosis, coagulation or carbonization (ii) moderate hyperthermia (41–46°C) affects both cellular and tissue (iii) diathermia (<41°C) for rheumatic diseases. Cellular effects of moderate hyperthermia include induction and regulation of apoptosis, signal transduction and MDR. Super-paramagnetic iron oxide particles induced therapeutic hyperthermia; liposomal nanocarrier revealed high intra-tumoral accumulation of magnetic particles on application of magnetic field (100–120 kHz) to attain temperatures 40–45°C. Folate receptor targeted Doxorubicin liposomes with hyperthermia reduced IC_{50} in cervical carcinoma cells. Temperature sensitive poly(N-isopropylacrylamide) nanocarriers release anticancer drugs in presence of specific temperature triggers. Hyperthermia enables magnetic nanoparticles to enter tumor cells by generating heat in tissues/cells and is utilized for selective targeting through cancer-specific binding agents and controlled drug delivery over conventional hyperthermia (Chicheł et al., 2007; Kumar and Faruq, 2011).

DRUG DELIVERY WITH ULTRASOUND THERAPY

Ultrasound induces thermal effects and helps nanocarrier's extravasation in tumor, enhance drug diffusion through tumor interstitium, release drug from nanocarriers within tumor and increase intracellular drug accumulation on irradiation to enhance treatment of MDR cancer. Howard et al. demonstrated that sonication enhanced uptake of Paclitaxel 20-fold from micellar system in breast cancer tumor cell line and inhibited 90% cell proliferation. Doxorubicin-pluronic® P105 micelles with ultrasound resulted in high intracellular drug accumulation in promyelocytic leukemia HL-60 cells, ovarian carcinoma drug sensitive and multidrug resistant cells (A2780 and A2780/ADR) and breast cancer (MCF-7) cells (Marin et al., 2002). Paclitaxel micelles of methoxy poly (ethylene glycol)-block-poly (D, L-lactide) enhanced intracellular drug accumulation 2-fold and cytotoxicity in drug-sensitive (MDCKII and MCF-7) and P-gp expressing (MDCKII-MDR and NCI-ADR) cell lines with ultrasound (Wan et al., 2012). Pure and mixed micelles of pluronic® P105, PEG2000-diacylphospholipid and poly (ethylene glycol)-co-poly(β-benzyl-L-aspartate) loaded Doxorubicin with ultrasound treatment enhanced intracellular drug accumulation in ovarian carcinoma tumor model in nu/nu mice and inhibited tumor growth rate (Gao et al., 2005). Ultrasound therapy downregulated levels of P-gp, MRP and lung resistance protein to 62.84 ± 3.42%, 10.26 ± 1.18%, and 3.05 ± 0.37% in HepG2/ADM cells from 96.97 ± 2.41%, 20.84 ± 3.12%, and 1.16 ± 0.59% levels, respectively. Ultrasound increased percent Bax in HepG2/ADM cells leading to cellular apoptosis and MDR reversal (Liu et al., 2001; Rapoport, 2004; Howard et al., 2006; Kedar et al., 2010; Milane et al., 2011; Wu et al., 2011; Gao et al., 2012). The studies indicate potential of ultrasound waves to disrupt nanocarrier core, form micropores in cell membrane allowing diffusion of drugs and modulate membrane drug efflux pumps function. However which mechanisms of ultrasound (heat, cavitation or microstreaming) are predominantly involved in modulating drug efflux transporter on cell membrane is still unclear. The studies on these aspects are underway in our lab.

DRUG DELIVERY WITH PHOTODYNAMIC THERAPY

Photodynamic therapy (PDT) has wide applications in cancer therapy due to its specificity and selectivity. PDT involves three components light, oxygen, and a photosensitizer (non-toxic drug) to achieve photocytotoxicity. PDT includes administration of a photosensitizer which specifically accumulates in cancer cells and when illuminated with red visible light (620–690 nm) generates reactive oxygen species in presence of tissue oxygen and causes cell death. Photofrin-2 (hematoporphyrin derivative) is the only PDT drug approved for clinical application in treatment of bladder, lung and esophageal cancer. Folic acid coated phospholipid-capped protoporphyrin IX (PpIX) loaded FITC-sensitized mesoporous silica nanocarriers (NanoPDT) effectively targeted receptors overexpressed on HeLa cells with high intracellular PpIX concentrations compared to free PpIX. NanoPDT on irradiation generated oxygen species, enhanced photocytotoxicity and inhibited 65% tumor growth in nude mice inoculated with B16F10 melanoma (Teng et al., 2013). Dendrimer phthalocyanine encapsulated polymeric micelle showed higher PDT efficacy in mice bearing human lung adenocarcinoma A549 cells, enhanced photocytotoxicity upon photoirradiation and accumulated in endolysosomes than Photofrin-2 (Nishiyama et al., 2009). However, polyethylene-glycol(PEG)-grafted transferrin-conjugated liposomes of second-generation photosensitizer 5, 10, 15, 20-tetra (*m*-hydroxyphenyl) chlorin (Foscan) did not improved the photocytotoxicity or intracellular accumulation of Foscan in esophageal cancer cell line when compared to unmodified liposomes (Paszko et al., 2013). Chitosan functionalized pluronic nanogel containing gold nanorod as photothermal therapy agent and chlorine e6 (Ce6) as photosensitizer for PDT enhanced tumor ablation *in-vivo* by combination of PDT followed by photothermal therapy compared to single therapy (Kim et al., 2013). Co-delivery of Docetaxel and photosensitizer zinc-phthalocyanine (ZnPc) loaded nanoparticles on irradiation decreased viability in HeLa cells after 72 h and enhanced antitumor activity in orthotopic amelanotic melanoma animal model compared to Docetaxel nanoparticles alone (Conte et al., 2013). Hyperbranched poly(ether-ester) (HPEE) loaded photosensitizer chlorin (e6) nanoparticles revealed better up taken by human oral tongue cancer CAL-27 cells after 4 h with cytoplasmic localization and higher phototoxicity compared to free ce6 after irradiation (Li et al., 2012c). Efficiency of second generation photosensitizers [2, 9, 17, 23-tetrakis-(1,6-hexanedithiol) phthalocyaninato] zinc (II) in PDT either free or encapsulated in gold nanoparticles/liposomes on photodamage of fibroblast and breast cancer cells revealed breast cancer cell damage with phthalocyanine liposomes while gold nanoparticles improved the effect with PDT (Nombona et al., 2012). Hematoporphyrin loaded liposomes revealed higher intratumoral accumulation of photosensitizer compared to free drug in MS-2 fibrosarcoma mouse model. Necrosis or apoptosis contributes to PDT mediated cell death in cancer and is due to generation of reactive oxygen species causing oxidative damage of cellular organelles. Thus, drug delivery in combination with PDT is a novel technique to selectively target cancer cells leading to cell lysis and overcome MDR in cancer therapy improving the efficacy.

NANOTHERANOSTICS

Nanotheranostics or quadrugnostic are third generation integrated nanovehicles comprising of four elements for diagnosis of tumor location/s, specific targeting to cancer cells, eradication of malignant cells with cytotoxic drug/s and neutralize drug resistance mechanism (**Figure 4**). Nanotheranostics serve dual roles as diagnostics and therapeutics thereby reducing chemotherapy dose, toxicity and side-effects to healthy tissues and increase therapeutic index (Ahmed et al., 2012). Superparamagnetic iron-oxide nanoparticles (SPIONs) with magnetic properties have excellent potential in tumor-targeting, diagnosis, monitoring and therapy (Santhosh and Ulrih, 2013). Polysorbate 80 coated Temozolomide-loaded PLGA superparamagnetic nanoparticles revealed higher intracellular uptake with antiproliferative effect on malignant brain glioma C6 cells compared to non-polysorbate 80 coated nanoparticles (Ling et al., 2012). Diagnostic, targeting and therapeutic potential of Doxorubicin loaded SPION and plasmonic gold nanoparticles have been evaluated in cancer treatment (Maeng et al., 2010). PEG and PEI-coated SPIONs increased intracellular concentration of Doxorubicin in resistant rat glioma C6-ADR cell line with IC_{50} values 3–5-fold lower

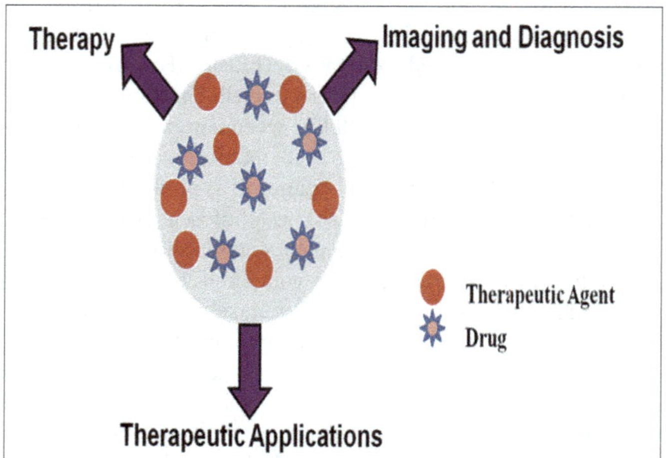

FIGURE 4 | Theragnostic agent.

compared to free Doxorubicin (Kievit et al., 2011). Fang et al. (2012) reported 3-fold lower IC_{50} with PBAE-coated SPIONs than free Doxorubicin in C6-ADR cells in accordance with Kievit et al. Gu et al. revealed that Doxorubicin loaded PEGylated gold nanoparticles were more cytotoxic on MDR cells compared to free Doxorubicin but less effective on sensitive cell lines (human hepatoma cells HepG2 and HepG2-R-a MDR subline). PEGylated Doxorubicin gold nanoparticles increased intracellular uptake and nuclear localization significantly up to 6 h by endocytosis (Gu et al., 2012). Theragnostic nanoparticles incorporating Doxorubicin or Paclitaxel for imaging and targeted chemotherapy were developed by Ahmed et al. (2012) and Kelkar and Reineke (2011). Paclitaxel loaded chitosan nanoparticles labeled with Cy5.5 (NIR fluorescence dye) were developed for imaging and cancer therapy in SCC7 tumor-bearing mouse models (Min et al., 2008; Kim et al., 2010b; Na et al., 2011; Ryu et al., 2011). Fluorescence property of Doxorubicin and photoluminescence of gold was utilized for imaging, monitoring drug uptake and tumor cells localization with folic acid decorated Doxorubicin gold nanorods (Newell et al., 2012). Chen et al. developed Doxorubicin encapsulated pH-responsive theragnostic nanoparticles with Cy5 for tissue targeting and imaging. Folate coated Doxorubicin SPIONs made of poly(ethylene oxide)-trimellitic anhydride chloride-folate increased anticancer efficacy in liver cancer, lowered expression of CD34 and Ki-67 markers of angiogenesis and cell proliferation respectively with 2- and 4-fold decrease in tumor volume compared to free Doxorubicin and Doxil® respectively (Maeng et al., 2010). Acetylated dendrimer-entrapped gold nanoparticles were taken by cell lysosomes and detected under X-ray after incubation *in-vitro* and in xenograft tumor model after intratumoral and intraperitoneal administration for imaging human lung adenocarcinoma cell line (SPC-A1 cell) (Wang et al., 2011b). Cetuximab conjugated magneto-fluorescent silica nanoparticles for targeting EGFR receptor and *in-vivo* colon cancer imaging revealed high tumor uptake with application of an external magnetic field and MRI signal changes in human colon cancer xenograft mouse model (Cho et al., 2010). Folic acid-conjugated PEG-SPIONs labeled with Cy5.5 for imaging and active targeting to lung cancer resulted in higher intracellular uptake in KB cells and lung cancer model compared to non-folic acid coated nanoparticles (Yoo et al., 2012). Butyl rhodamine B fluorescent nanoparticles conjugated with anti-Her-2 monoclonal antibody were developed successfully for imaging and targeting ovarian cancer (Hun et al., 2008). Paclitaxel SPIONs significantly increased intracellular uptake and induced regrowth delay *in-vivo* in CT-26 cells with no toxicity (Schleich et al., 2013). Folic acid decorated Tamoxifen magnetic nanoparticles were developed for imaging and detection of human breast cancer cells that over express folic acid receptors (Majd et al., 2013). Immuno-targeted gold-iron oxide nanoparticles selectively accumulated in SW1222 xenograft colorectal tumors compared to non-antigen-expressing tumor xenografts. Photothermal treatment with IR irradiation revealed >65% of antigen-expressing tumor cells presented corrupt extracellular matrix and cytoplasmic acidophilia suggesting effectiveness of nanoparticle-assisted thermal therapy (Xie et al., 2010; Lu et al., 2012; Luk et al., 2012; Kirui et al., 2013).

in cancer *in vitro*. *J. Control. Release* 152, 76–83. doi: 10.1016/j.jconrel.2011.01.024

Kim, E., Jung, Y., Choi, H., Yang, J., Suh, J., Huh, Y., et al. (2010a). Prostate cancer cell death produced by the co-delivery of Bcl-xL shRNA and doxorubicin using an aptamer-conjugated polyplex. *Biomaterials* 31, 4592–4599. doi: 10.1016/j.biomaterials.2010.02.030

Kim, J., Choi, W., Kim, M., and Tae, G. (2013). Tumor-targeting nanogel that can function independently for both photodynamic and photothermal therapy and its synergy from the procedure of PDT followed by PTT. *J. Control. Release* 171, 113–121. doi: 10.1016/j.jconrel.2013.07.006

Kim, K., Kim, J., Park, H., Kim, Y., Park, K., Nam, H., et al. (2010b). Tumor-homing multifunctional nanoparticles for cancer theragnosis: simultaneous diagnosis, drug delivery, and therapeutic monitoring. *J. Control. Release* 146, 219–227. doi: 10.1016/j.jconrel.2010.04.004

Kirui, D., Khalidov, I., Wang, Y., and Batt, C. (2013). Targeted near-IR hybrid magnetic nanoparticles for *in-vivo* cancer therapy and imaging. *Nanomed. Nanotech. Bio. Med.* 9, 702–711. doi: 10.1016/j.nano.2012.11.009

Kos, J., Obermajer, N., Doljak, B., Kocbek, P., and Kristl, J. (2009). Inactivation of harmful tumor associated proteolysis by nanoparticulate system. *Int. J. Pharm.* 381, 106–112. doi: 10.1016/j.ijpharm.2009.04.037

Koshkaryev, A., Piroyan, A., and Torchilin, V. (2012). Increased apoptosis in cancer cells *in vitro* and *in vivo* by ceramides in transferrin-modified liposomes. *Cancer Bio. Ther.* 13, 50–60. doi: 10.4161/cbt.13.1.18871

Kumar, A., and Liang, X. (2011). Gold nanoparticles: promising nanomaterials for the diagnosis of cancer and HIV/AIDS. *J. Nanomater.* 2011:202187. doi: 10.1155/2011/202187

Kumar, A., Ma, H., Zhang, X., Huang, K., Jin, S., Liu, J., et al. (2012). Gold nanoparticles functionalized with therapeutic and targeted peptides for cancer treatment. *Biomaterials* 33, 1180–1189. doi: 10.1016/j.biomaterials.2011.10.058

Kumar, A., Xu, Z., and Xing-Jie, L. (2013). Gold nanoparticles: emerging paradigm for targeted drug delivery system. *Biotech. Adv.* 31, 593–606. doi: 10.1016/j.biotechadv.2012.10.002

Kumar, C., and Faruq, M. (2011). Magnetic nanomaterials for hyperthermia-based therapy and controlled drug delivery. *Adv. Drug Deliv. Rev.* 63, 789–808. doi: 10.1016/j.addr.2011.03.008

Kuo, W., Ku, Y., Sei, H., Cheng, F., and Yeh, C. (2009). Paclitaxel-loaded stabilizer-free poly(D,L-lactide-co-glycolide) nanoparticles conjugated with quantum dots for reversion of anti-cancer drug resistance and cancer cellular imaging. *J. Chin. Chem. Soc.* 56, 923–934. doi: 10.1002/jccs.200900136

Lage, H. (2009). Therapeutic potential of RNA interference in drug-resistant cancers. *Future Oncol.* 5, 169–185. doi: 10.2217/14796694.5.2.169

Lee, D., Lockey, R., and Mohapatra, S. (2006). Folate receptor-mediated cancer cell specific gene delivery using folic acid-conjugated oligochitosans. *J. Nanosci. Nanotechnol.* 6, 2860–2866. doi: 10.1166/jnn.2006.465

Lee, E., Na, K., and Bae, Y. (2005). Doxorubicin loaded pH-sensitive polymeric micelles for reversal of resistant MCF-7 tumor. *J. Control. Release* 103, 405–418. doi: 10.1016/j.jconrel.2004.12.018

Lee, H., Kim, S., Choi, B., Park, M., Lee, J., Jeong, S., et al. (2011). Hyperthermia improves therapeutic efficacy of doxorubicin carried by mesoporous silica nanocontainers in human lung cancer cells. *Int. J. Hyperthermia* 27, 698–707. doi: 10.3109/02656736.2011.608217

Lee, R., and Low, P. (1995). Folate-mediated tumor cell targeting of liposome-entrapped doxorubicin *in-vitro*. *Biochim. Biophys. Acta Biomembranes* 1233, 134–144. doi: 10.1016/0005-2736(94)00235-H

Li, B., Xu, H., Li, Z., Yao, M., Xie, M., Shen, H., et al. (2012a). Bypassing multidrug resistance in human breast cancer cells with lipid/polymer particle assemblies. *Int. J. Nanomedicine* 7, 187–197. doi: 10.2147/IJN.S27864

Li, F., and Sethi, G. (2010). Targeting transcription factor NF-κB to overcome chemoresistance and radioresistance in cancer therapy. *Biochim. Biophys. Acta* 1805, 167–180. doi: 10.1016/j.bbcan.2010.01.002

Li, K., Chen, B., Xu, L., Feng, J., Xia, G., Cheng, J., et al. (2013a). Reversal of multidrug resistance by cisplatin-loaded magnetic Fe3O4 nanoparticles in A549/DDP lung cancer cells *in-vitro* and *in-vivo*. *Int. J. Nanomedicine* 8, 1867–1877. doi: 10.2147/IJN.S43752

Li, M.-H., Choi, S., Thomas, T., Desai, A., Lee, K.-H., Holl, M., et al. (2012b). Dendrimer-based multivalent methotrexates as dual acting nanoconjugates for cancer cell targeting. *Eur. J. Med. Chem.* 47, 560–572. doi: 10.1016/j.ejmech.2011.11.027

Li, P., Zhou, G., Zhu, X., Li, G., Yan, P., Shen, L., et al. (2012c). Photodynamic therapy with hyperbranched poly(ether-ester) chlorin(e6) nanoparticles on human tongue carcinoma CAL-27 cells. *Photodiagnosis Photodyn. Ther.* 9, 76–82. doi: 10.1016/j.pdpdt.2011.08.001

Li, X., Chen, Y., Wang, M., Ma, Y., Xia, W., and Gu, H. (2013b). A mesoporous silica nanoparticle – PEI – fusogenic peptide system for siRNA delivery in cancer therapy. *Biomaterials* 34, 1391–1401. doi: 10.1016/j.biomaterials.2012.10.072

Li, X., Xie, Q., Zhang, J., Xia, W., and Gua, H. (2011). The packaging of siRNA within the mesoporous structure of silica nanoparticles. *Biomaterials* 32, 9546–9556. doi: 10.1016/j.biomaterials.2011.08.068

Ling, Y., Wei, K., Zou, F., and Zhong, S. (2012). Temozolomide loaded PLGA-based superparamagnetic nanoparticles for magnetic resonance imaging and treatment of malignant glioma. *Int. J. Pharm.* 430, 266–275. doi: 10.1016/j.ijpharm.2012.03.047

Liu, Q., Zhang, J., Xia, W., and Gu, H. (2012). Magnetic field enhanced cell uptake efficiency of magnetic silica mesoporous nanoparticles. *Nanoscale* 4, 3415–3421. doi: 10.1039/c2nr30352c

Liu, X., Ryland, L., Yang, J., Liao, A., Aliaga, C., Watts, R., et al. (2010). Targeting of survivin by nanoliposomal ceramide induces complete remission in a rat model of NK-LGL leukemia. *Blood* 116, 4192–4201. doi: 10.1182/blood-2010-02-271080

Liu, X., and Sun, J. (2010). Endothelial cells dysfunction induced by silica nanoparticles through oxidative stress via JNK/P53 and NF-κB pathways. *Biomaterials* 31, 8198–8209. doi: 10.1016/j.biomaterials.2010.07.069

Liu, Y., Lillehei, K., Cobb, W., Christians, U., and Ng, K. (2001). Overcoming MDR by ultrasound-induced hyperthermia and P-glycoprotein modulation. *Biochem. Biophys. Res. Commun.* 289, 62–68. doi: 10.1006/bbrc.2001.5938

Lu, F., Doane, T., Zhu, J., and Burda, C. (2012). Gold nanoparticles for diagnostic sensing and therapy. *Inorg. Chim. Acta* 393, 142–153. doi: 10.1016/j.ica.2012.05.038

Lu, H., Syu, W., Nishiyama, N., Kataoka, K., and Lai, P. (2011). Dendrimer phthalocyanine-encapsulated polymeric micelle-mediated photochemical internalization extends the efficacy of photodynamic therapy and overcomes drug-resistance *in-vivo*. *J. Control. Release* 155, 458–464. doi: 10.1016/j.jconrel.2011.06.005

Luk, B., Fang, R., and Zhang, L., (2012). Lipid and polymer-based nanostructures for cancer theranostics. *Theranostics* 2, 1117–1126. doi: 10.7150/thno.4381

Luo, C., Zhu, Y., Jiang, T., Lu, X., Zhang, W., Jing, Q., et al. (2007). Matrine induced gastric cancer MKN45 cells apoptosis via increasing pro-apoptotic molecules of Bcl-2 family. *Toxicology* 229, 245–252. doi: 10.1016/j.tox.2006.10.020

Luqman, S., and Pezzuto, J. (2010). NF-κB: a promising target for natural products in cancer chemoprevention. *Phytother. Res.* 24, 949–963. doi: 10.1002/ptr.3171

Ma, P., Benhabbour, S., Feng, L., and Mumper, R. (2013). 2′-Behenoyl-paclitaxel conjugate containing lipid nanoparticles for the treatment of metastatic breast cancer. *Cancer Lett.* 334, 253–262. doi: 10.1016/j.canlet.2012.08.009

Ma, P., Dong, X., Swadley, C., Gupte, A., Leggas, M., Ledeburand, H., et al. (2009). Development of idarubicin and doxorubicin solid lipid nanoparticles to overcome P-gp mediated multiple drug resistance in leukemia. *J. Biomed. Nanotechnol.* 5, 151–161. doi: 10.1166/jbn.2009.1021

MacDiarmid, J., Amaro-Mugridge, N., Madrid-Weiss, J., Sedliarou, I., Wetzel, S., Kochar, K., et al. (2009). Sequential treatment of drug-resistant tumors with targeted minicells containing siRNA or a cytotoxic drug. *Nat. Biotechnol.* 27, 643–651. doi: 10.1038/nbt.1547

Maeng, J., Lee, D., Jung, K., Bae, Y., Park, I., Jeong, S., et al. (2010). Multifunctional doxorubicin loaded superparamagnetic iron oxide nanoparticles for chemotherapy and magnetic resonance imaging in liver cancer. *Biomaterials* 31, 4995–5006. doi: 10.1016/j.biomaterials.2010.02.068

Magné, N., Toillon, R., Bottero, V., Didelot, C., Van Houtte, P., Gérard, J., et al. (2006). NF-κB modulation and ionizing radiation: mechanisms and future directions for cancer treatment. *Cancer Lett.* 231, 158–168. doi: 10.1016/j.canlet.2005.01.022

Mai, W., and Meng, H. (2013). Mesoporous silica nanoparticles: a multifunctional nanotherapeutic system. *Integr. Biol. (Camb.)* 5, 19–28. doi: 10.1039/c2ib20137b

Majd, M., Asgari, D., Barar, J., Valizadeh, H., Kafil, V., Abadpour, A., et al. (2013). Tamoxifen loaded folic acid armed PEGylated magnetic nanoparticles for targeted imaging and therapy of cancer. *Colloids Surf. B Biointerfaces* 106, 117–125. doi: 10.1016/j.colsurfb.2013.01.051

Mamaeva, V., Sahlgren, C., and Lindén, M. (2013). Mesoporous silica nanoparticles in medicine-recent advances. *Adv. Drug Deliv. Rev.* 65, 689–702. doi: 10.1016/j.addr.2012.07.018

Marin, A., Sun, H., Husseini, G., Pitt, W., Christensen, D., and Rapoport, N. (2002). Drug delivery in pluronic micelles: effect of high-frequency ultrasound on drug release from micelles and intracellular uptake. *J. Control. Release* 84, 39–47. doi: 10.1016/S0168-3659(02)00262-6

Mei, L., Zhang, Y., Zheng, Y., Tian, G., Song, C., Yang, D., et al. (2009). A novel docetaxel-loaded poly (ε-Caprolactone)/Pluronic F68 nanoparticle overcoming multidrug resistance for breast cancer treatment. *Nanoscale Res. Lett.* 4, 1530–1539. doi: 10.1007/s11671-009-9431-6

Mendoza, A., Préat, V., Mollinedo, F., and Blanco-Prieto, M. (2011). *In-vitro* and *in-vivo* efficacy of edelfosine-loaded lipid nanoparticles against glioma. *J. Control. Release* 156, 421–426. doi: 10.1016/j.jconrel.2011.07.030

Miao, J., Du, Y., Yuan, H., Zhang, X., and Hu, F. (2013). Drug resistance reversal activity of anticancer drug loaded solid lipid nanoparticles in multi-drug resistant cancer cells. *Colloids Surf. B Biointerfaces* 110, 74–80. doi: 10.1016/j.colsurfb.2013.03.037

Miglietta, A., Cavalli, R., Bocca, C., Gabriel, L., and Gasco, M. (2000). Cellular uptake and cytotoxicity of solid lipid nanospheres (SLN) incorporating doxorubicin or paclitaxel. *Int. J. Pharm.* 210, 61–67. doi: 10.1016/S0378-5173(00)00562-7

Milane, L., Ganesh, S., Shah, S., Duan, Z., and Amiji, M. (2011). Multi-modal strategies for overcoming tumor drug resistance: hypoxia, the Warburg effect, stem cells and multifunctional nanotechnology. *J. Control. Release*155, 237–247. doi: 10.1016/j.jconrel.2011.03.032

Min, K., Park, K., Kim, Y., Bae, S., Lee, S., Jo, H., et al. (2008). Hydrophobically modified glycol chitosan nanoparticles-encapsulated camptothecin enhance the drug stability and tumor targeting in cancer therapy. *J. Control. Release* 127, 208–218. doi: 10.1016/j.jconrel.2008.01.013

Morad, S., Madigan, J., Levin, J., Abdelmageed, N., Karimi, R., Rosenberg, D., et al. (2013). Tamoxifen magnifies therapeutic impact of ceramide in human colorectal cancer cells independent of p53. *Biochem. Pharmacol.* 85, 1057–1065. doi: 10.1016/j.bcp.2013.01.015

Na, J., Koo, H., Lee, S., Min, K., Park, K., Yoo, H., et al. (2011). Real-time and non-invasive optical imaging of tumor-targeting glycol chitosan nanoparticles in various tumor models. *Biomaterials* 32, 5252–5261. doi: 10.1016/j.biomaterials.2011.03.076

Nadali, F., Pourfathollah, A., and Alimoghaddam, C. (2007). Multidrug resistance inhibition by antisense oligonucleotide against MDR1/mRNA in P-glycoprotein expressing leukemic cells. *Hematology* 12, 393–401. doi: 10.1080/10245330701283991

Nair, H., Anand, P., Sung, B., Kunnumakkara, A., Yadav, V., Tekmal, R., et al. (2010). Design of curcumin-loaded PLGA nanoparticles formulation with enhanced cellular uptake, and increased bioactivity *in vitro* and superior bioavailability *in vivo*. *Biochem. Pharmacol.* 79, 330–338. doi: 10.1016/j.bcp.2009.09.003

Némati, F., Dubernet, C., Fessi, H., Colin de Verdière, A., Poupon, M., Puisieux, F., et al. (1996). Reversion of multidrug resistance using nanoparticles in vitro: influence of the nature of the polymer. *Int. J. Pharm.* 138, 237–246. doi: 10.1016/0378-5173(96)04559-0

Newell, B., Wang, Y., and Irudayaraj, J. (2012). Multifunctional gold nanorod theragnostics probed by multi-photon imaging, *Eur. J. Med. Chem.* 48, 330–337. doi: 10.1016/j.ejmech.2011.12.036

Nieth, C., Priebsch, A., Stege, A., and Lage, H. (2003). Modulation of the classical multidrug resistance (MDR) phenotype by RNA interference (RNAi). *FEBS Lett.* 545, 144–150. doi: 10.1016/S0014-5793(03)00523-4

Nishiyama, N., Nakagishi, Y., Morimoto, Y., Lai, P., Miyazaki, K., Urano, K., et al. (2009). Enhanced photodynamic cancer treatment by supramolecular nanocarriers charged with dendrimer phthalocyanine. *J. Control. Release* 133, 245–251. doi: 10.1016/j.jconrel.2008.10.010

Noguchi, S., Hirashima, N., Furuno, T., and Nakanishi, M. (2003). Remarkable induction of apoptosis in cancer cells by a novel cationic liposome complexed with a bcl-2 antisense oligonucleotide. *J. Control. Release* 88, 313–320. doi: 10.1016/S0168-3659(02)00484-4

Nombona, N., Maduray, K., Antunes, E., Karsten, A., and Nyokong, T. (2012). Synthesis of phthalocyanine conjugates with gold nanoparticles and liposomes for photodynamic therapy. *J. Photochem. Photobiol. B Biol.* 107, 35–44. doi: 10.1016/j.jphotobiol.2011.11.007

O'Donnell, J., Joyce, M., Shannon, A., Harmey, J., Geraghty, J., and Bouchier-Hayes, D. (2006). Oncological implications of hypoxia inducible factor-1α (HIF-1α) expression. *Cancer Treat. Rev.* 32, 407–416. doi: 10.1016/j.ctrv.2006.05.003

Okayama, R., Noji, M., and Nakanishi, M. (1997). Cationic cholesterol with a hydroxyethylamino head group promotes significantly liposome-mediated gene transfection. *FEBS Lett.* 408, 232–234. doi: 10.1016/S0014-5793(97)00431-6

Otranto, M., Sarrazy, V., Bonte, F., Hinz, B., Gabbiani, G., and Desmouliere, A. (2012). The role of the myofibroblast in tumor stroma remodelling. *Cell Adh. Migr.* 6, 1–49. doi: 10.4161/cam.20377

Ozben, T. (2006). Mechanisms and strategies to overcome multiple drug resistance in cancer. *FEBS Lett.* 580, 2903–2909. doi: 10.1016/j.febslet.2006.02.020

Pan, L., Liu, J., He, Q., Wang, L., and Shi, J. (2013). Overcoming multidrug resistance of cancer cells by direct intranuclear drug delivery using TAT-conjugated mesoporous silica nanoparticles. *Biomaterials* 34, 2719–2730. doi: 10.1016/j.biomaterials.2012.12.040

Paszko, E., Vaz, G., Ehrhardt, C., and Senge, M. (2013). Transferrin conjugation does not increase the efficiency of liposomal Foscan during *in vitro* photodynamic therapy of oesophageal cancer. *Eur. J. Pharm. Sci.* 48, 202–210. doi: 10.1016/j.ejps.2012.10.018

Patil, Y., Sadhukh, T., Ma, L., and Panyam, T. (2009b). Nanoparticle-mediated simultaneous and targeted delivery of paclitaxel and tariquidar overcomes tumor drug resistance. *J. Control. Release* 136, 21–29. doi: 10.1016/j.jconrel.2009.01.021

Patil, Y., Swaminathan, S., Sadhukha, T., Ma, L., and Panyam, J. (2010). The use of nanoparticle-mediated targeted gene silencing and drug delivery to overcome tumor drug resistance. *Biomaterials* 31, 358–365. doi: 10.1016/j.biomaterials.2009.09.048

Patil, Y., Toti, U., Khdair, A., Ma, L., and Panyam, J. (2009a). Single step surface functionalization of polymeric nanoparticles for targeted drug delivery. *Biomaterials* 30, 859–866. doi: 10.1016/j.biomaterials.2008.09.056

Pettus, B., Chalfant, C., and Hannun, Y. (2002). Ceramide in apoptosis: an overview and current perspectives. *Biochim. Biophys. Acta* 1585, 114–125. doi: 10.1016/S1388-1981(02)00331-1

Pramanik, D., Campbell, N., Das, S., Gupta, S., Chenna, V., Bisht, S., et al. (2012). A composite polymer nanoparticle overcomes multidrug resistance and ameliorates doxorubicin-associated cardiomyopathy. *Oncotarget* 3, 640–650.

Prasad, P., Shuhendler, A., Cai, P., Rauth, A., and Wu, X. (2013). Doxorubicin and mitomycin C co-loaded polymer-lipid hybrid nanoparticles inhibit growth of sensitive and multidrug resistant human mammary tumor xenografts. *Cancer Lett.* 334, 263–273. doi: 10.1016/j.canlet.2012.08.008

Rapisarda, A., and Melillo, G. (2009). Role of the hypoxic tumor microenvironment in the resistance to anti-angiogenic therapies. *Drug Resist. Update* 12, 74–80. doi: 10.1016/j.drup.2009.03.002

Rapoport, N. (2004). Combined cancer therapy by micellar-encapsulated drug and ultrasound. *Int. J. Pharm.* 277, 155–162. doi: 10.1016/j.ijpharm.2003.09.048

Ren, Y., Wang, Y., Zhang, Y., and Wei, D. (2008). Overcoming multidrug resistance in human carcinoma cells by an antisense-oligodeoxynucleotide-doxorubicin conjugate *in vitro* and *in vivo*. *Mol. Pharm.* 5, 579–587. doi: 10.1021/mp800001j

Robey, R., Shukla, S., Finley, E., Oldham, R., Barnett, D., Ambudkar, S., et al. (2008). Inhibition of P-glycoprotein (ABCB1) - and multidrug resistance-associated protein 1 (ABCC1)-mediated transport by the orally administered inhibitor, CBT-1®. *Biochem. Pharmacol.* 75, 1302–1312. doi: 10.1016/j.bcp.2007.12.001

Rofstad, E. (2000). Microenvironment-induced cancer metastasis. *Int. J. Radiat. Biol.* 76, 589–605. doi: 10.1080/095530000138259

Ronaldson, P., Ashraf, T., and Bendayan, R. (2010). Regulation of multidrug resistance protein 1 by tumor necrosis factor alpha in cultured glial cells: involvement of nuclear factor-kappaB and c-Jun N-terminal kinase signaling pathways. *Mol. Pharmacol.* 77, 644–659. doi: 10.1124/mol.109.059410

Ryu, J., Kim, S., Koo, H., Yhee, J., Lee, A., Na, J., et al. (2011). Cathepsin B-sensitive nanoprobe for *in vivo* tumor diagnosis. *J. Mater. Chem.* 21, 17631–17634. doi: 10.1039/c1jm13064a

Saad, M., Garbuzenko, O., and Minko, T. (2008). Co-delivery of siRNA and an anti-cancer drug for treatment of multidrug-resistant cancer. *Nanomedicine (Lond)* 3, 761–776. doi: 10.2217/17435889.3.6.761

Sadeghi-Aliabadi, H., Mozaffari, M., Behdadfar, B., Raesizadeh, M., and Zarkesh-Esfahani, H. (2013). Preparation and cytotoxic evaluation of magnetite (Fe_3O_4) nanoparticles on breast cancer cells and its combinatory effects with doxorubicin used in hyperthermia. *Avicenna J. Med. Biotechnol.* 5, 96–103.

Sahay, G., Kim, J., and Kabanov, A. (2010). The exploitation of differential endocytic pathways in normal and tumor cells in the selective targeting of nanoparticulate chemotherapeutic agents. *Biomat* 31, 923–933. doi: 10.1016/j.biomaterials.2009.09.101

Santhosh, P., and Ulrih, N. (2013). Multifunctional superparamagnetic iron oxide nanoparticles: promising tools in cancer theranostics. *Cancer Lett.* 336, 8–17. doi: 10.1016/j.canlet.2013.04.032

Savla, R., Taratula, O., Garbuzenko, O., and Minko, T. (2011). Tumor targeted quantum dot-mucin 1 aptamer-doxorubicin conjugate for imaging and treatment of cancer. *J. Control Rel.* 153, 16–22. doi: 10.1016/j.jconrel.2011.02.015

Schleich, N., Sibret, P., Danhier, P., Ucakar, B., Laurent, S., Muller, R., et al. (2013). Dual anticancer drug/superparamagnetic iron oxide loaded PLGA-based nanoparticles for cancer therapy and magnetic resonance imaging. *Int. J. Pharm.* 447, 94–101. doi: 10.1016/j.ijpharm.2013.02.042

Schornack, P., and Gillies, R. (2003). Contributions of cell metabolism and H^+ diffusion to the acidic pH of tumors. *Neoplasia* 5, 135–145. doi: 10.1016/S1476-5586(03)80005-2

Schreck, R., Meier, B., Männel, D., Dröge, W., and Baeuerle, P. (1992). Dithiocarbamates as potent inhibitors of nuclear factor kappa B activation in intact cells. *J. Exp. Med.* 175, 1181–1194. doi: 10.1084/jem.175.5.1181

Schwartz, S., Hernandez, A., and Evers, B. (1999). The role of NF-κB/IκB proteins in cancer: implications for novel treatment strategies. *Surg. Oncol.* 8, 143–153. doi: 10.1016/S0960-7404(00)00012-8

Sekhon, B. (2012). Current scenario on impact of nanomedicine. *J. Pharm. Educ. Res.* 3, 71–76.

Shabbits, J., and Mayer, L. (2003). Intracellular delivery of ceramide lipids via liposomes enhances apoptosis *in vitro*. *Biochim. Biophys. Acta.* 1612, 98–106. doi: 10.1016/S0005-2736(03)00108-1

Sharma, A. K., Zhang, L., Li, S., Kelly, D. L., Alakhov, V. Y., Batrakova, E. V., et al. (2008). Prevention of MDR development in leukemia cells by micelle-forming polymeric surfactant. *J. Control Rel.* 131, 220–227. doi: 10.1016/j.jconrel.2008.07.031

Sharom, F. (1997). The P-glycoprotein efflux pump: how does it transport drugs? *J. Membr. Biol.* 160, 161–175. doi: 10.1007/s002329900305

Shen, J., He, Q., Gao, Y., Shi, J., and Li, Y. (2011). Mesoporous silica nanoparticles loading doxorubicin reverse multidrug resistance: performance and mechanism. *Nanoscale* 3, 4314–4322. doi: 10.1039/c1nr10580a

Shen, J., Yin, Q., Chen, L., Zhang, Z., and Li, Y. (2012). Co-delivery of paclitaxel and survivin shRNA by pluronic P85-PEI/TPGS complex nanoparticles to overcome drug resistance in lung cancer. *Biomaterials* 33, 8613–8624. doi: 10.1016/j.biomaterials.2012.08.007

Siddiqui, A., Patwardhan, G., Liu, Y., and Nazzal, S. (2010). Mixed backbone antisense glucosylceramide synthase oligonucleotide (MBO-asGCS) loaded solid lipid nanoparticles: *in vitro* characterization and reversal of multidrug resistance in NCI/ADR-RES cells. *Int. J. Pharm.* 400, 251–259. doi: 10.1016/j.ijpharm.2010.08.044

Siegal, T., Horowitz, A., and Gabizon, A. (1995). Doxorubicin encapsulated in sterically stabilized liposomes for the treatment of a brain tumor model: biodistribution and therapeutic efficacy. *J. Neurosurg.* 83, 1029–1037. doi: 10.3171/jns.1995.83.6.1029

Simon, S., Roy, D., and Schindler, M. (1994). Intracellular pH and the control of multi-drug resistance. *Proc. Natl. Acad. Sci. U.S.A.* 91, 1128–1132. doi: 10.1073/pnas.91.3.1128

Singh, A., Fahima, D., and Sahoo, S. (2011). Long circulating lectin conjugated paclitaxel loaded magnetic nanoparticles: a new theranostic avenue for leukemia therapy. *PLoS ONE* 6:e26803. doi: 10.1371/journal.pone.0026803

Singh, S., and Kaur, H. (in press). Tumor microenvironment: a review. *J. Oral Maxillofac. Surg. Med. Pathol.* doi: 10.1016/j.ajoms.2012.12.011

Song, X., Cai, Z., Zheng, Y., He, G., Cui, F., Gong, D., et al. (2009). Reversion of multidrug resistance by co-encapsulation of vincristine and verapamil in PLGA nanoparticles. *Eur. J. Pharm. Sci.* 37, 300–305. doi: 10.1016/j.ejps.2009.02.018

Stover, T., Kim, Y., Lowe, T., and Kester, M. (2008).Thermoresponsive and biodegradable linear-dendritic nanoparticles for targeted and sustained release of a pro-apoptotic drug. *Biomaterials* 29, 359–369. doi: 10.1016/j.biomaterials.2007.09.037

Susa, M., Iyer, A., Ryu, K., Choy, E., Hornicek, F., Mankin, H., et al. (2010). Inhibition of ABCB1 (MDR1) expression by a siRNA nanoparticulate delivery system to overcome drug resistance in osteosarcoma. *PLoS ONE* 5:10764. doi: 10.1371/journal.pone.0010764

Tang, M., Lei, L., Guo, S., and Huang, W. (2010). Recent progress in nanotechnology for cancer therapy. *Chin. J. Cancer* 29, 775–780. doi: 10.5732/cjc.010.10075

Taratula, O., Kuzmov, A., Shah, M., Garbuzenko, O., and Minko, T. (2013). Nanostructured lipid carriers as multifunctional nanomedicine platform for pulmonary co-delivery of anticancer drugs and siRNA. *J. Control. Release* 171, 349–357. doi: 10.1016/j.jconrel.2013.04.018

Tas, S., Vervoordeldonk, M., and Tak, P. (2009). Gene therapy targeting nuclear factor-κB: towards clinical application in inflammatory diseases and cancer. *Curr. Gene Ther.* 9,160–170. doi: 10.2174/156652309788488569

Teng, I., Chang, Y., Wang, L., Lu, H., Wu, L., Yang, C., et al. (2013). Phospholipid-functionalized mesoporous silica nanocarriers for selective photodynamic therapy of cancer. *Biomaterials* 34, 7462–7470. doi: 10.1016/j.biomaterials.2013.06.001

Teow, H., Zhou, Z., Najlah, M., Yusof, S., Abbott, N., and D'Emanuele, A. (2013). Delivery of Paclitaxel across cellular barriers using a dendrimer-based nanocarrier. *Int. J. Pharm.* 441, 701–711. doi: 10.1016/j.ijpharm.2012.10.024

Thakor, A., Jokerst, J., Zavaleta, C., Massoud, T., and Gambhir, S. (2011). Gold nanoparticles: a revival in precious metal administration to patients. *Nano Lett.* 11, 4029–4036. doi: 10.1021/nl202559p

Thomas, C., Ferris, D., Lee, J., Choi, E., Cho, M., Kim, E., et al. (2010). Noninvasive remote-controlled release of drug molecules *in vitro* using magnetic actuation of mechanized nanoparticles. *J. Am. Chem. Soc.* 132, 10623–10625. doi: 10.1021/ja1022267

Thomas, H., and Coley, H. (2003). Overcoming multidrug resistance in cancer: an update on the clinical strategy of inhibiting p-glycoprotein. *Cancer Control* 10, 159–165.

Tomida, A., and Tsuruo, T. (2002). "Drug resistance pathways as targets," in *Anticancer Drug Development*, Chapter 5, eds B. C. Baguley and D. J. Kerr (Tokyo: Academic Press), 77–90.

van Kempen, L., Ruiter, D., van Muijen, G., and Coussens, L. (2003). The tumor microenvironment: a critical determinant of neoplastic evolution. *Eur. J. Cell Biol.* 82, 539–548. doi: 10.1078/0171-9335-00346

van Vlerken, L., Duan, Z., Little, S., Seiden, M., and Amiji, M. (2008). Biodistribution and pharmacokinetic analysis of paclitaxel and ceramide administered in multifunctional polymer-blend nanoparticles in drug resistant breast cancer model. *Mol. Pharm.* 5, 516–526. doi: 10.1021/mp800030k

van Vlerken, L., Duan, Z., Little, S., Seiden, M., and Amiji, M. (2010). Augmentation of therapeutic efficacy in drug-resistant tumor models using ceramide coadministration in temporal-controlled polymer-blend nanoparticle delivery systems. *AAPS J.* 12, 171–180. doi: 10.1208/s12248-010-9174-4

Vekariya, K., Kaur, J., and Tikoo, K. (2012). ERα signaling imparts chemotherapeutic selectivity to selenium nanoparticles in breast cancer. *Nanomedicine* 8, 1125–1132. doi: 10.1016/j.nano.2011.12.003

Velingkar, V., and Dandekar, V. (2010). Modulation of P-glycoprotein mediated multidrug resistance (MDR) in cancer using chemosensitizers. *Int. J. Pharm. Sci. Res.*1, 104–111.

Venishetty, V., Komuravelli, R., Kuncha, M., Sistla, R., and Diwan, P. (2013). Increased brain uptake of docetaxel and ketoconazole loaded folate-grafted solid lipid nanoparticles. *Nanomed. Nanotechnol. Biol. Med.* 9, 111–121. doi: 10.1016/j.nano.2012.03.003

Vigderman, L., and Zubarev, E. (2012). Therapeutic platforms based on gold nanoparticles and their covalent conjugates with drug molecules. *Adv. Drug Deliv. Rev.* 65, 663–676. doi: 10.1016/j.addr.2012.05.004

Wan, C., Jackson, J., Pirmoradi, F., Chiao, M., and Burt, H. (2012). Increased accumulation and retention of micellar Paclitaxel in drug-sensitive and P-glycoprotein-expressing cell lines following ultrasound exposure. *Ultrasound Med. Bio.* 38, 736–744. doi: 10.1016/j.ultrasmedbio.2012.01.023

Wang, F., Zhang, D., Zhang, Q., Chen, Y., Zheng, D., Hao, L., et al. (2011a). Synergistic effect of folate-mediated targeting and verapamil-mediated P-gp inhibition with paclitaxel-polymer micelles to overcome multi-drug resistance. *Biomaterials* 32, 9444–9456. doi: 10.1016/j.biomaterials.2011.08.041

Wang, H., Zheng, L., Peng, C., Guo, R., Shen, M., Shi, X., et al. (2011b). Computed tomography imaging of cancer cells using acetylated dendrimer-entrapped gold nanoparticles. *Biomaterials* 32, 2979–2988. doi: 10.1016/j.biomaterials.2011.01.001

Wang, J., Tao, X., Zhang, Y., Wei, D., and Ren, Y. (2010). Reversion of multidrug resistance by tumor targeted delivery of antisense oligodeoxynucleotides in hydroxypropyl-chitosan nanoparticles. *Biomaterials* 31, 4426–4433. doi: 10.1016/j.biomaterials.2010.02.007

Wang, L., Zeng, R., Li, C., and Qiao, R. (2009). Self-assembled polypeptide block poly (vinylpyrrolidone) as prospective drug delivery systems. *Colloid Surf. B Biointerfaces* 74, 284–292. doi: 10.1016/j.colsurfb.2009.07.032

Wang, X., Zhang, R., Wu, C., Dai, Y., Song, M., Gutmann, S., et al. (2007). The application of Fe3O4 nanoparticles in cancer research: a new strategy to inhibit drug resistance. *J. Biomed. Mater. Res. A* 80, 852–860. doi: 10.1002/jbm.a.30901

Weber, C., and Kuo, P. (2012). The tumor microenvironment. *Surg. Oncol.* 21, 172–177. doi: 10.1016/j.suronc.2011.09.001

Wei, Z., Hao, J., Yuan, S., Li, Y., Juan, W., Shaa, X., et al. (2009). Paclitaxel-loaded Pluronic P123/F127 mixed polymeric micelles: formulation, optimization and *in vitro* characterization. *Int. J. Pharm.* 376, 176–185. doi: 10.1016/j.ijpharm.2009.04.030

Wei, Z., Yuan, S., Chen, Y., Yu, S., Hao, J., Luo, J., et al. (2010). Enhanced antitumor efficacy by Paclitaxel-loaded Pluronic P123/F127 mixed micelles against non-small cell lung cancer based on passive tumor targeting and modulation of drug resistance. *Eur. J. Pharm. Biopharm.* 75, 341–353. doi: 10.1016/j.ejpb.2010.04.017

Wong, H., Bendayan, R., Rauth, A., and Wu, X. (2006). Simultaneous delivery of doxorubicin and GG918 (Elacridar) by new polymer-lipid hybrid nanoparticles (PLN) for enhanced treatment of multidrug-resistant breast cancer. *J. Control. Release* 116, 275–284. doi: 10.1016/j.jconrel.2006.09.007

Wouters, B., Koritzinsky, M., Chiu, R., and Theys, J. (2003). Modulation of cell death in the tumor microenvironment. *Semin. Radiat. Oncol.* 13, 31–41. doi: 10.1053/srao.2003.50004

Wu, C., Calcagno, A., and Ambudkar, S. (2008). Reversal of ABC drug transporter-mediated multidrug resistance in cancer cells: evaluation of current strategies. *Curr. Mol. Pharmacol.* 1, 93–105. doi: 10.2174/1874467210801020093

Wu, F., Shao, Z., Zhai, B., Zhao, C., and Shen, D. (2011). Ultrasound reverses multidrug resistance in human cancer cells by altering gene expression of ABC transporter proteins and Bax protein. *Ultrasound Med. Biol.* 37, 151–159. doi: 10.1016/j.ultrasmedbio.2010.10.009

Wu, J., Lu, Y., Lee, A., Pan, X., Yang, X., Zhao, X., et al. (2007). Reversal of multidrug resistance by transferrin-conjugated liposomes co-encapsulating doxorubicin and verapamil. *J. Pharmacol. Pharm. Sci.* 10, 350–357.

Xiao, J., Duan, X., Yin, Q., Miao, Z., Yu, H., Chen, C., et al. (2013). The inhibition of metastasis and growth of breast cancer by blocking the NF-κB signaling pathway using bioreducible PEI-based/p65 shRNA complex nanoparticles. *Biomaterials* 34, 5381–5390. doi: 10.1016/j.biomaterials.2013.03.084

Xie, J., Lee, S., and Chen, X. (2010). Nanoparticle-based theranostic agents. *Adv. Drug Deliv. Rev.* 62, 1064–1079. doi: 10.1016/j.addr.2010.07.009

Xu, Z., Chen, L., Gu, W., Gao, Y., Lin, L., Zhang, Z., et al. (2009). The performance of docetaxel-loaded solid lipid nanoparticles targeted to hepatocellular carcinoma. *Biomaterials* 30, 226–232. doi: 10.1016/j.biomaterials.2008.09.014

Yabbarov, N., Posypanova, G., Vorontsov, E., Obydenny, S., and Severin, E. (2013). A new system for targeted delivery of doxorubicin into tumor cells. *J. Control. Release* 168, 135–141. doi: 10.1016/j.jconrel.2013.03.007

Yanan, W., Baoan, C., Jian, C., Feng, G., Wenlin, X., Jiahua, D., et al. (2009). Reversal of multidrug resistance by magnetic Fe_3O_4 nanoparticle copolymerisating daunorubicin and 5-bromotetrandrine in xenograft nude-mice. *Int. J. Nanomedicine* 4, 73–78.

Yang, W., Cheng, Y., Xu, T., Wang, X., and Wen, L. (2009a). Targeting cancer cells with biotin–dendrimer conjugates. *Eur. J. Med. Chem.* 44, 862–868. doi: 10.1016/j.ejmech.2008.04.021

Yang, X., Koh, C., Liu, S., Pan, X., Santhanam, R., Yu, B., et al. (2009b). Transferrin receptor-targeted lipid nanoparticles for delivery of an antisense oligodeoxyribonucleotide against Bcl-2. *Mol. Pharm.* 6, 221–230. doi: 10.1021/mp800149s

Yared, J., and Tkaczuk, K. (2012). Update on taxane development: new analogs and new formulations. *Drug Des. Devel. Ther.* 6, 371–384.

Yoo, M., Park, I., Lim, H., Lee, S., Jiang, H., Kim, Y., et al. (2012). Folate–PEG–superparamagnetic iron oxide nanoparticles for lung cancer imaging. *Acta Biomater.* 8, 3005–3013. doi: 10.1016/j.actbio.2012.04.029

Yu, D., Wu, F., Liu, Y., Liu, H., and Xia, Q. (2013). Bcl-2 gene silence enhances the sensitivity toward 5-Fluorouracil in gastric adenocarcinoma cells. *Biomed. Pharmacother.* 67, 615–617. doi: 10.1016/j.biopha.2013.03.007

Zhang, G., Shi, L., Selke, M., and Wang, X. (2011a). CdTe quantum dots with daunorubicin induce apoptosis of multidrug-resistant human hepatoma HepG2/ADM cells: *in vitro* and *in vivo* evaluation. *Nanoscale Res. Lett.* 6, 418. doi: 10.1186/1556-276X-6-418

Zhang, H., Yee, D., and Wang, C. (2008a). Quantum dots for cancer diagnosis and therapy: biological and clinical perspectives. *Nanomedicine (Lond.)* 3, 83–91. doi: 10.2217/17435889.3.1.83

Zhang, P., Ling, G., Pan, X., Sun, J., Zhang, T., Pu, X., et al. (2012). Novel nanostructured lipid-dextran sulfate hybrid carriers overcome tumor multidrug resistance of mitoxantrone hydrochloride. *Nanomed. Nanotech. Biol. Med.* 8, 185–193. doi: 10.1016/j.nano.2011.06.007

Zhang, P., Ling, G., Sun, J., Zhang, T., Yuan, Y., Sun, Y., et al. (2011b). Multifunctional nanoassemblies for vincristine sulfate delivery to overcome multidrug resistance by escaping P-glycoprotein mediated efflux. *Biomaterials* 32, 5524–5533. doi: 10.1016/j.biomaterials.2011.04.022

Zhang, T., Chen, J., Zhang, Y., Shen, Q., and Pan, W. (2011c). Characterization and evaluation of nanostructured lipid carrier as a vehicle for oral delivery of etoposide. *Eur. J. Pharm. Sci.* 43, 174–179. doi: 10.1016/j.ejps.2011.04.005

Zhang, X., Miao, J., Dai, Y., Du, Y., Yuan, H., and Hu, F. (2008b). Reversal activity of nanostructured lipid carriers loading cytotoxic drug in multi-drug resistant cancer cells. *Int. J. Pharm.* 361, 239–244. doi: 10.1016/j.ijpharm.2008.06.002

Zhang, X., Xu, X., Lam, R., Giljohann, D., Ho, D., and Mirkin, C. (2011d). Strategy for increasing drug solubility and efficacy through covalent attachment to polyvalent DNA nanoparticle conjugates. *ACS Nano* 5, 6962–6970. doi: 10.1021/nn201446c

Zhao, P., Wang, H., Gao, H., Li, C., and Zhang, Y. (2013). Reversal of multidrug resistance by magnetic chitosan$-Fe_3O_4$ nanoparticle−encapsulated MDR1 siRNA in glioblastoma cell line. *Neurol. Res.* 35, 821–828. doi: 10.1179/1743132813Y.0000000218

Zhou, R., Mazurchuk, R., and Straubinger, R. (2002). Antivasculature effects of doxorubicin containing liposomes in an intracranial rat brain tumor model. *Cancer Res.* 62, 2561–2566.

Zhou, Y., Shi, L., Li, Q., Jiang, H., Lv, G., Zhao, J., et al. (2010). Imaging and inhibition of multi-drug resistance in cancer cells via specific association with negatively charged CdTe quantum dots. *Biomaterials* 31, 4958–4963. doi: 10.1016/j.biomaterials.2010.02.053

Zingarelli, B., Sheehan, M., and Wong, H. (2003). Nuclear factor-[kappa] B as a therapeutic target in critical care medicine. *Crit. Care Med.* 31, S105–S111. doi: 10.1097/00003246-200301001-00015

Customizing the therapeutic response of signaling networks to promote antitumor responses by drug combinations

Alexey Goltsov[1]*, Simon P. Langdon[2], Gregory Goltsov[3], David J. Harrison[4] and James Bown[1]

[1] Centre for Research in Informatics and Systems Pathology (CRISP), University of Abertay Dundee, Dundee, UK
[2] Division of Pathology, Institute of Genetics and Molecular Medicine, Western General Hospital, University of Edinburgh, Edinburgh, UK
[3] Touch Surgery, London, UK
[4] School of Medicine, University of St Andrews, St Andrews, UK

Edited by:
Jan Trøst Jørgensen, Dx-Rx Institute, Denmark

Reviewed by:
Katarzyna Anna Rejniak, H. Lee Moffitt Cancer Center & Research Institute, USA
Andrea Degasperi, University College Dublin, Ireland

***Correspondence:**
Alexey Goltsov, Centre for Research in Informatics and Systems Pathology (CRISP), University of Abertay Dundee, Bell Street, Dundee DD1 1HG, UK
e-mail: a.goltsov@abertay.ac.uk

Drug resistance, *de novo* and acquired, pervades cellular signaling networks (SNs) from one signaling motif to another as a result of cancer progression and/or drug intervention. This resistance is one of the key determinants of efficacy in targeted anti-cancer drug therapy. Although poorly understood, drug resistance is already being addressed in combination therapy by selecting drug targets where SN sensitivity increases due to combination components or as a result of *de novo* or acquired mutations. Additionally, successive drug combinations have shown low resistance potential. To promote a rational, systematic development of combination therapies, it is necessary to establish the underlying mechanisms that drive the advantages of combination therapies, and design methods to determine drug targets for combination regimens. Based on a joint systems analysis of cellular SN response and its sensitivity to drug action and oncogenic mutations, we describe an *in silico* method to analyze the targets of drug combinations. Our method explores mechanisms of sensitizing the SN through a combination of two drugs targeting vertical signaling pathways. We propose a paradigm of SN response customization by one drug to both maximize the effect of another drug in combination and promote a robust therapeutic response against oncogenic mutations. The method was applied to customize the response of the ErbB/PI3K/PTEN/AKT pathway by combination of drugs targeting HER2 receptors and proteins in the down-stream pathway. The results of a computational experiment showed that the modification of the SN response from hyperbolic to smooth sigmoid response by manipulation of two drugs in combination leads to greater robustness in therapeutic response against oncogenic mutations determining cancer heterogeneity. The application of this method in drug combination co-development suggests a combined evaluation of inhibition effects together with the capability of drug combinations to suppress resistance mechanisms before they become clinically manifest.

Keywords: anti-cancer combination therapy, cancer drug resistance, pathway engineering, signaling networks, pertuzumab, PI3K/PTEN/AKT

INTRODUCTION

Anti-cancer combination therapies are an increasingly promising way to better treat patients, offering an increase in efficacy of drugs, and a means to overcome/avoid resistance to targeted drug therapy. An evidence base of successes of multidrug strategies in anti-cancer therapy is growing yearly, but typically the mechanism of synergy is not entirely understood. To promote a more directed and systematic development of combination therapies, it is necessary to clearly elucidate the underlying mechanisms that drive the advantages of drug combination effect. Exploration of these mechanisms can impact significantly on the determination and validation of advanced combination of targets in novel drug development strategies such as drug combination co-development (1) and drug-diagnostics co-development (2). With respect to a drug combination co-development strategy, novel compounds should be developed in a combinatorial context and not independently in order to gain those proven integrative benefits with respect to tumor growth inhibition, drug resistance, and toxicity. In the drug–diagnostic co-development model, the drug and the diagnostic assay are developed in conjunction. Companion diagnostic (CDx) assays as well as clinical trial strategies in the case of drug combination therapy should be adapted to multiple biomarkers and different drug combinations (2). Considering the risk of increasing toxicity by the use of drug combination therapy, the US food and drug administration (FDA) released drug co-development guidance, which proposed stringent regulatory recommendations for the use of combination strategies (1, 3). According to these recommendations, there should exist a strong biological rationale for the use of the combinations and proven significant advantages over the use of the drugs as individual agents.

Rational determination and validation of advanced targets for drug combination therapy are the main challenges for these strategies. The inherent complexities of signaling networks (SNs), including crosstalk logic and redundancy in their topology (4, 5) limit the relevance of genotype-based screening to identify and validate optimal drug combination targets among several hundred possible targets. In the face of these challenges, we need more sophisticated methods to design effective combination therapies (1).

Systems biology and computational bioinformatics may offer a key role in advancing drug combination co-development. These technologies are being developed to support rationalized screening of effective drug combinations, and to formulate quantitative criteria for drug combination target validation and specific properties of each drug in a combination context and in the face of different mutational statuses of different cancers (6–9). Such developments are motivated by the potential to reduce the size, duration, and cost of clinical trials as well as to accelerate regulatory approval. Our own studies to support drug combination co-development are described here. Our method is based on analysis of the response of a cellular SN to drug intervention, and its modification by drug combination to achieve high efficacy and reduce drug resistance potential. The approach developed here is founded on the two most attractive advantages of drug combination well established recently: (i) a drug combination suppresses *de novo* or acquired resistance to one of the drugs in the combination – a resistance suppression effect; and (ii) one drug in a combination sensitizes therapeutic response to a second drug – a sensitizing effect.

Resistance suppression effects arising from drug combination are used widely in clinics now, by manipulating pathway dynamics or by slowing down the cancer evolution. Some examples of pathway manipulations are summarized in Ref. (1) targeting different domains of the same protein with two drugs [for example, trastuzumab combined with pertuzumab for human epidermal growth factor receptor, HER2, in breast (10) and ovarian (11, 12) cancers]; horizontally targeting parallel signaling pathways [for example, combined MEK and PI3K/AKT inhibition (13, 14)], and vertically targeting up- and down-stream pathways in one SN [for example, targeting BRAF and MEK, HER2, and PI3K, PI3K/AKT and mTOR (15–17)]. An evolutionary approach (adaptive therapy) to treat drug resistance has been suggested, with the aim of lowering the cancer cell's capacity to evolve resistance mechanisms through adaptive combination therapy in order to hinder the emergence of resistance types (18). Beyond these approaches, the combination of chemotherapy and molecular targeted therapy demonstrates a complementary mechanism of efficacy and may suggest a route for next-generation cancer therapy (10, 19, 20). For example, a clinical trial of HER2-positive breast cancer progression following HER2 inhibitor trastuzumab therapy showed that trastuzumab in combination with chemotherapeutic agent (capecitabine) was more effective than capecitabine alone. It would seem that trastuzumab sensitizes cell response to other drugs despite the fact that cells are refractory to trastuzumab and that there is therapeutic benefit to continue trastuzumab therapy in combination with other drugs beyond progression (21).

The sensitizing effects of drug combinations are well established in combined therapies targeting different pathways, such as the PI3K/PTEN/AKT and MAPK networks (13, 14); EGFR, DNA-damaging apoptotic signaling pathways (22) as well as in drug combinations inhibiting different nodes in the same pathway: PI3K/PTEN/AKT/mTOR (23–25), Ras/RAF/MEK/ERK (26, 27). However, there are longer-term implications arising from drug combinations since they may lead to different mutations and negatively impact resistance potential. For example, comparison of pre- and post-trastuzumab treatment of tissue samples in metastatic HER2-amplified breast cancer from patients progressing on trastuzumab allowed determination of mutations in *PIK3CA* and *PTEN* arising during treatment (4). A significant reduction, or full loss, of PTEN expression was observed in trastuzumab refractory metastatic tumors compared to the cohort untreated by trastuzumab. It was suggested that PTEN expression reduction was acquired as a result of trastuzumab therapy, leading itself to trastuzumab resistance (4). In contrast, treatment by everolimus, an mTOR inhibitor, did not increase mutational load in pre/post treatment samples of renal carcinomas (28). Moreover, this phenomenon is context specific: for example, abiraterone alone and given in combination with other drugs to control side effects contributes to resistance by activating mutations in the hormone receptor genes; however, a different combination including abiraterone was reported to delay drug resistance (29).

These examples highlight the complexities of combination drug therapy design, including the change in sensitivity to mutation and resistance potential through combination action, and the attending challenges associated with validation. To help overcome these complexities and challenges, we propose a method for the *in vitro*/*in vivo*/*in silico* validation of the targets of drug combinations and quantitative estimation of the perturbations induced by drugs in SNs. Our method is based on the study of drug response characteristics of (i) a SN and its modification by different oncogenic mutations and drug action; and (ii) perturbation of SN sensitivity to drug action induced by mutations. Using sensitivity analysis (SA) of this signaling response, we show that inhibition of various targets by the first drug significantly sensitizes SN response to both compensating mutations leading to resistance and the second drug in combination. We present a scheme for customizing the SN response through drug combination to enhance the robustness of the therapeutic response due to weakening of the drug-sensitizing effect to compensation mutations. To demonstrate the method and to study in detail the drug/mutation modification of SN response, we used the kinetic model of drug combination targeting HER2 receptors and vertical PI3K/PTEN/AKT signaling pathway (30–32).

MATERIALS AND METHODS

The method is based on the analysis of input/output (I/O) responses of a cellular SN, $R_{SN} = C_{out}$ (C_{in}, P_{SN}, D, t), which describes the relation between output signal C_{out} and input signal C_{in} (see scheme in **Figure 1**). R_{SN} depends on molecular parameters, P_{SN}, of the SN components: specifically, kinetic parameters of the proteins/receptors, $K = k_1, \ldots, k_n$ (dissociation constants, catalytic rates), and their expression levels, $E = e_1, \ldots, e_m$. R_{SN} also depends on the concentrations of drugs, D, which inhibit proteins in the SN. Typically, R_{SN} is measured in experimental systems as the dose dependence of output signal on drug/ligand concentration at a defined time, t, following ligand/drug application in a cellular assay. The experimental dose dependence, $R_{SN} = C_{out}$

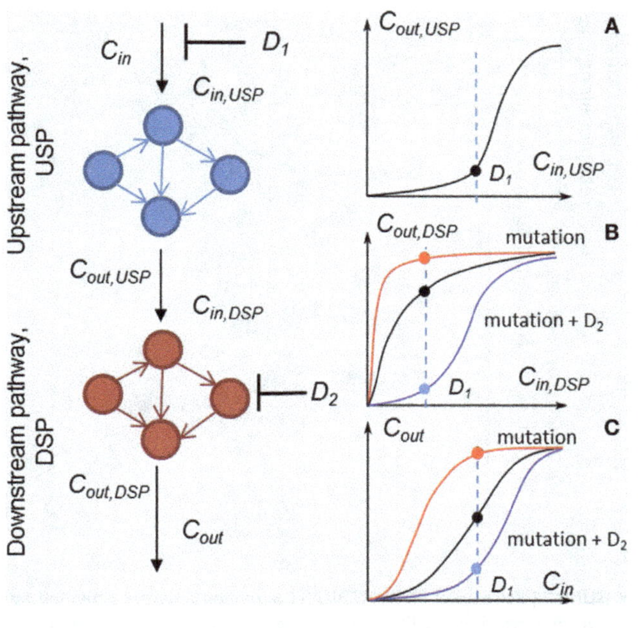

FIGURE 1 | Scheme of the method of customizing cellular signaling response by drug combination targeting upstream (drug D_1) and down-stream pathway (drug D_2). Plot sketches A, B, and C show responses, $R_{USP} = C_{out,USP}$ ($C_{in,USP}$, D_1), $R_{DSP} = C_{out,DSP}$ ($C_{in,DSP}$, D_2), and the whole SN $R_{SN} = C_{out}$ (C_{in}, D_1, D_2), respectively. Examples of the responses of unmodified DSP (black line), modified by a mutation in the DSP (red lines) and modified by the second drug D_2 (blue lines) in the presence of the mutation. Input signal C_{in} inhibited by drug D_1 is shown by the dashed lines.

(C_{in}, P_{SN}, D, t), on drug concentration allows the definition of the IC_{50} of drug D_1, which strongly depends on the target of drug D_2, the concentration of this second drug, and the mutational status of the SN determined by parameters, P_{SN}.

To analyze in detail the combination effect of two drugs at different mutations of the SN, we decompose the SN into up- and down-stream pathways that are the targets of drugs D_1 and D_2, respectively (see **Figure 1**). The response, R_{SN}, of the SN can be represented through the response R_{USP} of upstream pathway (USP) and the response, R_{DSP} of down-stream pathway (DSP) in the form, $R_{SN} = R_{DSP}(R_{USP})$, where $R_{USP} = C_{out,UPS}(C_{in}, P_{USP}, D_1, t)$ and $R_{DSP} = C_{out,DSP}(C_{in,DSP}, P_{DSP}, D_2, t)$. In this formulation, we took into account equivalences of I/O signals: $C_{in,DSP} = C_{out,USP}$ and $C_{out\_DSP} = C_{out}$ (see **Figure 1**). Theoretically, the I/O responses, R_{SN}, R_{USP}, and R_{DSP}, are readily calculated from the model of the SN. Experimentally, R_{DSP} can be extracted from two experimental dose dependencies: dose dependence of the whole SN, R_{SN}, and the receptor activation/inhibition dose dependence on activator/inhibitor concentration, R_{USP}, and represented in the form $R_{DSP} = C_{out}(R_{USP}, P_{DSP}, D_2, t)$.

Input/output response R_{DSP} determines the output signal amplitude of the DSP depending on input signals, which is controlled by the first drug D_1, the molecular parameters, P_{DSP}, and the action of the second drug D_2. Analysis of R_{DSP} allows us to study the effect of mutations, i.e., changes in kinetic properties and expression levels of proteins, P_{DSP}, on the change in R_{DSP} and how these changes determine a transition from drug sensitivity to drug resistance. Plots A, B, and C (black lines) in **Figure 1** show arbitrary responses, R_{USP}, R_{DSP}, and R_{SN}, corresponding to sensitivity of the SN to D_1. According to this type of smooth hyperbolic R_{DSP}, the output signal of the SN changes when the input signal changes under inhibitor D_1 (see black points in plots A, B, and C showing inhibited signal at drug concentration D_1 in **Figure 1**). The example of I/O response R_{DSP} modified by oncogenic mutations is shown in plot B in **Figure 1** (red line). This type of switch-like R_{DSP} corresponds to resistance of the SN to drug D_1 because the output signal of the SN does not change when the input signal changes under the action of inhibitor D_1 (see red lines and points in plots B and C in **Figure 1**). Our method provides a means to search for the protein target for drug D_2 to modify the response, R_{DSP}, in such a way as to reach two complementary effects: first, an increase in inhibition effectiveness of drug D_1 (see, e.g., R_{DSP} modified by drug D_2 in plot B, blue line in **Figure 1**); and second, to ensure robustness of this inhibition effect against different mutations in DSP (see below). One example of such a modified R_{DSP} is shown by the blue line in plot B in **Figure 1**.

To evaluate the robustness of the response R_{DSP}, we supplemented the analysis of the shape of the response curve with the SA of the DSP to both external and internal perturbations: i.e., changes in input signal and alterations of kinetic parameters and expression level of the proteins involved, P_{DSP}. We define the relative sensitivity, S_{DSP}, of the DSP to the input signal as the relative change of output signal $C_{out,DSP}$ in response to a relative change in input signal $C_{in,DSP}$, which can be written through changes in I/O responses, R_{USP} and R_{DPS}:

$$S_{DSP}(C_{in,DSP}, P_{DSP}, D_2, t) = \frac{\Delta C_{out,DSP}}{\Delta C_{in,DSP}} = \frac{\Delta R_{DSP}/R_{DSP}}{\Delta R_{USP}/R_{USP}}. \quad (1)$$

To analyze the sensitivity of the DSP response to different mutations causing changes in protein parameters (phosphorylation rate and expression level), we calculate an absolute value of relative sensitivity to changes in individual parameters p of proteins:

$$S_{DSP,p}(C_{in,DSP}, P_{DSP}, D_2, t) = \left|\frac{\Delta R_{DSP}/R_{DSP}}{\Delta p/p}\right|. \quad (2)$$

We base our local SA on the results of the application of SA to a study of the responses of various cellular signaling pathways to different mutations and drug actions. For the first time, the computational analysis of the change in sensitivity of SN depending on the protein expression level was carried out in the modeling of the apoptosis pathway (33). The SA revealed a sensitivity increase in the response of the apoptotic pathway to overexpression of Bcl-2 protein. It allowed prediction of selectivity of a Bcl-2 inhibitor for tumor cells with Bcl-2 overexpression against healthy cells with a normal level of Bcl-2. SA was first used to analyze the robustness of the MAPK cascade to oncogenic mutations in Ref. (34). The further application of the SA to an *in silico* study of the effects of the most frequent mutations in cancer (EGFR, Ras, BRaf) on the dynamics of MAPK response to receptors activation were analyzed in Refs. (35–39). An application of the SA to a study of SN response to drug action was first studied in Refs. (40, 41).

Sensitivity analysis of the I/O response allows us to: (i) determine the resistance potential of a single drug and drug combination to protein mutations in the DSP; and (ii) determine whether the DSP response to a specific drug combination is robust against various mutations in the DSP and suggest more robust combinations, which enhance the therapeutic effect in the face of mutations.

RESULTS

CHARACTERIZING SIGNALING NETWORK RESPONSE TO DIFFERENT ONCOGENIC MUTATIONS

We illustrate this method by application to the analysis of the response of PI3K/PTEN/AKT signaling to a drug combination targeting the HER2 receptor and a protein in the DSP, PI3K, which were established to be promising drug targets in both mono- and combination therapy in different cancers (1, 15, 42). The aim of the analysis of known drugs and targets is to elucidate the mechanism underlying high efficacy of their combination against different oncogenic mutations in cancer (43, 44).

The analysis is based on the kinetic model of Ras/RAF/MEK/ERK and PI3K/PTEN/AKT signaling developed in Ref. (30). This model describes the response kinetics of the SN to heregulin (HRG)-induced HER3/HER2 receptor heterodimerization and the effect of HER2 inhibitor, pertuzumab (2C4 antibody), on ERK and AKT activation in the human ovarian carcinoma cell line PE04. The scheme of the PI3K/PTEN/AKT SN that corresponds to the SN undertaken here is shown in **Figure 2**. The ordinary differential equations (ODEs) of the model and set of the model parameters are given in the Supplementary Information. In the model, we neglected other ErbB receptor heterodimers because HER2/HER3 heterodimerization activation was found to be the most mitogenic signal and induces cellular growth in the PE04 cell line (45). The model of the SN including 56 ODEs, 58 reactions, and almost 100 parameters (kinetic constants and protein concentrations) was parameterized by experimental data on the phosphorylation kinetics of HER2, ERK, AKT, and PTEN in the absence and presence of pertuzumab (30). Considering incomplete identifiability of model parameters based on the limited set of experimental data used in model calibration, we validated the model on independent experimental data on the different combination effects of PTEN, PI3K, and HER2 inhibition on the ErbB/PI3K/PTEN/AKT pathway activation (30, 32, 40, 41, 46). Model validation evidenced a good account of sensitivity of the SN to single drug action (pertuzumab) and drug combinations targeting different nodes of the SN (pertuzumab and inhibitors of PI3K, PDK1, and PTEN) (32, 40, 41, 46).

According to our method, we decomposed the ErbB/PI3K/PTEN/AKT network into two sub-networks: an upstream signaling system – the receptor system constituting HER2/HER3 receptor signaling (USP); and a down-stream pathway constituting PI3K/PTEN/AKT pathway (DSP). We used the phospho-heterodimer HER23 signal (pHER23) as the output signal of USP and input signal of the DSP (see **Figure 2**). The I/O response, R_{USP}, of USP was defined as the dependence of pHER23 concentration on the concentration of HER2 inhibitor, 2C4: $R_{HER} = p\text{HER23}(\text{HRG}, P_{USP}, 2\text{C4}, t)$. The I/O response of DSP, R_{AKT}, is the dependence of pAKT on

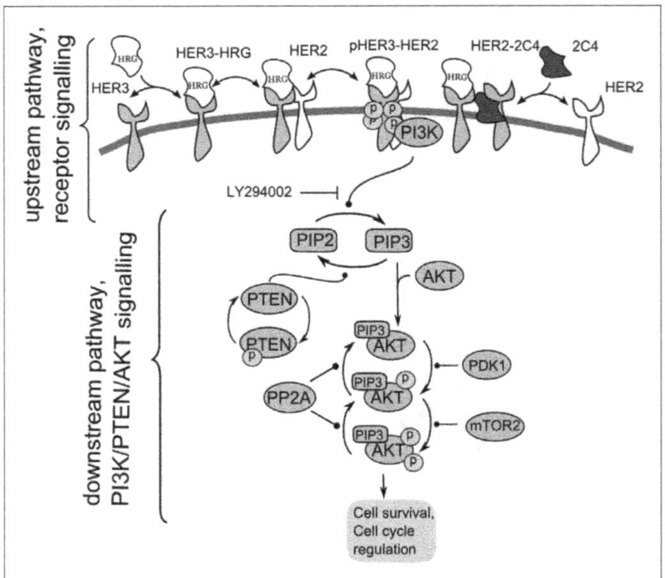

FIGURE 2 | Scheme of PI3K/PTEN/AKT signaling network activated by heterodimerization of HER2/HER3 receptors induced by heregulin (HRG) and inhibited by pertuzumab, 2C4. Decomposition of the signaling network to upstream pathway (receptor signaling pathway) and down-stream pathway (PI3K/PTEN/AKT network) is shown.

concentration of phospho-heterodimer HER3/HER2, pHER23: $R_{AKT} = p\text{AKT}(p\text{HER23}, P_{AKT}, D_2, t)$. The input signal of PI3K/PTEN/AKT is the receptor phosphorylation signal, pHER23, which is changed in the calculation by varying the concentrations of the HER2 inhibitor, 2C4, in the physiological region from zero to saturated value, 1 μM (47). The dose dependence, R_{AKT}, was calculated at time $t = 30$ min after HRG and 2C4 addition that corresponds to saturation of pHER23 and pAKT signals both in modeling and experiment (30, 32).

To show how the I/O response R_{AKT} depends on mutations in the PI3K/PTEN/AKT pathway, we compared the theoretical response, $R_{AKT} = p\text{AKT}(p\text{HER23}, P_{AKT}, D_2, t)$ for the unperturbed DSP (see black line in **Figure 3A**) with the response R_{AKT} modified by oncogenic mutations in the PI3K/PTEN/AKT pathway: PTEN loss (50 and 70%), variation of PI3K activity (**Figure 3B**), and 50% overexpression of AKT (see red lines in **Figures 3A–C**).

Comparing the shapes of unmodified and modified responses curves R_{AKT}, we defined sensitive and resistance modes in the DSP. In sensitive mode, an increase in pHER23 signal causes a gradual increase in pAKT signal from 0 to its saturated value (black line in **Figure 3A**). In resistance mode, the R_{AKT} curve becomes steeper and transforms to a switch-like response curve at the activation mutations (red lines in **Figures 3A,B**). The pAKT output signal is unresponsive to input pHER23 signal controlled by D_1: e.g., pAKT signal does not change when pHER23 changes in the range from 0.04 to 1 at 70% PTEN loss and activated mutation in PI3K (see red lines 3 and 4 in **Figures 3A,B**, respectively). In the case of AKT overexpression, pAKT signal significantly exceeds the basal activation level of pAKT in the range of pHER23 signal from 0.04 to 1 (see red line in **Figure 3C**). This lack of AKT response to input signal at

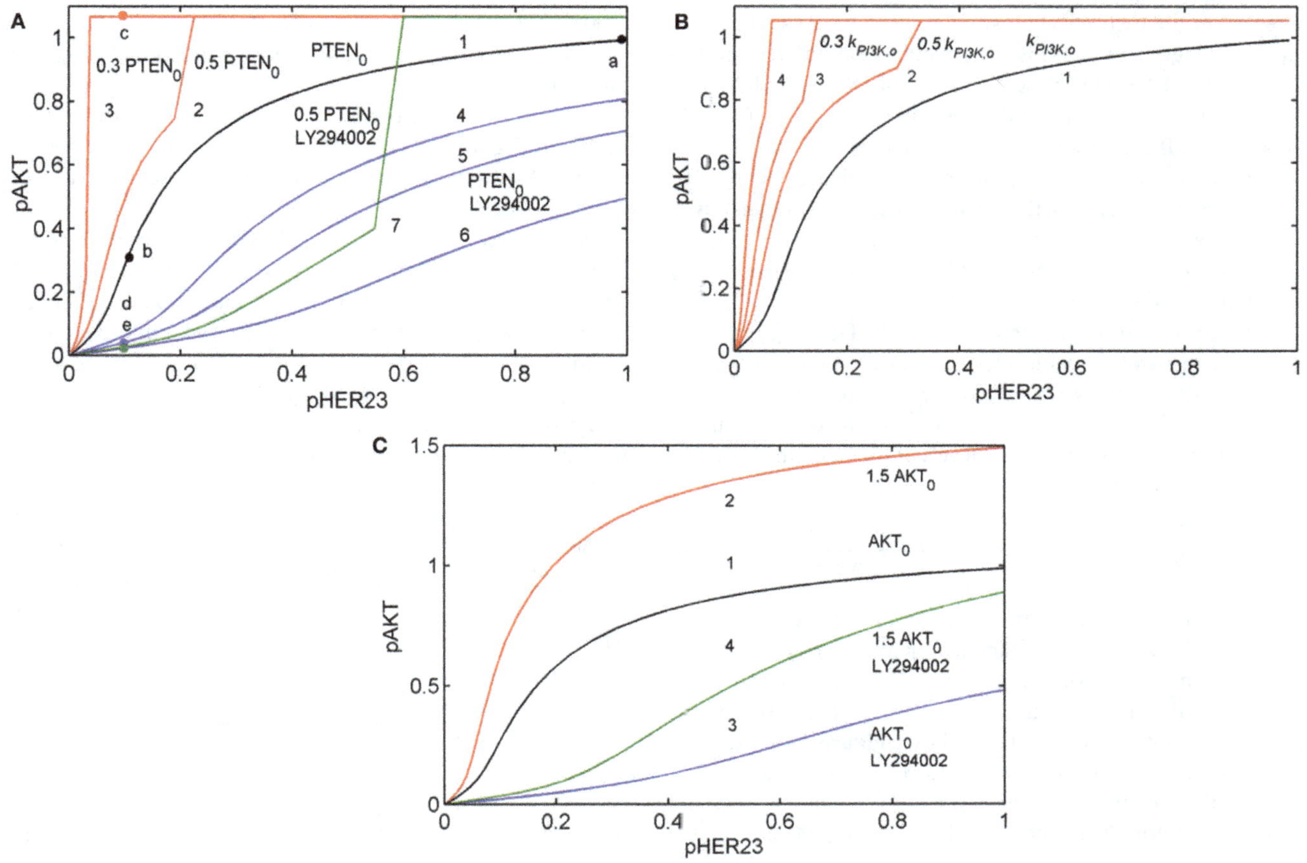

FIGURE 3 | Input/output response of the PI3K/PTEN/AKT pathway R_{AKT} to *p*HER23 input signal and its modification by activation mutations of PTEN, PI3K, and AKT proteins and inhibition of PI3K by LY294002 inhibitor. **(A)** Modification of R_{AKT} by a change of initial concentration of PTEN: response curve at the reference concentration of $PTEN_0 = 40\,\mu M$ (line 1), 50% PTEN loss (line 2), 70% PTEN loss (line 3). Modification of R_{AKT} by PI3K inhibition: 0.3 μM LY294002 (line 4), 0.5 μM LY294002 (line 5), and 1 μM LY294002 (line 6). Modification of R_{AKT} by 50% PTEN loss and inhibition of PI3K by 3 μM LY294002 (line 7). Points a, b, c, d, and e correspond to saturated *p*AKT signal (*p*HER23 = 1), its inhibition by 100 nM 2C4 (*p*HER23 = 0.1), resistance to 2C4 at 50% PTEN loss (*p*HER23 = 0.1), combined inhibition by 2C4 and LY294002 in the absence and presence of 50% PTEN loss (*p*HER23 = 0.1), respectively. **(B)** Modification of R_{AKT} by a change of PI3K activities, k_{PI3K}: reference $k_{PI3K,0}$ (line 1), 0.5 $k_{PI3K,0}$ (line 2), 0.3 $k_{PI3K,0}$ (line 3), and 0.1 $k_{PI3K,0}$ (line 4). **(C)** Modification of R_{AKT} by 50% overexpression of AKT: reference concentration AKT_0 (line 1) and 1.5 AKT_0 (line 2). Modification of R_{AKT} by 1 μM LY294002 at reference concentration of AKT_0 (line 3) and 50% overexpression of AKT (line 4).

pathway modification by mutations corresponds to the resistance of *p*AKT signal to HER2 inhibition by pertuzumab. Amongst the modifications of response R_{AKT} shown in **Figures 3A–C**, the most pronounced transition from a graded to a steep switch-like shape was observed at PTEN loss. In the model, this effect is due to the post-translational regulation of PTEN activity by its phosphorylation (see **Figure 2**) leading to the additional loss of PTEN activity (31, 48).

Analysis of R_{AKT} shows how receptor inhibition of *p*HER23 signal by D_1 transforms the functioning state of the DSP from its normal function at saturated receptor signal (*p*HER23 = 1) to non-saturated inhibited signal at low *p*HER23 <0.3 (points a and b in **Figure 3A**, respectively). When the DSP functions in non-saturation mode, the inhibited input signal differs from that in (normal) saturation mode in both a decrease in *p*AKT signal and an increase in sensitivity of the DSP to both input signal *p*HER23 and mutations causing changes in kinetic parameters and expression level of the proteins involved. To study the second effect, we analyzed the behavior of sensitivities of the DSP S_{DSP} Eq. 1 and $S_{DSP,p}$ Eq. 2 at different internal (mutations) and external (inhibition) modifications of the DSP.

The relative sensitivity of the PI3K/PTEN/AKT pathway is defined as the relative response (change) of the output signal of DSP, ΔpAKT, to a relative change in its input signal, ΔpHER23:

$$S_{AKT}(pHER23, P_{AKT}, D_2, t) = \frac{\Delta pAKT/pAKT}{\Delta pHER23/pHER23}. \quad (3)$$

Sensitivity S_{AKT} (Eq. 3) was calculated at time $t = 30$ min after HRG and 2C4 addition that corresponds to the saturation of both *p*HER23 and *p*AKT signals. Information on S_{AKT} can be obtained based on an analysis of the tangent of the response curve R_{AKT}: the steeper the response behaviors, the more sensitive the system responses to the external signal. Commonly, sensitivity increases at low input signal and this corresponds in our case to receptor signal inhibition by the first drug (see **Figure 3A**). At high receptor signal, S_{AKT} decreases at saturated signal, $p\text{HER23} \cong 1$. We represent the theoretical sensitivity S_{AKT} (Eq. 3) as the upper heatmap in **Figure 4** (columns 1–4) calculated at different perturbations of the DSP: (1) at the activation of DSP ($p\text{HER23} = 1$); (2) at the presence of 100 nM 2C4 ($p\text{HER23} = 0.1$); (3) 50% PTEN loss ($p\text{HER23} = 1$); and (4) 50% PTEN loss with 100 nM 2C4 ($p\text{HER23} = 0.1$). According to the shape change in response curve under these perturbations (see **Figure 3A**), the sensitivity S_{AKT} increases under 2C4 treatment in sensitive mode (compare columns 1 and 2) and decreases at 50% PTEN loss, corresponding to resistance mode (compare columns 1 with 3 and 4).

We also observed that the sensitivity of the DSP $S_{AKT,p}$ to protein parameters and expression level increases in the same region of pHER23 signal (40). Relative sensitivities $S_{AKT,p}$ (Eq. 2) of the PI3K/PTEN/AKT pathway to a specific parameter p (including kinetic parameters and expression levels of the signaling proteins) were determined as follows:

$$S_{AKT,p}(p\text{HER23}, P_{AKT}, D_2, t) = \left| \frac{\Delta p\text{AKT}/p\text{AKT}}{\Delta p/p} \right|. \quad (4)$$

To show how drug and protein mutations change sensitivity, $S_{AKT,p}$ (Eq. 4), we calculated and compared $S_{AKT,p}$ for kinetic parameters and initial concentrations of proteins involved in the PI3K/PTEN/AKT network under a normal functioning of the DPS and the mutations considered above. **Figure 4** (middle and lower heatmaps, columns 1–4) shows $S_{STS,p}$ calculated at: (1) HER23 activation by HRG ($p\text{HER23} = 1$); (2) in the presence of HER2 inhibitor, 2C4, when pHER23 signal is 90% inhibited ($p\text{HER23} = 0.1$); (3) at 50% PTEN loss ($p\text{HER23} = 1$); and (4) at 50% PTEN loss in the presence of 2C4 ($p\text{HER23} = 0.1$) (see columns 1–4 in **Figure 4**, respectively). Analysis of $S_{AKT,p}$ at normal signaling in the PI3K/PTEN/AKT network ($p\text{HER23} = 1$) revealed the most sensitive modules within this network (see column 1 in **Figure 4**). The results obtained in our model are in agreement with the results of local and global sensitivity analyses of other models of the PI3K/PTEN/AKT pathway (41, 49, 50).

We observed a two-to-four orders of magnitude increase in $S_{AKT,p}$ in response to changes in the kinetic parameters and initial concentrations of the proteins at 90% inhibition of pHER23 signal by 100 nM 2C4 (compare columns 1 and 2 in **Figure 4**, lower heatmap). This increase correlates with an increase in sensitivity, S_{AKT}, at an inhibited signal of pHER23 (see upper heatmap in **Figure 4**). The increase in sensitivities S_{AKT} and $S_{STS,p}$ at low pHER23 signals corresponds to the transition of the DSP from functioning in saturated mode ($p\text{HER23} \cong 1$) to functioning at HER2 inhibition (non-saturation). This correlation in the behavior of S_{AKT} and $S_{STS,p}$ can be readily understood: sensitivity, $S_{AKT,p}(p\text{HER23}, P_{AKT})$, to a change in P_{AKT} varies in accordance with sensitivity S_{AKT} ($pHER2$, P_{AKT}) to a change in input signal, pHER23:

$$\frac{\Delta S_{AKT}(p\text{HER23}, P_{AKT})}{\Delta p} = \frac{\Delta S_{AKT,p}(p\text{HER23}, P_{AKT})}{\Delta p\text{HER23}}, \quad (5)$$

where ΔS_{AKT} and $\Delta S_{AKT,p}$ denote sensitivity changes. Equation 5 can be derived from well-known equality of mixed derivatives

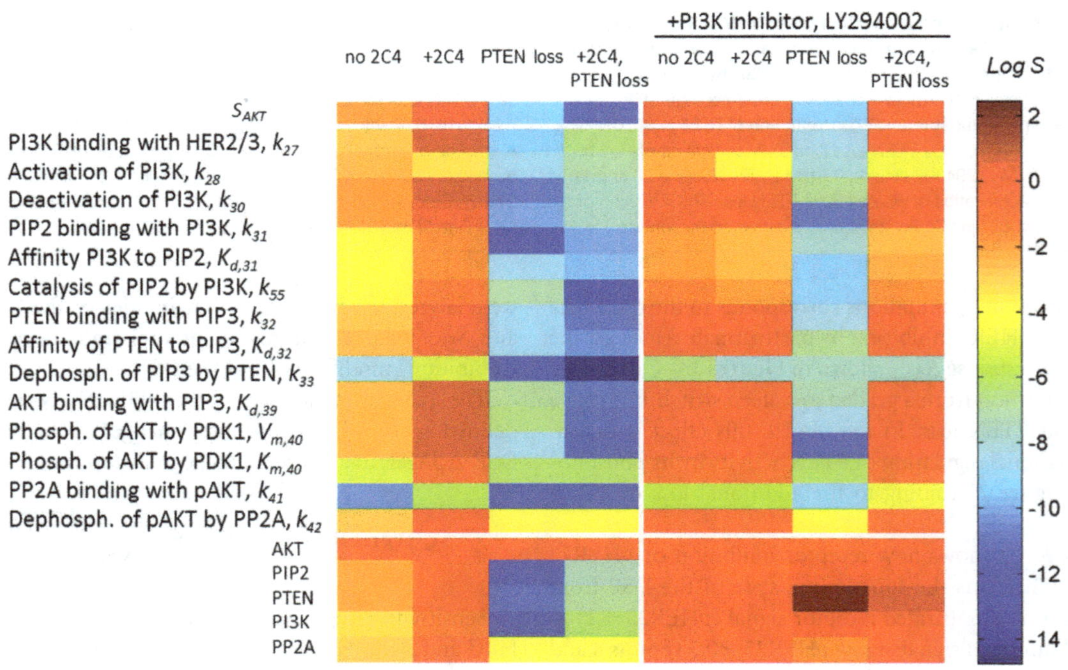

FIGURE 4 | A change in sensitivities S_{AKT} and $S_{AKT,p}$ following different perturbations in the PI3K/PTEN/AKT network. Heatmap of sensitivity S_{AKT} to pHER23 signal (upper heatmap) and sensitivity $S_{AKT,p}$ to kinetic parameters (middle heatmap) and initial protein concentrations (lower heatmap) at normal functioning of the SN (column 1), in the presence of 100 nM 2C4 (column 2), and at 50% PTEN loss in the absence (column 3) and presence of 100 nM 2C4 (column 4). Columns 5–8 show $S_{ATP,p}$ as per columns 1–4 in the presence of 3 μM LY294002. The relative change of the parameters in sensitivity analysis was 0.01% (see Eq. 4) and sensitivity values were taken at time $t = 30$ min after HRG and 2C4 addition.

for continuous function of many variables, turning to infinitesimal increments Δ in Eq. 5 – in our case for I/O response function pAKT(pHER23, P_{AKT}) depending on variables pHER23 and P_{AKT} taken at fixed time t.

We applied the results of this analysis to study the change in SN sensitivity to oncogenic mutations in the PI3K/PTEN/AKT pathway. Given an increase in sensitivity $S_{AKT,p}$ to all the parameters and expression levels of the proteins of the DSP to external perturbation (+2C4) (see column 2 in **Figure 4**, lower heatmap), we calculated sensitivity $S_{AKT,p}$ at internal perturbations: 50% PTEN loss (column 3 in **Figure 4**, lower heatmap), variation of PI3K catalytic rate, and 50% overexpression of AKT (data not shown). For all perturbations, we observed the same dramatic fall in sensitivity, $S_{STS,p}$, over almost all parameters and this drop in $S_{STS,p}$ endows the DSP with insensitivity to any further changes in kinetic parameters of proteins and their abundances. The fall of $S_{STS,p}$ correlates with the shape change of the response curve pAKT(pHER23, P_{AKT}) (red lines in **Figure 3**) and the loss of sensitivity S_{AKT} to input receptor signal pHER23 inhibited by 2C4. In contrast to a sensitive network, this insensitive DSP cannot be sensitized by drug D_1 inhibiting the input signal: the calculation of $S_{AKT,p}$ at 100 nM 2C4 showed no change in sensitivity following 50% PTEN loss (see column 4, lower heatmap in **Figure 4**). Thus, drug D_1 (2C4) acts in very different ways on unmodified and modified DSPs: it sensitizes the unmodified network (sensitive mode), but does not change sensitivity and inhibition level in the mutated DSP. Further D_1, inhibiting the input signal, shifts the DSP to a state with more sensitivity to compensation mutations, which may in turn cause the restoration of the initially activated signal and also lower network sensitivities to other external and internal perturbations.

CUSTOMIZING SIGNALING NETWORK RESPONSE THROUGH DRUG COMBINATION

Our analysis of the sensitivity of the PI3K/PTEN/AKT pathway showed that inhibition of input signal pHER23 sensitizes the response of the DSP to protein perturbations such as a change in protein expression level. Such perturbations can be also exerted by inhibition of protein phosphorylation activity. Here, we use the observed drug-induced sensitizing effect to enhance the action of the second drug D_2 targeting the DSP. Specifically, we considered PI3K inhibition by LY294002 and calculated the response of PI3K/PTEN/AKT pathway, $R_{AKT} = p$AKT(pHER23, P_{AKT}, D_2, t) to pHER23 signal at different concentrations of this inhibitor. Inhibition of PI3K modifies the response curve from hyperbolic to a smooth sigmoid form with high inhibition effect (see blue lines in **Figures 3A,C**). This modified response has a most pronounced inhibition effect of the second drug D_2 in the region of low pHER23 signal (0–0.2) where the sensitizing effect of drug D_1 is maximal (see black lines in **Figures 3A,C** and column 2 in **Figure 4**). This observation confirms that the effective and synergistic effect of the HER2 inhibitor (D_1) in combination with PI3K inhibitor (D_2) is due to a sensitizing effect of D_1 at low pHER23 signals. The key indicator of the synergistic effect of D_1 and D_2 is a change in the curvature of the response curve from convex to concave at low pHER23 signal (0.1–0.3). We assume that modification of the response curve defines the synergistic effect of HER2 and PI3K inhibitor combination (D_1 and D_2). Below, we show that this effect corresponds to a significant decrease of the IC_{50} of pertuzumab in the presence of LY294002 (see Modification of the Dose Response and its Sensitivity by Drug Combination in the Presence of Mutations).

The additional benefit of this transformation of the response curve is an insensitivity of the modified response (smooth sigmoidal shape) to oncogenic mutations in the PI3K/PTEN/AKT pathway at low pHER23 signals. To show the acquired robustness of the network in the face of these mutations, we calculated the response, $R_{AKT} = p$AKT(pHER23, P_{AKT}), at 50% PTEN loss and AKT overexpression in the presence of 3 μM LY294002 (green lines in **Figures 3A,C**). As can be seen, PTEN loss and AKT overexpression did not change significantly the inhibited signal pAKT in the range of inhibited input signal, pHER23 < 0.3 (compare state d and e in **Figure 3A** and points on lines 3 and 4 at pHER23 = 0.1 in **Figure 3C**, respectively). Thus, in contrast to our results on resistance to 2C4 induced by PTEN loss and AKT overexpression, these abnormalities in the context of PI3K inhibition did not result in resistance to HER2 inhibition by 2C4. Note that the advantages of that drug combination vanish at higher signals pHER23 > 0.4 where mutations and protein overexpression significantly increase pAKT signal (see lines 6 and 7 in **Figure 3A** and lines 3 and 4 in **Figure 3C**). Therefore, the response is more robust than an unmodified hyperbolic one with respect to the activation of mutations in the PI3K/PTEN/AKT pathway at inhibited pHER23 signal (pHER23 < 0.3).

This advantage of a modified smooth sigmoidal response curve was confirmed by the calculation of sensitivities, S_{AKT} and $S_{AKT,p}$, carried out in the presence of PI3K inhibitor (columns 5–8 in **Figure 4**). As can be seen, at this modification, 90% inhibition of pHER23 by pertuzumab causes a decrease in sensitivities, S_{AKT} and $S_{AKT,p}$, in contrast to their increase at the pertuzumab treatment alone (compare columns 2 and 6 in **Figure 4**). A decrease in sensitivity S_{AKT} at low pHER23 concentrations (row 1 in column 6 in **Figure 4**) confers robustness of 90% pAKT inhibition in a wider range of inhibited pHER23 signal (up to 0.3; see lines 4–6 in **Figure 3A** and lines 3 and 4 in **Figure 3C**) than in the case of hyperbolic response in the absence of the second drug. A slight decrease in $S_{AKT,p}$ in turn leads to less sensitivity to oncogenic mutations in the PI3K/PTEN/AKT pathway and suppression of drug resistance in contrast to the case of pertuzumab treatment alone. As can been seen from the I/O response curve, the robust inhibition of pAKT at low pHER23 signal is independent of the oncogenic mutations (mainly 50% PTEN loss and AKT overexpression) (compare points d and e in **Figure 3A** and points on lines 3 and 4 in **Figure 3C** at pHER23 = 0.1). Note this insensitivity to mutations at this drug combination vanishes at higher input signals pHER23 > 0.4, where mutations and protein overexpression significantly increase pAKT signal (see, e.g., pAKT values at pHER23 = 0.6 on lines 6 and 7 in **Figure 3A** and lines 3 and 4 in **Figure 3C**). Thus, the combination of HER2 inhibitor with PI3K inhibition endows the DSP with robustness against activation mutations in PI3K/PTEN/AKT pathway only at inhibited pHER23 signal in the range up to pHER23 = 0.3.

Note that in the model, drug D_2 causes an increase in the sensitivity $S_{AKT,p}$ to the protein parameters in comparison with the unperturbed SN that can sensitize the DSP to compensatory mutations (see columns 1 and 5 in **Figure 4**). This discrepancy may be due to the fact that in the calculation we compared the sensitivity at inhibited (pHER23 = 0.1) and saturated (pHER23 = 1) pHER23 signals (points d and a in **Figure 3A**, respectively). Here we assumed that the activation growth factor signal (1 nM HRG) is saturated (point a in **Figure 3A**). However, if we assume ligand concentration to be lower than the saturation level (e.g., 0.6–0.8) (51) and compare the sensitivities at inhibited and this pHER23 signal, we find that drug D_2 does not change the sensitivity in comparison with the unperturbed DSP (data not shown).

MODIFICATION OF THE DOSE RESPONSE AND ITS SENSITIVITY BY DRUG COMBINATION IN THE PRESENCE OF MUTATIONS

To show how the modifications of I/O response of the AKT subsystem, R_{AKT}, effect on the dose dependence of the whole ErbB/PI3K/PTEN/AKT network for drug D_1, we calculated pAKT and $S_{AKT,p}$ dose dependencies for pertuzumab at different perturbations of the PI3K/PTEN/AKT subsystem discussed above (see solid and dashed lines in **Figure 5**, respectively). Specifically, we calculated sensitivity $S_{AKT,k31}$ to the rate constant of the reaction of PI3K binding with PIP2, k_{31} (see **Figure 2** and model description in Supplementary Information). The calculation for other parameters p was shown to effect the same results (as guaranteed by the general behavior of $S_{AKT,p}$ for all p, according to the discussion of Eq. 5). In the case of an unperturbed DSP, sensitivity $S_{AKT,k31}$ increases by approximately 20 times (relative to its level in the absence of pertuzumab) and has a peak at 80% inhibition of pAKT (IC_{80} for pertuzumab) (see black circle and square on the dashed and solid black lines at 100 nM pertuzumab in **Figure 5**, respectively). Key features of the dose dependence $S_{AKT,k31}$ calculated with the unperturbed PI3K/AKT module are the presence of maximum in the range of IC_{80}, a non-zero limit at high drug concentrations, and a limiting value at low drug concentration, which corresponds to the sensitivity of the signaling system in the absence of the drug (see heatmap in **Figure 4**). The detailed analysis of these features is given in Supplementary Information (see Figures S1 and S2 in Supplementary Material).

The calculation of the pAKT dose dependencies for pertuzumab in the presence of PI3K inhibitor showed the shift of the dose dependence curve to lower drug concentrations and a decrease of IC_{50} for pertuzumab from 30 nM to 1 nM at an increase in LY294002 concentration up to 3 μM (see solid blue line in **Figure 5** and Figure S2 in Supplementary Material). In contrast to dose dependence, calculation of relative sensitivity $S_{AKT,k31}$ revealed a complex behavior that only moves to low pertuzumab concentrations at increasing LY294002 concentration: the maximum near IC_{80} disappears and sensitivity behavior becomes almost monotonically decreasing with a slight minimum (see Figure S2A in Supplementary Material). We assume that a shape change of $S_{AKT,k31}$ at the shift of the dose dependence is the manifestation of transformation of the DSP response curve (**Figure 3A**). Sensitivity $S_{AKT,k31}$ at 3 μM LY294002 does not have maximum at IC_{80} and decreases from its initial value at low 2C4 concentration to approximately its limit value at high pertuzumab concentration (see blue circle and square on the dashed and solid blue lines, respectively at 6 nM pertuzumab in **Figure 5**). This dose dependence corresponds to the modified response curve (line 6 in **Figure 3A**). We predict a significant decrease of IC_{50} for pertuzumab in the presence of 3 μM LY294002 due to the synergistic combination of these two drugs and explain this effect by modification of the response of PI3K/PTEN/AKT pathway at low input signals (line 6 in **Figure 3A**).

Calculation of absolute sensitivity, $S_{AKT,k31}$ (Eq. S2.1 in Supplementary Material), showed that it possesses similar features except for a zero limiting value at high drug concentration (see Figure S2B in Supplementary Material). Similarly, at 3 μM LY294002, absolute sensitivity loses its maximum in the range of IC_{80} and

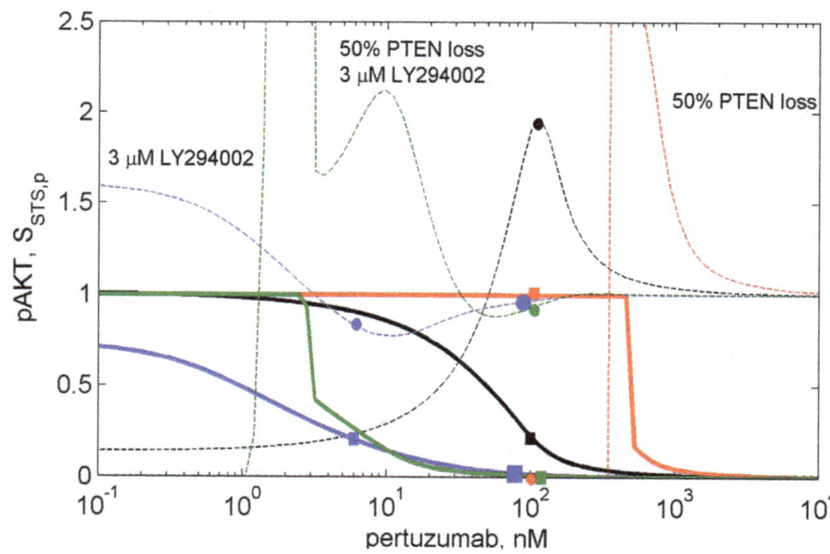

FIGURE 5 | The dose dependences of pAKT inhibition (solid lines) and sensitivity $S_{AKT,k31}$(2C4,p) of the PI3K/PTEN/AKT network to the rate constant of the reaction of PI3K binding with PIP2, k_{31} (dash lines) at different drug combinations. The dose dependencies of inhibition and sensitivity on pertuzumab concentration (black lines), at 50% PTEN loss (red lines), at 3 μM LY294002 (blue lines), at 50% PTEN loss and 3 μM LY294002 (green lines).

monotonically decreases when drug concentration increases. We consider this transformation of sensitivity behavior as the results of modification of the DSP dose response from hyperbolic to smooth sigmoid shape (**Figure 3**). This transformation, and the range of second drug concentration where it occurs, can be used in optimization of drug composition to inhibit signaling, so avoiding a significant increase in sensitivity of the SNs to mutations. Below we consider one such optimization.

Transformation of the response of the DSP module leads to *p*AKT inhibition by two drugs to exceed 80% in the wide range of LY294002 concentrations (0.3–3 μM) at a significantly lower concentration of pertuzumab (6 nM) in comparison with *p*AKT inhibition by pertuzumab alone, 100 nM (see **Figure 5**; Figure S2 in Supplementary Material). This allows optimization of drug concentrations with respect to both inhibition of *p*AKT signal and sensitivity of the SN to mutations. Since these two characteristics are interlinked and change correlatively in the same region of the response curve (**Figure 3A**) and dose dependence (**Figure 5**), the problem of trade-off between them arises. It is possible to disentangle inhibition and sensitivity characteristics from each other by optimal manipulation of two drugs in the concentration range discussed above. One can establish two optimized conditions of drug combination action with high inhibition and low sensitivity. The first optimum condition is to decrease 2C4 concentration to maintain 80% inhibition of *p*AKT ($IC_{80} = 6$ nM) with low sensitivity at 2–3 μM LY294002 (see blue square and circle on solid and dashed blue lines respectively in **Figure 5** and lines 5 and 6 in Figure S2 in Supplementary Material). The second optimum is full inhibition of *p*AKT with 100 nM pertuzumab and a minimal increase (six times) of sensitivity at 3 μM LY294002 (see large blue square and circle on solid and dashed blue lines respectively in **Figure 5**).

To demonstrate the sensitivity to resistance transition in response to HER2 inhibition at PTEN loss, we calculated the dose dependences of *p*AKT and $S_{AKT,p}$ at 50% PTEN loss (see red solid and dashed lines in **Figure 5** and corresponding I/O response of the *p*AKT, line 2 in **Figure 3A**). PTEN loss leads to a 10-fold shift of *p*AKT dependence to a higher pertuzumab concentration, so causing resistance to HER2 inhibition in the range of physiological pertuzumab concentration (100 nM). In this region of drug concentration, both inhibition of *p*AKT and sensitivity $S_{AKT,p}$ are approximately zero (see red square and circle on solid and dashed red lines in **Figure 5**, respectively). Sensitivity to HER2 inhibition is restored through modification of the network by PI3K inhibitor, LY294002. This modification causes approximately full inhibition of *p*AKT (green square on green solid line in **Figure 5**) while sensitivity $S_{AKT,p}$ (green circle on green dashed line in **Figure 5**) is at approximately the same level as for normal PTEN concentration.

Joint analysis of the I/O response of the PI3K/PTEN/AKT pathway and *p*AKT dose dependence for pertuzumab (drug D_1) revealed a trade-off between inhibition and sensitivity, which can be formulated as follows. If the concentration of drug D_1 is high (low *p*HER23 signal), *p*AKT inhibition is strong and sensitivity to protein parameters is low: this is of a benefit with respect to signal inhibition and suppression of compensatory mutations. If the concentration of D_1 is low (high *p*HER23 signal), *p*AKT concentration increases while sensitivity decreases, which gives advantages with respect to mutation suppression but leads to a decrease in inhibition effect of the drug, D_1. If the concentration of drug D_1 is in the region of its IC_{50}, sensitivity increases which affords the use of the second drug more effectively (drug-sensitizing effect), and a disadvantage with respect to increasing sensitivity of the SN to compensation mutations. This analysis showed the inhibition-sensitivity trade-off decision can be optimized by customizing the I/O response of the SN through manipulation of the concentrations of the two drugs. Optimization of drug concentration allows the separation of the regions with high inhibition and high sensitivity, which overlap each other in single drug treatment.

DISCUSSION

We have shown that the sensitivity of the SN to drug action is attended by an increase in sensitivity $S_{DSP,p}$ of the DSP to the kinetic parameters and expression levels of the proteins involved in this pathway. As a result, the DSP is sensitized by drug action and may be more fragile with respect to mutations, which change protein kinetic properties (catalytic or/and dissociation constants) and their expression level (overexpression or suppression of gene expression). In particular, an increasing sensitivity may result in an adverse effect of inhibitor action since a high sensitivity endows the SN with fragility with respect to mutations that can compensate for the intended inhibitor effect by restoring a high output signal as well as initial low sensitivity of the SN to external perturbations. It follows that increasing SN sensitivity can be one of the causes of resistance potential to drug action. We suggest that this effect should be taken into account at drug target validation, and the drug resistance potential linked with this sensitizing effect should be evaluated in drug combination co-development. We present a method to design drug combination strategies that modify the I/O response of the SN to minimize any drug-sensitizing effect, enhance robustness of drug inhibition effect, and improve drug resistance potential by vertically targeting the SN.

The method is based on the modularity approach to analyzing the efficacy of combination therapy developed by Fitzgerald et al. (52). According to this approach, we divide the signaling system into up- and down-stream pathways, which are the targets of the first and second drugs, respectively (see scheme in **Figure 1**). In this work, we focused on the I/O response characteristics of the down-stream pathways, DSP, which is a signal transduction module in the whole signaling pathway. As shown in Ref. (52), the effect of drug combination significantly depends on the I/O response properties of the receptor systems, and mainly receptor expression level, that shifts the IC_{50} concentration of drug, D_1. To exclude the effects determined by the I/O response properties of the receptor system, we considered only the output signal of the USP which is varied from zero to a saturated level. In this modularity approach, the effect of drug D_1 defines only the input signal for the I/O response curve of the DSP (see **Figures 1** and **3A**). We expanded this approach developed by Fitzgerald et al. (52) to investigate the modification of the I/O response of the down-stream pathways as a result of external and internal perturbations such as inhibition of signaling proteins and protein mutations. The analysis of the responsiveness of the whole system to the first drug was shown to depend significantly on the I/O response characteristic of the down-stream signaling module. We suggest that the response curve, R_{DSP}, can be considered as a biomarker (characteristic signature) of a particular cancer signaling pathways (e.g., MAPK, PI3K/AKT, Wnt, and others (53) in specific cancer cell lines. To illustrate this, we have extracted the I/O response R_{DSP} of the PI3K/PTEN/AKT and MAPK pathways for different cancer cell lines using experimental data on the dose dependence of receptor activation (EGFR and PDGFR) and output signal (*p*AKT and *p*ERK) on ligand concentrations (EGF and PDGF) (49, 54, 55). The characteristic I/O response curves obtained for different activating input signals in various cell lines are shown in **Figure 6**. The experimental data on I/O responses were fitted by the Hill function with a Hill constant, *n*, which characterizes that response as switch-like (higher *n*) or more graded (lower *n*). As shown, AKT responses are more varied compared with the more conserved set of ERK responses that are typically switch-like ($n = 2.65–12.8$). *p*AKT responses range from switch-like for HBL and AU565 cells (**Figures 6A,B**) to graded hyperbolic for T47 and PE04 cells (**Figures 6C,E,F**) and smooth sigmoidal for MCF7 cells (**Figure 6D**) responses. We assume that such variety in the responses of the PI3K/PTEN/AKT pathway results from a variation in the internal parameters of the networks caused by mutations and different expression levels of signaling proteins. We suggest that I/O responses can be considered as a biomarker of mutation and protein expression status of specific cancer cells.

The *in silico* analysis of the I/O response of the PI3K/PTEN/AKT pathway confirmed that the SN can possess a smooth hyperbolic response, which corresponds to the sensitivity mode in signal transduction, and this response can be transformed into a switch-like response by changing protein parameters, which corresponds to activating mutations of the proteins involved (PTEN, PI3K, and AKT). This transformation relates to the transition from sensitivity to resistance of the SN to drug inhibiting receptor signals (32). Joint analysis of the I/O response of the PI3K/PTEN/AKT pathway and its sensitivity showed that these two key characteristics of the cellular SN are interconnected and they both significantly depend on the protein parameters and their expression levels. We observed from *in silico* experiments that perturbations of protein parameters corresponding either to 50% decreases in PTEN concentration (PTEN loss), PI3K activation mutation, or AKT overexpression significantly changes in the I/O response of the PI3K/PTEN/AKT pathway and its sensitivity. The transformation of the I/O response from smooth hyperbolic to switch-like at PTEN loss significantly endows the SN with hypersensitivity (56) that is assumed to be typical for the signaling cascade in cells at decreasing phosphatase activity (38). The steep switch response observed at PTEN loss is assumed to be due to a post-translational regulation of PTEN activity by its phosphorylation leading to the additional loss of PTEN activity (31, 48) considered in our model.

We showed that PTEN loss, or *PIK3CA* activation mutation, AKT and PI3K overexpression (40) decreased sensitivity $S_{AKT,p}$ by four to six orders of magnitude for all protein parameters and this corresponds to the transformation of the I/O response from smooth hyperbolic to switch-like. At this mutation, the PI3K/PTEN/AKT pathway acquires insensitivity to further

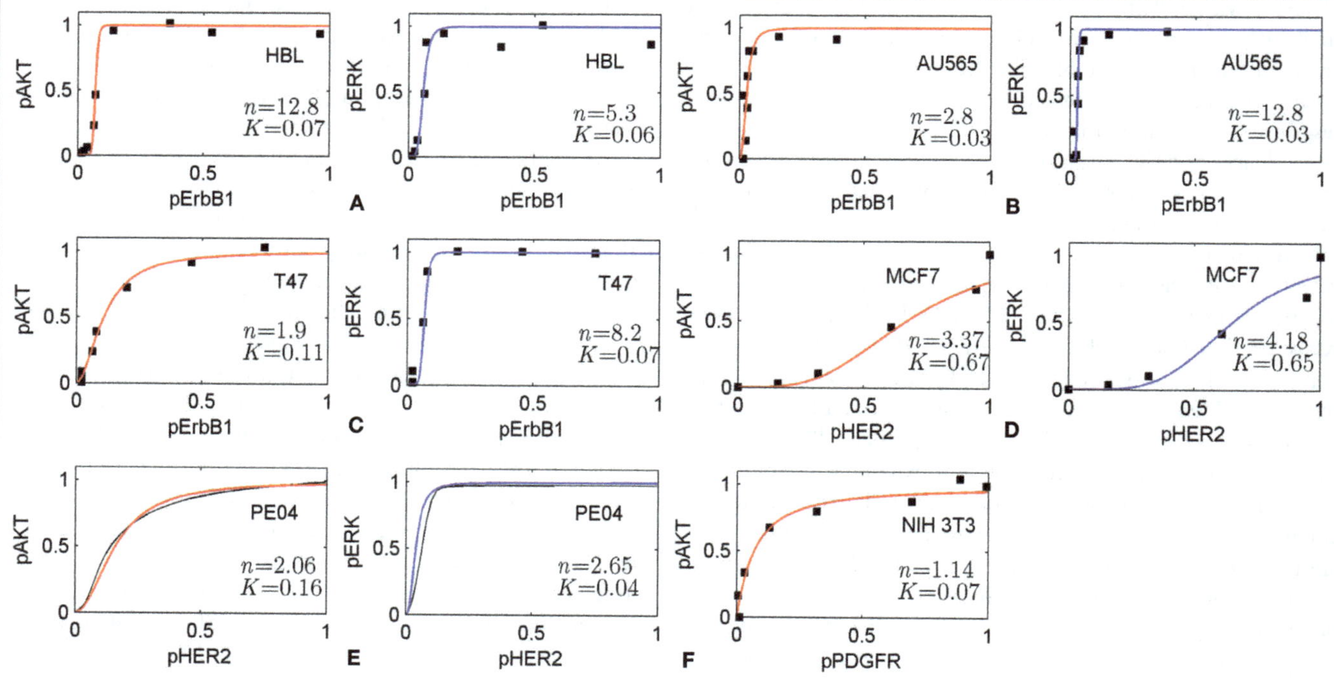

FIGURE 6 | Input/output responses of PI3K/AKT and MAPK pathways to the activation of growth factor receptors in different cells. The dependences of *p*AKT and *p*ERK on the activation level of ErbB1 receptors in HBL100 **(A)**, AU565 **(B)**, T47 **(C)** cells; on the level of HER2 receptors in MCF7 **(D)** and PE04 **(E)** cells; and platelet-derived growth factor receptor (PDGF) in NIH 3T3 fibroblasts **(F)**. Data on I/O response were extracted from experimental dose dependences [**(A–C)** (49), **(D)** (54), and **(F)** (55)] and normalized at maximal values of input/output signals. *p*AKT, *p*ERK dose dependencies for PE04 cells **(E)** are theoretical data (40) (black lines). Experimental data were fitted by Hill function: $y = x^n/(x^n + K^n)$ with Hill constant, *n*, and half-maximum constant, *K*, which are given in Figures. Hill function is depicted by red lines for *p*AKT and blue lines for *p*ERK. Experimental data were kindly allowed to be used by PK Sorger **(A–C)**, M Hatakeyama **(D)**, and JM Haugh **(E)**.

perturbation of the SN: it becomes robust in the face of both external perturbations (inhibition of input signal) and internal aberrations (mutations). PTEN loss leads to resistance to drug action (resistance to HER2 inhibition) and causes robust activation of the AKT output signal (57). Note that the observed decrease in sensitivity of the SN at either PTEN loss or PI3K aberration suggests that PTEN loss and *PIK3CA* mutation are mutually exclusive. Clinical study of oncogenic mutations in the PI3K/PTEN/AKT pathway reported both the data on mutually exclusive of PTEN loss and *PIK3CA* mutation in human breast (58) and gastric (59) carcinomas and frequently concordant in breast cancer (43, 44). As both mutations activate AKT and each decreases sensitivity of the DSP to another mutation, our finding suggests either redundancy in mutations, the need for two alterations in the single module to activate AKT, or that PTEN loss and *PIK3CA* mutation contribute differently to carcinogenesis (60).

Combining analysis of the I/O response with SA, we showed that a hyperbolic response in sensitivity mode is robust at high input (saturated receptor signals) and loses its robustness against activation mutations of the proteins at low *p*HER23 signals. Importantly, the I/O response can be modified through drug combination action, here through customization of the I/O response of the DSP by drug D_2 to reach high robustness of the inhibition response to drug D_1 against oncogenic protein mutations in the pathway, leading to the transformation of a hyperbolic response to a graded sigmoidal response curve (see blue lines in **Figure 3A**). The first benefit of that modification is an effective inhibition of output signal, *p*AKT. The most pronounced inhibition effect of the second drug is at low *p*HER23 region (0–0.2), where the sensitizing effect by the first drug, pertuzumab, is at a maximum. We exploit a synergistic interaction between these two drugs, specifically the sensitizing effect of one drug on the action of another. A second benefit of that modification is a decrease in the sensitivity of this response in the range of low *p*HER23 signal (0–0.2) (see blue lines in **Figure 3A**). We hypothesized that the modified response is more robust against oncogenic mutation than the hyperbolic type of the response. To check this, we carried out robustness screening of this response with respect to the following aberrations in the PI3K/PTEN/AKT pathway: PTEN loss, activation mutation of PI3K, and overexpression of AKT. In all these cases we observed effective inhibition of *p*AKT and so a high degree of robustness in the modified response to common oncogenic mutations in the PI3K/PTEN/AKT pathway (see green lines in **Figures 3A,C**). We showed that a hyperbolic response is more adapted to signal discrimination and signal transaction while a modified graded sigmoidal response close to linear response is more adapted to therapeutic inhibition of signaling pathway activated by oncogenic mutations.

Note, a similar transformation from hyperbole to switch-like response was observed *in silico* and *in vitro* experiments in Raf/MEK/ERK pathway as a result of deletion of negative feedbacks from ppERK to Son of Sevenless protein (SOS) and Raf (26). This finding and other theoretical and experimental studies show that multiple feedback and gene regulation can significantly control drug efficacy (4, 5, 52). An extension of the modularity approach used in our work should be performed to explore the consequences of feedback and gene regulation networks, which control the robustness of SNs in normal and malignant conditions (61, 62). For example, to develop more reliable model of SN response to drug combination, it is necessary to take into account the negative feedback in the PI3K/PTEN/AKT pathway which includes phosphorylation (inactivation) of GSK3β by *p*AKT which phosphorylates (inactivates) PTEN, and therefore increases AKT phosphorylation (31).

As discussed in the Section "Introduction," many experiments and clinical trials confirm the suppression of drug resistance and the robustness response of drug combinations acting on the vertical signaling pathways in different cancers. For example, complementary inhibition of the vertical targets in the PI3K/PTEN/AKT/mTOR pathway restores the inhibition effect of trastuzumab and pertuzumab (15, 17). Moreover, the experimental study of the combination of PI3K inhibition (GDC-0941) with HER2 inhibitors (trastuzumab, pertuzumab) showed that the high efficacy of this combination therapy is a general effect for different breast cancer cell lines despite the fact that different cell lines have different susceptibilities/resistance to each drug separately (42).

Our *in silico* experiments indicate that anti-cancer response robustness to drug action emerges due to a smooth sigmoid response of the SN when modified by drug combination. Experimentally, the robustness of the modified response to a change in expression level of signaling proteins can be measured in RNA interference (RNAi) screening with respect to repression of protein expression. RNAi screening has been applied successfully to a study of resistance mechanisms and development of effective combination therapy by determining drug targets (60, 63), and allows estimation of the robustness of the therapeutic response to the perturbations in expression of the proteins (isomers or catalytic/regulatory protein subunits) surrounding drug targets in a SN (both vertical and horizontal targeted pathways). Robustness screening with respect to overexpression of the proteins surrounding targeted proteins can be measured using isogenic cell clones customized to genomic status involved in screening (64). Most critical experimental validations are assumed to be carried out with heterogeneous tumor samples. Here we suggest that designing into a combination therapy regime, an unchanged landscape of sensitivity across a mutation spectrum, such as that shown in heatmap in **Figure 4** (columns 5, 6, and 8), may slow down the evolution of subpopulations of cancer cells under a selection pressure of drug therapy and suppresses the development of drug-resistant clones (28, 65). Further, effecting this slowing down in resistance evolution may require a longer-term engineered drug combination regime that accounts for a drift in cell signaling behavior over many cellular generations.

The method of investigation of the I/O response of the SN modules developed here can be considered as a supplementary tool for the analysis of the dose dependence for drug D_1 and the mechanism of IC_{50} changes at oncogenic mutations and combination therapy. To show the link between response dynamics properties of the PI3K/PTEN/AKT pathway and the dose response of the whole SN, we calculated the dose dependence of *p*AKT on concentration of pertuzumab (drug D_1): $R_{SN} = C_{out}(C_{in}, D, P_{SN}, t)$, and showed how the modification of the DSP response by mutations and drugs changes IC_{50} for pertuzumab (**Figure 5**). In the calculation, we observed a decrease of IC_{50} for pertuzumab in the presence of PI3K inhibitor, LY294002, suggesting lower concentrations to be effective. These results supplement the analysis of the drug-induced shift in dose dependence and the synergetic effect of two drugs targeting vertical pathways discussed by Fitzgerald et al. (52). Additionally, we showed that drug-induced sensitivity to the second drug modify both response curve and dose dependence for the first drug that significantly enhances synergetic effect of two drugs in combination.

We showed that the sensitivity of the DSP without customization increases significantly in the range of IC_{80} of pertuzumab (see solid and dashed black lines in **Figure 5**). The simplest way to reach the goal of high inhibition and low sensitivity is to increase the drug concentration and go far beyond the range of maximal sensitivity (>1 μM pertuzumab, **Figure 5**). In practice, this is often not a realistic solution for toxicity reasons, although there is evidence that drug concentrations that are twice the IC_{50} can suppress acquired resistance due to mutations following drug therapy (29). A more realistic approach is to customize the network response to inhibition through combination therapy, manipulating the inhibition and sensitivity dose dependencies through the action of the second drug, which modifies the I/O response of the DSP. Additionally, our calculation showed that a significantly lower IC_{50} for pertuzumab in combination with the PI3K inhibitor can be a basis for decreasing a dose of drug D_1 to reduce its toxicity.

We applied the method to two well-known targets and drugs and investigated the mechanism of their effectiveness. We demonstrated that the drug-induced sensitivity of the DSP to changes in protein parameters and their expression levels has the potential to sensitize this pathway to mutations that compensate for drug action, i.e., low output signal at inhibited input signal. Moreover, such mutations can effect a decrease in sensitivity of the DSP to further external and internal perturbations leading to an increase in DSP robustness. It is thus possible that drug action may significantly perturb DSP functioning, stimulating the activation of compensatory response mechanisms in the cell.

We then demonstrated a method of minimizing the drug-sensitizing effect while maintaining the intended effect of drug action by customizing the I/O response of the DSP response. The goal of this customization was to reach a high inhibition of input signal without sensitizing the SN to mutations leading to an increased potential for resistance, specifically PTEN loss and AKT overexpression. Our focus was the modification of the I/O response of the PI3K/PTEN/AKT pathway to inhibition of pHER2 by pertuzumab.

These results suggest that the I/O response of signaling modules can be used as biomarker to select advantaged drug targets for mono- and combination therapy. To illustrate this concept, we considered different strategies of drug selection depending on the response of the PI3K/PTEN/AKT signaling module of the different cells represented in **Figure 6.** We assume that in the case of switch-like response with low threshold of activation (low parameter K) such as represented in **Figure 6A** (HBL cells) and **Figure 6B** (AU565 cells), a rational strategy is to use drug combination in which one drug targets the DSP and modifies the response curve to more graded or sigmoid form while another drug in combination inhibits input and output signals according to that modified response curve. In the case of responses of smooth hyperbolic type like represented in **Figure 6C** (T47), **Figure 6E** (PE04), and **Figure 6F** (NIH 3T3), the drug targeting USP effectively inhibits *p*AKT in the 80–90% range of inhibited receptor signal but sensitizes down-stream module to compensation mutations. To avoid the latter effect, we suggest modifying the response of the down-stream module to a smooth sigmoid curve by a second drug targeting the DSP. The I/O smooth sigmoid response of the type given in **Figure 6D** (MCF7) is assumed to endow the signaling module with high sensitivity to the drug inhibiting its input signal and low sensitivity to compensatory mutations. In this case, inhibition of the USP by one drug is effective with respect to both signal inhibition and sensitivity suppression. The use of the second drug targeting down-stream pathway is redundant from the viewpoint of the response modification and toxicity. These analyses indicate the strategy of drug–diagnostic co-development (2, 66) when drug therapies (mono- or combination) are selected based on the integrative biomarker corresponding to the I/O response of signaling modules. Stratification of patients according to different I/O response curves can help identify patients who are most likely to benefit from selected therapy. Constant monitoring of the transformation of the I/O response curve during treatment can indicate at compensatory gene regulation (12, 45, 67, 68) and acquired mutations as a result of the selected therapy and so can serve as a guide for changing therapeutic regime. The obtained results showed that it is desirable to introduce an additional characteristic of drugs to support this strategy – drug-induced sensitivity of the SN or resistance potential of drugs, which significantly depends on the I/O response of targeted SN.

The joint analysis, the I/O response of the PI3K/PTEN/AKT pathway, and *p*AKT dose response for pertuzumab revealed the challenge of the trade-off between high sensitivity to drug action and oncogenic mutations. The proposed method of modification of the I/O response of the PI3K/PTEN/AKT pathway and manipulating separately by the inhibition and sensitivity dose dependencies through action of a second drug resolved this problem partially. Despite PI3K inhibition causing the loss of relative sensitivity at different perturbations (pHER2 inhibition and the different mutations in PI3K/PTEN/AKT pathway), it increased the overall level of sensitivity of the DSP to protein parameters that is assumed to sensitize the SN to the compensation mutations (compare columns 1 and 5 in **Figure 4**). To further optimize this trade-off at the combination design stage, we propose that other means of customizing the I/O response to improve drug resistance potential are needed, e.g., by using the methods and results of synthetic biology in signaling pathway engineering to customize their I/O responses (69–71). For example, using some modulators it is possible to alter/reshape dose dependence from a graded to a sharply sensitive, switch-like response and a time dependence from sustained to pulse or delayed responses in MAPK pathway signaling (71). It has been shown that modification of cellular response obtained by genetic engineering can also be reached through drug action. For example, cellular responses were engineered by dynamic rewiring of SN topology (22, 72) and controlling negative feedback circuits in SN by drug combination (26). Ultimately the application of this arsenal of engineering methods in network and synthetic biology, underpinned by integrative systems biology, can be a powerful tool for adaptation of signaling response to effective combination therapy and rational drug combinations co-development.

ACKNOWLEDGMENTS

This work was supported by grants from Breakthrough Breast Cancer and Scottish Funding Council (SRDG), and personal support to Alexey Goltsov from Scottish Informatics and Computer Science Alliance (SICSA) and to James Bown from The Northwood Trust. We also acknowledge the Reviewers for detailed analysis of the method proposed and valuable comments.

REFERENCES

1. Yap TA, Omlin A, de Bono JS. Development of therapeutic combinations targeting major cancer signaling pathways. *J Clin Oncol* (2013) **31**:1592–605. doi:10.1200/JCO.2011.37.6418
2. Jørgensen JT. Companion diagnostics in oncology – current status and future aspects. *Oncology* (2013) **85**:59–68. doi:10.1159/000353454
3. US Food and Drug Administration. *New Guidance for Industry: Codevelopment of Two or More Unmarketed Investigational Drugs for Use in Combination.* Available from: http://www.fda.gov/ForConsumers/ByAudience/ForPatientAdvocates/ucm237264.htm
4. Chandarlapaty S. Negative feedback and adaptive resistance to the targeted therapy of cancer. *Cancer Discov* (2012) **2**:311–9. doi:10.1158/2159-8290.CD-12-0018
5. Carracedo A, Pandolfi PP. The PTEN-PI3K pathway: of feedbacks and cross-talks. *Oncogene* (2008) **27**:5527–41. doi:10.1038/onc.2008.247
6. Azmi AS, Wang Z, Philip PA, Mohammad RM, Sarkar FH. Proof of concept: network and systems biology approaches aid in the discovery of potent anticancer drug combinations. *Mol Cancer Ther* (2010) **9**:3137–44. doi:10.1158/1535-7163.MCT-10-0642
7. Boran AD, Iyengar R. Systems approaches to polypharmacology and drug discovery. *Curr Opin Drug Discov Devel* (2010) **13**:297–309.
8. Nelander S, Wang W, Nilsson B, She Q-B, Pratilas C, Rosen N, et al. Models from experiments: combinatorial drug perturbations of cancer cells. *Mol Syst Biol* (2008) **4**:216. doi:10.1038/msb.2008.53
9. Tang J, Karhinen L, Xu T, Szwajda A, Yadav B, Wennerberg K, et al. Target inhibition networks: predicting selective combinations of druggable targets to block cancer survival pathways. Roth FP, editor. *PLoS Comput Biol* (2013) **9**:e1003226. doi:10.1371/journal.pcbi.1003226
10. Baselga J, Cortés J, Kim S-B, Im S-A, Hegg R, Im Y-H, et al. Pertuzumab plus trastuzumab plus docetaxel for metastatic breast cancer. *N Engl J Med* (2012) **366**:109–19. doi:10.1056/NEJMoa1113216
11. Faratian D, Zweemer AJM, Nagumo Y, Sims AH, Muir M, Dodds M, et al. Trastuzumab and pertuzumab produce changes in morphology and estrogen receptor signaling in ovarian cancer xenografts revealing new treatment strategies. *Clin Cancer Res* (2011) **17**:4451–61. doi:10.1158/1078-0432.CCR-10-2461
12. Sims AH, Zweemer AJM, Nagumo Y, Faratian D, Muir M, Dodds M, et al. Defining the molecular response to trastuzumab, pertuzumab and combination therapy in ovarian cancer. *Br J Cancer* (2012) **106**:1779–89. doi:10.1038/bjc.2012.176
13. Hoeflich KP, Merchant M, Orr C, Chan J, Den Otter D, Berry L, et al. Intermittent administration of MEK inhibitor GDC-0973 plus PI3K inhibitor GDC-0941 triggers robust apoptosis and tumor growth inhibition. *Cancer Res* (2012) **72**:210–9. doi:10.1158/0008-5472.CAN-11-1515
14. Haagensen EJ, Kyle S, Beale GS, Maxwell RJ, Newell DR. The synergistic interaction of MEK and PI3K inhibitors is modulated by mTOR inhibition. *Br J Cancer* (2012) **106**:1386–94. doi:10.1038/bjc.2012.70
15. Sharial M, Crown J, Hennessy BT. Overcoming resistance and restoring sensitivity to HER2-targeted therapies in breast cancer. *Ann Oncol* (2012) **23**:3007–16. doi:10.1093/annonc/mds200
16. Zheng J, Hudder A, Zukowski K, Novak RF. Rapamycin sensitizes Akt inhibition in malignant human breast epithelial cells. *Cancer Lett* (2010) **296**:74–87. doi:10.1016/j.canlet.2010.03.018
17. Morrow PK, Wulf GM, Ensor J, Booser DJ, Moore JA, Flores PR, et al. Phase I/II study of trastuzumab in combination with everolimus (RAD001) in patients with HER2-overexpressing metastatic breast cancer who progressed on trastuzumab-based therapy. *J Clin Oncol* (2011) **29**:3126–32. doi:10.1200/JCO.2010.32.2321
18. Gillies RJ, Verduzco D, Gatenby RA. Evolutionary dynamics of carcinogenesis and why targeted therapy does not work. *Nat Rev Cancer* (2012) **12**:487–93. doi:10.1038/nrc3298
19. Masui K, Gini B, Wykosky J, Zanca C, Mischel PS, Furnari FB, et al. A tale of two approaches: complementary mechanisms of cytotoxic and targeted therapy resistance may inform next-generation cancer treatments. *Carcinogenesis* (2013) **34**:725–38. doi:10.1093/carcin/bgt086
20. Cesca M, Bizzaro F, Zucchetti M, Giavazzi R. Tumor delivery of chemotherapy combined with inhibitors of angiogenesis and vascular targeting agents. *Front Oncol* (2013) **3**:259. doi:10.3389/fonc.2013.00259
21. von Minckwitz G, du Bois A, Schmidt M, Maass N, Cufer T, de Jongh FE, et al. Trastuzumab beyond progression in human epidermal growth factor receptor 2-positive advanced breast cancer: a German breast group 26/breast international group 03-05 study. *J Clin Oncol* (2009) **27**:1999–2006. doi:10.1200/JCO.2008.19.6618
22. Lee MJ, Ye AS, Gardino AK, Heijink AM, Sorger PK, MacBeath G, et al. Sequential application of anticancer drugs enhances cell death by rewiring apoptotic signaling networks. *Cell* (2012) **149**:780–94. doi:10.1016/j.cell.2012.03.031
23. Wallin JJ, Edgar KA, Guan J, Berry M, Prior WW, Lee L, et al. GDC-0980 is a novel class I PI3K/mTOR kinase inhibitor with robust activity in cancer models driven by the PI3K pathway. *Mol Cancer Ther* (2011) **10**:2426–36. doi:10.1158/1535-7163.MCT-11-0446
24. Nahta R, O'Regan RM. Evolving strategies for overcoming resistance to HER2-directed therapy: targeting the PI3K/Akt/mTOR pathway. *Clin Breast Cancer* (2010) **10**(Suppl 3):S72–8. doi:10.3816/CBC.2010.s.015
25. Junttila TT, Akita RW, Parsons K, Fields C, Lewis Phillips GD, Friedman LS, et al. Ligand-independent HER2/HER3/PI3K complex is disrupted by trastuzumab and is effectively inhibited by the PI3K inhibitor GDC-0941. *Cancer Cell* (2009) **15**:429–40. doi:10.1016/j.ccr.2009.03.020
26. Sturm OE, Orton R, Grindlay J, Birtwistle M, Vyshemirsky V, Gilbert D, et al. The mammalian MAPK/ERK pathway exhibits properties of a negative feedback amplifier. *Sci Signal* (2010) **3**:ra90. doi:10.1126/scisignal.2001212
27. Flaherty KT, Infante JR, Daud A, Gonzalez R, Kefford RF, Sosman J, et al. Combined BRAF and MEK inhibition in melanoma with BRAF V600 mutations. *N Engl J Med* (2012) **367**:1694–703. doi:10.1056/NEJMoa1210093
28. Gerlinger M, Rowan AJ, Horswell S, Larkin J, Endesfelder D, Gronroos E, et al. Intratumor heterogeneity and branched evolution revealed by multiregion sequencing. *N Engl J Med* (2012) **366**:883–92. doi:10.1056/NEJMoa1113205
29. Richards J, Lim AC, Hay CW, Taylor AE, Wingate A, Nowakowska K, et al. Interactions of abiraterone, eplerenone, and prednisolone with wild-type and mutant androgen receptor: a rationale for increasing abiraterone exposure or combining with MDV3100. *Cancer Res* (2012) **72**:2176–82. doi:10.1158/0008-5472.CAN-11-3980
30. Faratian D, Goltsov A, Lebedeva G, Sorokin A, Moodie S, Mullen P, et al. Systems biology reveals new strategies for personalizing cancer medicine and confirms the role of PTEN in resistance to trastuzumab. *Cancer Res* (2009) **69**:6713–20. doi:10.1158/0008-5472.CAN-09-0777
31. Goltsov A, Deeni Y, Khalil H, Idowu M, Kyriakidis S, Goltsov G, et al. Role of post-translational regulation of PTEN activity in cancer cell addiction to heterozygous PTEN mutations. In: Xu K, editor. *PTEN Structure, Mechanism of Action, Role Cell Signalling and Regulation.* Hauppauge, NY: Nova Science Publishers (2013). p. 173–210.
32. Goltsov A, Faratian D, Langdon SP, Bown J, Goryanin I, Harrison DJ. Compensatory effects in the PI3K/PTEN/AKT signaling network following receptor tyrosine kinase inhibition. *Cell Signal* (2011) **23**:407–16. doi:10.1016/j.cellsig.2010.10.011
33. Hua F, Cornejo MG, Cardone MH, Stokes CL, Lauffenburger DA. Effects of Bcl-2 levels on Fas signaling-induced caspase-3 activation: molecular genetic tests of computational model predictions. *J Immunol* (2005) **175**:985–95.
34. Wolf J, Dronov S, Tobin F, Goryanin I. The impact of the regulatory design on the response of epidermal growth factor receptor-mediated signal transduction towards oncogenic mutations. *FEBS J* (2007) **274**:5505–17. doi:10.1111/j.1742-4658.2007.06066.x
35. Orton RJ, Adriaens ME, Gormand A, Sturm OE, Kolch W, Gilbert DR. Computational modelling of cancerous mutations in the EGFR/ERK signalling pathway. *BMC Syst Biol* (2009) **3**:100. doi:10.1186/1752-0509-3-100
36. Yoon J, Deisboeck TS. Investigating differential dynamics of the MAPK signaling cascade using a multi-parametric global sensitivity analysis. *PLoS One* (2009) **4**:e4560. doi:10.1371/journal.pone.0004560

37. Dana S, Nakakuki T, Hatakeyama M, Kimura S, Raha S. Computation of restoration of ligand response in the random kinetics of a prostate cancer cell signaling pathway. *Comput Methods Programs Biomed* (2011) **101**:1–22. doi:10.1016/j.cmpb.2010.04.001
38. Nguyen LK, Matallanas D, Croucher DR, von Kriegsheim A, Kholodenko BN. Signalling by protein phosphatases and drug development: a systems-centred view. *FEBS J* (2013) **280**:751–65. doi:10.1111/j.1742-4658.2012.08522.x
39. Zou X, Liu M, Pan Z. Robustness analysis of EGFR signaling network with a multi-objective evolutionary algorithm. *Biosystems* (2008) **91**:245–61. doi:10.1016/j.biosystems.2007.10.001
40. Goltsov A, Faratian D, Langdon SP, Mullen P, Harrison DJ, Bown J. Features of the reversible sensitivity-resistance transition in PI3K/PTEN/AKT signalling network after HER2 inhibition. *Cell Signal* (2012) **24**:493–504. doi:10.1016/j.cellsig.2011.09.030
41. Lebedeva G, Sorokin A, Faratian D, Mullen P, Goltsov A, Langdon SP, et al. Model-based global sensitivity analysis as applied to identification of anti-cancer drug targets and biomarkers of drug resistance in the ErbB2/3 network. *Eur J Pharm Sci* (2012) **46**:244–58. doi:10.1016/j.ejps.2011.10.026
42. Yao E, Zhou W, Lee-Hoeflich ST, Truong T, Haverty PM, Eastham-Anderson J, et al. Suppression of HER2/HER3-mediated growth of breast cancer cells with combinations of GDC-0941 PI3K inhibitor, trastuzumab, and pertuzumab. *Clin Cancer Res* (2009) **15**:4147–56. doi:10.1158/1078-0432.CCR-08-2814
43. Stemke-Hale K, Gonzalez-Angulo AM, Lluch A, Neve RM, Kuo W-L, Davies M, et al. An integrative genomic and proteomic analysis of PIK3CA, PTEN, and AKT mutations in breast cancer. *Cancer Res* (2008) **68**:6084–91. doi:10.1158/0008-5472.CAN-07-6854
44. Cheung LWT, Hennessy BT, Li J, Yu S, Myers AP, Djordjevic B, et al. High frequency of PIK3R1 and PIK3R2 mutations in endometrial cancer elucidates a novel mechanism for regulation of PTEN protein stability. *Cancer Discov* (2011) **1**:170–85. doi:10.1158/2159-8290.CD-11-0039
45. Nagumo Y, Faratian D, Mullen P, Harrison DJ, Hasmann M, Langdon SP. Modulation of HER3 is a marker of dynamic cell signaling in ovarian cancer: implications for pertuzumab sensitivity. *Mol Cancer Res* (2009) **7**:1563–71. doi:10.1158/1541-7786.MCR-09-0101
46. Hu H, Goltsov A, Bown JL, Sims AH, Langdon SP, Harrison DJ, et al. Feedforward and feedback regulation of the MAPK and PI3K oscillatory circuit in breast cancer. *Cell Signal* (2013) **25**:26–32. doi:10.1016/j.cellsig.2012.09.014
47. Franklin MC, Carey KD, Vajdos FF, Leahy DJ, de Vos AM, Sliwkowski MX. Insights into ErbB signaling from the structure of the ErbB2-pertuzumab complex. *Cancer Cell* (2004) **5**:317–28. doi:10.1016/S1535-6108(04)00083-2
48. Leslie NR, Foti M. Non-genomic loss of PTEN function in cancer: not in my genes. *Trends Pharmacol Sci* (2011) **32**:131–40. doi:10.1016/j.tips.2010.12.005
49. Chen WW, Schoeberl B, Jasper PJ, Niepel M, Nielsen UB, Lauffenburger DA, et al. Input-output behavior of ErbB signaling pathways as revealed by a mass action model trained against dynamic data. *Mol Syst Biol* (2009) **5**:239. doi:10.1038/msb.2008.74
50. Schoeberl B, Pace EA, Fitzgerald JB, Harms BD, Xu L, Nie L, et al. Therapeutically targeting ErbB3: a key node in ligand-induced activation of the ErbB receptor-PI3K axis. *Sci Signal* (2009) **2**:ra31. doi:10.1126/scisignal.2000352
51. Stoica GE, Franke TF, Wellstein A, Morgan E, Czubayko F, List H-J, et al. Heregulin-beta1 regulates the estrogen receptor-alpha gene expression and activity via the ErbB2/PI 3-K/Akt pathway. *Oncogene* (2003) **22**:2073–87. doi:10.1038/sj.onc.1206769
52. Fitzgerald JB, Schoeberl B, Nielsen UB, Sorger PK. Systems biology and combination therapy in the quest for clinical efficacy. *Nat Chem Biol* (2006) **2**:458–66. doi:10.1038/nchembio817
53. Kessler T, Hache H, Wierling C. Integrative analysis of cancer-related signaling pathways. *Front Physiol* (2013) **4**:124. doi:10.3389/fphys.2013.00124
54. Nagashima T, Shimodaira H, Ide K, Nakakuki T, Tani Y, Takahashi K, et al. Quantitative transcriptional control of ErbB receptor signaling undergoes graded to biphasic response for cell differentiation. *J Biol Chem* (2007) **282**:4045–56. doi:10.1074/jbc.M608653200
55. Park CS, Schneider IC, Haugh JM. Kinetic analysis of platelet-derived growth factor receptor/phosphoinositide 3-kinase/Akt signaling in fibroblasts. *J Biol Chem* (2003) **278**:37064–72. doi:10.1074/jbc.M304968200
56. Goldbeter A, Koshland DE. An amplified sensitivity arising from covalent modification in biological systems. *Proc Natl Acad Sci U S A* (1981) **78**:6840–4. doi:10.1073/pnas.78.11.6840
57. Marty B, Maire V, Gravier E, Rigaill G, Vincent-Salomon A, Kappler M, et al. Frequent PTEN genomic alterations and activated phosphatidylinositol 3-kinase pathway in basal-like breast cancer cells. *Breast Cancer Res* (2008) **10**:R101. doi:10.1186/bcr2204
58. Saal LH, Holm K, Maurer M, Memeo L, Su T, Wang X, et al. PIK3CA mutations correlate with hormone receptors, node metastasis, and ERBB2, and are mutually exclusive with PTEN loss in human breast carcinoma. *Cancer Res* (2005) **65**:2554–9. doi:10.1158/0008-5472-CAN-04-3913
59. Byun D-S, Cho K, Ryu B-K, Lee M-G, Park J-I, Chae K-S, et al. Frequent monoallelic deletion of PTEN and its reciprocal association with PIK3CA amplification in gastric carcinoma. *Int J Cancer* (2003) **104**:318–27. doi:10.1002/ijc.10962
60. Berns K, Bernards R. Understanding resistance to targeted cancer drugs through loss of function genetic screens. *Drug Resist Updat* (2012) **15**:268–75. doi:10.1016/j.drup.2012.10.002
61. Kitano H. Cancer as a robust system: implications for anticancer therapy. *Nat Rev Cancer* (2004) **4**:227–35. doi:10.1038/nrc1300
62. Stelling J, Sauer U, Szallasi Z, Doyle FJ, Doyle J. Robustness of cellular functions. *Cell* (2004) **118**:675–85. doi:10.1016/j.cell.2004.09.008
63. Lee AJX, Swanton C. Tumour heterogeneity and drug resistance: personalising cancer medicine through functional genomics. *Biochem Pharmacol* (2012) **83**:1013–20. doi:10.1016/j.bcp.2011.12.008
64. Hengel SM, Murray E, Langdon S, Hayward L, O'Donoghue J, Panchaud A, et al. Data-independent proteomic screen identifies novel tamoxifen agonist that mediates drug resistance. *J Proteome Res* (2011) **10**:4567–78. doi:10.1021/pr2004117
65. Cooke SL, Ng CKY, Melnyk N, Garcia MJ, Hardcastle T, Temple J, et al. Genomic analysis of genetic heterogeneity and evolution in high-grade serous ovarian carcinoma. *Oncogene* (2010) **29**:4905–13. doi:10.1038/onc.2010.245
66. Simon R. Drug-diagnostics co-development in oncology. *Front Oncol* (2013) **3**:315. doi:10.3389/fonc.2013.00315
67. Chakrabarty A, Sánchez V, Kuba MG, Rinehart C, Arteaga CL. Feedback upregulation of HER3 (ErbB3) expression and activity attenuates antitumor effect of PI3K inhibitors. *Proc Natl Acad Sci U S A* (2012) **109**:2718–23. doi:10.1073/pnas.1018001108
68. Narayan M, Wilken JA, Harris LN, Baron AT, Kimbler KD, Maihle NJ. Trastuzumab-induced HER reprogramming in "resistant" breast carcinoma cells. *Cancer Res* (2009) **69**:2191–4. doi:10.1158/0008-5472.CAN-08-1056
69. Pryciak PM. Systems biology. Customized signaling circuits. *Science* (2008) **319**:1489–90. doi:10.1126/science.1156414
70. Brandman O, Meyer T. Feedback loops shape cellular signals in space and time. *Science* (2008) **322**:390–5. doi:10.1126/science.1160617
71. Bashor CJ, Helman NC, Yan S, Lim WA. Using engineered scaffold interactions to reshape MAP kinase pathway signaling dynamics. *Science* (2008) **319**:1539–43. doi:10.1126/science.1151153
72. Behar M, Barken D, Werner SL, Hoffmann A. The dynamics of signaling as a pharmacological target. *Cell* (2013) **155**:448–61. doi:10.1016/j.cell.2013.09.018

13

In situ protein detection for companion diagnostics

Gabriela Gremel, Karin Grannas, Lesley Ann Sutton, Fredrik Pontén and Agata Zieba*

Science for Life Laboratory, Department of Immunology, Genetics and Pathology, Uppsala University, Uppsala, Sweden

Edited by:
Jan Trøst Jørgensen, Dx-Rx Institute, Denmark

Reviewed by:
Todd Skaar, Indiana University Medical Center, USA
Tove Kirkegaard, Danish Cancer Society, Denmark

***Correspondence:**
Agata Zieba, Department of Immunology, Genetics and Pathology, Uppsala University, Dag Hammarskjölds väg 20, Rudbecklaboratoriet, 751 85 Uppsala, Sweden
e-mail: agata.zieba@igp.uu.se; agata.e.zieba@gmail.com

The emergence of targeted therapies for cancer has created a need for the development of companion diagnostic tests. Assays developed in recent years are aimed at determining both the effectiveness and safety of specific drugs for a defined group of patients, thus, enabling the more efficient design of clinical trials and also supporting physicians when making treatment-related decisions. Immunohistochemistry (IHC) is a widely accepted method for protein expression analyses in human tissues. Immunohistochemical assays, used to localize and quantitate relative protein expression levels within a morphological context, are frequently used as companion diagnostics during clinical trials and also following drug approval. Herein, we describe established immunochemistry-based methods and their application in routine diagnostics. We also explore the possibility of using IHC to detect specific protein mutations in addition to DNA-based tests. Finally, we review alternative protein binders and proximity ligation assays and discuss their potential to facilitate the development of novel, targeted therapies against cancer.

Keywords: companion diagnostics, immunohistochemistry, Her2, alternative binders, proximity ligation assays

INTRODUCTION

Throughout recent decades, our understanding of the molecular basis of cancer development has dramatically improved. This is reflected in the growing number of targeted cancer therapies and significantly affects today's standard of care in oncology. Nevertheless, a prerequisite for an effective, targeted cancer treatment concerns the selection of patient, which creates a growing demand for reliable companion diagnostic devices. The rationale behind such developments is to ensure that treatment is not withheld from patients whom it may benefit while at the same time protecting them from overtreatment, the risk of unnecessary side effects and, most importantly, a delay in receiving treatment with a more suitable agent.

Companion diagnostics also play an important role during the pre-clinical stages of drug testing. A potent effect observed in a small patient population may be missed by the absence of a reliable companion diagnostic test. Conversely, a novel subset of patients may be found to benefit from treatment or no difference in efficiency may be detected, regardless of biomarker positivity. These issues pose a challenge to the parallel development of drug and companion diagnostic tests and consequently, the latter should be fully validated before the initiation of clinical trials and the trial design adjusted accordingly (1). Despite much advances, the corresponding regulatory framework is still incomplete and while the US Food and Drug Administration (FDA) dictates a stringent premarket approval procedure for all companion diagnostic devices, similar legislation is still under review in Europe (1). Currently, only 19 companion diagnostic devices have been approved by the FDA, 10 of which are intended for the detection of the human epidermal growth factor receptor 2 (ERBB2, also referred to as HER2)[1].

Most companion diagnostic tests used in a clinical setting are based on immunohistochemistry (IHC), real-time reverse transcription PCR (qRT-PCR), or *in situ* hybridization (ISH). With regard to ISH, assay systems based on either fluorescent (FISH) or colorimetric (CISH) signal detection have been established and each testing modality is associated with a number of advantages and disadvantages (**Table 1**).

While the scope of companion diagnostics is broad, with this review we will focus on techniques designed to detect proteins in formalin-fixed, paraffin-embedded (FFPE) tissue. We will discuss currently applied companion diagnostic tests which use IHC and also novel developments regarding mutation-specific antibodies, *in situ* proximity ligation assays (PLA), and alternative protein binders.

APPLICATION OF IMMUNOHISTOCHEMISTRY IN CLINICALLY USED COMPANION DIAGNOSTICS

ESTROGEN RECEPTOR

The introduction of tamoxifen, a selective estrogen receptor (ER) modulator, over 30 years ago has revolutionized the clinical management of breast cancer. However, since significant treatment benefits were only observed in ER-positive patients (2, 3), companion diagnostic testing became imperative. Originally, various ligand binding assays (LBAs) were used to quantify the expression of ER, however, they required homogenization of fresh frozen tumor material and were thus laborious in their execution. With the development of monoclonal antibodies targeting the ER and antigen retrieval methods for the use of FFPE tissue, LBAs were soon replaced and IHC became the standard diagnostic tool. Several grading systems were subsequently introduced to describe IHC-based ER expression levels, including (1) Allred score (range: 0–8) (4), (2) Quick score (range: 0–7) (5) (both of which are based on the sum of fraction and intensity units of the stained cells), (3) *J*-score (range: 0–3, based on the fraction of stained cells) (6)

[1]http://www.fda.gov/MedicalDevices/ProductsandMedicalProcedures/InVitroDiagnostics/ucm301431.htm

Table 1 | Advantages and disadvantages of currently used companion diagnostic techniques.

Technique	Advantage	Disadvantage
IHC	Routinely performed; low technological requirements; time and cost effective; preservation of histological information; suitable for small tumor samples	Semi-quantitative; subjective interpretation of results; variability dependent on fixation procedure, staining protocol, and antibody selection
qRT-PCR	Quantitative; large dynamic range	No histological information retained; contamination of test results by stromal/normal tissue possible; increased technological requirements; increased time and cost requirements; variability dependent on tissue quality, RNA extraction/processing procedures and primer/probe selection
ISH	Quantitative for genetic alterations; higher reproducibility	Increased technological requirements (especially for FISH); increased time and cost requirements; added expertise in result interpretation necessary

IHC, immunohistochemistry; qRT-PCR, quantitative real-time PCR; ISH, in situ hybridization; FISH, fluorescent in situ hybridization; CISH, colorimetric in situ hybridization.

and (4) H-score (range: 0–300, based on the product of fraction and the intensity unit of stained cells) (7). Differences between positive/negative definitions together with variations regarding antibody clones, tissue fixation, antigen retrieval, and detection protocols, all contributed to a significant rate of variability in ER detection (8–10). For instance, a study headed by the UK National External Quality Assessment Scheme for Immunocytochemistry (NEQAS-ICC) reported false negativity rates ranging from 30 to 60% following the testing of a standardized sample with low ER expression by 200 laboratories throughout 26 countries (8).

Due to the historic nature of ER testing, there are currently no FDA-approved companion diagnostic devices available. To minimize inter-laboratory variation, the American Society of Clinical Oncology and the College of American Pathologists (ASCO/CAP) have recently published a document outlining their recommendations for the immunohistochemical testing of ER in breast cancer (11). The optimal testing conditions and tissue handling requirements were defined together with guidelines for both the internal and external quality assurance procedure. The same guidelines were also applicable to the detection of the progesterone receptor (PR) via IHC. PR is located downstream of ER and a positive PR test result may be indicative of an intact estrogen signaling cascade (12). This line of thinking was corroborated by the finding that patients with PR positive tumors had a better prognosis than patients with ER-positive/PR negative breast cancers (13). Alternative methods for the detection of ER and PR are continuously under investigation and Oncotype DX is one such example. This is a qRT-PCR-based assay system designed to estimate the probability of distant tumor recurrence in tamoxifen-treated, node-negative breast cancers (14) and measures the expression PR and ER, together with 19 other genes, in mRNA extracted from FFPE tissue. Proof-of-concept studies on the applicability of Oncotype DX as a companion diagnostic tool for tamoxifen treatment reported varying conclusions. In a study supported by Genomic Health Inc., Badve and colleagues reasoned that ER/PR determination using Oncotype DX performed comparably well to IHC-based detection systems (15). This was in contrast to an independent evaluation by Kraus et al. who concluded that IHC was superior to the Oncotype DX qRT-PCR-based test, not only due to higher sensitivity but also the lower cost, the ease of application and the preservation of morphological information (16).

HUMAN EPIDERMAL GROWTH FACTOR RECEPTOR 2

Overexpression of the HER2 protein and/or amplification of the HER2-encoding gene have been associated with an unfavorable prognosis in several types of cancer, including breast, gastric, and pancreatic cancer (17–19). Trastuzumab (Herceptin), an antibody-based inhibitor, was the first HER2-targeted drug to be approved for the treatment of breast cancer and has since been shown to significantly improve survival in a metastatic and adjuvant setting (20, 21). Numerous studies support the close relationship between HER2 positivity and trastuzumab responsiveness (20, 22) and bearing in mind that a HER2-amplification rate of approximately 25% occurs in breast cancer, initial clinical trials may not have yielded significant data had no pre-selection of patients according to HER2 status taken place (23). Since gene-amplification is the primary cause of HER2 overexpression (24), both FISH- (or CISH-) and IHC-based companion diagnostic devices have been approved by the FDA. Nevertheless, the initial evaluation of HER2 status is usually performed using an IHC-based method and only ambiguous (or equivocal) cases are subjected to FISH reflex testing.

Substantial inter-laboratory variations in test results are an inherent problem when considering IHC-based tests. Similar to the guidelines established for ER, ASCO/CAP has produced recommendations for HER2 testing in breast cancer (25, 26). In contrast to the instructions for the commonly used FDA-approved HercepTest (Dako), which states that a finding of more than 10% of cells with strong, uniform membrane staining qualifies as a positive result, the ASCO/CAP guidelines require complete intense membrane staining in >30% of cells in order to qualify as a positive test result following IHC testing. In addition, unlike the FDA-approved cut-off ratio of 2.0 for HER2/Chromosome 17 centromere (CEP17) testing via FISH (or four HER2 copies in assays without internal CEP17 probes), ASCO/CAP considered the range of ratios between 1.8 and 2.2 (or four to six HER2 copies) as equivocal and stated that only cases with HER2/CEP17 ratios >2.2

(or more than six copies of HER2) could be deemed to be positive based on FISH analysis. The aim of the new ASCO/CAP guidelines was to reduce the number of inconclusive cases and although some groups were positive to these new definitions (27, 28), others saw no added benefit (29). While high concordance between IHC- and FISH-based HER2 testing was demonstrated by several studies, thus justifying the use of routine IHC as an initial test (30), critics are keen to highlight the technical superiority of FISH over IHC and consequently advocate FISH as the gold standard for HER2 testing (31). Hence, it is evident that more conclusive studies on the clinical significance of both testing modality are required.

EPIDERMAL GROWTH FACTOR RECEPTOR

The epidermal growth factor receptor (EGFR) is a prominent therapeutic target in both colorectal and non-small cell lung cancer (NSCLC). In colorectal cancer, it is primarily targeted by the monoclonal antibody-based drugs cetuximab and panitumumab. These drugs target the extracellular domain of the EGFR and block down-stream signaling. Clinical trials for both agents initially required the pre-selection of patients based on positive expression of the EGFR protein, as determined by IHC, however, it soon became evident that IHC-based protein expression levels did not correlate with therapy outcome (32, 33) and that even patients with EGFR-negative tumors may benefit from EGFR-targeted therapy (34, 35). The causes for this discrepancy may be of a technical nature and connected to the variability/sensitivity of immunohistochemical techniques, or they may be a direct consequence of biological determinants. For instance, metastatic tumors may have lost the expression of EGFR, rendering them unresponsive to therapy (36). In addition, Chung and co-workers reasoned that antibodies used within IHC-based detection systems were unable to discriminate between high- and low-affinity EGFRs. Consequently, the relative distribution of such high- and low-affinity EGFRs within colorectal cancer tissue may be crucial in determining the response to therapy (34). Furthermore, it has been noted that therapeutic antibodies that target EGFR may induce antibody-dependent, cell-mediated cytotoxicity, resulting in an indirect beneficial effect owing to the recruitment of cytotoxic immune cells such as monocytes and natural killer cells to the tumor (34).

While the immunohistochemical detection of EGFR expression did not prove to be decisive in determining the clinical response, promising data has been generated in support of using the EGFR gene copy number as a predictive biomarker for EGFR-targeted therapy (37). Nevertheless, in order to achieve definitive proof and to facilitate the development of standardized testing modalities further investigation is required. In NSCLC, EGFR is targeted primarily using the small molecule inhibitors gefitinib and erlotinib. In contrast to colorectal cancer, mutations within the EGFR in NSCLC are common and mutational testing is recommended for all NSCLC cases (38). The application of mutation-specific antibodies for this purpose is discussed below. A further distinguishing feature regarding the testing of EGFR in colorectal cancer and NSCLC is that in the latter, IHC positivity or high EGFR gene copy numbers showed no conclusive correlation with treatment response (38).

V-KIT HARDY-ZUCKERMAN 4 FELINE SARCOMA VIRAL ONCOGENE HOMOLOG

Immunohistochemistry provides an excellent tool for the differential diagnosis of gastrointestinal stromal tumors (GIST). This is largely due to the fact that greater than 85% of GIST test positive for v-kit Hardy-Zuckerman 4 feline sarcoma viral oncogene homolog (KIT), in contrast to the negative result generated by most other mesenchymal tumors (39, 40). Imatinib mesylate (Gleevec, Novartis, Basel, Switzerland) is a specific tyrosine kinase inhibitor that exhibits high therapeutic activity in patients with chronic myeloid leukemia by targeting the fusion protein BCR-ABL (41). Additional targets of imatinib mesylate include the platelet-derived growth factor receptor (PDGFR) and KIT. For patients with unresectable or metastatic GIST, a positive immunohistochemical staining for KIT was initially required as an entry criteria into clinical trials investigating the efficacy of imatinib mesylate (42, 43). Significant clinical responses were recorded and this revolutionized the management of advanced GIST, a malignancy that had previously failed to respond to conventional chemotherapy. Activating mutations within the KIT gene and, to a lesser degree, PDGFR, are commonly found in patients with GIST and depending on their location within the coding region of the respective gene, they are highly correlated with the likelihood of a response to imatinib mesylate treatment (44, 45). That notwithstanding, since a small percentage of patients with GIST do not express detectable levels of KIT or do not harbor mutations within KIT/PDGFR (44–46) IHC or mutational analysis should not be used to deny treatment with imatinib mesylate since these patients may still be sensitive to this therapy.

ANAPLASTIC LYMPHOMA KINASE REARRANGEMENTS

In addition to EGFR, the anaplastic lymphoma kinase (ALK) represents a second therapeutic target in NSCLC. Chromosomal rearrangements involving the associated gene have been detected in approximately 5% of cases, most frequently resulting in the fusion to echinoderm microtubule-associated protein-like 4 (EML4) and the constitutive expression of a chimeric tyrosine kinase protein (47, 48). Second-line treatment of NSCLC patients with confirmed ALK rearrangements, using the small molecule inhibitor crizotinib, has recently been shown to significantly prolong progression-free survival compared to standard chemotherapy (49). The current "gold standard" for ALK rearrangement testing is dual-color break-apart FISH. However, interpretation of test results may be challenging since EML4 and ALK are located on the same chromosome, resulting in limited separation of the 5′ and 3′ probes. To define a positive test result, only signals separated by more than two signal diameters and/or single 3′ signals (correlating to the ALK kinase domain) should be counted. In addition, at least 50 cells should be reviewed with a positive signal detectable in at least 15% (50). The immunohistochemical detection of ALK has been considered as an attractive addition to routine FISH testing. Since ALK is not expressed in lung tissue unless driven by promoter rearrangement, a good correlation between IHC and FISH results and low IHC background staining have been reported. In addition, a number of studies confirm that IHC-negative cases are almost exclusively negative in FISH analysis and therefore indicate that IHC could be applicable as a quick and cost-effective screening tool for ALK rearrangements (51–54). FISH reflex testing for all IHC positive cases has been proposed, somewhat similar to the evaluation strategy for HER2 (55). Interestingly, the percentage of ALK rearrangement positive cells during FISH evaluation did not significantly correlate with the response to crizotinib (56). Nonetheless, comprehensive data on the correlation between the intensity of ALK staining as determined by IHC and treatment response is still lacking.

MUTATION-SPECIFIC ANTIBODIES

The selection of patients for a targeted cancer treatment frequently relies on the detection of specific gene mutations. The routinely applied techniques are generally based on the isolation of chromosomal DNA from fresh, frozen or FFPE material and analysis can involve various techniques such as mutation-specific real-time PCR, direct sequencing, mass spectrometry, mismatch ligation assays, high-resolution melting curve assays, or denaturating high-performance liquid chromatography, among others. A common drawback relates to the fact that information on tissue morphology is lost and also that "contamination" of tumor material with normal cells may hamper detection or obscure the results. In addition, increased demands on sample size and quality and extra requirements regarding technology and expertise, associated with higher cost and expenditure of time, frequently apply. The development of mutation-specific antibodies and their application in routine IHC may provide a convenient addition to DNA-based profiling techniques.

BRAF V600E

The v-raf murine sarcoma viral oncogene homolog B1 (BRAF) represents an outstanding target for the development of a mutation-specific antibody. Mutations of the associated gene occur in a range of human malignancies including cutaneous melanoma, colorectal cancer, NSCLC, papillary thyroid cancer, and hairy-cell leukemia (57–59). By far, the most common BRAF mutation results in the substitution of valine for glutamic acid at position 600 (V600E), leading to the constitutive activation of the protein's kinase domain. In human cutaneous melanoma, mutated BRAF has been detected in 40–50% of cases, with up 90% of these alterations concerning the V-E substitution at codon 600 (60). Vemurafenib and dabrafenib are two potent small molecule inhibitor drugs that specifically target BRAF V600E and have demonstrated remarkable response rates in metastatic melanoma patients (61, 62). Mutational testing of the patient tumor material is required before commencement of treatment and is to date commonly based on the detection of genomic alterations. As an addition to DNA testing, Capper et al. recently proposed a mutation-specific antibody for the detection of BRAF V600E in FFPE tissue specimens by means of IHC (**Figure 1**) (63). The results obtained from using this antibody to determine the BRAF mutational status in melanoma and thyroid cancer samples were identical to those achieved following DNA sequencing-based profiling. These results have since been substantiated by numerous studies with similarly high levels of specificity and sensitivity (up to 100%, respectively) (64–68).

In samples where the number of tumor cells is low, IHC-based BRAF testing was suggested to be more sensitive than direct DNA sequencing or high-resolution melting curve analysis (64, 65). In addition, IHC-based staining results showed low inter-observer variability (68). Nevertheless, despite the benefits of using IHC-based methods for determining the presence/absence of mutations within the BRAF gene, the presence of (non-specific) strong,

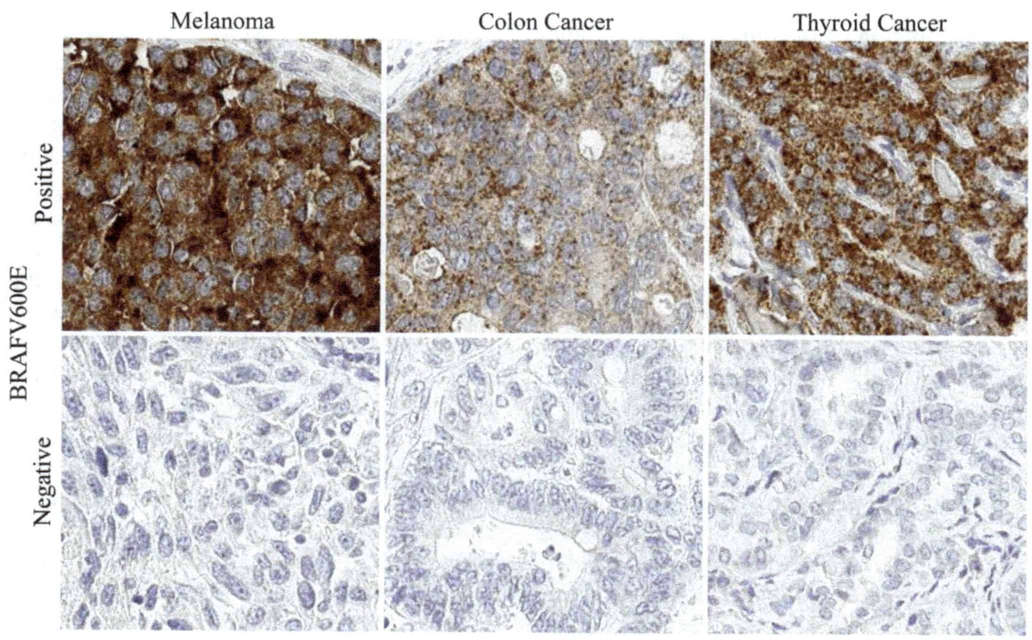

FIGURE 1 | BRAFV600E mutation-specific antibody staining. Immunohistochemical staining examples of the BRAFV600E mutation-specific antibody VE1 are presented for a BRAFV600E-positive and a BRAFV600E-negative case of melanoma, colon cancer, and thyroid cancer, respectively. BRAFV600E-positive staining is generally detected as a granular, cytoplasmic signal that can easily be distinguished from BRAFV600E-negative cases. In the presented example images, 3,3′-Diaminobenzidine (DAB) was used as a chromogen.

nuclear staining may complicate the assessment of staining results. In addition, false-negative IHC results may occur due to unsuitable or incomplete tissue fixation, the presence of necrotic or pre-necrotic tissue areas or low levels of total protein expression (63, 64). The latter may be controlled for through the use of an additional antibody capable of detecting total BRAF protein expression. With regard to the intra-tumor heterogeneity of BRAF V600E, only few cases with non-homogenous expression have been observed following immunohistochemical detection (67, 69). These results are in direct contrast to previous reports describing significant variability of BRAF mutational status among individual cells within a tumor and warrant further investigation (70, 71). Regarding the possible relationship between BRAF V600E protein expression and clinical outcome, no significant correlation was seen between the percentage of BRAF V600E positive tumor cells and the response to treatment with either dabrafenib or vemurafenib (72). Similarly, the total intensity of mutation-specific antibody staining did not significantly correlate with patient outcome.

EGFR L858R AND E746_A750del

Epidermal growth factor receptor mutations have been detected in 2–17% of NSCLC patients from Europe and the United States, however, the mutational frequency increases to 30% when analyzing cases from East Asia (73–75). Specific mutations, in particular those affecting the EGFR kinase domain, have been associated with response to gefitinib and erlotinib treatment (76, 77). The two most common types of EGFR mutations are in-frame deletions of exon 19 and a leucine to arginine substitution at codon 858 (L858R) in exon 21. Taken together, alterations at these sites account for up to 90% of all EGFR mutations (78). Exon 19 deletions may affect a varying number of nucleotides. For example, E746_A750del results in a five amino acid deletion in the corresponding protein and is the most common deletion detected, occurring in approximately 70% of cases (79). The application of mutation-specific antibodies designed to target L858R and the E746_A750del modification, have yielded varying levels of detection specificity and sensitivity. For L858R, several studies reported sensitivity values in the range of 70–100% and specificities exceeding 95% (79–83). While these results were promising, sensitivities as low as 36 and 40% have also been described for the same antibody clone (84, 85). Similarly, regarding the E746_A750del-specific antibody, the same studies published sensitivity and specificity values of 40–100% and 95–100%, respectively. The possible sources of variation are numerous and include the application of different scoring systems, discrepancy between the definitions of positivity/negativity, different DNA-based reference techniques, different tissue fixation methods, and the types of specimens analyzed. While initial attempts to determine optimal tissue preparation and staining evaluation have been presented (86), additional steps toward a standardized protocol for the detection of EGFR mutations using IHC should be undertaken.

The overall high levels of specificity associated with IHC-based EGFR-mutational testing imply that IHC may be suitable as a pre-screening tool for the identification of NSCLC patients that are eligible for EGFR-inhibitor treatment. Since a number of mutations are not currently detectable by antibody-based profiling, the additional testing of IHC-negative cases using direct DNA sequencing or similar assays is necessary (79, 81). The applicability of IHC in predicting response to EGFR-targeted therapy remains controversial. Confirming the importance of EGFR-mutational status for treatment response, positive IHC staining has been associated with longer progression-free survival compared to IHC-negative or -equivocal cases (83, 87). In addition, high mutant EGFR expression (as defined by the sum of scores for fraction and intensity) was significantly related to elevated progression-free survival but not overall survival (88) and a fraction of positive tumor cells exceeding 50% of all cells predicted better response to EGFR inhibition treatment in univariate but not multivariate analysis (89). Despite the aforementioned results, a study by Kato and co-workers could not detect a significant correlation between IHC staining and treatment response or survival (82). Shortcomings in the significance of IHC-based detection methods in predicting survival benefit, in particular when compared to DNA-based techniques, may occur due to the limited mutation spectrum detected via IHC. Furthermore, EGFR-mutation-specific antibodies have been shown to occasionally detect mutations associated with EGFR-inhibitor resistance via mechanisms that are not yet fully understood (84).

ALTERNATIVE PROTEIN BINDERS

In situ affinity-based detection of proteins remains one of the best sources of information about either the healthy status of an individual tissue or potential pathological changes, and is thus applicable within several medical settings. Molecular imaging allows for the early detection and classification of many human diseases and, when specific, permits improved, target-directed therapies. Molecules generated through immunization such as polyclonal, monospecific polyclonal, and monoclonal antibodies continue to be the best established and most widely used binders in diagnostics (90, 91). Methods for the detection of proteins based on antibody recognition often encounter problems due to poor selectivity and/or sensitivity (92). Poorly characterized antibodies and/or insufficient quality control often render them as unsuitable for demanding applications such as companion diagnostics (93). Commercially available antibodies frequently perform very differently within various laboratories and often do not perform as advertised, thus raising doubts regarding their reliability when incorporated into assays requiring high specificity (94). Antibodies can be biochemically and physiologically modified and use of their derivatives, such as single chain variable fragments (scFv) or Fab fragments, may result in the improved detection of a wide range of target molecules (**Figure 2**) (95). Currently only a few antibodies and recombinant proteins are used within clinical settings, largely due to the reasons outlined above. Recombinant binders that are generated in immune-free, *in vitro*-based approaches, hold the potential of taking priority over conventional antibodies (96). Stability, specificity, ease of manipulation, low cost, high throughput, and reproducibility of production are some of the advantages that make novel scaffold molecules highly desirable (97). Alternative binders are promising molecules for novel approaches in individualized medicine (**Figure 2**). They can serve as personalized molecular imaging tools for *in vivo*, live diagnostics of the changes occurring in the expression of markers following treatment (95).

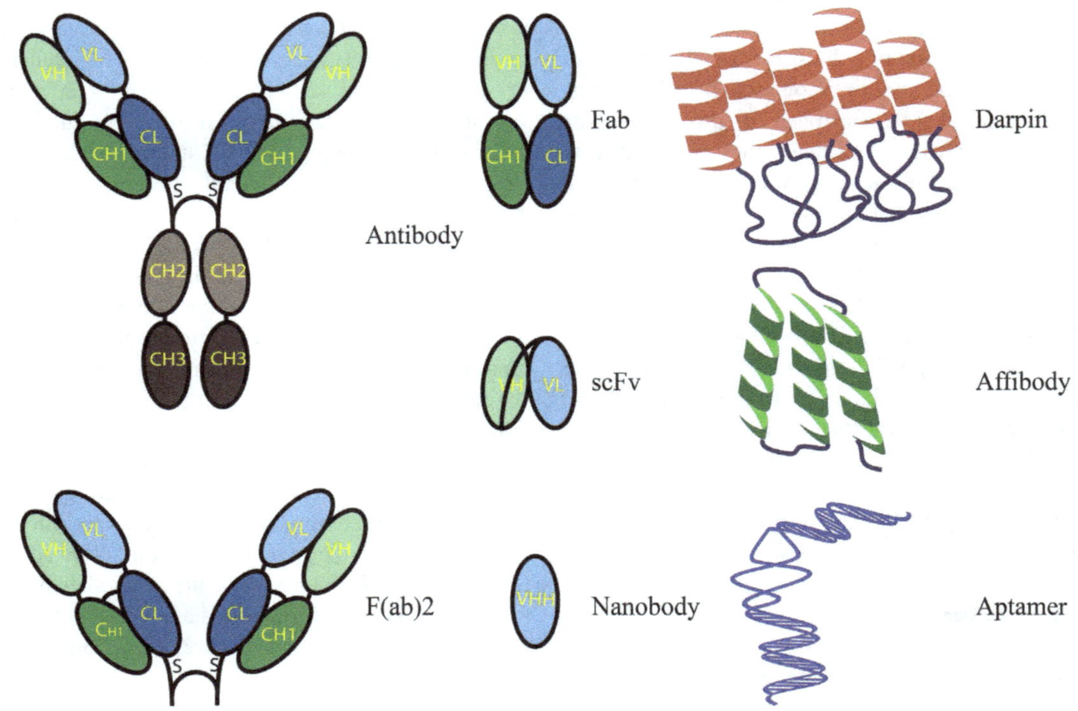

FIGURE 2 | Schematic representation of binder formats.

RECOMBINANT ANTIBODY FRAGMENTS

Antibody fragments are generated in order to obtain binders with improved characteristics, compared to conventional antibodies, but similar functional and recognition properties. Fab and $F(ab)_2$ fragments are antigen-binding fragments generated after proteolysis of full length antibodies. Single chain variable fragments (scFvs) are smaller than Fab fragments and are composed of genetically linked light and heavy chains containing variable regions. These molecules can also exist as dimers (98). Another class of antibody-derived antigen-binding molecules, termed nanobodies, are small, single-domain polypeptides derived from the variable part of the heavy chain (VHH) of light-chain deficient antibodies that were originally discovered in camelids (camels, llamas) (99, 100). Their reduced size, greater stability and solubility, and antibody-like binding characteristics make nanobodies ideal for use in the targeting and imaging of antigens in live cells, protein precipitation *in vivo*, and targeted enzymes modulations (101–103). As a result of their smaller size (only 15 kDa), nanobodies can bind to epitopes that are hidden or shielded and reach affinities within the range of nanomolar to picomolar. Nanobodies are highly specific for their targets and have no known cross-reactivity to structurally related proteins, which makes them excellent tools for targeting kinases and tyrosine phosphatases. In addition, nanobodies have technological advantages that render them superior to conventional antibodies. They are easily modified to avoid chemically reactive groups such a primary amines or to alter the primary amine number to allow more selective and controlled chemical conjugation. The selection of binders for certain applications is usually based on their performance in experimental settings and depends on their preference for particular epitopes and the accessibility of binding sites.

AFFIBODY MOLECULES

Affibody molecules are small (~7 kDa), alpha-helical *Z*-domain of Staphylococcal protein A, immune-independent affinity molecules that target a wide range of proteins (104, 105). They can be produced in functional form both via recombinant expression in *Escherichia coli* or peptide synthesis. They possess picomolar affinities, are highly soluble and stable. In addition, they are cysteine-free which prevents non-specific binding events when applied to tissues. Furthermore, the lack of cysteine provides an opportunity for site-specific labeling through the introduction of unique cysteine molecules. High affinity affibodies were engineered against targets such as the IL2 receptor, Alzheimer's amyloid-beta peptide or EGFR (106–108). They have been used in various types of experiments and are intended for both *in vivo* and *in vitro* imaging and also therapeutic applications including the detection of HER2 within different experimental settings (109, 110).

DESIGNED ANKYRIN REPEAT PROTEINS

Designed ankyrin repeat proteins (DARPins) are potent alternatives to conventional antibodies. They detect antigens with high specificity and picomolar affinity, are independent of target immunogenicity and possess attractive molecular properties such as small size and high stability (111). They are synthetic, non-immunoglobulin binding proteins that form scaffolds containing tandem repeats of an elementary, structural motif, typically composed of 33 amino acid residues folded into a β-turn followed by two antiparallel α-helices. A single protein may contain up to 29 repeats of this motif. The production of DARPins does not require the use of animals at any step, therefore permitting the large scale, parallel production of variable binders. DARPins are correctly folded in both prokaryotes and eukaryotes, due to the absence of disulfide bonds, which enables their use in a variety of functional assays (112). They can easily be genetically modified to form fusion proteins and site-specifically targeted for chemical conjugation. DARPins against a wide range of protein targets, including extracellular, intracellular, and membrane proteins, were generated with high yield from synthetic libraries and successfully used as replacements for conventional antibodies. One such example is the DARPins generated against HER2; these displayed higher specificity and similar sensitivity when compared to FDA-approved antibodies for the *in situ* identification of HER2 expression status in FFPE breast cancer tissue (113). DARPins can easily be made functional for use in various biomedical applications through the introduction of site-specific, clickable modifications. Such alterations do not affect their physical properties (114).

APTAMERS

Aptamers are a class of small, synthetic, self-folding, and single-stranded RNA or DNA molecules that form secondary and tertiary structures and specifically bind to proteins, small molecules, or other cellular targets such as nucleic acids (115, 116). They are comparable to antibodies in terms of their target recognition capabilities, their binding affinities, and the diversity of applications that they can be used in; however, they possess numerous significant characteristics that render them advantageous over their protein equivalents. Aptamers are highly specific, non-immunogenic, redox-insensitive, and temperature- and pH-tolerant. In addition, they do not have hydrophobic cores which are usual in proteins and, therefore, they do not aggregate. In order to select aptamers, information on protein conformation is not required, a feature which can be useful for screening for unidentified disease biomarkers. Aptamers can be generated through cell-based aptamer selection that utilizes differences between the molecular signatures of any two different cell types. The selected aptamers selectively bind to an unknown protein within one cell type only, are cross-linked to their targets and once the complex is purified the targets can be analyzed by mass spectrometry (117). Therefore, the cell-based selection of aptamer molecules has great potential for the development of specific probes suitable for biomarker discovery and companion diagnostics development. Since chemical synthesis is a process that is well defined and highly reproducible, the production of aptamers can easily be scaled up. They can be synthesized with specific, custom tailored functional groups attached to 5′ or 3′ termini which creates an easy approach to conjugation and multiplexing *in situ* assays. Furthermore, aptamer conjugations do not generally alter their binding affinity. With advances in imaging techniques, aptamers are already considered as prospective reagents for *in situ* targeting. To date, several aptamers have been developed against important clinical targets such as PDGF, von Willebrand factor (vWF), E-selectin, vascular endothelial growth factor (VEGF), and prostate specific membrane antigen (PSMA) and their applicability within a clinical setting is currently being investigated (118–121).

IN SITU PROXIMITY LIGATION ASSAY

Using traditional IHC techniques, the level of protein expression can easily be determined. However, the functional status of a cell cannot be evaluated by the level of expressed protein alone. The activity of signaling pathways, as assessed by the analysis of post-translation modifications (PTMs) and protein interactions, needs to be determined and taken into consideration (122). Cancer does not consist of a homologous mass of cells but of complex, heterogeneous cell populations that are affected by interactions with each other and the surrounding environment. Therefore, the analysis of cancer tissue at single cell resolution provides a much better understanding of the differences in signaling status and activity (123). *In situ* PLA enables a localized and specific detection by utilizing oligonucleotide-conjugated antibodies to determine the proximity between one or more targeted epitopes. This makes it a suitable method for detecting molecular events in cells and tissue, for example the status of a signaling pathway. The use of two independent binders and the additional requirement of proximity for reporting enable the specific detection of proteins, protein–protein interactions, and PTMs (124). Proximity ligation converts the recognition of a protein, protein complex, or PTM by two or more antibodies into an amplifiable, circular DNA molecule (**Figure 3**). Upon proximal binding of a pair of oligonucleotide-conjugated antibodies (PLA probes), the oligonucleotides guide the formation of a circle after applying two additional, single-stranded DNA molecules. This circular DNA molecule is then ligated and amplified by phi29 polymerase within a rolling-circle amplification (RCA) reaction, resulting in a localized, concatameric product. The latter is visualized by hybridization of detection oligonucleotides labeled with fluorophores or horse radish peroxidase (**Figure 3**) (125). Due to the environment of fixed cells and tissue the amplification product will collapse into a bundle with a diameter of approximately 1 μM (126) that can then be visualized as a bright dot that is quantifiable and easily distinguished from the background (127).

Heterogeneity within a sample increases the demands on the dynamic range of a method in order to allow for the detection of both abundant and scarce targets within the same sample. *In situ* PLA uses an amplifiable DNA circle as a reporter molecule and by using reagents that give rise to three variants of the reporter DNA circles and adding them at decreasing concentrations the dynamic range of the PLA is increased. By labeling the circles with different fluorophores, the readout can be adjusted to the fluorophore whose concentration gives rise to quantifiable and easily distinguishable signals. In a heterogeneous sample, different readout fluorophores can be used for different parts of the sample, enabling the detection of a target that varies greatly within the sample without the risk of signal saturation. As the size of a patient sample is often limited, this approach reduces the need to optimize the binder concentration and enables the evaluation of patient samples where knowledge on the expected results is limited (128).

Multiplex *in situ* PLA permits the parallel analyses of multiple protein complexes involved in signaling pathways directly in tissue and cells thus making it possible to compare levels of

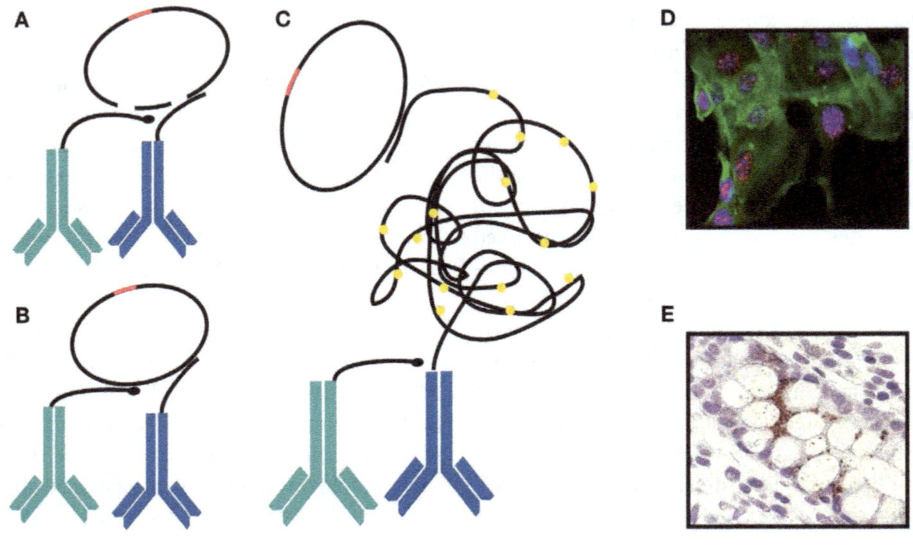

FIGURE 3 | Proximity ligation assay. (A) Two probes stay in close proximity by binding to a protein or two proteins present in one complex. **(B)** They are joined and circularized by DNA ligation upon introduction of linear connector oligonucleotides. After ligation, rolling-circle amplification (RCA) is initiated. One of the proximity probes is used as a primer. **(C)** The single-stranded RCA products are hybridized with labeled detection oligonucleotide complementary to a multiplied motif in the sequence of the RCA product. The detection oligonucleotide can be labeled with fluorophore **(D)** or a horse radish peroxidase **(E)**.

protein complexes between individual cells and also providing information regarding the spatial distributions of these complexes. A tag-specific sequence within the PLA probe targeting a protein gives rise to a DNA circular molecule that carries information on the identity of the target protein. The amplified tags in the RCA products can then be visualized using oligonucleotides labeled with different fluorophores, to uniquely recognize the tag sequences corresponding to a certain target (129). *In situ* PLA has been shown to provide valuable information about the status of signaling pathways by detecting molecular events such as dimerizations, the formation of protein complexes and PTMs. It enables the detection of activity at different levels within a signaling pathway, thereby enabling specific aberrations to be pinpointed. *In situ* PLA has been utilized in studies investigating both EGFR dimerization and receptor activation, which has been proposed to play a crucial role during tumor progression, and also the development of drug resistance. Dimerization and aberrant activity has been shown to be independent of EGFR expression, explaining why the deregulated expression of the EGFR in several types of human malignancies was shown to have limited value as a prognostic or diagnostic marker. Receptor dimerization events detected by mutation-specific PLA appeared to be more suitable for the selection of patients for EGFR-targeted treatment (130).

Similarly, the overexpression of human epidermal growth factor receptors (HERs) has been linked to poor prognosis in patients with early breast cancer. Dimers containing the HER2 isoform were shown to be more stable and have prolonged active signaling compared to HER2 deficient dimers. Elevated levels of HER2-HER2 and HER2-HER3 complexes detected by PLA showed a significant association with decreased recurrent-free survival and a reduction in overall survival of breast cancer patients, proving that PLA and the detection of cellular signaling processes can be successfully implemented in studies on prognostic markers in clinical specimens (131). Through the application of *in situ* PLA, it is now possible to screen for the effects of a drug treatment on intracellular signaling, providing information on the specific level of signaling pathways. Being able to study primary cell lines and patient tissue sample gives valuable information of the signaling status within a specific tumor and allows to predict the response to a certain therapy (132). PLA technologies have been used to address a variety of biomedical problems and demonstrated the potential to address some difficulties, both concerning the validation of biomarkers and the applicability for clinical diagnostics. Implementing PLA techniques as an alternative to IHC in everyday laboratory practice allows for a more precise and quantitative evaluation of antibody performance characteristics and their suitability for an anticipated analytical use. Application of the PLA technique provides an opportunity to develop a high-quality procedure for *in situ* detection of proteins and signaling pathways in companion diagnostics. This will offer the medical industry powerful, universally applicable tools for clinical research and routine diagnostics.

CONCLUSION

Affinity proteomics for the analysis of proteins as companion diagnostics requires access to reagents that can be used in specific detection reactions. The comprehensive validation and improvement of existing and newly generated antibodies to obtain well characterized, high-quality, and well-controlled resources as tools for large scale studies of the human proteome in health and disease is a widely acknowledged demand. In many routine clinical, diagnostic, and life science applications, antibodies have proven to be the reagents of choice. IHC is routinely performed in the majority of clinical laboratories and widely acknowledged as superior to other analysis techniques regarding time- and cost-effective application. In selected cases, IHC and mutation-specific antibodies may even provide an attractive alternative to DNA-based testing methods. As a highly valuable resource documenting the availability and identification of novel biomarker candidates, the Human Protein Atlas[2] project has generated antibodies targeting proteins from over 15,000 genes, corresponding to about 75% of all human protein-coding genes (133, 134). All antibodies are routinely subjected to a series of validation steps, including protein arrays, western blots, and immunofluorescence and used to assess protein expression patterns in a broad spectrum of normal and cancer tissues through application of IHC. Nevertheless, efforts to detect proteins when high specificity is required often fail. Hence, there is a strong need for better methods and reagents for assessing protein expression in tissues as means of companion diagnostics and alternative binders or PLA in combination with existing antibodies represent promising candidate alternatives.

ACKNOWLEDGMENTS

This work was supported by grants from the Knut and Alice Wallenberg Foundation, from the Swedish Cancer Society and from the European Union Seventh Framework Program under grant agreement 241481 (Affinomics).

REFERENCES

1. Jorgensen JT. Companion diagnostics in oncology – current status and future aspects. *Oncology* (2013) **85**:59–68. doi:10.1159/000353454
2. Fisher B, Redmond C, Brown A, Wolmark N, Wittliff J, Fisher ER, et al. Treatment of primary breast cancer with chemotherapy and tamoxifen. *N Engl J Med* (1981) **305**:1–6. doi:10.1056/NEJM198107023050101
3. Fisher B, Redmond C, Brown A, Wickerham DL, Wolmark N, Allegra J, et al. Influence of tumor estrogen and progesterone receptor levels on the response to tamoxifen and chemotherapy in primary breast cancer. *J Clin Oncol* (1983) **1**:227–41.
4. Allred DC, Harvey JM, Berardo M, Clark GM. Prognostic and predictive factors in breast cancer by immunohistochemical analysis. *Mod Pathol* (1998) **11**:155–68.
5. Barnes DM, Harris WH, Smith P, Millis RR, Rubens RD. Immunohistochemical determination of oestrogen receptor: comparison of different methods of assessment of staining and correlation with clinical outcome of breast cancer patients. *Br J Cancer* (1996) **74**:1445–51. doi:10.1038/bjc.1996.563
6. Umemura S, Kurosumi M, Moriya T, Oyama T, Arihiro K, Yamashita H, et al. Immunohistochemical evaluation for hormone receptors in breast cancer: a practically useful evaluation system and handling protocol. *Breast Cancer* (2006) **13**:232–5. doi:10.2325/jbcs.13.232
7. Kinsel LB, Szabo E, Greene GL, Konrath J, Leight GS, McCarty KS Jr. Immunocytochemical analysis of estrogen receptors as a predictor of prognosis in breast cancer patients: comparison with quantitative biochemical methods. *Cancer Res* (1989) **49**:1052–6.
8. Rhodes A, Jasani B, Barnes DM, Bobrow LG, Miller KD. Reliability of immunohistochemical demonstration of oestrogen receptors in routine practice: interlaboratory variance in the sensitivity of detection and evaluation of scoring systems. *J Clin Pathol* (2000) **53**:125–30. doi:10.1136/jcp.53.2.125
9. Rhodes A, Jasani B, Balaton AJ, Barnes DM, Miller KD. Frequency of oestrogen and progesterone receptor positivity by immunohistochemical analysis in 7016 breast carcinomas: correlation with patient age, assay sensitivity, threshold value, and mammographic screening. *J Clin Pathol* (2000) **53**:688–96. doi:10.1136/jcp.53.9.688
10. Francis GD, Dimech M, Giles L, Hopkins A. Frequency and reliability of oestrogen receptor, progesterone receptor and HER2 in breast carcinoma determined by immunohistochemistry in Australasia: results of the RCPA Quality Assurance Program. *J Clin Pathol* (2007) **60**:1277–83. doi:10.1136/jcp.2006.044701
11. Hammond ME, Hayes DF, Dowsett M, Allred DC, Hagerty KL, Badve S, et al. American Society of Clinical Oncology/College of American Pathologists guideline recommendations for immunohistochemical testing of estrogen and progesterone receptors in breast cancer (unabridged version). *Arch Pathol Lab Med* (2010) **134**:e48–72. doi:10.1043/1543-2165-134.7.e48
12. Horwitz KB, McGuire WL. Predicting response to endocrine therapy in human breast cancer: a hypothesis. *Science* (1975) **189**:726–7. doi:10.1126/science.168640
13. Clark GM, McGuire WL, Hubay CA, Pearson OH, Marshall JS. Progesterone receptors as a prognostic factor in Stage II breast cancer. *N Engl J Med* (1983) **309**:1343–7. doi:10.1056/NEJM198312013092240
14. Paik S, Shak S, Tang G, Kim C, Baker J, Cronin M, et al. A multigene assay to predict recurrence of tamoxifen-treated, node-negative breast cancer. *N Engl J Med* (2004) **351**:2817–26. doi:10.1056/NEJMoa041588
15. Badve SS, Baehner FL, Gray RP, Childs BH, Maddala T, Liu ML, et al. Estrogen- and progesterone-receptor status in ECOG 2197: comparison of immunohistochemistry by local and central laboratories and quantitative reverse transcription polymerase chain reaction by central laboratory. *J Clin Oncol* (2008) **26**:2473–81. doi:10.1200/JCO.2007.13.6424
16. Kraus JA, Dabbs DJ, Beriwal S, Bhargava R. Semi-quantitative immunohistochemical assay versus oncotype DX(R) qRT-PCR assay for estrogen and progesterone receptors: an independent quality assurance study. *Mod Pathol* (2012) **25**:869–76. doi:10.1038/modpathol.2011.219
17. Press MF, Bernstein L, Thomas PA, Meisner LF, Zhou JY, Ma Y, et al. HER-2/neu gene amplification characterized by fluorescence in situ hybridization: poor prognosis in node-negative breast carcinomas. *J Clin Oncol* (1997) **15**:2894–904.
18. Lei S, Appert HE, Nakata B, Domenico DR, Kim K, Howard JM. Overexpression of HER2/neu oncogene in pancreatic cancer correlates with shortened survival. *Int J Pancreatol* (1995) **17**:15–21.
19. Nakajima M, Sawada H, Yamada Y, Watanabe A, Tatsumi M, Yamashita J, et al. The prognostic significance of amplification and overexpression of c-met and c-erb B-2 in human gastric carcinomas. *Cancer* (1999) **85**:1894–902. doi:10.1002/(SICI)1097-0142(19990501)85:93.0.CO;2-J
20. Slamon DJ, Leyland-Jones B, Shak S, Fuchs H, Paton V, Bajamonde A, et al. Use of chemotherapy plus a monoclonal antibody against HER2 for metastatic breast cancer that overexpresses HER2. *N Engl J Med* (2001) **344**:783–92. doi:10.1056/NEJM200103153441101
21. Joensuu H, Kellokumpu-Lehtinen PL, Bono P, Alanko T, Kataja V, Asola R, et al. Adjuvant docetaxel or vinorelbine with or without trastuzumab for breast cancer. *N Engl J Med* (2006) **354**:809–20. doi:10.1056/NEJMoa053028
22. Mass RD, Press MF, Anderson S, Cobleigh MA, Vogel CL, Dybdal N, et al. Evaluation of clinical outcomes according to HER2 detection by fluorescence in situ hybridization in women with metastatic breast cancer treated with trastuzumab. *Clin Breast Cancer* (2005) **6**:240–6. doi:10.3816/CBC.2005.n.026
23. Maitland ML, Schilsky RL. Clinical trials in the era of personalized oncology. *CA Cancer J Clin* (2011) **61**:365–81. doi:10.3322/caac.20135
24. Slamon DJ, Godolphin W, Jones LA, Holt JA, Wong SG, Keith DE, et al. Studies of the HER-2/neu proto-oncogene in human breast and ovarian cancer. *Science* (1989) **244**:707–12. doi:10.1126/science.2470152
25. Wolff AC, Hammond ME, Schwartz JN, Hagerty KL, Allred DC, Cote RJ, et al. American Society of Clinical Oncology/College of American Pathologists guideline recommendations for human epidermal growth factor receptor 2 testing in breast cancer. *Arch Pathol Lab Med* (2007) **131**:18–43. doi:10.1043/1543-2165(2007)131
26. Hammond ME, Hayes DF, Wolff AC. Clinical Notice for American Society of Clinical Oncology-College of American Pathologists guideline recommendations on ER/PgR and HER2 testing in breast cancer. *J Clin Oncol* (2011) **29**:e458. doi:10.1200/JCO.2011.35.2245
27. Middleton LP, Price KM, Puig P, Heydon LJ, Tarco E, Sneige N, et al. Implementation of American Society of Clinical Oncology/College of American Pathologists HER2 Guideline Recommendations in a tertiary care facility increases HER2 immunohistochemistry and fluorescence in situ hybridization concordance and decreases the number of inconclusive cases. *Arch Pathol Lab Med* (2009) **133**:775–80. doi:10.1043/1543-2165-133.5.775

[2]www.proteinatlas.org

28. Shah SS, Ketterling RP, Goetz MP, Ingle JN, Reynolds CA, Perez EA, et al. Impact of American Society of Clinical Oncology/College of American Pathologists guideline recommendations on HER2 interpretation in breast cancer. *Hum Pathol* (2010) **41**:103–6. doi:10.1016/j.humpath.2009.07.001
29. Vergara-Lluri ME, Moatamed NA, Hong E, Apple SK. High concordance between HercepTest immunohistochemistry and ERBB2 fluorescence in situ hybridization before and after implementation of American Society of Clinical Oncology/College of American Pathology 2007 guidelines. *Mod Pathol* (2012) **25**:1326–32. doi:10.1038/modpathol.2012.93
30. Jorgensen JT, Moller S, Rasmussen BB, Winther H, Schonau A, Knoop A. High concordance between two companion diagnostics tests: a concordance study between the HercepTest and the HER2 FISH pharmDx kit. *Am J Clin Pathol* (2011) **136**:145–51. doi:10.1309/AJCPJPJ8ZWGDTTWC
31. Sauter G, Lee J, Bartlett JM, Slamon DJ, Press MF. Guidelines for human epidermal growth factor receptor 2 testing: biologic and methodologic considerations. *J Clin Oncol* (2009) **27**:1323–33. doi:10.1200/JCO.2007.14.8197
32. Van Cutsem E, Peeters M, Siena S, Humblet Y, Hendlisz A, Neyns B, et al. Open-label phase III trial of panitumumab plus best supportive care compared with best supportive care alone in patients with chemotherapy-refractory metastatic colorectal cancer. *J Clin Oncol* (2007) **25**:1658–64. doi:10.1200/JCO.2006.08.1620
33. Cunningham D, Humblet Y, Siena S, Khayat D, Bleiberg H, Santoro A, et al. Cetuximab monotherapy and cetuximab plus irinotecan in irinotecan-refractory metastatic colorectal cancer. *N Engl J Med* (2004) **351**:337–45. doi:10.1056/NEJMoa033025
34. Chung KY, Shia J, Kemeny NE, Shah M, Schwartz GK, Tse A, et al. Cetuximab shows activity in colorectal cancer patients with tumors that do not express the epidermal growth factor receptor by immunohistochemistry. *J Clin Oncol* (2005) **23**:1803–10. doi:10.1200/JCO.2005.08.037
35. Lenz HJ, Van Cutsem E, Khambata-Ford S, Mayer RJ, Gold P, Stella P, et al. Multicenter phase II and translational study of cetuximab in metastatic colorectal carcinoma refractory to irinotecan, oxaliplatin, and fluoropyrimidines. *J Clin Oncol* (2006) **24**:4914–21. doi:10.1200/JCO.2006.06.7595
36. Scartozzi M, Bearzi I, Berardi R, Mandolesi A, Fabris G, Cascinu S. Epidermal growth factor receptor (EGFR) status in primary colorectal tumors does not correlate with EGFR expression in related metastatic sites: implications for treatment with EGFR-targeted monoclonal antibodies. *J Clin Oncol* (2004) **22**:4772–8. doi:10.1200/JCO.2004.00.117
37. Custodio A, Feliu J. Prognostic and predictive biomarkers for epidermal growth factor receptor-targeted therapy in colorectal cancer: beyond KRAS mutations. *Crit Rev Oncol Hematol* (2013) **85**:45–81. doi:10.1016/j.critrevonc.2012.05.001
38. Ellis PM, Blais N, Soulieres D, Ionescu DN, Kashyap M, Liu G, et al. A systematic review and Canadian consensus recommendations on the use of biomarkers in the treatment of non-small cell lung cancer. *J Thorac Oncol* (2011) **6**:1379–91. doi:10.1097/JTO.0b013e318220cb8e
39. Sarlomo-Rikala M, Kovatich AJ, Barusevicius A, Miettinen M. CD117: a sensitive marker for gastrointestinal stromal tumors that is more specific than CD34. *Mod Pathol* (1998) **11**:728–34.
40. Hirota S, Isozaki K, Moriyama Y, Hashimoto K, Nishida T, Ishiguro S, et al. Gain-of-function mutations of c-kit in human gastrointestinal stromal tumors. *Science* (1998) **279**:577–80. doi:10.1126/science.279.5350.577
41. Goldman JM, Melo JV. Chronic myeloid leukemia – advances in biology and new approaches to treatment. *N Engl J Med* (2003) **349**:1451–64. doi:10.1056/NEJMra020777
42. van Oosterom AT, Judson I, Verweij J, Stroobants S, Donatodi Paola E, Dimitrijevic S, et al. Safety 740 and efficacy of imatinib (STI571) in metastatic gastrointestinal stromal tumours: a 741 phase I study. *Lancet* (2001) **358**:1421–3. doi:10.1016/S0140-6736(01)06535-7
43. Demetri GD, von Mehren M, Blanke CD, Van den Abbeele AD, Eisenberg B, Roberts PJ, et al. Efficacy and safety of imatinib mesylate in advanced gastrointestinal stromal tumors. *N Engl J Med* (2002) **347**:472–80. doi:10.1056/NEJMoa020461
44. Debiec-Rychter M, Dumez H, Judson I, Wasag B, Verweij J, Brown M, et al. Use of c-KIT/PDGFRA mutational analysis to predict the clinical response to imatinib in patients with advanced gastrointestinal stromal tumours entered on phase I and II studies of the EORTC Soft Tissue and Bone Sarcoma Group. *Eur J Cancer* (2004) **40**:689–95. doi:10.1016/j.ejca.2003.11.025
45. Heinrich MC, Corless CL, Demetri GD, Blanke CD, von Mehren M, Joensuu H, et al. Kinase mutations and imatinib response in patients with metastatic gastrointestinal stromal tumor. *J Clin Oncol* (2003) **21**:4342–9. doi:10.1200/JCO.2003.04.190
46. Medeiros F, Corless CL, Duensing A, Hornick JL, Oliveira AM, Heinrich MC, et al. KIT-negative gastrointestinal stromal tumors: proof of concept and therapeutic implications. *Am J Surg Pathol* (2004) **28**:889–94. doi:10.1097/00000478-200407000-00007
47. Soda M, Choi YL, Enomoto M, Takada S, Yamashita Y, Ishikawa S, et al. Identification of the transforming EML4-ALK fusion gene in non-small-cell lung cancer. *Nature* (2007) **448**:561–6. doi:10.1038/nature05945
48. Rodig SJ, Mino-Kenudson M, Dacic S, Yeap BY, Shaw A, Barletta JA, et al. Unique clinicopathologic features characterize ALK-rearranged lung adenocarcinoma in the western population. *Clin Cancer Res* (2009) **15**:5216–23. doi:10.1158/1078-0432.CCR-09-0802
49. Shaw AT, Kim DW, Nakagawa K, Seto T, Crino L, Ahn MJ, et al. Crizotinib versus chemotherapy in advanced ALK-positive lung cancer. *N Engl J Med* (2013) **368**:2385–94. doi:10.1056/NEJMoa1214886
50. Thunnissen E, Bubendorf L, Dietel M, Elmberger G, Kerr K, Lopez-Rios F, et al. EML4-ALK testing in non-small cell carcinomas of the lung: a review with recommendations. *Virchows Arch* (2012) **461**:245–57. doi:10.1007/s00428-012-1281-4
51. Park HS, Lee JK, Kim DW, Kulig K, Kim TM, Lee SH, et al. Immunohistochemical screening for anaplastic lymphoma kinase (ALK) rearrangement in advanced non-small cell lung cancer patients. *Lung Cancer* (2012) **77**:288–92. doi:10.1016/j.lungcan.2012.03.004
52. Yi ES, Boland JM, Maleszewski JJ, Roden AC, Oliveira AM, Aubry MC, et al. Correlation of IHC and FISH for ALK gene rearrangement in non-small cell lung carcinoma: IHC score algorithm for FISH. *J Thorac Oncol* (2011) **6**:459–65. doi:10.1097/JTO.0b013e318209edb9
53. Paik JH, Choe G, Kim H, Choe JY, Lee HJ, Lee CT, et al. Screening of anaplastic lymphoma kinase rearrangement by immunohistochemistry in non-small cell lung cancer: correlation with fluorescence in situ hybridization. *J Thorac Oncol* (2011) **6**:466–72. doi:10.1097/JTO.0b013e31820b82e8
54. Selinger CI, Rogers TM, Russell PA, O'Toole S, Yip P, Wright GM, et al. Testing for ALK rearrangement in lung adenocarcinoma: a multicenter comparison of immunohistochemistry and fluorescent in situ hybridization. *Mod Pathol* (2013). doi:10.1038/modpathol.2013.87
55. Rothschild SI, Gautschi O. Crizotinib in the treatment of non-small-cell lung cancer. *Clin Lung Cancer* (2013) **14**:473–80. doi:10.1016/j.cllc.2013.04.006
56. Camidge DR, Theodoro M, Maxson DA, Skokan M, O'Brien T, Lu X, et al. Correlations between the percentage of tumor cells showing an anaplastic lymphoma kinase (ALK) gene rearrangement, ALK signal copy number, and response to crizotinib therapy in ALK fluorescence in situ hybridization-positive nonsmall cell lung cancer. *Cancer* (2012) **118**:4486–94. doi:10.1002/cncr.27411
57. Davies H, Bignell GR, Cox C, Stephens P, Edkins S, Clegg S, et al. Mutations of the BRAF gene in human cancer. *Nature* (2002) **417**:949–54. doi:10.1038/nature00766
58. Nikiforov YE, Nikiforova MN. Molecular genetics and diagnosis of thyroid cancer. *Nat Rev Endocrinol* (2011) **7**:569–80. doi:10.1038/nrendo.2011.142
59. Tiacci E, Trifonov V, Schiavoni G, Holmes A, Kern W, Martelli MP, et al. BRAF mutations in hairy-cell leukemia. *N Engl J Med* (2011) **364**:2305–15. doi:10.1056/NEJMoa1014209
60. Platz A, Egyhazi S, Ringborg U, Hansson J. Human cutaneous melanoma; a review of NRAS and BRAF mutation frequencies in relation to histogenetic subclass and body site. *Mol Oncol* (2008) **1**:395–405. doi:10.1016/j.molonc.2007.12.003
61. Flaherty KT, Puzanov I, Kim KB, Ribas A, McArthur GA, Sosman JA, et al. Inhibition of mutated, activated BRAF in metastatic melanoma. *N Engl J Med* (2010) **363**:809–19. doi:10.1056/NEJMoa1002011
62. Hauschild A, Grob JJ, Demidov LV, Jouary T, Gutzmer R, Millward M, et al. Dabrafenib in BRAF-mutated metastatic melanoma: a multicentre, open-label, phase 3 randomised controlled trial. *Lancet* (2012) **380**:358–65. doi:10.1016/S0140-6736(12)60868-X
63. Capper D, Preusser M, Habel A, Sahm F, Ackermann U, Schindler G, et al. Assessment of BRAF V600E mutation status by immunohistochemistry with

a mutation-specific monoclonal antibody. *Acta Neuropathol* (2011) **122**:11–9. doi:10.1007/s00401-011-0841-z
64. Capper D, Berghoff AS, Magerle M, Ilhan A, Wohrer A, Hackl M, et al. Immunohistochemical testing of BRAF V600E status in 1,120 tumor tissue samples of patients with brain metastases. *Acta Neuropathol* (2012) **123**:223–33. doi:10.1007/s00401-011-0887-y
65. Long GV, Wilmott JS, Capper D, Preusser M, Zhang YE, Thompson JF, et al. Immunohistochemistry is highly sensitive and specific for the detection of V600E BRAF mutation in melanoma. *Am J Surg Pathol* (2013) **37**:61–5. doi:10.1097/PAS.0b013e31826485c0
66. Colomba E, Helias-Rodzewicz Z, Von Deimling A, Marin C, Terrones N, Pechaud D, et al. Detection of BRAF p.V600E mutations in melanomas: comparison of four methods argues for sequential use of immunohistochemistry and pyrosequencing. *J Mol Diagn* (2013) **15**:94–100. doi:10.1016/j.jmoldx.2012.09.001
67. Busam KJ, Hedvat C, Pulitzer M, von Deimling A, Jungbluth AA. Immunohistochemical analysis of BRAF(V600E) expression of primary and metastatic melanoma and comparison with mutation status and melanocyte differentiation antigens of metastatic lesions. *Am J Surg Pathol* (2013) **37**:413–20. doi:10.1097/PAS.0b013e318271249e
68. Marin C, Beauchet A, Capper D, Zimmermann U, Julie C, Ilie M, et al. Detection of BRAF p.V600E mutations in melanoma by immunohistochemistry has a good interobserver reproducibility. *Arch Pathol Lab Med* (2013). doi:10.5858/arpa.2013-0031-OA
69. Yeh I, von Deimling A, Bastian BC. Clonal BRAF mutations in melanocytic nevi and initiating role of BRAF in melanocytic neoplasia. *J Natl Cancer Inst* (2013) **105**:917–9. doi:10.1093/jnci/djt119
70. Yancovitz M, Litterman A, Yoon J, Ng E, Shapiro RL, Berman RS, et al. Intra- and inter-tumor heterogeneity of BRAF(V600E) mutations in primary and metastatic melanoma. *PLoS ONE* (2012) **7**:e29336. doi:10.1371/journal.pone.0029336
71. Lin J, Goto Y, Murata H, Sakaizawa K, Uchiyama A, Saida T, et al. Polyclonality of BRAF mutations in primary melanoma and the selection of mutant alleles during progression. *Br J Cancer* (2011) **104**:464–8. doi:10.1038/sj.bjc.6606072
72. Wilmott JS, Menzies AM, Haydu LE, Capper D, Preusser M, Zhang YE, et al. (V600E) protein expression and outcome from BRAF inhibitor treatment in BRAF(V600E) metastatic melanoma. *Br J Cancer* (2013) **108**:924–31. doi:10.1038/bjc.2013.29
73. Rosell R, Moran T, Queralt C, Porta R, Cardenal F, Camps C, et al. Screening for epidermal growth factor receptor mutations in lung cancer. *N Engl J Med* (2009) **361**:958–67. doi:10.1056/NEJMoa0904554
74. Paez JG, Janne PA, Lee JC, Tracy S, Greulich H, Gabriel S, et al. EGFR mutations in lung cancer: correlation with clinical response to gefitinib therapy. *Science* (2004) **304**:1497–500. doi:10.1126/science.1099314
75. Tanaka T, Matsuoka M, Sutani A, Gemma A, Maemondo M, Inoue A, et al. Frequency of and variables associated with the EGFR mutation and its subtypes. *Int J Cancer* (2010) **126**:651–5. doi:10.1002/ijc.24746
76. Lynch TJ, Bell DW, Sordella R, Gurubhagavatula S, Okimoto RA, Brannigan BW, et al. Activating mutations in the epidermal growth factor receptor underlying responsiveness of non-small-cell lung cancer to gefitinib. *N Engl J Med* (2004) **350**:2129–39. doi:10.1056/NEJMoa040938
77. Eberhard DA, Johnson BE, Amler LC, Goddard AD, Heldens SL, Herbst RS, et al. Mutations in the epidermal growth factor receptor and in KRAS are predictive and prognostic indicators in patients with non-small-cell lung cancer treated with chemotherapy alone and in combination with erlotinib. *J Clin Oncol* (2005) **23**:5900–9. doi:10.1200/JCO.2005.02.857
78. Sharma SV, Bell DW, Settleman J, Haber DA. Epidermal growth factor receptor mutations in lung cancer. *Nat Rev Cancer* (2007) **7**:169–81. doi:10.1038/nrc2088
79. Brevet M, Arcila M, Ladanyi M. Assessment of EGFR mutation status in lung adenocarcinoma by immunohistochemistry using antibodies specific to the two major forms of mutant EGFR. *J Mol Diagn* (2010) **12**:169–76. doi:10.2353/jmoldx.2010.090140
80. Fan X, Liu B, Xu H, Yu B, Shi S, Zhang J, et al. Immunostaining with EGFR mutation-specific antibodies: a reliable screening method for lung adenocarcinomas harboring EGFR mutation in biopsy and resection samples. *Hum Pathol* (2013) **44**:1499–507. doi:10.1016/j.humpath.2012.12.002
81. Ho HL, Chang FP, Ma HH, Liao LR, Chuang YT, Chang-Chien YC, et al. Molecular diagnostic algorithm for epidermal growth factor receptor mutation detection in Asian lung adenocarcinomas: comprehensive analyses of 445 Taiwanese cases with immunohistochemistry, PCR-direct sequencing and Scorpion/ARMS methods. *Respirology* (2013). doi:10.1111/resp.12148
82. Kato Y, Peled N, Wynes MW, Yoshida K, Pardo M, Mascaux C, et al. Novel epidermal growth factor receptor mutation-specific antibodies for non-small cell lung cancer: immunohistochemistry as a possible screening method for epidermal growth factor receptor mutations. *J Thorac Oncol* (2010) **5**:1551–8. doi:10.1097/JTO.0b013e3181e9da60
83. Wu SG, Chang YL, Lin JW, Wu CT, Chen HY, Tsai MF, et al. Including total EGFR staining in scoring improves EGFR mutations detection by mutation-specific antibodies and EGFR TKIs response prediction. *PLoS ONE* (2011) **6**:e23303. doi:10.1371/journal.pone.0023303
84. Kitamura A, Hosoda W, Sasaki E, Mitsudomi T, Yatabe Y. Immunohistochemical detection of EGFR mutation using mutation-specific antibodies in lung cancer. *Clin Cancer Res* (2010) **16**:3349–55. doi:10.1158/1078-0432.CCR-10-0129
85. Angulo B, Conde E, Suarez-Gauthier A, Plaza C, Martinez R, Redondo P, et al. A comparison of EGFR mutation testing methods in lung carcinoma: direct sequencing, real-time PCR and immunohistochemistry. *PLoS ONE* (2012) **7**:e43842. doi:10.1371/journal.pone.0043842
86. Xiong Y, Bai Y, Leong N, Laughlin TS, Rothberg PG, Xu H, et al. Immunohistochemical detection of mutations in the epidermal growth factor receptor gene in lung adenocarcinomas using mutation-specific antibodies. *Diagn Pathol* (2013) **8**:27. doi:10.1186/1746-1596-8-27
87. Kawahara A, Taira T, Azuma K, Tominaga M, Hattori S, Kawahara M, et al. A diagnostic algorithm using EGFR mutation-specific antibodies for rapid response EGFR-TKI treatment in patients with non-small cell lung cancer. *Lung Cancer* (2012) **78**:39–44. doi:10.1016/j.lungcan.2012.07.002
88. Azuma K, Okamoto I, Kawahara A, Taira T, Nakashima K, Hattori S, et al. Association of the expression of mutant epidermal growth factor receptor protein as determined with mutation-specific antibodies in non-small cell lung cancer with progression-free survival after gefitinib treatment. *J Thorac Oncol* (2012) **7**:122–7. doi:10.1097/JTO.0b013e31822eeba2
89. Kozu Y, Tsuta K, Kohno T, Sekine I, Yoshida A, Watanabe S, et al. The usefulness of mutation-specific antibodies in detecting epidermal growth factor receptor mutations and in predicting response to tyrosine kinase inhibitor therapy in lung adenocarcinoma. *Lung Cancer* (2011) **73**:45–50. doi:10.1016/j.lungcan.2010.11.003
90. Wootla B, Denic A, Rodriguez M. Polyclonal and monoclonal antibodies in clinic. *Methods Mol Biol* (2014) **1060**:79–110. doi:10.1007/978-1-62703-586-6_5
91. Saito M, Sakurai S, Motegi A, Saito K, Sano T, Nakajima T. Comparative study using rabbit-derived polyclonal, mouse-derived monoclonal, and rabbit-derived monoclonal antibodies for KIT immunostaining in GIST and other tumors. *Pathol Int* (2007) **57**:200–4. doi:10.1111/j.1440-1827.2007.02081.x
92. Michel MC, Wieland T, Tsujimoto G. How reliable are G-protein-coupled receptor antibodies? *Naunyn Schmiedebergs Arch Pharmacol* (2009) **379**:385–8. doi:10.1007/s00210-009-0395-y
93. Skliris GP, Parkes AT, Limer JL, Burdall SE, Carder PJ, Speirs V. Evaluation of seven oestrogen receptor beta antibodies for immunohistochemistry, western blotting, and flow cytometry in human breast tissue. *J Pathol* (2002) **197**:155–62. doi:10.1002/path.1077
94. Bordeaux J, Welsh A, Agarwal S, Killiam E, Baquero M, Hanna J, et al. Antibody validation. *Biotechniques* (2010) **48**:197–209. doi:10.2144/000113382
95. Romer T, Leonhardt H, Rothbauer U. Engineering antibodies and proteins for molecular in vivo imaging. *Curr Opin Biotechnol* (2011) **22**:882–7. doi:10.1016/j.copbio.2011.06.007
96. Lofblom J, Frejd FY, Stahl S. Non-immunoglobulin based protein scaffolds. *Curr Opin Biotechnol* (2011) **22**:843–8. doi:10.1016/j.copbio.2011.06.002
97. Wurch T, Lowe P, Beck A, Corvaia N. Protein scaffolds as alternatives to whole antibodies: from discovery research to clinical development. *Med Sci (Paris)* (2009) **25**:1169–72. doi:10.1051/medsci/200925121169
98. Holliger P, Hudson PJ. Engineered antibody fragments and the rise of single domains. *Nat Biotechnol* (2005) **23**:1126–36. doi:10.1038/nbt1142
99. Hamers-Casterman C, Atarhouch T, Muyldermans S, Robinson G, Hamers C, Songa EB, et al. Naturally occurring antibodies devoid of light chains. *Nature* (1993) **363**:446–8. doi:10.1038/363446a0

100. Arbabi Ghahroudi M, Desmyter A, Wyns L, Hamers R, Muyldermans S. Selection and identification of single domain antibody fragments from camel heavy-chain antibodies. *FEBS Lett* (1997) **414**:521–6. doi:10.1016/S0014-5793(97)01062-4
101. Jobling SA, Jarman C, Teh MM, Holmberg N, Blake C, Verhoeyen ME. Immunomodulation of enzyme function in plants by single-domain antibody fragments. *Nat Biotechnol* (2003) **21**:77–80. doi:10.1038/nbt772
102. Rothbauer U, Zolghadr K, Tillib S, Nowak D, Schermelleh L, Gahl A, et al. Targeting and tracing antigens in live cells with fluorescent nanobodies. *Nat Methods* (2006) **3**:887–9. doi:10.1038/nmeth953
103. Muyldermans S. Single domain camel antibodies: current status. *J Biotechnol* (2001) **74**:277–302. doi:10.1016/S1389-0352(01)00021-6
104. Nilsson FY, Tolmachev V. Affibody molecules: new protein domains for molecular imaging and targeted tumor therapy. *Curr Opin Drug Discov Devel* (2007) **10**:167–75.
105. Lofblom J, Feldwisch J, Tolmachev V, Carlsson J, Stahl S, Frejd FY. Affibody molecules: engineered proteins for therapeutic, diagnostic and biotechnological applications. *FEBS Lett* (2010) **584**:2670–80. doi:10.1016/j.febslet.2010.04.014
106. Friedman M, Nordberg E, Hoiden-Guthenberg I, Brismar H, Adams GP, Nilsson FY, et al. Phage display selection of Affibody molecules with specific binding to the extracellular domain of the epidermal growth factor receptor. *Protein Eng Des Sel* (2007) **20**:189–99. doi:10.1093/protein/gzm011
107. Hoyer W, Gronwall C, Jonsson A, Stahl S, Hard T. Stabilization of a beta-hairpin in monomeric Alzheimer's amyloid-beta peptide inhibits amyloid formation. *Proc Natl Acad Sci U S A* (2008) **105**:5099–104. doi:10.1073/pnas.0711731105
108. Gronwall C, Snelders E, Palm AJ, Eriksson F, Herne N, Stahl S. Generation of Affibody ligands binding interleukin-2 receptor alpha/CD25. *Biotechnol Appl Biochem* (2008) **50**:97–112. doi:10.1042/BA20070261
109. Kramer-Marek G, Kiesewetter DO, Martiniova L, Jagoda E, Lee SB, Capala J. [18F]FBEM-Z(HER2:342)-Affibody molecule-a new molecular tracer for in vivo monitoring of HER2 expression by positron emission tomography. *Eur J Nucl Med Mol Imaging* (2008) **35**:1008–18. doi:10.1007/s00259-007-0658-0
110. Tran T, Orlova A, Sivaev I, Sandstrom M, Tolmachev V. Comparison of benzoate- and dodecaborate-based linkers for attachment of radioiodine to HER2-targeting Affibody ligand. *Int J Mol Med* (2007) **19**:485–93.
111. Stumpp MT, Amstutz P. DARPins: a true alternative to antibodies. *Curr Opin Drug Discov Devel* (2007) **10**:153–9.
112. Boersma YL, Pluckthun A. DARPins and other repeat protein scaffolds: advances in engineering and applications. *Curr Opin Biotechnol* (2011) **22**:849–57. doi:10.1016/j.copbio.2011.06.004
113. Theurillat JP, Dreier B, Nagy-Davidescu G, Seifert B, Behnke S, Zurrer-Hardi U, et al. Designed ankyrin repeat proteins: a novel tool for testing epidermal growth factor receptor 2 expression in breast cancer. *Mod Pathol* (2010) **23**:1289–97. doi:10.1038/modpathol.2010.103
114. Simon M, Zangemeister-Wittke U, Pluckthun A. Facile double-functionalization of designed ankyrin repeat proteins using click and thiol chemistries. *Bioconjug Chem* (2012) **23**:279–86. doi:10.1021/bc200591x
115. Ni X, Castanares M, Mukherjee A, Lupold SE. Nucleic acid aptamers: clinical applications and promising new horizons. *Curr Med Chem* (2011) **18**:4206–14. doi:10.2174/092986711797189600
116. Hu M, Zhang K. The application of aptamers in cancer research: an up-to-date review. *Future Oncol* (2013) **9**:369–76. doi:10.2217/fon.12.201
117. Shangguan D, Li Y, Tang Z, Cao ZC, Chen HW, Mallikaratchy P, et al. Aptamers evolved from live cells as effective molecular probes for cancer study. *Proc Natl Acad Sci U S A* (2006) **103**:11838–43. doi:10.1073/pnas.0602615103
118. Gilbert JC, DeFeo-Fraulini T, Hutabarat RM, Horvath CJ, Merlino PG, Marsh HN, et al. First-in-human evaluation of anti von Willebrand factor therapeutic aptamer ARC1779 in healthy volunteers. *Circulation* (2007) **116**:2678–86. doi:10.1161/CIRCULATIONAHA.107.724864
119. Green LS, Jellinek D, Bell C, Beebe LA, Feistner BD, Gill SC, et al. Nuclease-resistant nucleic acid ligands to vascular permeability factor/vascular endothelial growth factor. *Chem Biol* (1995) **2**:683–95. doi:10.1016/1074-5521(95)90032-2
120. Green LS, Jellinek D, Jenison R, Ostman A, Heldin CH, Janjic N. Inhibitory DNA ligands to platelet-derived growth factor B-chain. *Biochemistry* (1996) **35**:14413–24. doi:10.1021/bi961544+
121. Lupold SE, Hicke BJ, Lin Y, Coffey DS. Identification and characterization of nuclease-stabilized RNA molecules that bind human prostate cancer cells via the prostate-specific membrane antigen. *Cancer Res* (2002) **62**:4029–33.
122. Casado P, Alcolea MP, Iorio F, Rodriguez-Prados JC, Vanhaesebroeck B, Saez-Rodriguez J, et al. Phosphoproteomics data classify hematological cancer cell lines according to tumor type and sensitivity to kinase inhibitors. *Genome Biol* (2013) **14**:R37. doi:10.1186/gb-2013-14-4-r37
123. Hanahan D, Weinberg RA. Hallmarks of cancer: the next generation. *Cell* (2011) **144**:646–74. doi:10.1016/j.cell.2011.02.013
124. Soderberg O, Leuchowius KJ, Gullberg M, Jarvius M, Weibrecht I, Larsson LG, et al. Characterizing proteins and their interactions in cells and tissues using the in situ proximity ligation assay. *Methods* (2008) **45**:227–32. doi:10.1016/j.ymeth.2008.06.014
125. Soderberg O, Gullberg M, Jarvius M, Ridderstrale K, Leuchowius KJ, Jarvius J, et al. Direct observation of individual endogenous protein complexes in situ by proximity ligation. *Nat Methods* (2006) **3**:995–1000. doi:10.1038/nmeth947
126. Fredriksson S, Gullberg M, Jarvius J, Olsson C, Pietras K, Gustafsdottir SM, et al. Protein detection using proximity-dependent DNA ligation assays. *Nat Biotechnol* (2002) **20**:473–7. doi:10.1038/nbt0502-473
127. Zieba A, Wahlby C, Hjelm F, Jordan L, Berg J, Landegren U, et al. Bright-field microscopy visualization of proteins and protein complexes by in situ proximity ligation with peroxidase detection. *Clin Chem* (2010) **56**:99–110. doi:10.1373/clinchem.2009.134452
128. Clausson CM, Allalou A, Weibrecht I, Mahmoudi S, Farnebo M, Landegren U, et al. Increasing the dynamic range of in situ PLA. *Nat Methods* (2011) **8**:892–3. doi:10.1038/nmeth.1743
129. Leuchowius KJ, Clausson CM, Grannas K, Erbilgin Y, Botling J, Zieba A, et al. Parallel visualization of multiple protein complexes in individual cells in tumor tissue. *Mol Cell Proteomics* (2013) **12**:1563–71. doi:10.1074/mcp.O112.023374
130. Gajadhar AS, Bogdanovic E, Munoz DM, Guha A. In situ analysis of mutant EGFRs prevalent in glioblastoma multiforme reveals aberrant dimerization, activation, and differential response to anti-EGFR targeted therapy. *Mol Cancer Res* (2012) **10**:428–40. doi:10.1158/1541-7786.MCR-11-0531
131. Spears M, Taylor KJ, Munro AF, Cunningham CA, Mallon EA, Twelves CJ, et al. In situ detection of HER2:HER2 and HER2:HER3 protein-protein interactions demonstrates prognostic significance in early breast cancer. *Breast Cancer Res Treat* (2012) **132**:463–70. doi:10.1007/s10549-011-1606-z
132. Leuchowius KJ, Jarvius M, Wickstrom M, Rickardson L, Landegren U, Larsson R, et al. High content screening for inhibitors of protein interactions and post-translational modifications in primary cells by proximity ligation. *Mol Cell Proteomics* (2010) **9**:178–83. doi:10.1074/mcp.M900331-MCP200
133. Uhlen M, Oksvold P, Fagerberg L, Lundberg E, Jonasson K, Forsberg M, et al. Towards a knowledge-based Human Protein Atlas. *Nat Biotechnol* (2010) **28**:1248–50. doi:10.1038/nbt1210-1248
134. Ponten F, Schwenk JM, Asplund A, Edqvist PH. The Human Protein Atlas as a proteomic resource for biomarker discovery. *J Intern Med* (2011) **270**:428–46. doi:10.1111/j.1365-2796.2011.02427.x

14

miR-21 expression in cancer cells may not predict resistance to adjuvant trastuzumab in primary breast cancer

Boye Schnack Nielsen[1]*, Eva Balslev[2], Tim Svenstrup Poulsen[2], Dorte Nielsen[3], Trine Møller[1], Christiane Ehlers Mortensen[3], Kim Holmstrøm[1] and Estrid Høgdall[2]

[1] *Bioneer A/S, Hørsholm, Denmark*
[2] *Department of Pathology, Herlev Hospital, University of Copenhagen, Herlev, Denmark*
[3] *Department of Oncology, Herlev Hospital, University of Copenhagen, Herlev, Denmark*

Edited by:
Jan Trøst Jørgensen, Dx-Rx Institute, Denmark

Reviewed by:
Revati Wani, Pfizer Inc., USA
Ricardo Martinez, Eli Lilly, USA

Correspondence:
Boye Schnack Nielsen, Molecular Histology, Bioneer A/S, Kogle Allé 2, Hørsholm 2970, Denmark
e-mail: bsn@bioneer.dk

Trastuzumab is established as standard care for patients with HER2-positive breast cancer both in the adjuvant and metastatic setting. However, 50% of the patients do not respond to the trastuzumab therapy, and therefore new predictive biomarkers are highly warranted. MicroRNAs (miRs) constitute a new group of biomarkers and their cellular expression can be determined in tumor samples by *in situ* hybridization (ISH) analysis. miR-21 is highly prevalent and up-regulated in breast cancer and has been linked to drug resistance in clinical and *in vitro* settings. To determine expression patterns of miR-21 in high-grade breast cancers, we examined miR-21 expression in 22 HER2-positive tumors and 15 HER2-negative high-grade tumors by ISH. The histological examination indicated that patient samples could be divided into three major expression patterns: miR-21 predominantly in tumor stroma, predominantly in cancer cells, or in both stromal and cancer cells. There was no obvious difference between the HER2-positive and HER2-negative tumors in terms of the miR-21 expression patterns and intensities. To explore the possibility that miR-21 expression levels and/or cellular localization could predict resistance to adjuvant trastuzumab in HER2-positive breast cancer patients, we analyzed additional 16 HER2-positive tumors from patients who were treated with trastuzumab in the adjuvant setting. Eight of the 16 patients showed clinical recurrence and were considered resistant. Examination of the miR-21 expression patterns and intensities revealed no association between the miR-21 scores in the cancer cell population ($p = 0.69$) or the stromal cells population ($p = 0.13$) and recurrent disease after adjuvant trastuzumab. Thus, our findings show that elevated miR-21 expression does not predict resistance to adjuvant trastuzumab.

Keywords: biomarker, breast cancer, HER2, miR-21, prediction, response, trastuzumab

INTRODUCTION

The human epidermal growth factor receptor-2 (HER2, NEU, and c-ERBB-2) is a cell surface receptor tyrosine kinase that is strongly up-regulated in more than 15% of all breast cancers (1), and breast cancer patients with HER2 overexpressing tumors have poor prognosis (2, 3). HER2-directed therapy using the humanized monoclonal antibody, trastuzumab in combination with conventional chemotherapy, improves overall survival in patients with HER2-positive breast cancers (4). However, only half of the HER2-positive breast cancer patients respond to the HER2-directed therapy (5). The lack of therapeutic efficacy and high cost of the therapeutic agent urges identification and development of predictive markers as companion diagnostics. So far, no clinically validated predictive markers for response to trastuzumab have been reported.

MicroRNAs (miRs) are short non-coding RNAs that regulate protein synthesis at the post-transcriptional level by binding to the 3'UTR of mRNAs causing mRNA destabilization or degradation. miRs can be measured in tissues and body fluids by *in situ* hybridization (ISH), qPCR, and microarray or high-throughput sequencing, and as such, miRs constitute a relatively novel group of biomarkers. One of the most abundant miRs in solid tumors is miR-21. miR-21 expression is highly increased in malignant tumors, including breast, colon, lung, and brain cancer (6, 7), and high expression levels are associated with poor prognosis (8–11). Solid tumors, including breast cancers, are complex tissues consisting of the malignant epithelial cells and a surrounding stroma consisting of fibroblasts, inflammatory cells, and vascular cells. ISH studies of tissue from breast, colon, brain, pancreas, and esophagus cancer (10–14) have shown that miR-21 is predominantly expressed in the stromal cells; however, subpopulations of miR-21 positive cancer cells are also reported (10, 11, 15).

Some miRs are found to be indicators of drug resistance and some even to confer drug resistance to a variety of cancer drugs (16–18). miR-21 is one the most studied and has been found to confer drug resistance to trastuzumab (19), 5-fluorouracil (20, 21), doxorubicin (22, 23), cisplatin (24, 25), and paclitaxel (26). Gong et al. (19) reported that high miR-21 levels in breast cancer biopsies before and after neoadjuvant trastuzumab were associated with trastuzumab resistance, and that blocking the action of miR-21 re-sensitized resistant breast cancer cell lines to trastuzumab (19). The authors suggested that miR-21 may function through the tumor suppressor phosphatase and tensin homolog (PTEN), a well-described miR-21 target protein (27–29), which has been reported to be a potential predictor for trastuzumab resistance (30). Thus, miR-21 may play an important role in multi-drug resistance mechanisms.

Recent studies have indicated that drug resistance in cancer therapy is not only related to the malignant cancer cells, but also to cells in the stromal compartment (31–34). For example, in the study by Alkhateeb et al. (34), high levels of inflammation markers measured in serum from HER2-positive breast cancer patients were associated with poor response to trastuzumab-containing therapy. Thus, molecular biomarkers derived from the breast cancer stroma should also be considered in the search for novel predictive biomarkers.

In this paper, we addressed whether miR-21 ISH analysis in primary breast cancers can help to predict trastuzumab resistance in HER2-positive breast cancer patients treated with trastuzumab in the adjuvant setting, and whether the miR-21 expression pattern correlated with HER2 status or other known clinical markers.

MATERIALS AND METHODS

PATIENTS

Tissue samples were separated into two sample groups, here named reference group and study group (see also **Table 1**). The reference group included 36 breast cancer samples from patients diagnosed 1999–2009 with high-grade invasive ductal carcinoma (IDC). Among them, 21 cases were HER2-positive and 15 cases were HER2-negative. The study group included samples from 16 HER2-positive ethnic Danish breast cancers patients. These patients were diagnosed from 2005 to 2008 and had their primary tumor surgically removed and received adjuvant trastuzumab (trastuzumab/Herceptin was obtained from Roche). After surgery, the patients received adjuvant chemotherapy, irradiation, and anti-hormonal treatment according to national standards, and eventually trastuzumab. All patients received trastuzumab every third week for one year. None of the patients had been treated for breast cancer previously. Eight patients developed recurrent disease with distant metastases after 5–8 years of follow up. In the present study, we considered these patients as resistant to trastuzumab. Patients without recurrence were considered sensitive. All samples were obtained from the local tissue bank (Herlev Hospital, Copenhagen, Denmark) as formalin-fixed paraffin-embedded (FFPE, here fixed within 1 h of surgery by 24–72 h incubation in formalin at room temperature). Tumor grade was based on HE stained sections. The study was performed in accordance with permission given by The Regional Scientific-Ethical Committee for Copenhagen, Denmark (J. nr. H-3-2014-010).

Table 1 | Patients included in this study.

	n	Age (range)	Diagnosis year	HER2 neg (*n*)	HER2 pos (*n*)
Reference group	36	62 (36–92)	1999–2009	15	21
Study group	16	51 (33–68)	2005–2008	0	16

Age range and year range of diagnosis are indicated for the reference group and study group.

IMMUNOHISTOCHEMISTRY

Immunoperoxidase staining for clinical biomarkers included staining for ER (mAb clone SP1, Dako, Glostrup, Denmark), PR (mAb clone PqR636, Dako), P53 (mAb clone DO7, Dako), Ki67 (mAb clone Mib1, Dako), and HER2 (mAb clone 4B5, Roche). For ER (RTU), PR (mAb diluted 1:100), P53 (mAb diluted 1:200), and Ki67 (mAb diluted 1:200), 3–5 μm tissue sections were pre-treated using DakoLink and stained in a Dako immunostainer, whereas HER2 staining was performed using a Ventana instrument (Ventana) according to the manufacturers guidelines. Scores of ER, PR, p53, and Ki67 were the percentage of positive cancer cells. The IHC scores of HER2 were performed in accordance with the HercepTest™ Interpretation Manual – Breast (Dako, Glostrup, Denmark).

HER2 FISH

Cases that scored 2 in HER2 immunoperoxidase staining were additionally tested by FISH analysis using the HER2 FISH pharmDx™ Kit-K331 (Dako, Glostrup, Denmark) according to the manufacturers' instructions.

MicroRNA-21 *IN SITU* HYBRIDIZATION AND SCORING

Automated miR-21 ISH was performed on a Tecan Genepaint instrument (Tecan, Switzerland) essentially as described previously (10). In brief, deparaffinized sections were treated with proteinase-K (25 μg/mL for 8 min at 37°C). Double-FAM-labeled miR-21 and scrambled LNA™ probes (Exiqon, Vedbæk, Denmark) were incubated at 30 nM for 1 h in Exiqon hybridization buffer (Exiqon) at 57°C. The probes were detected with alkaline-phosphatase conjugated anti-FAM (1:800, Roche) for 30 min at 30°C and then incubated with freshly prepared NBT-BCIP substrate containing 0.2 nM levamisole for 1 h at 30°C. For scoring of the miR-21 ISH staining, we obtained digital whole slides using a Hamamatsu scanner (20× objective). The miR-21 staining was scored at the level of cellular tissue compartments, stromal vs. cancer cells, and at the level of staining intensity/density (0, 1, 2, or 3). Score 0, indicated no staining or similar staining as background level, score 1 indicated staining in a subset of cells that could be weak or intense (up to 10%), score 2 indicated staining in a larger subset of cells (10–50% of the cells) that could be weak or intense, and score 3 indicated intense staining in virtually all cells of the tissue compartment (examples of miR-21 scores are shown in **Figure 1**). Scoring was performed independently blinded by two observers (Eva Balslev and Boye Schnack Nielsen). If the difference between scores was more than one, a consensus score was determined. The averages of the two scores are presented.

MicroRNA-21/HER2 DOUBLE STAINING

MicroRNA-21 ISH combined with immunohistochemical staining for HER2 was performed essentially as described (35). After proteinase-K treatment, sections were hybridized with 20 nM

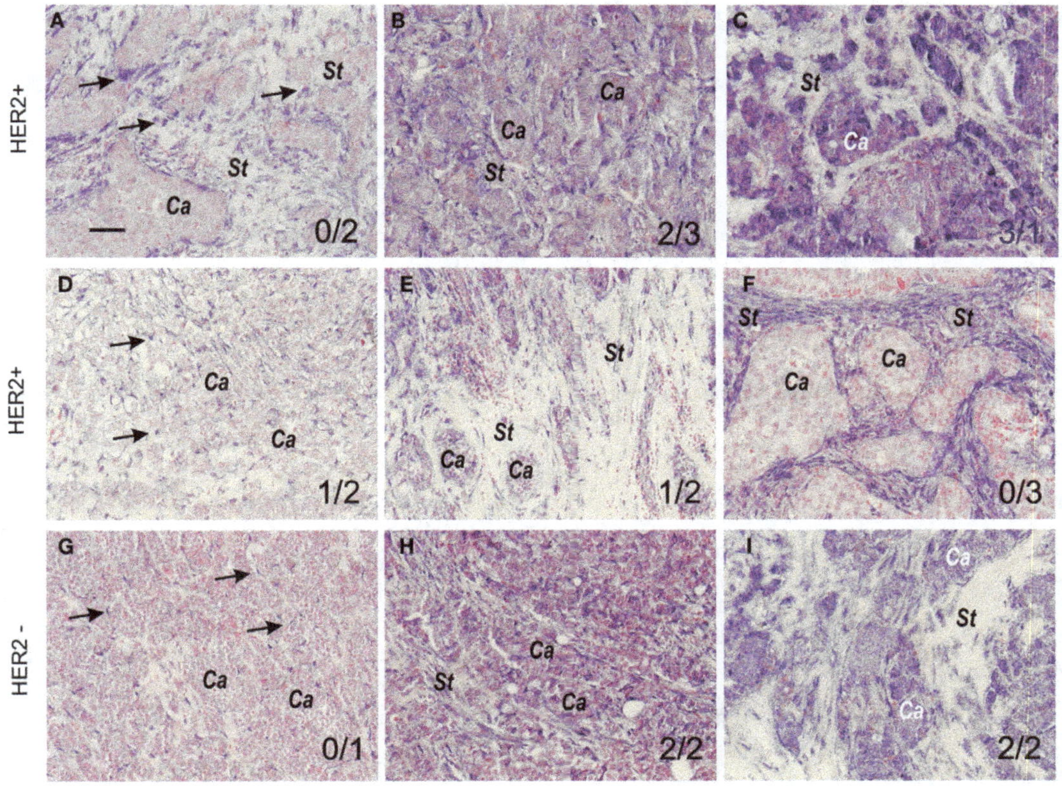

FIGURE 1 | MicroRNA-21 expression patterns and scoring in grade 3 breast cancers. Representative miR-21 ISH expression patterns and intensities in HER2-positive **(A–F)** and HER2-negative tumors **(G–I)**. The miR-21 ISH signal (dark blue staining, examples indicated by arrows in **(A)**) is seen exclusively in stromal cells **(A,D,F,** and **G)**, or in both stromal cells and cancer cells **(B,C,E,H,** and **I)**. Stromal and cancer cell tissue compartments are indicated by *St* and *Ca*, respectively. In **(D,G,** and **H)**, arrows indicate miR-21 positive stromal cells. The variations in miR-21 ISH signal intensity and prevalence of positive cells were scored 0, 1, 2, or 3 by two observers (see Material and Methods section) in both cancer and stromal cells. The miR-21^{CC} and miR-21St scores are indicated (miR-21^{CC}/miR-21St). All sections were counter stained with nuclear fast red. The examples are from tumors in the reference group and are representative for the individual tumors. Bar: 50 μm.

miR-21 LNA probe for 1 h, and the probe was detected with peroxidase-conjugated anti-FAM (Roche) followed by incubation tyramine-signal-amplification (TSA)-Cy5 substrate for 5 min at room temperature. Polyclonal rabbit anti-ErbB-2 (ab2428, AbCam, Cambridge, UK) was incubated at room temperature and detected with Cy3-conjugated goat anti rabbit (Jackson ImmunoResearch, West Grove, PA, USA). Slides were mounted with Antifade Gold with DAPI (Invitrogen).

STATISTICS

Spearman's rank correlation analyses of miR-21 scores and known clinical parameters were conducted to obtain Spearman rank correlation coefficients, *r*. The differences in miR-21 scores between HER2-positive and HER2-negative, and trastuzumab-sensitive and -resistant patient groups were evaluated using the non-parametric Mann–Whitney *U* test. Statistical significance was considered at the 5% probability level ($p < 0.05$). All statistical analyses and calculations were performed with GraphPad Prism 5 (GraphPad Sofware, La Jolla, CA, USA).

RESULTS

PATIENTS

The patient material is briefly described in **Table 1**. The patient samples in the reference group were used to delineate miR-21 expression patterns and intensities in high-grade breast cancers and to establish a miR-21 scoring system. The miR-21 scores were compared with known clinical parameters, including the HER2 status. The samples in the study group were used to evaluate the miR-21 expression patterns and intensities, to obtain miR-21 scores for correlation with recurrence of disease after adjuvant trastuzumab.

MicroRNA-21 EXPRESSION PATTERNS AND SCORING

MicroRNA-21 ISH was performed in parallel on the 36 samples on an automated platform. miR-21 ISH signal was seen in all cases with variation both in staining intensity and in localization. Among the 36 tumors, all showed staining in tumor stromal cells, mostly fibroblasts, but probably also inflammatory and endothelial cells were positive. The stromal miR-21 staining varied from confined focal staining, with most intense staining in the fibroblastic cells surrounding islands of cancer cells, to staining involving most of or the whole tumor stroma. Using a semiquantitative approach, we scored the miR-21 stroma staining (miR-21st) gradually 1, 2, or 3 as described in Material and Methods section (examples in **Figure 1**). miR-21 ISH signal was also prevalent in cancer cells (miR-21^{CC}) in 23 of the cases, and the positive reaction was scored 0, 1, 2, or 3 in terms of staining intensity

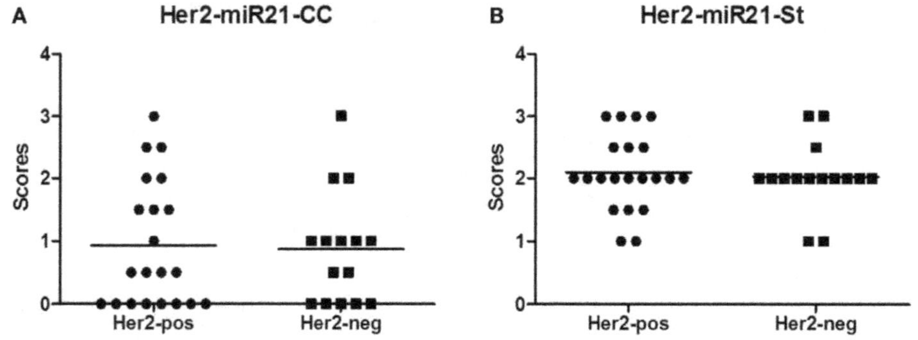

FIGURE 2 | MicroRNA (miR)-21 scores in the HER2 reference group. The miR-21 scoring was performed as described in Material and Methods section, here presented as average scores of two observers: miR-21^{CC} **(A)** and miR-21^{St} **(B)**.

Table 2 | Correlation analyses.

		n	miR-21^{St}	ER	PR	Ki67	P53
miR-21^{CC}	HER2 pos	21	−0.31	−0.07	0.03	−0.24	0.03
	HER2 neg	15	−0.14	0.38	0.56*	−0.04	0.35
	All	36	−0.22	0.07	0.22	−0.15	0.15
		n	**miR-21^{CC}**	**ER**	**PR**	**Ki67**	**P53**
miR-21^{St}	HER2 pos	21	−0.31	0.11	0.19	−0.19	−0.24
	HER2 neg	15	−0.14	−0.26	0.13	−0.17	−0.37
	All	36	−0.22	−0.07	0.14	−0.22	−0.26

*Spearman correlation analyses of miR-21 scores (cancer cell expression, miR-21^{CC} and stromal expression, miR-21^{St}) and available clinical parameters here separated into HER2-negative and positive tumors (Spearman correlations, *$p < 0.05$).*

(examples in **Figure 1**). In general, miR-21 ISH signal was equally intense in all stained tumor cells in the same tumor, however, some variations were observed. Most dramatic variation was seen in two cases (both HER2-negative) in which one tumor cell compartment showed strong staining, whereas an adjacent tumor cell compartment showed virtually no staining (data not shown). In these two cases the scores presented are those with highest staining intensity. Intensely stained myoepithelial cells surrounding foci of carcinoma *in situ* (CIS) were seen in 8 of the 36 cases (data not shown). No ISH signal was obtained with the scramble probe in any of the samples. Additional specificity analyses of the miR-21 ISH probe in breast cancer samples have been performed previously (12).

MicroRNA-21 LOCALIZATION AND HER2 STATUS AND OTHER CLINICAL PARAMETERS

There was no obvious difference in the miR-21^{CC} expression pattern or miR-21^{St} expression pattern when comparing HER2-positive with HER2-negative cases (**Figure 2**), suggesting that the miR-21 expression pattern is independent of the HER2 status. A series of additional molecular parameters were obtained from the cohort by immunohistochemistry: ER, PR, Ki67, and p53 and then correlated with the miR-21 scores (**Table 2**). In HER2-negative tumors, we noted a significant positive correlation ($p = 0.04$) between miR-21^{CC} and elevated PR. Otherwise, none of these parameters showed significant correlation with the two miR-21 scores, miR-21^{CC} and miR-21^{St}. We have previously reported that increased stromal miR-21 levels in grade 1 and 2 lesions are associated with increased cancer cell proliferation as measured by the Ki67 index (12). We did not see a similar correlation in these grade 3 lesions.

MicroRNA-21 CO-LOCALIZES WITH HER2

In order to perform double fluorescence analysis of HER2 and miR-21, we employed a polyclonal antibody, which was compatible with the proteinase-K-directed antigen retrieval needed for miR ISH on FFPE samples. Six samples from the reference group were selected for miR-21/HER2 double immunofluorescence based on (1) the intense staining for HER2 with the polyclonal antibody and (2) the miR-21^{CC} and/or miR-21^{St} positive staining. As expected, we found miR-21 ISH signal in HER2-positive cancer cells (**Figure 3**). We noted that the miR-21 staining intensity in HER2-positive cancer cells varied from absent to strongly positive. For comparison, in a case with prevalent stromal miR-21, we found miR-21 positive stromal cells surrounding HER2-positive clusters of cancers cells (**Figure 3**).

MicroRNA-21 STAINING PATTERNS AND RECURRENCE AFTER HER2-DIRECTED THERAPY

MicroRNA-21 ISH was then performed in parallel on the 16 HER2-positive cases with known disease status after adjuvant trastuzumab. Eight of the patients experienced no recurrent disease after treatment within the 5–8 years follow-up period (sensitive tumors), whereas the other eight patients experienced recurrent disease (resistant tumors). Examination of the miR-21 staining patterns in these samples indicated expression patterns similar to those observed in the *reference group*, thus both tumors with predominant miR-21^{CC} and miR-21^{St} were present (**Figure 4**). However, there was no significant difference in the miR-21^{CC} and miR-21^{St} as well as in the summarized total average miR-21 scores, when comparing resistant and sensitive tumors (Mann–Whitney *U* test). Thus, we found no indications that miR-21 expression patterns could help to identify HER2-positive patients resistant to adjuvant trastuzumab in this study group.

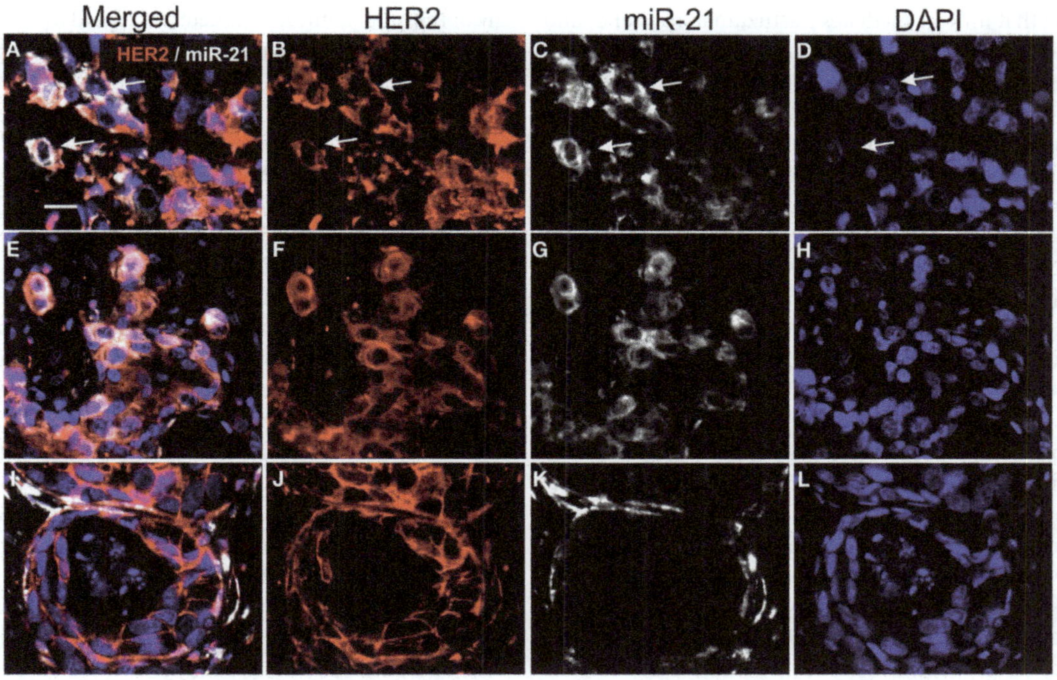

FIGURE 3 | Double staining for miR-21 and HER2 in HER2-positive breast cancers. Tissue sections were processed first for miR-21 ISH and subsequently for HER2 IHC. The figure shows three cases **(A–D)**, **(E–H)** and **(I–L)**. miR-21 was detected using TSA-Cy5 substrate (white) and HER2 with Cy3-conjugated anti-rabbit antibody (red). All sections were counterstained with DAPI (blue). miR-21 ISH signal is seen in HER2-positive cancer cells in cases **(A–D)** and **(E–H)** [examples are indicated by arrows in **(A–D)**], whereas HER2-positive cancer cells in case **(I–L)** are miR-21-negative. The examples are from tumors in the reference group and are representative for the three tumors. Bars: 20 μm.

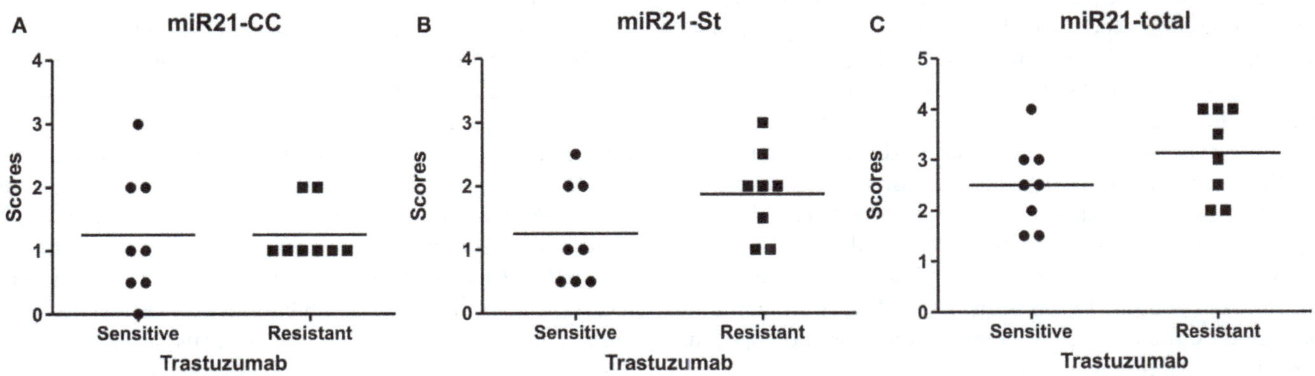

FIGURE 4 | MicroRNA-21 scores in the HER2 study group. The miR-21 scores for cancer cell-associated miR-21 expression, miR-21^{CC} **(A)**, miR-21 stromal expression, miR-21St **(B)**, and the total summarized miR-21 scores **(C)**. The scores are averages of two observers and here presented in scatter grams. Mann–Whitney *U* test: $p = 0.69$ for miR-21^{CC}, $p = 0.13$ for miR-21St, and $p = 0.20$ for total miR-21.

DISCUSSION

MicroRNA-21 is one of the most prevalent miRs in solid tumors, and increased expression levels are associated with poor prognosis both in untreated early-stage colon cancer patients (8, 10, 15) and in breast and colon cancer patients treated with chemotherapy (8, 9, 36, 37). In addition, several recent studies have suggested that miR-21 confers drug resistance to cancer cells *in vitro* (38, 39), including resistance to trastuzumab treatment of HER2-positive patients (19). We assumed that if miR-21 indeed confers drug resistance in HER2 breast cancer patients, knowing the specific cellular origin of miR-21 in the tumors may help to predict response to HER2-directed therapy. In this study, we show that miR-21 is highly expressed in high-grade breast cancers, both in HER2-positive and negative cases, and that miR-21 ISH signal can be seen in both stromal cells and cancer cells in varying expression levels.

Gong et al. (19) found increased miR-21 ISH signal in resistant tumors before and after trastuzumab-directed therapy, and showed that miR-21 antisense oligonucleotides could restore trastuzumab sensitivity in resistant cells by inducing PTEN expression, suggesting that miR-21 mediates trastuzumab resistance and that antagonizing miR-21 in a therapeutic setting could sensitize cancer cells to HER2-directed therapy. Indeed, we found that both miR-21 ISH signal and HER2 immunoreactivity are seen in the same cancer cells, which would be a prerequisite for successful combination of anti-miR-21 and HER2-directed therapy. In order to assess if miR-21^{CC} expression could predict the response to trastuzumab therapy, we examined the cellular expression of miR-21^{CC} in 16 HER2-positive tumors, half of which relapsed within the 5–8 years follow-up period after adjuvant trastuzumab. However, since we also found miR-21^{CC} expression in trastuzumab-sensitive tumors at the same frequency, our findings do not indicate that high miR-21^{CC} can predict recurrence. Based on our studies of 16 patients treated in the adjuvant setting, our observations imply that miR-21 did not confer trastuzumab resistance, a finding which appears inconsistent with the conclusion drawn by Gong et al. (19), who investigated 32 patients treated in the neoadjuvant setting. However, the major difference in treatment protocols of the two studies does not justify a direct comparison of the results.

Although the relatively small sample size offered little statistical strength to our observations, it should be noted that the concomitant adjuvant chemotherapy may have been a confounding factor that prevented identification of a direct link between miR-21 expression and trastuzumab resistance. Likewise, small patient groups will be relatively sensitive to genetic variation, which in our case may also have contributed to cover the impact of miR-21 as a predictive biomarker. Another parameter that may have prevented identification of a direct link between miR-21 and trastuzumab resistance is the semiquantitative scoring approach employed. In order to minimize experimental variation in staining intensities, all sections, both in the reference group and in the study group, were processed identically and stained in parallel on an automated platform. Manual scoring was then performed on digital whole slides by two observers, and since considerable variation between samples could easily be discriminated, we assumed that our scoring approach was not a limiting factor. Furthermore, a manual scoring approach could potentially be implemented in the daily diagnosis. In previous studies, we used image analysis to obtain quantitative estimates of miR-21 expression (10, 12, 15), but common for those studies, the expression patterns were more homogenous. Here, the cellular origin of expression was a key parameter. It cannot be excluded that alternative semiquantitative approaches may have classified the cases better. For example, RT-qPCR analyses of microdissected tissue compartments, stroma and cancer cells, may potentially provide useful quantitative estimates of the miR-21 expression. Thus, more studies, including examination of the primary and recurrent tumors in both the adjuvant and neoadjuvant settings, are needed to better address how the miR-21^{CC} (and miR-21St) parameters potentially can be used as predictive biomarkers.

In our previous study of miR-21 in grade 1–2 breast cancers (12), none of the 24 included cases showed noteworthy expression in the cancer cells. In the current study, 9 of the 36 cases (25%) showed intense miR-21^{CC} (miR-21^{CC} score 2 or above). These miR-21^{CC} cases included both hormone receptor-positive and -negative cases. Furthermore, miR-21^{CC} did not correlate with any of the other clinical parameters analyzed in the HER2-positive tumors. In HER2-negative tumors, we found a significant positive correlation between miR-21^{CC} and PR. The significance of this association will need to be further explored. Because miR-21 was found strongly expressed in myoepithelial cells surrounding occasional CIS structures in some of the lesions, it is tempting to speculate whether the miR-21^{CC} cases were all of the basal subtype. However, this is unlikely since some of the miR-21^{CC} cases were ER-positive. Thus, our data suggest that the miR-21^{CC} lesions represent an independent group of grade 3 breast cancers. The apparent variation in the cellular expression pattern of miR-21 is an important feature that may impact on targeted therapy since miR-21 in different cell populations may have different (mRNA) targets. Sempere et al. (40) analyzed breast cancers of various grades and hormone receptor status and reported frequent expression in cancer cells as well as expression in the breast cancer-associated fibroblast in some cases. More studies are needed to better establish whether high miR-21 expression in cancer cells is confined to grade 3 breast cancers.

As mentioned above, increased miR-21 expression levels are associated with adverse prognosis in several types of cancer. Experimental studies of tumor models in mice support these findings. In a K-ras-dependent lung cancer model, overexpression of miR-21 caused increased tumor formation, whereas miR-21 deficiency reduced the tumor formation (41). In a skin carcinogenesis model, miR-21 deficiency resulted in reduced papilloma formation (42). In addition, mice lacking the tumor suppressor p53 showed reduced tumor incidence if also lacking miR-21 (43). Thus, based on both clinical and experimental findings, miR-21 is likely a positive driver in the oncogenic process.

Two of the best described miR-21 targets are the tumor suppressors PDCD4 and PTEN. In the context of this study, it is notable that Huang et al. (44) found that activation of HER2 up-regulates miR-21 in breast cancer cell lines and causes successive down-regulation of PDCD4 preventing the tumor cells to enter apoptosis. However, PDCD4 is likely a multifunctional protein, whose role in cancer is only partly understood. PDCD4 was originally found as a nuclear antigen of proliferating cells (45), while others found PDCD4 associated with apoptosis (46, 47). In addition, PDCD4 was reported to be an inhibitor of neoplastic transformation and metastasis (48, 49). In breast cancer tissue, PDCD4 is seen in both normal and malignant epithelial cells and localizes to the nuclei and/or the cytoplasm (50). It remains to be established if miR-21 is involved in the regulation of all of these pivotal functions of PDCD4. Like PDCD4, PTEN has been found in relation to cell proliferation and apoptosis (51), and its presence has been linked to drug resistance (30). Lack of PTEN in breast tumor stroma has, in model systems, been found to strongly enhance transformation of the mammary epithelium (52, 53). In our study, high levels of miR-21 in the breast cancer stroma, which would cause miR-21-directed loss of stromal PTEN, were weakly ($p = 0.13$) associated with resistance to adjuvant trastuzumab. Trastuzumab resistance was reported in patients with breast cancers that were PTEN-negative in immunohistochemistry (30), however, a systematic delineation of the presence of PTEN in different cellular compartments in breast cancer lesions is highly warranted, particularly in the light of recent studies implying that drug resistance can be generated through tumor stroma (31–34).

In our previous study of grade 1 and 2 breast cancers (12), we found that high stromal miR-21 levels determined by image analysis correlated significantly with increased Ki67 proliferation index. Quantitative assessment by image analysis of the miR-21 ISH signal in the current grade 3 samples was not accomplished due to the complex expression patterns as discussed above. However, our analysis of the miR-21 expression scores in the stroma or cancer cells in the current grade 3 cancers did not reveal correlation with the Ki67 index.

In conclusion, we have shown that the miR-21 expression patterns in HER2-positive breast cancers are highly variable being present in cancer and/or stromal cells, and not linked to known clinical parameters. In the relatively small group of HER2-positive tumors studied, our miR-21 ISH analyses did not contribute significantly to the identification of patients with recurrent disease after adjuvant trastuzumab. We noted that both miR-21^{CC} and miR-21^{St} were independent of ER, PR, Ki67, and p53, suggesting that more extensive studies on trastuzumab resistance are warranted across additional subgroups of breast cancer. Molecular markers of trastuzumab resistance like the serum-derived inflammatory biomarkers (34), or expression of PTEN (30), or truncated HER2 (54) have so far not successfully showed to be clinically valuable predictive biomarkers.

ACKNOWLEDGMENTS

The Danish CancerBiobank (DCB) is acknowledged for biological material and for the data regarding handling and storage.

REFERENCES

1. Dowsett M, Dunbier AK. Emerging biomarkers and new understanding of traditional markers in personalized therapy for breast cancer. *Clin Cancer Res* (2008) **14**(24):8019–26. doi:10.1158/1078-0432.ccr-08-0974
2. Antoniotti S, Taverna D, Maggiora P, Sapei ML, Hynes NE, De Bortoli M. Oestrogen and epidermal growth factor down-regulate erbB-2 oncogene protein expression in breast cancer cells by different mechanisms. *Br J Cancer* (1994) **70**(6):1095–101. doi:10.1038/bjc.1994.454
3. Ravdin PM, Chamness GC. The c-erbB-2 proto-oncogene as a prognostic and predictive marker in breast cancer: a paradigm for the development of other macromolecular markers – a review. *Gene* (1995) **159**(1):19–27. doi:10.1016/0378-1119(94)00866-Q
4. Slamon DJ, Leyland-Jones B, Shak S, Fuchs H, Paton V, Bajamonde A, et al. Use of chemotherapy plus a monoclonal antibody against HER2 for metastatic breast cancer that overexpresses HER2. *N Engl J Med* (2001) **344**(11):783–92. doi:10.1056/NEJM200103153441101
5. Nielsen DL, Kumler I, Palshof JA, Andersson M. Efficacy of HER2-targeted therapy in metastatic breast cancer. Monoclonal antibodies and tyrosine kinase inhibitors. *Breast* (2013) **22**(1):1–12. doi:10.1016/j.breast.2012.09.008
6. Fu X, Han Y, Wu Y, Zhu X, Lu X, Mao F, et al. Prognostic role of microRNA-21 in various carcinomas: a systematic review and meta-analysis. *Eur J Clin Invest* (2011) **41**(11):1245–53. doi:10.1111/j.1365-2362.2011.02535.x
7. Kumarswamy R, Volkmann I, Thum T. Regulation and function of miRNA-21 in health and disease. *RNA Biol* (2011) **8**(5):706–13. doi:10.4161/rna.8.5.16154
8. Schetter AJ, Leung SY, Sohn JJ, Zanetti KA, Bowman ED, Yanaihara N, et al. MicroRNA expression profiles associated with prognosis and therapeutic outcome in colon adenocarcinoma. *JAMA* (2008) **299**(4):425–36. doi:10.1001/jama.299.4.425
9. Qian B, Katsaros D, Lu L, Preti M, Durando A, Arisio R, et al. High miR-21 expression in breast cancer associated with poor disease-free survival in early stage disease and high TGF-beta1. *Breast Cancer Res Treat* (2009) **117**(1):131–40. doi:10.1007/s10549-008-0219-7
10. Nielsen BS, Jorgensen S, Fog JU, Sokilde R, Christensen IJ, Hansen U, et al. High levels of microRNA-21 in the stroma of colorectal cancers predict short disease-free survival in stage II colon cancer patients. *Clin Exp Metastasis* (2011) **28**(1):27–38. doi:10.1007/s10585-010-9355-7
11. Hermansen SK, Dahlrot RH, Nielsen BS, Hansen S, Kristensen BW. miR-21 expression in the tumor cell compartment holds unfavorable prognostic value in gliomas. *J Neurooncol* (2013) **111**(1):71–81. doi:10.1007/s11060-012-0992-3
12. Rask L, Balslev E, Jorgensen S, Eriksen J, Flyger H, Moller S, et al. High expression of miR-21 in tumor stroma correlates with increased cancer cell proliferation in human breast cancer. *APMIS* (2011) **119**(10):663–73. doi:10.1111/j.1600-0463.2011.02782.x
13. Kadera BE, Li L, Toste PA, Wu N, Adams C, Dawson DW, et al. MicroRNA-21 in pancreatic ductal adenocarcinoma tumor-associated fibroblasts promotes metastasis. *PLoS One* (2013) **8**(8):e71978. doi:10.1371/journal.pone.0071978
14. Nouraee N, Van Roosbroeck K, Vasei M, Semnani S, Samaei NM, Naghshvar F, et al. Expression, tissue distribution and function of miR-21 in esophageal squamous cell carcinoma. *PLoS One* (2013) **8**(9):e73009. doi:10.1371/journal.pone.0073009
15. Kjaer-Frifeldt S, Hansen TF, Nielsen BS, Joergensen S, Lindebjerg J, Soerensen FB, et al. The prognostic importance of miR-21 in stage II colon cancer: a population-based study. *Br J Cancer* (2012) **107**(7):1169–74. doi:10.1038/bjc.2012.365
16. Hummel R, Hussey DJ, Haier J. MicroRNAs: predictors and modifiers of chemo- and radiotherapy in different tumour types. *Eur J Cancer* (2010) **46**(2):298–311. doi:10.1016/j.ejca.2009.10.027
17. Haenisch S, Cascorbi I. miRNAs as mediators of drug resistance. *Epigenomics* (2012) **4**(4):369–81. doi:10.2217/epi.12.39
18. Kanakkanthara A, Miller JH. MicroRNAs: novel mediators of resistance to microtubule-targeting agents. *Cancer Treat Rev* (2013) **39**(2):161–70. doi:10.1016/j.ctrv.2012.07.005
19. Gong C, Yao Y, Wang Y, Liu B, Wu W, Chen J, et al. Up-regulation of miR-21 mediates resistance to trastuzumab therapy for breast cancer. *J Biol Chem* (2011) **286**(21):19127–37. doi:10.1074/jbc.M110.216887
20. Valeri N, Gasparini P, Braconi C, Paone A, Lovat F, Fabbri M, et al. MicroRNA-21 induces resistance to 5-fluorouracil by down-regulating human DNA MutS homolog 2 (hMSH2). *Proc Natl Acad Sci U S A* (2010) **107**(49):21098–103. doi:10.1073/pnas.1015541107
21. Tomimaru Y, Eguchi H, Nagano H, Wada H, Tomokuni A, Kobayashi S, et al. MicroRNA-21 induces resistance to the anti-tumour effect of interferon-alpha/5-fluorouracil in hepatocellular carcinoma cells. *Br J Cancer* (2010) **103**(10):1617–26. doi:10.1038/sj.bjc.6605958
22. Wang ZX, Lu BB, Wang H, Cheng ZX, Yin YM. MicroRNA-21 modulates chemosensitivity of breast cancer cells to doxorubicin by targeting PTEN. *Arch Med Res* (2011) **42**(4):281–90. doi:10.1016/j.arcmed.2011.06.008
23. Tao J, Lu Q, Wu D, Li P, Xu B, Qing W, et al. MicroRNA-21 modulates cell proliferation and sensitivity to doxorubicin in bladder cancer cells. *Oncol Rep* (2011) **25**(6):1721–9. doi:10.3892/or.2011.1245
24. Chen Y, Tsai YH, Fang Y, Tseng SH. Micro-RNA-21 regulates the sensitivity to cisplatin in human neuroblastoma cells. *J Pediatr Surg* (2012) **47**(10):1797–805. doi:10.1016/j.jpedsurg.2012.05.013
25. Yang SM, Huang C, Li XF, Yu MZ, He Y, Li J. miR-21 confers cisplatin resistance in gastric cancer cells by regulating PTEN. *Toxicology* (2013) **306**:162–8. doi:10.1016/j.tox.2013.02.014
26. Mei M, Ren Y, Zhou X, Yuan XB, Han L, Wang GX, et al. Downregulation of miR-21 enhances chemotherapeutic effect of taxol in breast carcinoma cells. *Technol Cancer Res Treat* (2010) **9**(1):77–86.
27. Meng F, Henson R, Wehbe-Janek H, Ghoshal K, Jacob ST, Patel T. MicroRNA-21 regulates expression of the PTEN tumor suppressor gene in human hepatocellular cancer. *Gastroenterology* (2007) **133**(2):647–58. doi:10.1053/j.gastro.2007.05.022
28. Roy S, Khanna S, Hussain SR, Biswas S, Azad A, Rink C, et al. MicroRNA expression in response to murine myocardial infarction: miR-21 regulates fibroblast metalloprotease-2 via phosphatase and tensin homologue. *Cardiovasc Res* (2009) **82**(1):21–9. doi:10.1093/cvr/cvp015
29. Correia NC, Girio A, Antunes I, Martins LR, Barata JT. The multiple layers of non-genetic regulation of PTEN tumour suppressor activity. *Eur J Cancer* (2014) **50**(1):216–25. doi:10.1016/j.ejca.2013.08.017
30. Nagata Y, Lan KH, Zhou X, Tan M, Esteva FJ, Sahin AA, et al. PTEN activation contributes to tumor inhibition by trastuzumab, and loss of PTEN

predicts trastuzumab resistance in patients. *Cancer Cell* (2004) **6**(2):117–27. doi:10.1016/j.ccr.2004.06.022
31. Ostman A. The tumor microenvironment controls drug sensitivity. *Nat Med* (2012) **18**(9):1332–4. doi:10.1038/nm.2938
32. Shree T, Olson OC, Elie BT, Kester JC, Garfall AL, Simpson K, et al. Macrophages and cathepsin proteases blunt chemotherapeutic response in breast cancer. *Genes Dev* (2011) **25**(23):2465–79. doi:10.1101/gad.180331.111
33. Nakasone ES, Askautrud HA, Kees T, Park JH, Plaks V, Ewald AJ, et al. Imaging tumor-stroma interactions during chemotherapy reveals contributions of the microenvironment to resistance. *Cancer Cell* (2012) **21**(4):488–503. doi:10.1016/j.ccr.2012.02.017
34. Alkhateeb AA, Leitzel K, Ali SM, Campbell-Baird C, Evans M, Fuchs EM, et al. Elevation in inflammatory serum biomarkers predicts response to trastuzumab-containing therapy. *PLoS One* (2012) **7**(12):e51379. doi:10.1371/journal.pone.0051379
35. Nielsen BS, Holmstrom K. Combined microRNA *in situ* hybridization and immunohistochemical detection of protein markers. *Methods Mol Biol* (2013) **986**:353–65. doi:10.1007/978-1-62703-311-4_22
36. Yan LX, Huang XF, Shao Q, Huang MY, Deng L, Wu QL, et al. MicroRNA miR-21 overexpression in human breast cancer is associated with advanced clinical stage, lymph node metastasis and patient poor prognosis. *RNA* (2008) **14**(11):2348–60. doi:10.1261/rna.1034808
37. Ozgun A, Karagoz B, Bilgi O, Tuncel T, Baloglu H, Kandemir EG. MicroRNA-21 as an indicator of aggressive phenotype in breast cancer. *Onkologie* (2013) **36**(3):115–8. doi:10.1159/000348678
38. Hong L, Han Y, Zhang Y, Zhang H, Zhao Q, Wu K, et al. MicroRNA-21: a therapeutic target for reversing drug resistance in cancer. *Expert Opin Ther Targets* (2013) **17**(9):1073–80. doi:10.1517/14728222.2013.819853
39. Pan X, Wang ZX, Wang R. MicroRNA-21: a novel therapeutic target in human cancer. *Cancer Biol Ther* (2010) **10**(12):1224–32. doi:10.4161/cbt.10.12.14252
40. Sempere LF, Martinez P, Cole C, Baguna J, Peterson KJ. Phylogenetic distribution of microRNAs supports the basal position of acoel flatworms and the polyphyly of platyhelminthes. *Evol Dev* (2007) **9**(5):409–15. doi:10.1111/j.1525-142X.2007.00180.x
41. Hatley ME, Patrick DM, Garcia MR, Richardson JA, Bassel-Duby R, van Rooij E, et al. Modulation of K-Ras-dependent lung tumorigenesis by microRNA-21. *Cancer Cell* (2010) **18**(3):282–93. doi:10.1016/j.ccr.2010.08.013
42. Ma X, Kumar M, Choudhury SN, Becker Buscaglia LE, Barker JR, Kanakamedala K, et al. Loss of the miR-21 allele elevates the expression of its target genes and reduces tumorigenesis. *Proc Natl Acad Sci U S A* (2011) **108**(25):10144–9. doi:10.1073/pnas.1103735108
43. Ma X, Choudhury SN, Hua X, Dai Z, Li Y. Interaction of the oncogenic miR-21 microRNA and the p53 tumor suppressor pathway. *Carcinogenesis* (2013) **34**(6):1216–23. doi:10.1093/carcin/bgt044
44. Huang TH, Wu F, Loeb GB, Hsu R, Heidersbach A, Brincat A, et al. Up-regulation of miR-21 by HER2/neu signaling promotes cell invasion. *J Biol Chem* (2009) **284**(27):18515–24. doi:10.1074/jbc.M109.006676
45. Yoshinaga H, Matsuhashi S, Fujiyama C, Masaki Z. Novel human PDCD4 (H731) gene expressed in proliferative cells is expressed in the small duct epithelial cells of the breast as revealed by an anti-H731 antibody. *Pathol Int* (1999) **49**(12):1067–77. doi:10.1046/j.1440-1827.1999.00995.x
46. Shibahara K, Asano M, Ishida Y, Aoki T, Koike T, Honjo T. Isolation of a novel mouse gene MA-3 that is induced upon programmed cell death. *Gene* (1995) **166**(2):297–301. doi:10.1016/0378-1119(95)00607-9
47. Jurisicova A, Latham KE, Casper RF, Casper RF, Varmuza SL. Expression and regulation of genes associated with cell death during murine preimplantation embryo development. *Mol Reprod Dev* (1998) **51**(3):243–53. doi:10.1002/(SICI)1098-2795(199811)51:3<243::AID-MRD3>3.0.CO;2-P
48. Yang HS, Jansen AP, Nair R, Shibahara K, Verma AK, Cmarik JL, et al. A novel transformation suppressor, Pdcd4, inhibits AP-1 transactivation but not NF-kappaB or ODC transactivation. *Oncogene* (2001) **20**(6):669–76. doi:10.1038/sj.onc.1204137
49. Nieves-Alicea R, Colburn NH, Simeone AM, Tari AM. Programmed cell death 4 inhibits breast cancer cell invasion by increasing tissue inhibitor of metalloproteinases-2 expression. *Breast Cancer Res Treat* (2009) **114**(2):203–9. doi:10.1007/s10549-008-9993-5
50. Wen YH, Shi X, Chiriboga L, Matsahashi S, Yee H, Afonja O. Alterations in the expression of PDCD4 in ductal carcinoma of the breast. *Oncol Rep* (2007) **18**(6):1387–93.
51. Blanco-Aparicio C, Renner O, Leal JF, Carnero A. PTEN, more than the AKT pathway. *Carcinogenesis* (2007) **28**(7):1379–86. doi:10.1093/carcin/bgm052
52. Trimboli AJ, Cantemir-Stone CZ, Li F, Wallace JA, Merchant A, Creasap N, et al. Pten in stromal fibroblasts suppresses mammary epithelial tumours. *Nature* (2009) **461**(7267):1084–91. doi:10.1038/nature08486
53. Wallace JA, Li F, Leone G, Ostrowski MC. Pten in the breast tumor microenvironment: modeling tumor-stroma coevolution. *Cancer Res* (2011) **71**(4):1203–7. doi:10.1158/0008-5472.CAN-10-3263
54. Anido J, Scaltriti M, Bech Serra JJ, Santiago Josefat B, Todo FR, Baselga J, et al. Biosynthesis of tumorigenic HER2 C-terminal fragments by alternative initiation of translation. *EMBO J* (2006) **25**(13):3234–44. doi:10.1038/sj.emboj.7601191

15

ABC transporters in CSCs membranes as a novel target for treating tumor relapse

Laura Zinzi[1], Marialessandra Contino[1]*, Mariangela Cantore[2], Elena Capparelli[1], Marcello Leopoldo[1,2] and Nicola A. Colabufo[1,2]

[1] *Dipartimento di Farmacia-Scienze del Farmaco, Università degli Studi di Bari "A. Moro," Bari, Italy*
[2] *Dipartimento di Farmacia-Scienze del Farmaco, Biofordrug srl, Spin-off of University of Bari, Bari, Italy*

Edited by:
Stefania Nobili, University of Florence, Italy

Reviewed by:
Nathan Thomas Ihle, Pfizer, USA
Andrea Lapucci, University of Florence, Italy

****Correspondence:***
Marialessandra Contino, Dipartimento di Farmacia-Scienze del Farmaco, Università degli Studi di Bari "A. Moro," Via Orabona 4, 70125 Bari, Italy
e-mail: marialessandra.contino@uniba.it

CSCs are responsible for the high rate of recurrence and chemoresistance of different types of cancer. The current antineoplastic agents able to inhibit bulk replicating cancer cells and radiation treatment are not efficacious toward CSCs since this subpopulation has several intrinsic mechanisms of resistance. Among these mechanisms, the expression of ATP-Binding Cassette (ABC) transporters family and the activation of different signaling pathways (such as Wnt/β-catenin signaling, Hedgehog, Notch, Akt/PKB) are reported. Therefore, considering ABC transporters expression on CSCs membranes, compounds able to modulate MDR could induce cytotoxicity in these cells disclosing an exciting and alternative strategy for targeting CSCs in tumor therapy. The next challenge in the cure of cancer relapse may be a *multimodal strategy*, an approach where specific CSCs targeting drugs exert simultaneously the ability to circumvent tumor drug resistance (ABC transporters modulation) and cytotoxic activity toward CSCs and the corresponding differentiated tumor cells. The efficacy of suggested multimodal strategy could be probed by using several scaffolds active toward MDR pumps on CSCs isolated by tumor specimens.

Keywords: CSCs, MDR, TICs markers, HTS, P-gp

INTRODUCTION

The emerging concept about tumorigenesis is that cancer lesions are organized in a hierarchy of heterogeneous cell populations displaying different biological properties and tumorigenic potentials (Lorico and Rappa, 2011). Among these populations, only a small portion, the cancer stem cell or tumor-initiating cell (CSC/TIC) subpopulation is able to induce tumor formation and growth, leading to differentiated cells, the bulk of the tumor. In 1977 Hamburger and Salmon suggested the "*CSC theory*" by hypothesizing that cancer originates from uncommon cells, CSCs, showing pluripotency and self-renewal (Hamburger and Salmon, 1977; Boman and Wicha, 2008). In 1997 Lapidot and coworkers identified CSCs in leukemia on the basis of cell-surface-markers expression (Lapidot et al., 1994). The discovery of CSCs in leukemia and in several solid tumors, such as breast carcinoma (Al-Hajj et al., 2003; Hemmati et al., 2003; Singh et al., 2003; Carla et al., 2005; Fang et al., 2005; Xin et al., 2005; Lawson et al., 2007; Li et al., 2007; Ricci-Vitiani et al., 2007), was the proof of the *CSC theory* in cancer development.

CSC/TICs are characterized by the following properties: (a) production of all types of cells in a tumor, including CSC/TICs and non-CSC/TICs; (b) unlimited self-renewal and division capacity; (c) quiescence or slow proliferation, and (d) resistance to conventional antineoplastic therapy (Clevers, 2011). Moreover, recent studies have demonstrated that CSC/TIC phenotypes such as self-renewal and pluripotency are acquired by the activation of oncogenic genes or the inactivation of tumor suppressor genes (Baccelli and Trumpp, 2012). Since CSCs are characterized by specific surface markers, this subpopulation of cells can be isolated from mixed tumorigenic and non-tumorigenic tumor cells, by different methods of immune selection. CD44 targeting is used in the treatment of acute myeloid leukemia (AML) (Jin et al., 2006), CD24 targeting is for the treatment of colon and pancreatic cancer (Sagiv et al., 2008) and CD133 is targeted for the treatment of hepatocellular and gastric cancer (Smith et al., 2008). The current antineoplastic agents, able to inhibit bulk replicating cancer cells, and radiation treatment are not efficacious toward CSCs and, therefore, targeting these cells could be an helpful strategy for eradicating tumors more efficiently.

However, CSCs possess several intrinsic mechanisms of resistance to current chemotherapeutic drugs. Among these mechanisms, the expression of ATP-Binding Cassette (ABC) transporters family (An and Ongkeko, 2009; Calcagno et al., 2010; Fuchs et al., 2010; Clevers, 2011; Moitra et al., 2011; Pietras, 2011) and the activation of different signaling pathways such as Wnt/β-catenin signaling (Teng et al., 2010; Yeung et al., 2010; Takebe et al., 2011; Janikowa and Skarda, 2012), Hedgehog (Hh), Notch (Kobune et al., 2009; Wang et al., 2009; Zhao et al., 2009; Takebe et al., 2011; Janikowa and Skarda, 2012; Jiang et al., 2012), Akt/PKB, ATR/CHK1 survival pathways (Ma et al., 2008; Korkaya et al., 2009; Jiang et al., 2012) and constitutive activation of NF-κB are reported (Zhou et al., 2008; Liu et al., 2010).

The first of these mechanisms is the overexpression of ABC transporters such as P-glycoprotein (P-gp), Breast Cancer

Resistance Protein (BCRP), and Multidrug Resistance-associated Proteins (MRPs) that use the energy of ATP hydrolysis to extrude compounds out of cells (Colabufo et al., 2010). These proteins are overexpressed in several tumors and, since responsible for drug efflux, are the main cause of MultiDrug Resistance (MDR) (Colabufo et al., 2010). Among these transporters, P-gp is the mostly studied and is localized in the luminal membrane of endothelial cells constituting the Blood-Brain Barrier (BBB), Blood-CerebroSpinal Fluid Barrier (B-CSF), and Blood-Testis Barrier (BTB); thus P-gp exerts a protective function in our body (Pharm et al., 2008; Colabufo et al., 2010). BCRP as P-gp monomer, is considered a "half-transporter" and it effluxes the same P-gp substrates (Pharm et al., 2008; Colabufo et al., 2010). MRPs differ from P-gp for the presence of an additional and specific five transmembrane domain and it efflux organic ions with high molecular weight (Pharm et al., 2008; Colabufo et al., 2010).

Since several antineoplastic drugs are substrates of ABC transporters, one of the strategy to reverse MDR is the use of inhibitors toward these pumps and their co-administration with antineoplastic agents (Perez-Tomas, 2006; Teodori et al., 2006; Gimenez-Bonafe et al., 2008). However, when antineoplastic drugs and P-gp inhibitors are co-administrated, an increased toxicity has been observed because, at the same time, the protective role of P-gp is abolished (Coley, 2010).

Over the last decade, our research group has developed P-gp ligands with different scaffolds displaying different P-gp intrinsic activities (Colabufo et al., 2008a,b, 2009, 2013; Contino et al., 2012, 2013a,b; Nesi et al., 2014). Therefore, considering ABC transporters expression on CSCs membranes, compounds able to modulate MDR activity could induce cytotoxicity in these cells disclosing an exciting and alternative strategy for targeting CSCs in tumors therapy.

CSCs BIOMARKERS

CSCs display several cell surface markers and their detection is useful for the identification of CSCs in tumors. In addition, the development of antibodies or antibody constructs toward these markers is also suggested as a therapeutic strategy to target CSCs (Kwon and Shin, 2013).

CD133 AND ALDH1

CD133 and ALDH1 have been identified as markers of TICs in primary human ovarian tumors (Landen et al., 2010). CD133 has been also identified as surface marker to characterize adult stem/progenitor cells in human thyroid glands (Thomas et al., 2006). ALDH1 and CD133 are also markers for the identification of CSCs in colorectal carcinoma (CRC) (Zhou et al., 2014). CD133, together with CD44, is a specific cell-surface marker of prostate cancer (Wang et al., 2013a).

CD44, CD117, CD24

The hyaluronic acid (HA) receptor CD44 and the stem cell factor receptor CD117 are specific surface markers of ovarian CSC/TICs (Zhang et al., 2008). CD44+CD117+ cells isolated from human ovarian adenocarcinomas represent a subpopulation with an ovarian tumor-initiating capacity, that, injected in mice, induce original tumors from which they are derived (Zhang et al., 2008). CD24+ cells, isolated from patient tumor specimens, are enriched in ovarian CSC/TICs and have stem-like properties, such as chemoresistance, self-renewal and differentiation (Gao et al., 2010).

METHODS FOR THE ISOLATION OF CSCs

Fluorescence-Activated Cell Sorting (FACS) is a magnetic cell separation method used to isolate CSCs based on the expression of specific cell surface markers, such as CD24, CD44, and CD133 (Wright et al., 2008; Takaishi et al., 2009). The detection can be performed with specific antibodies in flow cytometry, competitive ELISA (cELISA) or magnetic beads (Dobbin and Landen, 2013). Xia and coworkers have developed humanized antibodies toward the surface marker CD133 that was detected by cELISA (Xia et al., 2013). However the limitation of surface markers recognition is that the results can be ascribed to the specific studied population. Therefore, a second method, represented by the detection of the activity of a specific protein such as the membrane pump ABCG2 or ALDH1A1 enzyme, seems to be more useful than markers recognition alone. The first technique uses the DNA-binding dye Hoechst 33342, originally developed for bone marrow cells (Goodell et al., 1996). This fluorescent dye, used to identify a Hoechst-negative CSC "side population" (Kondo et al., 2004), has been successfully employed to isolate stem cells from solid tissues such as skeletal muscle, lung, liver, testis, kidney, skin, mammary gland and brain (Challen and Little, 2006). This method allows to select the cells displaying an increase in the Hoechst 33342 efflux, ABCG2-mediated, from the nucleus. The limitation of this method is due to the dye toxicity (Siemann and Keng, 1986; Erba et al., 1988).

The high ALDH activity described for CSCs suggested also this enzyme as a probe to isolate these cells. Aldefluor, an ALDH1 substrate, initially used for the isolation of hematopoietic stem cells by FACS (Storms et al., 1999; Cheung et al., 2007) and for CSCs separation in tumor tissue and cancer cell lines (Moreb, 2008; Jiang et al., 2009), has been successfully used for ALDH1 activity detection of CSCs in lung (Jiang et al., 2009), prostate (Li et al., 2010), breast (Charafe-Jauffret et al., 2010), colon (Huang et al., 2009a), and bladder (Su et al., 2010). Aldefluor contains the ALDH1 substrate BODIPY-aminoacetaldehyde (BAAA), that is converted into the fluorescent metabolite BODIPY-aminoacetate (BAA) by ALDH1 (Storms et al., 1999). BAA is then retained in living cells, because of its charge and also because Aldefluor inhibits the multidrug-resistance transporters. Therefore, Aldefluor-treated cells, with high ALDH1 activity, display high fluorescence and can be isolated by FACS into two subpopulations: ALDH-hi and ALDH-low (Moreb, 2008). This method has been validated for some cancers but it has not been widely employed because of some limitations due to cells handling that can induce stress, disrupt gene expression, and lead to altered cell physiology (Orfao and Ruiz-Arguelles, 1996). To overcome these limitations, the use of Adelfluor staining has been assessed in adherent cell cultures, that resulted in the attached-cell Aldefluor method (ACAM). ACAM displays several advantages since single-cell imaging of physiological processes in CSCs is easier in monolayers than in cells suspension or tumorsphere cultures that are usually used for growing CSCs (Fael Al-Mayhani et al., 2009; Pollard et al., 2009; Hirschhaeuser et al., 2010).

CSCs have also been usually sorted into SP cells using UV excitation ($\lambda = 350$ nm) but the limitation of this method was the cell damage caused by UV radiation exposure. Tomiyasu et al. reported a new method in which CSCs have been sorted by a violet laser ($\lambda = 407$ nm) to avoid DNA damage (Tomiyasu et al., 2014).

Another method to select CSCs is the use of molecular probes, termed aptamers, that are produced by the iterative *in vitro* selection process SELEX (Systematic Evolution of Ligands by EXponential enrichment) (Ellington and Szostak, 1990; Tuerk and Gold, 1990). Aptamers are short single-stranded oligonucleotides of DNA or RNA sequences that fold into unique secondary and tertiary structures that selectively bind the target proteins and other small molecules with high affinity and selectivity. They can be synthesized *in vitro* and therefore do not require animal or bacterial hosts for production. In recent years, in order to improve aptamers qualities and reducing time and cost of production, a number of new SELEX variants have been performed and among them, cell-SELEX uses whole living cells as target to select DNA aptamers (Shangguan et al., 2006; Sefah et al., 2010). Aptamers have many appealing features: low molecular weight, easy chemical modifications, low toxicity and immunogenicity, long shelf-life, high affinity (K_d value is in the picomolar to nanomolar range) and high specificity. They can be used in diagnosis, for purification processes, in drug discovery and in therapy (Proske et al., 2005). In particular, the therapeutic perspectives involve the targeting of chemotherapeutic agents, nanoparticles, drug-encapsulated liposomes and radioactive materials on cell specific biomarkers. Aptamers bind their targets with high affinity and specificity discriminating very closely related targets. The anti-theophylline aptamer is able to distinguish theophylline from caffeine, and the anti L-arginine RNA aptamer binds more strongly L-arginine than D-arginine (Jenison et al., 1994; Geiger et al., 1996). Aptamers are also useful in drug delivery strategy: 2′-fluoro- RNA aptamers have effect toward the highly expressed prostate specific membrane antigene (PSMA) (Lupold et al., 2002) and Docetaxel-encapsulated nanoparticles functionalized with a specific aptamer (A10) target PSMA expressing cells (Farokhzad et al., 2006). Another interesting example is AS1411 aptamer that recognizes Nucleolin (NCL), a multifactorial protein involved in many cellular pathways of cancer. AS1411 has been functionalized with cisplatin-liposome and evaluated in MCF-7 (NCL positive) and LNCaP (NCL negative) cell lines. The cytotoxic effects were higher in MCF-7 cells as compared to LNCaP cells (Cao et al., 2009). Moreover, specific aptamers are used in several assays to isolate, enrich and identify CSCs and for the characterization of specific markers for CSCs such as aptamers toward HA domain of CD4, RNA aptamers targeting CD133, a cell surface glycoprotein considered a universal marker of normal hematopoietic and organ-specific stem cells and aptamers identifying brain CSCs (Griguer et al., 2008; Kim et al., 2013).

STRATEGIES TO ERADICATE CSCs

CSCs are responsible for tumor re-growth and potentially resistant to antitumor therapies. Therefore, the development of strategies that can act effectively against this subpopulation of cells has been envisaged, such as (**Figure 1**):

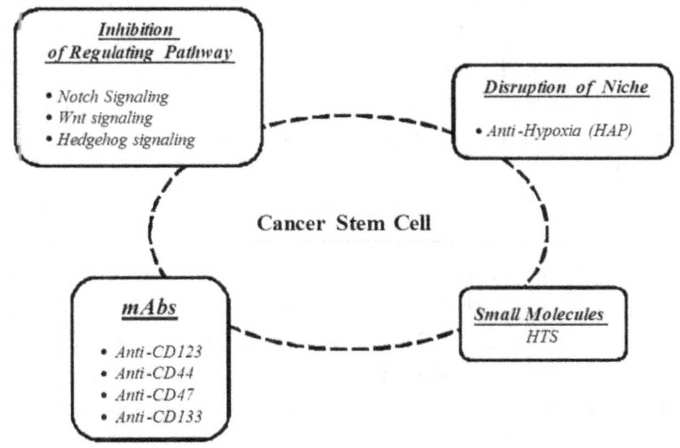

FIGURE 1 | Cancer stem cells targeting strategies.

- Immunological therapies;
- Evaluation of genes and pathways pivotal in CSCs regulation;
- High-throughput screening (HTS) of potential inhibitory compounds;
- Regulation of tumor microenvironment.

IMMUNOLOGICAL THERAPIES

Since current cancer therapies fail to eradicate CSCs, causing cancer recurrence and progression, the use of monoclonal antibodies (mAbs) and antibody constructs selective for CSCs is a novel cancer therapeutic strategy. Several studies have been performed on cell surface markers that are associated with CSCs. These markers have been suggested as targets for antibodies, for antibody-drug conjugates (ADCs) in immunological therapies to overcome the side effects and the limitations of current cancer chemotherapies (Naujokat, 2014). Several mAbs, directed toward specific surface markers (Anti-CD123, Anti-CD44, Anti-CD47, Anti-CD133) or toward protein of CSCs (Anti-Notch1 and Anti-Frizzled) have been reported (Naujokat, 2014). Antibody constructs can be classified as bispecific antibodies (BsAb), targeting two different surface markers (such as BsAb-CD123 and -CD3) or as trispecific antibodies when they target three different markers (such as CD123, CD33, CD16) (Naujokat, 2014). The use of mAbs or mAbs constructs had high efficacy in tumor xenografts mice and in some clinical trials and since these markers or proteins are expressed in CSCs, they can be specifically targeted by mAbs or constructs without collateral tissue damage. Moreover, it is also possible to conjugate antineoplastic drugs to mAbs leading to ADCs. As example, Lou et al. have developed a dual-targeting drug delivery system displaying an outer layer of polymers and traditional anti-cancer drugs such as doxorubicin dispersed in the polymer (Lou et al., 2012). The internal part is represented by the ADCs since includes mAbs directed to the specific marker of CSCs (such as anti-CD133 mAb or anti-CD44 mAb), highly cytotoxic drugs (such as calicheamicin) and linkers. The inner ADCs can be released from the delivery system in tumor cells where CSCs are recognized by the specific mAb of the system and ADCs are endocytosed. Some ADCs have displayed good antitumor effects and have entered preclinical trials (Iyer and Kadambi, 2011).

PhotoChemical Internalization (PCI) is a another innovative drug delivery technology based on light-controlled cytosolic release of drugs entrapped in endosomes or lysosomes (Stratford et al., 2013).

The combination of CD133-targeting therapeutics with PCI technology, where light-activation is constrained to the tumor, has been performed to develop an immunotoxin consisting of a biotinylated anti-CD133 mAb bound to streptavidin-saporin system (Stratford et al., 2013). This combined strategy has been used in a sarcoma model system (harboring CSCs within the CD133 high population) and the results have demonstrated that PCI-based drug delivery by the CD133-receptor inhibited cells viability and growth, and the ability to form tumors *in vivo*. Since CD133 overexpression is also found in different tumors, the study performed on sarcoma model can be transferable to treatment of all solid tumors expressing CD133 (Smith et al., 2008; Waldron et al., 2011; Bostad et al., 2013).

REGULATING PATHWAYS

The inhibition of biological pathways crucial in the regulation of the renew and the maintenance of CSCs, in combination with traditional chemotherapies, is a promising strategy for the treatment of CSCs and to circumvent MDR.

Notch pathway

The Notch pathway is important in gene regulation and in cell differentiation processes. This pathway is involved in the pathogenesis of several human tumors such as ovarian cancer (Park et al., 2006). There are four members of the mammalian Notch receptor family (Notch 1–4) activated through a series of cleavage events. The mature Notch receptors are composed of two subunits generated from an initial cleavage event by furin-like convertase. Blaumueller et al. (1997) Notch signaling pathway activation occurs when a Notch receptor binds to ligands. This binding causes a receptor conformational change allowing a second cleavage by tumor necrosis-factor-alpha converting enzyme (TACE) (Brou et al., 2000). The following cleavage is carried out by preselenin (a γ-secretase) releasing Notch intracellular domain and activating target genes expression. Notch plays a significant role in ovarian CSCs regulation and in platinum resistance (Park et al., 2006; Takebe et al., 2011). Also, Notch 3 inhibitors increase the sensitivity of ovarian cancer to cisplatin, reducing the ovarian CSC population (McAuliffe et al., 2012).

Wnt pathway

The Wnt signaling pathway, regulating several processes fundamental in embryogenesis such as proliferation, differentiation, polarity, adhesion and motility, plays key roles in tumorigenesis. Indeed, the progression of several cancers is associated with specific mutations in Wnt pathway components resulting in dysregulated β-catenin-mediated gene transcription. There are two distinct pathways for transduction of Wnt signals: the "canonical" Wnt/β-catenin pathway and the "non-canonical" β-catenin-independent pathway (Clevers and Nusse, 2012). The "canonical" pathway is activated by several Wnt ligands through the binding to Frizzled (FZD) receptors and to low-density lipoprotein receptor-related proteins-5/6 (LRP5/6) co-receptors. As a result, β-catenin accumulates in the cytoplasm, translocates to the nucleus and regulates transcription of Wnt/β-catenin target genes by binding to the T-cell factor/lymphoid enhancer factor (TCF/LEF) (MacDonald et al., 2009). In the absence of Wnt signaling, β-catenin levels are regulated by a cytoplasmic destruction complex (DC). DC is a multiproteins complex composed of protein Axin, the tumor suppressor adenomatous polyposis coli protein (APC), casein kinase α (CK1α), glycogen synthase kinase 3 β (GSK3) and additional associated proteins such as the members of the PARP-family of poly-ADP-ribosylation enzymes (Tankyrases, TNKSs). Axin, the concentration-limiting component of DC, is pivotal for the stability of the β-catenin-DC. By destabilizing Axin, TNKSs directly control the levels of this protein. Therefore, TNKSs inhibition, promoting Axin stabilization, leads to β-catenin phosphorylation and degradation, attenuating Wnt signaling (Liu et al., 2002; Lee et al., 2003). For this reason, in recent years, considerable efforts have been made to identify drugs that inhibit Wnt/β-catenin signaling. Another factor exerting a fundamental role in the biogenesis of Wnt pathway is represented by a member of the Membrane-Bound O-Acyl Transferase (MBOAT) family, Porcupine (PORCN) (Tanaka et al., 2000). PORCN is an integral membrane enzyme resident in the endoplasmic reticulum, required for the lipid modification of Wnt proteins. Acylation by PORCN is essential for the proper secretion and activity of Wnt signaling and, therefore, its inhibition is an attractive therapeutic strategy in diseases with increased Wnt signaling (Chen et al., 2009).

Hedgehog pathway

The Hh pathway is involved in several developmental processes of cells: determination of cell fate, patterning, proliferation, survival, and differentiation (Varjosalo and Taipale, 2008). In mammals, three Hh proteins (Sonic Hh, Indian Hh, and Desert Hh) are derived from proteolysis of inactive precursor that contains its own autoprocessing domain. Hh acts by binding to 12 transmembrane glycoprotein components Patched (Ptch). In the absence of ligand, Ptch constitutively represses the activity of Smoothened (Smo), a 7-pass transmembrane spanning protein with homology to G-protein coupled receptors. When Hh ligand binds to Ptch, the repression of Smo is released and the expression and/or post-translational processing of the three GLI zinc-finger transcription factors, inducing the expression of several target genes, is modulated (Sasaki et al., 1999). Overactivation of Hh pathway is associated with cancer and emerging data from many human tumors, including glioblastoma, breast cancer, pancreatic cancer, and chronic myeloid leukemia (CML), have suggested that Hh signaling regulates CSCs (Liu et al., 2006; Bar et al., 2007; Feldmann et al., 2007; Zhao et al., 2009). The Hh signaling pathway interacts also with other pathways commonly activated in human cancers, such as the phosphatidylinositol-3-kinase (PI3K)/Akt pathway (Riobo et al., 2006).

PI3K/AKT pathway

PI3K/AKT is important for pluripotency maintenance of stem cells. PI3K enzymes are normally regulated by growth factors and are useful to phosphorylate phospholipids on the plasma membrane (Hennessy et al., 2005). In addition, it has been suggested that PI3K/Akt activation pathway is required for CSCs maintenance and viability in breast cancer, prostate cancer, and brain tumor (Zhou et al., 2007; Hambardzumyan et al., 2008; Dubrovska et al., 2009). The PI3K/Akt pathway can also modulate functions of ABC transporters through various mechanisms. Inhibition of the PI3K/Akt pathway causes BCRP internalization in hematopoietic stem cells and glioma stem-like cells. Hence, the PI3K/Akt pathway can be an attractive target for cancer therapy (Mogi et al., 2003; Bleau et al., 2009).

HIGH-THROUGHPUT SCREENING (HTS)

The development of agents active toward CSCs population may be useful in the treatment of patients with recurrent cancer. HTS allows to identify potential compounds targeting specifically CSCs. In recent years, several studies have been carried out and in one of these studies the chemical library Microsource Spectrum collection of 2000 compounds has been screened to identify therapeutic agents inhibiting Glioblastome Multiforme stem cells (GSCs). This library has been selected based on the structural and biological diversity and consisted of FDA approved drugs, compounds in the late-phase clinical trials, experimental drugs and natural products. Among these, Disulfiram, a clinically approved drug for the treatment of alcoholism, was identified as a potent inhibitor of multiple patient-derived GSCs (Germain et al., 2013).

Another study has been carried out in order to identify agents able to selectively inhibit a cell-line model of breast CSCs screening over 300,000 compounds of the Molecular Libraries Small Molecules Repository (MLSMR) from the National Institute of Health (NIH). Among these compounds, a cinnamide analog displayed 20-fold selective inhibition of the breast CSC-line cell (HMLE_sh_Ecad) over the control (HMLE_sh_eGFP) (Hothi et al., 2012).

In another study, HTS of 825 potential drugs (the National Cancer Institute's "Mechanistic Set" library) toward ovarian CSCs and the subsequent identification of compounds displaying potential activity as ovarian CSC therapeutic agents is reported. Several compounds were classified as inhibitors and, among these, 5 compounds FDA-approved (dactinomycin, plicamycin, vinblastine, vincristine, and mepacrine) were identified as anticancer drugs (Mezencev et al., 2012).

TUMOR MICROENVIRONMENT

It has been proposed that CSCs are maintained by their surrounding microenvironment called "niche." Niche, important for CSCs sustaining, is composed by immune and stromal cells, blood vessels and extracellular matrix components. Biological processes, such as inflammation, hypoxia and angiogenesis, are important for CSCs, and signaling from this microenvironment is crucial for the activation of pathways involved in the maintenance of TICs functions (Cabarcas et al., 2011; Hanahan and Weinberg, 2011). Tumor hypoxia is implicated in the development of resistance to many conventional chemotherapeutic agents. It induces a decreased sensitivity to apoptotic and other cell-death signals, and increased signaling promoting angiogenesis, proliferation and systemic metastasis capacity (Feldmann, 2001; Kunz and Ibrahim, 2003). The initial response of cancer cells to hypoxia is the activation of hypoxia responsive transcription factors (HIFs) that regulate a number of genes involved in glucose metabolism, cell survival, erythropoiesis, stem cell maintenance, angiogenesis and resistance to chemotherapy and radiotherapy (Majmundar et al., 2010). Molecules like langkamide, piplartine and 3,4,5-trimethoxycinnamic acid (**Chart 1**), displaying HIF-2 inhibitory activity, may be used for targeting HIFs mediated regulation of CSCs (Bokesch et al., 2011). Another important transcription factor, involved in tumor growth, progression, and in the resistance to chemotherapy, is NFkB: this factor and HIF1α together regulate transcription of thousand genes controlling vital cellular processes (Gupta et al., 2010).

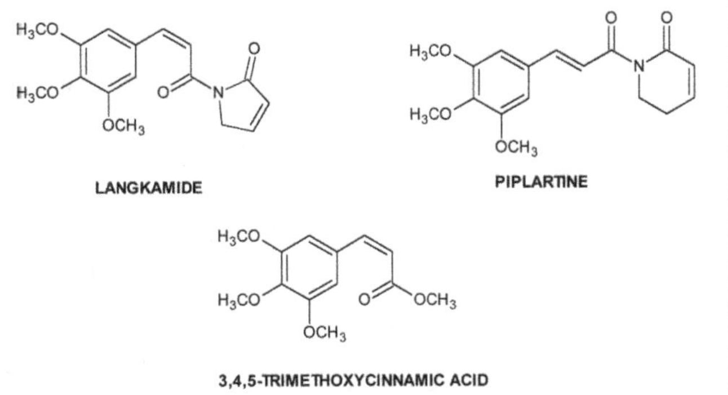

Chart 1 | Natural HIF inhibitors.

MOLECULES ACTIVE TOWARD CSCs

PORCUPINE AND TANKSs INHIBITORS

In the last years, considerable efforts have been made to identify drugs able to inhibit Wnt/β-catenin signaling, either by blocking Wnt secretion (PORCN inhibitors) or by interfering with β-catenin, by binding its transcription factor targets (TANKSs inhibitors).

Starting from four IWP ligands, additional PORCN inhibitors have been identified, that are characterized by two structural motifs of IWPs (phthalazinone and pyrimidinone moieties) interacting with PORCN and important for the activity. The lead optimization step led to a significant improvement in activity and to the identification of IWP-L6 (**Chart 2**) as a new sub-nanomolar PORCN inhibitor (Chen et al., 2009; Wang et al., 2013b). The first TANKSs inhibitor, identified by Huang et al. through a chemical genetic screen, was XAV-939 (**Chart 2**) (Huang et al., 2009b). It selectively affects β-catenin-mediated transcription, by stimulating its degradation by stabilizing Axin. By HTS, JW55, IWR-1, and WIKI4 (**Chart 2**) as specific tankyrases inhibitors have been discovered (Chen et al., 2009; James et al., 2012; Waaler et al., 2012).

HAP: HYPOXIA-ACTIVATED BIOREDUCTIVE PRODRUGS

The hypoxic microenvironment of solid tumors has attracted significant attention as target for the development of novel therapeutics for cancer treatment. A new class of drugs, the

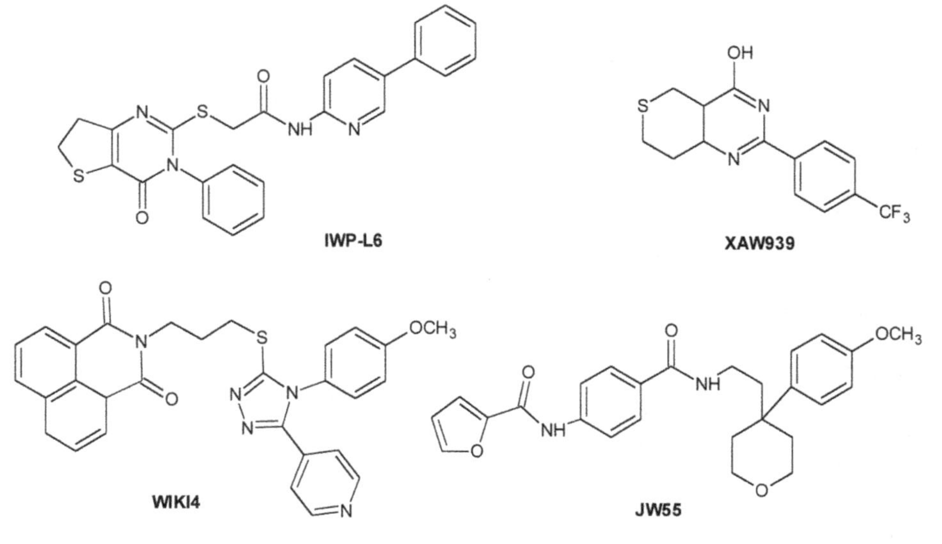

Chart 2 | Porcupine and Tankyrase inhibitors.

hypoxia activated prodrugs (HAP), has been designed for selective activation under low oxygen conditions, typical of many solid tumors. These are prodrugs that are enzymatically converted into active metabolites (effectors) by endogenous enzymes under the hypoxic conditions that prevail in tumors (Rauth et al., 1998). Taking into account the different activation profile, HAP could be classified into two groups: (1) Class I HAP (such as benzotriazine *N*-oxides tirapazamine and SN30000), activated under relatively mild hypoxia; (2) Class II HAP (such as the nitro compounds PR-104A or TH-302), activated only under extreme hypoxia (Yin et al., 2012; Foehrenbacher et al., 2013). Several hypoxia-specific prodrugs are in various stages of clinical development, although no registered agents have been used in clinical therapy. Moreover, the bioreductive compounds are classified in five classes: (1) aromatic *N*-oxides; (2) aliphatic *N*-oxides; (3) nitro(hetero)cyclic compounds; (4) quinones; (5) metal complexes.

The *N*-oxide tirapazamine (TPZ, SR4233) (**Chart 3**) has been the most extensively evaluated compound in the clinic to date. TPZ exhibited up to 300-fold higher toxicity under anoxic conditions than aerobic conditions *in vitro* (Zeman et al., 1986). TPZ undergoes one-electron reduction to generate the corresponding radical able to produce DNA breaks and lesions (Shinde et al., 2010). Although TPZ has been evaluated in a number of phase II clinical trials (Marcu and Olver, 2006), the results have not been translated into increased efficacy over conventional treatment in phase III clinical trials (Rischin et al., 2010). SN30000 (**Chart 3**) is a TPZ analog with improved pharmacokinetic properties and is presently scheduled to enter phase I clinical trials (Hicks et al., 2010).

N-oxide banoxantrone (AQ4N) (**Chart 3**) is metabolized under hypoxia giving a high affinity DNA intercalating agent, AQ4, that inhibits topoisomerase II (Patterson et al., 1994). In preclinical studies, AQ4N, combined with radio- or chemotherapy, demonstrated significant increasing activity (Patterson et al., 2000).

PR-104 (**Chart 3**), currently in phase II clinical trials, is a water-soluble phosphate ester pre-prodrug that rapidly is hydrolyzed *in vivo* to the prodrug PR-104A, a dinitrobenzamide mustard that is reduced to *p*-hydroxylamine and *p*-amine metabolites by various oxidoreductases (Singleton et al., 2009). Another promising compound, TH-302 (**Chart 3**), is a 2-nitroimidazole-based nitrogen mustard prodrug. The reduction in hypoxic cells to 2-nitroimidazole and the subsequent bromoisophosphoramide mustard affects DNA repair pathways (Meng et al., 2012). TH-302, in combination with chemotherapy, is currently in phase II and III clinical trials.

Quinone compounds (porfiromycin, RH1, and apaziquone EO9) (**Chart 3**) show greater selectivity toward hypoxic cells where their activation under hypoxia is carried out by one-electron reductases (Saunders et al., 2000; Phillips et al., 2013; Guise et al., 2014). Finally, although metal complexes could be potentially used as hypoxia-selective agents, none have been developed for clinical use so far.

MISCELLANEOUS

Several molecules, with unrelated chemical structures, are active toward CSCs. Among these, the antihelmintic niclosamide (**Chart 4**) selectively targets ovarian CSCs, and its effect is associated with the inhibition of metabolic pathways related to redox regulation (Yo et al., 2012). Metformin (**Chart 4**), an anti-diabetic drug, selectively targets CSCs in multiple types of cancer including prostate, lung and breast (Hirsch et al., 2009; Shank et al., 2012) and, in combination with chemotherapeutic agents (such as doxorubicin, paclitaxel, and carboplatinum) inhibits tumor growth (Gotlieb et al., 2008). This drug also displays an anti-proliferative and pro-apoptotic effects on ovarian CSCs *in vitro* (Yasmeen et al., 2011). Retinoids, in co-administration with cis-platinum, affect ovarian CSCs, whereas carboplatinum alone is not active (Whitworth et al., 2012). Ericalyxin B, a diterpenoid isolated from *Isodon eriocalyx* displaying antitumor

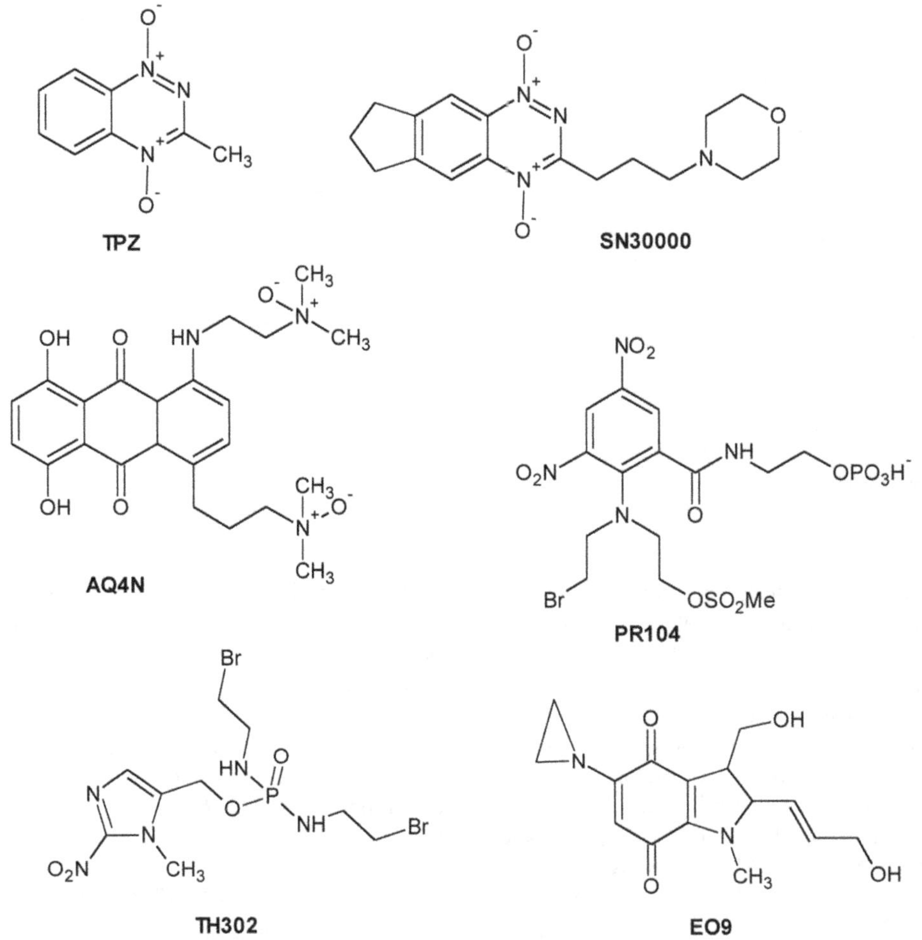

Chart 3 | Hypoxia Activated Prodrugs (HAP).

effects *via* multiple pathways, and 3-Bromopiruvate target ovarian CSCs inducing cell death (Leizer et al., 2011; Wintzell et al., 2012). Dactinomycin and Plicamycin, two FDA-approved CSCs-inhibitory compounds, are used in the treatment of several cancers including gestational trophoblastic neoplasia, Wilms' tumor, testicular cancer and hypercalcemia associated with advanced malignancy (Kennedy, 1970; Perlia et al., 1970; Lewis et al., 1972; Frei, 1974; Fraschini et al., 2005; Lee et al., 2006). Disulfiram (**Chart 4**), used in alcoholism treatment, is able to reduce cell growth and self-renewal of glioblastoma stem cells resistant to temozolomide *in vitro* by activating apoptotic pathways that modulate Bcl-2 family (Liu et al., 2012). DECA-14 (**Chart 4**), an analog of dequalinium (DECA-10), an antimicrobial agent and Rapamycin were identified as neuroblastoma (NB) TIC-selective agents. Both compounds induce CSCs death *in vitro*, reduce NB xenograft tumor weight *in vivo* and decrease self-renewal in treated tumors (Smith et al., 2010). Furthermore, NV-128 (**Chart 4**), an isoflavone derivative, induces cell death in chemoresistant CSCs population by inhibiting mitochondrial function and activating cell death pathways (Alvero et al., 2011).

CSC AND MDR: REPOSITIONING STRATEGY

The failure of cancer therapy is often due to tumor recurrence after chemotherapy because in several cancers a residual pool of CSCs remains (Dean et al., 2005). TICs that survive after therapy evolve in a population of chemoresistant cells able to sustain the growth of a more aggressive tumor. Among all the protective mechanisms for CSCs, ABC proteins overexpression is one of the mostly reported (An and Ongkeko, 2009; Calcagno et al., 2010; Fuchs et al., 2010; Clevers, 2011; Moitra et al., 2011; Pietras, 2011). There are two models useful to explain the connection between MDR and CSCs: (i) the original MDR model and (ii) the acquired MDR model (Holohan et al., 2013). The first model proposes that, after exposure to the chemotherapeutic agent, only CSCs expressing ABC transporters repopulate the tumor. The second suggests that, after chemotherapy, only CSCs survive and this population of survival cells, after mutations, originates new and more aggressive drug-resistant cell phenotypes (Holohan et al., 2013). The combination of CSCs targeting agents with novel or conventional cytotoxic drugs could lead to a potentiated effect. Flavonoids, a large family of polyphenolic molecules, modulate MDR transporters and inhibit CSCs growth (Colabufo et al.,

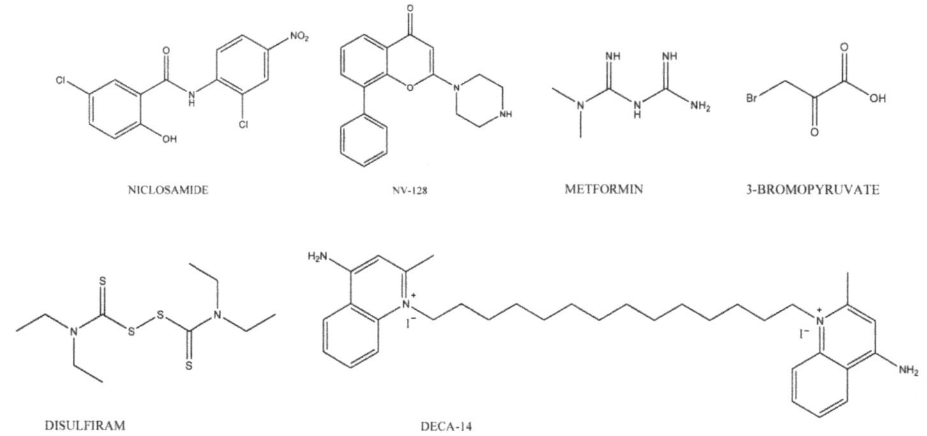

Chart 4 | Agents targeting CSCs.

2008c). Flavonoids anticancer properties are due to their antimitotic activity and to the inhibition of several enzymes. Recently, it has been suggested that flavonoids inhibit the function of ABC transporters such as P-gp, MRPs, and BCRP. Structural requirements for the interaction with these pumps are hydrophobic character and planarity. Flavonoids show low toxicity but, in the meantime, display a broad spectrum of biological activities (Colabufo et al., 2008c). Moreover, several studies have pointed out that flavonoids are able to affect CSCs. Luteolin, Casticin and 8-Bromo-7-methoxychrysin (BrMC) are active on glioma stem-like cells (Feng et al., 2012). BrMC is active on hepatocellular carcinoma (Hep-G2 cell line) where it induces apoptotic cell death by involving ROS products (Yang et al., 2010). LY294002, a PI3K specific inhibitor, blocks osteosarcoma CSCs cell cycle (G0/G1) in a dose-dependent manner inducing apoptosis by preventing phosphorylation of PKB/Akt *via* PI3K phosphorylation inhibition. Several studies show that this compound also inhibits BCRP, P-gp, and MRP1 highly expressed in stem cells. LY294002 reverses MDR in CSCs overexpressing BCRP by internalizing this pump (Imai et al., 2012). LY294002 competitively inhibits MRP1-mediated doxorubicin efflux in drug-resistant HT29RDB colon carcinoma cells. Sensitization was not restricted to doxorubicin, but it was also observed in cells treated with cisplatin, topotecan, and mitoxantron (Abdul-Ghani et al., 2006). Moreoever, LY294002 antagonizes transport activity of P-gp by reducing the degree of vincristine resistance in L1210/VCR mouse leukemic cell lines in a concentration-dependent manner (Barancík et al., 2006). However, the simultaneous inhibition of several cellular signaling pathways, transporters and channels may cause severe side effects.

Salinomycin, a polyether ionophore antibiotic isolated from *Streptomyces albus*, is able to affect CSCs in gastric cancer, lung adenocarcinoma, osteosarcoma, colorectal cancer, squamous cell carcinoma (SCC) and prostate by interfering with ABC transporters and CSC crucial pathways (Dong et al., 2011). The combination of salinomycin and the antibody for the anti-human epidermal growth factor receptor 2 (anti-HER2), trastuzumab, was found more efficacious than trastuzumab single-treatment in MCF-7-derived breast CSCs and HER2-expressing breast cancer cells. In colorectal cancer and in SCC, salinomycin, but not oxaliplatin or cisplatin, is able to reduce the portion of CSCs (Basu et al., 2011; Dong et al., 2011; Tang et al., 2011; Wang, 2011; Zhi et al., 2011; Ketola et al., 2012; Oak et al., 2012). Moreover, salinomycin is active toward human AML CSCs, because it overcomes ABC transporter-mediated MDR and apoptosis resistance and inhibits P-gp/MDR1 in different cancer cells (Fuchs et al., 2010; Riccioni et al., 2010).

CONCLUSIONS AND PERSPECTIVES

Although several items about CSCs theory remain open, there is a large evidence demonstrating that CSCs are essential to initiate and maintain tumors. CSCs are involved in tumor re-growth and are resistant to conventional anti-cancer therapy because of several mechanisms. Among them, the overexpression of ABC transporters in CSCs membranes represents a novel target for eradicating tumor relapse. To date, several strategies have been employed to isolate, target CSCs and circumvent MDR: (i) the development of sensitive biomarkers and targeted-aptamers; (ii) the evaluation of CSCs microenvironment; (iii) the study of the genes and pathways involved in CSCs regulation; (iv) evaluation of known and new molecules able to affect both TIC populations and ABC transporters. Therefore, the next challenge in this field may be a *multimodal strategy*, an approach in which specific CSCs targeting drugs exert simultaneously the ability to circumvent tumor drug resistance (ABC transporters modulation) and cytotoxic activity toward CSCs and the corresponding differentiated tumor cells. The efficacy of this suggested multimodal strategy will be probed by using several scaffolds active toward MDR pumps on CSCs isolated by tumor specimens.

REFERENCES

Abdul-Ghani, R., Serra, V., Györffy, B., Jürchott, K., Solf, A., and Schäfer, R. (2006). The PI3K inhibitor LY294002 blocks drug export from resistant colon carcinoma cells overexpressing MRP1. *Oncogene* 25, 1743–1752. doi: 10.1038/sj.onc.1209201

Al-Hajj, M., Wicha, M. S., Benito-Hernandez, A., Morrison, S. J., and Clarke, M. F. (2003). Prospective identification of tumorigenic breast cancer cells. *Proc. Natl. Acad. Sci. U.S.A.* 100, 3983–3988. doi: 10.1073/pnas.0530291100

Alvero, A. B., Montagna, M. K., Holmberg, J. C., Craveiro, V., Brown, D., and Mor, G. (2011). Targeting the mitochondria activates two independent cell death pathways in ovarian cancer stem cells. *Mol. Cancer Ther.* 10, 1385–1393. doi: 10.1158/1535-7163.MCT-11-0023

An, Y., and Ongkeko, W. M. (2009). ABCG2: the key to chemoresistance in cancer stem cells? *Expert Opin. Drug Metab. Toxicol.* 5, 1529–1542. doi: 10.1517/17425250903228834

Baccelli, I., and Trumpp, A. (2012). The evolving concept of cancer and metastasis stem cells. *J. Cell Biol.* 198, 281–293. doi: 10.1083/jcb.201202014

Bar, E. E., Chaudhry, A., Lin, A., Fan, X., Schreck, K., Matsui, W., et al. (2007). Cyclopamine-mediated Hedgehog pathway inhibition depletes stem-like cancer cells in glioblastoma. *Stem Cells* 25, 2524–2533. doi: 10.1634/stemcells.2007-0166

Barancík, M., Boháсová, V., Sedlák, J., Sulová, Z., and Breier, A. (2006). LY294,002, a specific inhibitor of PI3K/Akt kinase pathway, antagonizes P-glycoprotein mediated multidrug resistance. *Eur. J. Pharm. Sci.* 29, 426–434. doi: 10.1016/j.ejps.2006.08.006

Basu, D., Montone, K. T., Wang, L. P., Gimotty, P. A., Hammond, R., Diehl, J. A., et al. (2011). Detecting and targeting mesenchymal-like subpopulations within squamous cell carcinomas. *Cell Cycle* 10, 12008–12016. doi: 10.4161/cc.10.12.15883

Blaumueller, C. M., Qi, H., Zagouras, P., and Artavanis-Tsakonas, S. (1997). Intracellular cleavage of Notch leads to a heterodimic receptor on plasma membrane. *Cell* 90, 281–291. doi: 10.1016/S0092-8674(00)80336-0

Bleau, A. M., Hambardzumyan, D., Ozawa, T., Fomchenko, E. I., Huse, J. T., Brennan, C. W., et al. (2009). PTEN/PI3K/Akt pathway regulates the side population phenotype and ABCG2 activity in glioma tumor stem-like cell. *Cell Stem Cell* 4, 226–235. doi: 10.1016/j.stem.2009.01.007

Bokesch, H. R., Gardella, R. S., Rabe, D. C., Bottaro, D. P., Linehan, W. M., McMahon, J. B., et al. (2011). A new hypoxia inducible factor-2 inhibitory pyrrolinone alkaloid from roots and stems of Piper sarmentosum. *Chem. Pharm. Bull.* 59, 1178–1179. doi: 10.1248/cpb.59.1178

Boman, B. M., and Wicha, M. S. (2008). Cancer stem cells: a step toward the cure. *J. Clin. Oncol.* 26, 2795–2799. doi: 10.1200/JCO.2008.17.7436

Bostad, M., Berg, K., Høgset, A., Skarpen, E., Stenmark, H., and Selbo, P. K. (2013). Photochemical internalization (PCI) of immunotoxins targeting CD133 is specific and highly potent at femtomolar levels in cells with cancer stem-cell properties. *J. Control. Release* 168, 317–326. doi: 10.1016/j.jconrel.2013.03.023

Brou, C., Loget, F., Gupta, N., Bessia, C., LeBail, O., Doedens, J. R., et al. (2000). A novel proteolytic cleavage involved in Notch signaling: the role of the disintegrin-metalloprotease TACE. *Mol. Cell* 5, 207–216. doi: 10.1016/S1097-2765(00)80417-7

Cabarcas, S. M., Mathews, L. A., and Farrar, W. L. (2011). The cancer stem cell niche-there goes the neighborhood? *Int. J. Cancer* 129, 2315–2327. doi: 10.1002/ijc.26312

Calcagno, A. M., Salcido, C. D., Gillet, J. P., Wu, C. P., Fostel, J. M., Mumau, M. D., et al. (2010). Prolonged drug selection of breast cancer cells and enrichment of cancer stem cell characteristics. *J. Natl. Cancer Inst.* 102, 1637–1652. doi: 10.1093/jnci/djq361

Cao, Z., Tong, R., Mishra, A., Xu, W., Whong, G. C., Cheng, J., et al. (2009). Reversible cell-specific drug delivery with aptamer-funcionalized liposomes. *Angew. Chem. Int. Ed. Engl.* 48, 6494–6498. doi: 10.1002/anie.200901452

Carla, F., Kim, B., Jackson, E. L., Woolfenden, A. E., Lawrence, S., Babar, I., et al. (2005). Identification of bronchioalveolar stem cells in normal lung and lung cancer. *Cell* 121, 823–835. doi: 10.1016/j.cell.2005.03.032

Challen, G. A., and Little, M. H. (2006). A side order of stem cells: the SP phenotype. *Stem Cells* 24, 3–12. doi: 10.1634/stemcells.2005-0116

Charafe-Jauffret, E., Ginestier, C., Iovino, F., Tarpin, C., Diebel, M., Esterni, B., et al. (2010). Aldehyde dehydrogenase 1-positive cancer stem cells mediate metastasis and poor clinical outcome in inflammatory breast cancer. *Clin. Cancer Res.* 16, 45–55. doi: 10.1158/1078-0432.CCR-09-1630

Chen, B., Dodge, M. E., Tang, W., Lu, J., Ma, Z., Fan, C. W., et al. (2009). Small moleculemediated disruption of Wnt dependent signaling in tissue regeneration and cancer. *Nat. Chem. Biol.* 5, 100–107. doi: 10.1038/nchembio.137

Cheung, A. M., Wan, T. S., Leung, J. C., Chan, L. Y., Huang, H., Kwong, Y. L., et al. (2007). Aldehyde dehydrogenase activity in leukemic blasts defines a subgroup of acute myeloid leukemia with adverse prognosis and superior NOD/SCID engrafting potential. *Leukemia* 21, 1423–1430. doi: 10.1038/sj.leu.2404721

Clevers, H. (2011). The cancer stem cell: premises, promises and challenges. *Nat. Med.* 17, 313–319. doi: 10.1038/nm.2304

Clevers, H., and Nusse, R. (2012). Wnt/beta-catenin signaling and disease. *Cell* 149, 1192–1205. doi: 10.1016/j.cell.2012.05.012

Colabufo, N. A., Berardi, F., Cantore, M., Contino, M., Inglese, C., Niso, M., et al. (2010). Perspectives of P-glycoprotein modulating agents in oncology and neurodegenerative diseases: pharmaceutical, biological, and diagnostic potentials. *J. Med. Chem.* 53, 1883–1897. doi: 10.1021/jm900743c

Colabufo, N. A., Berardi, F., Cantore, M., Perrone, M. G., Contino, M., Inglese, C., et al. (2008a). Small P-gp modulating molecules: SAR studies on tetrahydroisoquinoline derivatives. *Bioorg. Med. Chem.* 16, 362–373. doi: 10.1016/j.bmc.2007.09.039

Colabufo, N. A., Berardi, F., Cantore, M., Perrone, M. G., Contino, M., Inglese, C., et al. (2008b). 4-Biphenyl and 2-naphthyl substituted 6,7-dimethoxytetrahydroisoquinoline derivatives as potent P-gp modulators. *Bioorg. Med. Chem.* 16, 3732–3743. doi: 10.1016/j.bmc.2008.01.055

Colabufo, N. A., Berardi, F., Cantore, M., Perrone, M. G., Contino, M., Inglese, C., et al. (2009). Multi-drug-resistance-reverting agents: 2-aryloxazole and 2-arylthiazole derivatives as potent BCRP or MRP1 inhibitors. *ChemMedChem* 4, 188–195. doi: 10.1002/cmdc.200800329

Colabufo, N. A., Berardi, F., Contino, M., Inglese, C., and Perrone, R. (2008c). *Multidrug Resistance: Biological and Pharmaceutical Advance in the Antitumour Treatment.* Kerala: Research Signpost.

Colabufo, N. A., Contino, M., Cantore, M., Capparelli, E., Perrone, M. G., Cassano, G., et al. (2013). Naphthalenyl derivatives for hitting P-gp/MRP1/BCRP transporters. *Bioorg. Med. Chem.* 21, 1322–1330. doi: 10.1016/j.bmc.2012.12.021

Coley, H. M. (2010). Overcoming multidrug resistance in cancer: clinical studies of p-glycoprotein inhibitors. *Methods Mol. Biol.* 596, 341–358. doi: 10.1007/978-1-60761-416-6_15

Contino, M., Cantore, M., Capparelli, E., Perrone, M. G., Niso, M., Inglese, C., et al. (2012). A benzopyrane derivative as P-glycoprotein stimulator: a potential agent to decrease β-amyloid accumulation in Alzheimer's disease. *ChemMedChem* 7, 391–395. doi: 10.1002/cmdc.201100469

Contino, M., Zinzi, L., Cantore, M., Perrone, M. G., Leopoldo, M., Berardi, F., et al. (2013b). Activity-Lipophilicity relationship studies on P-gp ligands designed as simplified Tariquidar bulky fragments. *Bioorg. Med. Chem. Lett.* 23, 3728–3731. doi: 10.1016/j.bmcl.2013.05.019

Contino, M., Zinzi, L., Perrone, M. G., Leopoldo, M., Berardi, F., Perrone, R., et al. (2013a). Potent and selective tariquidar bioisosters as potential PET radiotracers for imaging P-gp. *Bioorg. Med. Chem. Lett.* 23, 1369–1373. doi: 10.1016/j.bmcl.2012.12.084

Dean, M., Fojo, T., and Bates, S. (2005). Tumour stem cells and drug resistance. *Nat. Rev. Cancer* 5, 275–284. doi: 10.1038/nrc1590

Dobbin, Z. C., and Landen, C. N. (2013). Isolation and characterization of potential cancer stem cells from solid human tumors–potential applications. *Curr. Protoc. Pharmacol.* 63, Unit 14.28. doi: 10.1002/0471141755.ph1428s63

Dong, T. T., Zhou, H. M., Wang, L. L., Feng, B., Lv, B., and Zheng, M. H. (2011). Salinomycin selectively targets'CD133+' cell subpopulations and decreases malignant traits in colorectal cancer lines. *Ann. Surg. Oncol.* 18, 6797–1804. doi: 10.1245/s10434-011-1561-2

Dubrovska, A., Kim, S., Salamone, R. J., Walker, J. R., Maira, S. M., García-Echeverría, C., et al. (2009). The role of PTEN/Akt/PI3K signaling in the maintenance and viability of prostate cancer stem-like cell populations. *Proc. Natl. Acad. Sci. U.S.A.* 106, 268–273. doi: 10.1073/pnas.0810956106

Ellington, A. D., and Szostak, J. W. (1990). *In vitro* selection of RNA molecules that bind specific ligands. *Nature* 346, 818–822. doi: 10.1038/346818a0

Erba, E., Ubezio, P., Broggini, M., Ponti, M., and D'Incalci, M. (1988). DNA damage, cytotoxic effect and cell-cycle perturbation of Hoechst 33342 on L1210 cells *in vitro*. *Cytometry* 9, 1–6. doi: 10.1002/cyto.990090102

Fael Al-Mayhani, T. M., Ball, S. L., Zhao, J. W., Fawcett, J., Ichimura, K., Collins, P. V., et al. (2009). An efficient method for derivation and propagation of glioblastoma cell lines that conserves the molecular profile of their original tumours. *J. Neurosci. Methods* 176, 192–199. doi: 10.1016/j.jneumeth.2008.07.022

Fang, D., Nguyen, T. K., Leishear, K., Finko, R., Kulp, A. N., Hotz, S., et al. (2005). A tumorigenic subpopulation with stem cell properties in melanomas. *Cancer Res.* 65, 9328–9337. doi: 10.1158/0008-5472.CAN-05-1343

Farokhzad, O. C., Cheng, J., Teply, B. A., Sherifi, I., Jon, S., Kantoff, P. W., et al. (2006). Targeted nanoparticle-aptamer bioconjugates for cancer chemotherapy *in vivo*. *Proc. Natl. Acad. Sci. U.S.A.* 103, 6315–6320. doi: 10.1073/pnas.0601755103

Feldmann, G., Dhara, S., Fendrich, V., Bedja, D., Beaty, R., Mullendore, M., et al. (2007). Blockade of hedgehog signaling inhibits pancreatic cancer invasion and metastases: a new paradigm for combination therapy in solid cancers. *Cancer Res.* 67, 2187–2196. doi: 10.1158/0008-5472.CAN-06-3281

Feldmann, H. J. (2001). Oxygenation of human tumors–implications for combined therapy. *Lung Cancer* 33, S77–S83. doi: 10.1016/S0169-5002(01)00306-3

Feng, X., Zhou, Q., Liu, C., and Tao, M. (2012). Drug screening study using glioma stem-like cells. *Mol. Med. Rep.* 6, 1117–1120. doi: 10.3892/mmr.2012.1040

Foehrenbacher, A., Patel, K., Abbattista, M., Guise, C. P., Secomb, T. W., Wilson, W. R., et al. (2013). The role of by stander effects in the antitumor activity of the hypoxia-activated prodrug PR-104. *Front. Oncol.* 3:263. doi: 10.3389/fonc.2013.00263

Fraschini, A., Bottone, M. G., Scovassi, A. I., Denegri, M., Risueño, M. C., Testillano, P. S., et al. (2005). Changes in extranucleolar transcription during actinomycin D-induced apoptosis. *Histol. Histopathol.* 20, 107–117.

Frei, E. 3rd. (1974). The clinical use of actinomycin. *Cancer Chemother. Rep.* 58, 49–54.

Fuchs, D., Daniel, V., Sadeghi, M., Opelz, G., and Naujokat, C. (2010). Salinomycin overcomes ABC transporter-mediated multidrug and apoptosis resistance in human leukemia stem cell-like KG-1a cells. *Biochem. Biophys. Res. Commun.* 394, 1098–1104. doi: 10.1016/j.bbrc.2010.03.138

Gao, M. Q., Choi, Y. P., Kang, S., Youn, J. H., and Cho, N. H. (2010). CD24+ cells from hierarchically organized ovarian cancer are enriched in cancer stem cells. *Oncogene* 29, 2672–2680. doi: 10.1038/onc.2010.35

Geiger, A., Burgstaller, P., von der Eltz, H., Roeder, A., and Famulok, M. (1996). RNA aptamers that bind L-arginine with sub-micromolar dissociation constants and high enantioselectivity. *Nucleic Acids Res.* 24, 1029–1036. doi: 10.1093/nar/24.6.1029

Germain, A. R., Carmody, L. C., Nag, P. P., Morgan, B., VerPlank, L., Fernandez, C., et al. (2013). Cinnameds as selectiva small-molecule inhibitors of a cellular model of breast cancer stem cells. *Bioorg. Med. Chem. Lett.* 23, 1834–1838. doi: 10.1016/j.bmcl.2013.01.025

Gimenez-Bonafe, P., Guillen Canovas, A., Ambrosio, S., Tortosa, A., and Perez-Tomas, R. (2008). "Drugs modulating MDR," in *Multidrug Resistance: Biological and Pharmaceutical Advance in the Antitumour Treatment*, ed N. A. Colabufo (Kerala: Research Signpost), 63–99.

Goodell, M. A., Brose, K., Paradis, G., Conner, A. S., and Mulligan, R. C. (1996). Isolation and functional properties of murine hematopoietic stem cells that are replicating *in vivo*. *J. Exp. Med.* 183, 1797–1806. doi: 10.1084/jem.183.4.1797

Gotlieb, W. H., Saumet, J., Beauchamp, M. C., Gu, J., Lau, S., Pollak, M. N., et al. (2008). *In vitro* metformin anti-neoplastic activity in epithelial ovarian cancer. *Gynecol. Oncol.* 110, 246–250. doi: 10.1016/j.ygyno.2008.04.008

Griguer, C. E., Oliva, C. R., Gobin, E., Marcorelles, P., Benos, D. J., Lancaster, J. R. Jr., et al. (2008). CD133 is a marker of bioenergetic stress in human glioma. *PLoS ONE* 3:e3655. doi: 10.1371/journal.pone.0003655

Guise, C. P., Mowday, A. M., Ashoorzadeh, A., Yuan, R., Lin, W. H., Wu, D. H., et al. (2014). Bioreductive prodrugs as cancer therapeutics: targeting tumor hypoxia. *Chin. J. Cancer* 33, 80–86. doi: 10.5732/cjc.012.10285

Gupta, S. C., Sundaram, C., Reuter, S., and Aggarwal, B. B. (2010). Inhibiting NF-κB activation by small molecules as a therapeutic strategy. *Biochim. Biophys. Acta* 1799, 775–787. doi: 10.1016/j.bbagrm.2010.05.004

Hambardzumyan, D., Becher, O. J., Rosenblum, M. K., Pandolfi, P. P., Manova-Todorova, K., and Holland, E. C. (2008). PI3K pathway regulates survival of cancer stem cells residing in the perivascular niche following radiation in medulloblastoma *in vivo*. *Genes Dev.* 22, 436–448. doi: 10.1101/gad.1627008

Hamburger, A. W., and Salmon, S. E. (1977). Primary bioassay of human tumor stem cells. *Science* 197, 461–463. doi: 10.1126/science.560061

Hanahan, D., and Weinberg, R. A. (2011). Hallmarks of cancer: the next generation. *Cell* 144, 646–674. doi: 10.1016/j.cell.2011.02.013

Hemmati, H. D., Nakano, I., Lazareff, J. A., Masterman-Smith, M., Geschwind, D. H., Bronner-Fraser, M., et al. (2003). Cancerous stem cells can arise from pediatric brain tumors. *Proc. Natl. Acad. Sci. U.S.A.* 100, 15178–15183. doi: 10.1073/pnas.2036535100

Hennessy, B. T., Smith, D. L., Ram, P. T., Lu, Y., and Mills, G. B. (2005). Exploiting the PI3K/AKT pathway for cancer drug discovery. *Nat. Rev. Drug Discov.* 4, 988–1004. doi: 10.1038/nrd1902

Hicks, K. O., Siim, B. G., Jaiswal, J. K., Pruijn, F. B., Fraser, A. M., Patel, R., et al. (2010). Pharmacokinetic/pharmacodynamic modeling identifies SN30000 and SN29751 as tirapazamine analogues with improved tissue penetration and hypoxic cell killing in tumors. *Clin. Cancer Res.* 16, 20946–20957. doi: 10.1158/1078-0432.CCR-10-1439

Hirsch, H. A., Iliopoulos, D., Tsichlis, P. N., and Struhl, K. (2009). Metformin selectively targets cancer stem cells, and acts togheter with chemotherapy in block tumor growth and prolong remission. *Cancer Res.* 69, 7507–7511. doi: 10.1158/0008-5472.CAN-09-2994

Hirschhaeuser, F., Menne, H., Dittfeld, C., West, J., Mueller-Klieser, W., and Kunz-Schughart, L. A. (2010). Multicellular tumor spheroids: an underestimated tool is catching up again. *J. Biotechnol.* 148, 3–15. doi: 10.1016/j.jbiotec.2010.01.012

Holohan, C., Van Schaeybroeck, S., Longley, D. B., and Johnston, P. G. (2013). Cancer drug resistance: an evolving paradigm. *Nat. Rev. Cancer* 13, 714–726. doi: 10.1038/nrc3599

Hothi, P., Martins, T. J., Chen, L., Deleyrole, L., Yoon, J.-G., Reynolds, B., et al. (2012). High-throughput chemical screens identify Disulfiram as an inhibitor of human glioblastoma stem cells. *Oncotarget* 3, 1124–1136.

Huang, E. H., Hynes, M. J., Zhang, T., Ginestier, C., Dontu, G., Appelman, H., et al. (2009a). Aldehyde dehydrogenase 1 is a marker for normal and malignant human colonic stem cells (SC) and tracks SC overpopulation during colon tumorigenesis. *Cancer Res.* 69, 3382–3389. doi: 10.1158/0008-5472.CAN-08-4418

Huang, S. M., Mishina, Y. M., Liu, S., Cheung, A., Stegmeier, F., Michaud, G. A., et al. (2009b). Tankyrase inhibition stabilizes axin and antagonizes Wnt signaling. *Nature* 461, 614–620. doi: 10.1038/nature08356

Imai, Y., Yamagishi, H., Ono, Y., and Ueda, Y. (2012). Versatile inhibitory effects of the flavonoid-derived PI3K/Akt inhibitor, LY294002, on ATP-binding cassette transporters that characterize stem cells. *Clin. Transl. Med.* 1, 24–28. doi: 10.1186/2001-1326-1-24

Iyer, U., and Kadambi, V. J. (2011). Antibody drug conjugates-Trojan horses in the war on cancer. *J. Pharmacol. Toxicol. Methods* 64, 207–212. doi: 10.1016/j.vascn.2011.07.005

James, R. G., Davidson, K. C., Bosch, K. A., Biechele, T. L., Robin, N. C., Taylor, R. J., et al. (2012). WIKI4, a novel inhibitor of Tankyrase and Wnt/ß-Catenin signaling. *PLoS ONE* 7:e50457. doi: 10.1371/journal.pone.0050457

Janikowa, M., and Skarda, J. (2012). Differentiation pathways in carcinogenesis and in chemo- and radioresistance. *Neoplasma* 59, 6–17. doi: 10.4149/neo_2012_002

Jenison, R. D., Gill, S. C., Pardi, A., and Polisky, B. (1994). High-resolution molecular discrimination by RNA. *Science* 263, 1425–1429. doi: 10.1126/science.7510417

Jiang, F., Qiu, Q., Khanna, A., Todd, N. W., Deepak, J., Xing, L., et al. (2009). Aldehyde dehydrogenase 1 is a tumor stem cell-associated marker in lung cancer. *Mol. Cancer Res.* 7, 330–338. doi: 10.1158/1541-7786.MCR-08-0393

Jiang, W., Peng, J., Zhang, Y., Cho, W. C., and Jin, K. (2012). The implications of cancer stem cells for cancer therapy. *Int. J. Mol. Sci.* 13, 16636–16657. doi: 10.3390/ijms131216636

Jin, L., Hope, J. K., Zhai, Q., Smadja-Joffe, F., and Dick, J. E. (2006). Targeting of CD44 eradicates human acute myeloid leukemic stem cells. *Nat. Med.* 12, 1167–1174. doi: 10.1038/nm1483

Kennedy, B. J. (1970). Mithramycin therapy in advanced testicular neoplasms. *Cancer* 26, 755–766. doi: 10.1002/1097-0142(197010)26:4<755::AID-CNCR2820260403>3.0.CO;2-U

Ketola, K., Hilvo, M., Hyotylainen, T., Vuoristo, A., Ruskeepää, A. L., Orešić, M., et al. (2012). Salinomycin inhibits prostate cancer growth and migration via induction of oxidative stress. *Br. J. Cancer* 106, 19–106. doi: 10.1038/bjc.2011.530

Kim, Y., Wu, Q., Hamerlik, P., Hitomi, M., Sloan, A. E., Barnett, G. H., et al. (2013). Aptamer identification of brain tumor-initiating cells. *Cancer Res.* 73, 4923–4936. doi: 10.1158/0008-5472.CAN-12-4556

Kobune, M., Takimoto, R., Murase, K., Iyama, S., Sato, T., Kikuchi, S., et al. (2009). Drug resistance is dramatically restored by hedgehog inhibitors in CD34+ leukemic cells. *Cancer Sci.* 100, 948–955. doi: 10.1111/j.1349-7006.2009.01111.x

Kondo, T., Setoguchi, T., and Taga, T. (2004). Persistence of a small subpopulation of cancer stem-like cells in the C6 glioma cell line. *Proc. Natl. Acad. Sci. U.S.A.* 101, 781–786. doi: 10.1073/pnas.0307618100

Korkaya, H., Paulson, A., Charafe-Jauffret, E., Ginestier, C., Brown, M., Dutcher, J., et al. (2009). Regulation of mammary stem/progenitor cells by PTEN/Akt/β-catenin signaling. *PLoS Biol.* 7:e1000121. doi: 10.1371/journal.pbio.1000121

Kunz, M., and Ibrahim, S. M. (2003). Molecular responses to hypoxia in tumor cells. *Mol. Cancer* 2:23. doi: 10.1186/1476-4598-2-23

Kwon, M. J., and Shin, Y. K. (2013). Regulation of ovarian cancer stem cells or tumor-initiating cells. *Int. J. Mol. Sci.* 14, 6624–6648. doi: 10.3390/ijms14046624

Landen, C. N. Jr., Goodman, B., Katre, A. A., Steg, A. D., Nick, A. M., Stone, R. L., et al. (2010). Targeting aldehyde dehydrogenase cancer stem cells in ovarian cancer. *Mol. Cancer Ther.* 9, 3186–3199. doi: 10.1158/1535-7163.MCT-10-0563

Lapidot, T., Sirard, C., Vormoor, J., Murdoch, B., Hoang, T., Caceres-Cortes, J., et al. (1994). A cell initiating human acute myeloid leukaemia after transplantation into SCID mice. *Nature* 367, 645–648. doi: 10.1038/367645a0

Lawson, D. A., Xin, L. I., Lukacs, R. U., Cheng, D., and Witte, O. N. (2007). Isolation and functional characterization of murine prostate stem cells. *Proc. Natl. Acad. Sci. U.S.A.* 104, 181–186. doi: 10.1073/pnas.0609684104

Lee, E., Salic, A., Kruger, R., Heinrich, R., and Kirschner, M. W. (2003). The roles of APC and Axin derived from experimental and theoretical analysis of the Wnt pathway. *PLoS Biol.* 1:E10. doi: 10.1371/journal.pbio.0000010

Lee, T. J., Jung, E. M., Lee, J. T., Kim, S., Park, J. W., Choi, K. S., et al. (2006). Mithramycin A sensitizes cancer cells to TRAIL-mediated apoptosis by down-regulation of XIAP gene promoter through Sp1 sites. *Mol. Cancer Ther.* 5, 2737–2746. doi: 10.1158/1535-7163.MCT-06-0426

Leizer, A. L., Alvero, A. B., Fu, H. H., Holmberg, J. C., Cheng, Y. C., Silasi, D. A., et al. (2011). Regulation of inflammation by the NF-kappa B pathway in ovarian cancer stem cells. *Am. J. Reprod. Immunol.* 65, 438–447. doi: 10.1111/j.1600-0897.2010.00914.x

Lewis, J. L. Jr. (1972). Chemotherapy of gestational choriocarcinoma. *Cancer* 30, 1517–1521. doi: 10.1002/1097-0142(197212)30:6<1517::AID-CNCR2820300616>3.0.CO;2-8

Li, C., Heidt, D. G., Dalerba, P., Burant, C. F., Zhang, L., Adsay, V., et al. (2007). Identification of pancreatic cancer stem cells. *Cancer Res.* 67, 1030–1037. doi: 10.1158/0008-5472.CAN-06-2030

Li, T., Su, Y., Mei, Y., Leng, Q., Leng, B., Liu, Z., et al. (2010). ALDH1A1 is a marker for malignant prostate stem cells and predictor of prostate cancer patients' outcome. *Lab. Invest.* 90, 234–244. doi: 10.1038/labinvest.2009.127

Liu, C., Li, Y., Semenov, M., Han, C., Baeg, G. H., Tan, Y., et al. (2002). Control of beta-catenin phosphorylation/degradation by a dual-kinase mechanism. *Cell* 108, 837–847. doi: 10.1016/S0092-8674(02)00685-2

Liu, M., Sakamaki, T., Casimiro, M. C., Willmarth, N. E., Quong, A. A., Ju, X., et al. (2010). The canonical NF-κB pathway governs mammary tumorigenesis in transgenic mice and tumor stem cell expansion. *Cancer Res.* 70, 10464–10473. doi: 10.1158/0008-5472.CAN-10-0732

Liu, P., Brown, S., Goktug, T., Channathodiyil, P., Kannappan, V., Hugnot, J. P., et al. (2012). Cytotoxic effect of disulfiram/copper on human glioblastoma cell lines and ALDH positive cancer-stem-like cells. *Br. J. Cancer* 9, 1488–1497. doi: 10.1038/bjc.2012.442

Liu, S., Dontu, G., Mantle, I. D., Patel, S., Ahn, N. S., Jackson, K. W., et al. (2006). Hedgehog signaling and Bmi-1 regulate self-renewal of normal and malignant human mammary stem cells. *Cancer Res.* 66, 6063–6071. doi: 10.1158/0008-5472.CAN-06-0054

Lorico, A., and Rappa, G. (2011). Phenotypic heterogeneity of breast cancer stem cells. *J. Oncol.* 2011:135039. doi: 10.1155/2011/135039

Lou, D., Wang, B., Wang, Y., and Cao, Y. (2012). Selective killing of cancer stem cells by a novel dual-targeting strategy. *Med. Hypotheses* 79, 430–432. doi: 10.1016/j.mehy.2012.06.012

Lupold, S. E., Hicke, B. J., Lin, Y., and Coffet, D. S. (2002). Identification and characterization of nuclease-stabilized RNA molecules that bind human prostate cancer cells via the prostate-specific membrane antigen. *Cancer Res.* 62, 4029–4033.

Ma, S., Lee, T. K., Zheng, B. J., Chan, K. W., and Guan, X. Y. (2008). CD133+ HCC cancer stem cells confer chemoresistance by preferential expression of the Akt/PKB survival pathway. *Oncogene* 27, 1749–1758. doi: 10.1038/sj.onc.1210811

MacDonald, B. T., Tamai, K., and He, X. (2009). Wnt/beta-catenin signaling: components, mechanisms, and diseases. *Dev. Cell* 17, 9–26. doi: 10.1016/j.devcel.2009.06.016

Majmundar, A. J., Wong, W. J., and Simon, M. C. (2010). Hypoxia-inducible factors and the response to hypoxic stress. *Mol. Cell* 40, 294–309. doi: 10.1016/j.molcel.2010.09.022

Marcu, L., and Olver, I. (2006). Tirapazamine: from bench to clinical trials. *Curr. Clin. Pharmacol.* 1, 71–79. doi: 10.2174/157488406775268192

McAuliffe, S. M., Morgan, S. L., Wyant, G. A., Tran, L. T., Muto, K. W., Chen, Y. S., et al. (2012). Targeting Notch, a key pathway for ovarian cancer stem cells, sensitizes tumors to platinum therapy. *Proc. Natl. Acad. Sci. U.S.A.* 109, E2939–E2948. doi: 10.1073/pnas.1206400109

Meng, F., Evans, J. W., Bhupathi, D., Banica, M., Lan, L., Lorente, G., et al. (2012). Molecular and cellular pharmacology of the hypoxia-activated prodrug TH-302. *Mol. Cancer Ther.* 11, 740–751. doi: 10.1158/1535-7163.MCT-11-0634

Mezencev, R., Wang, L., and McDonald, J. F. (2012). Identification of inhibitors of ovarian cancer stem-like cells by high-throughput screening. *J. Ovarian Res.* 5, 30–41. doi: 10.1186/1757-2215-5-30

Mogi, M., Yang, J., Lambert, J. F., Colvin, G. A., Shiojima, I., Skurk, C., et al. (2003). Akt signaling regulates side population cell phenotype via Bcrp translocation. *J. Biol. Chem.* 278, 39068–39075. doi: 10.1074/jbc.M306362200

Moitra, K., Lou, H., and Dean, M. (2011). Multidrug efflux pumps and cancer stem cells: insights into multidrug resistance and therapeutic development. *Clin. Pharmacol. Ther.* 89, 491–502. doi: 10.1038/clpt.2011.14

Moreb, J. S. (2008). Aldehyde dehydrogenase as a marker for stem cells. *Curr. Stem Cell Res. Ther.* 3, 237–246. doi: 10.2174/157488808786734006

Naujokat, C. (2014). Monoclonal antibodies against human cancer stem cells. *Immunotherapy* 6, 290–308. doi: 10.2217/imt.14.4

Nesi, G., Colabufo, N. A., Contino, M., Perrone, M. G., Digiacomo, M., Perrone, R., et al. (2014). SAR study on Arylmethyloxyphenyl scaffold: looking for a P-gp nanomolar affinity. *Eur. J. Med. Chem.* 76, 558–566. doi: 10.1016/j.ejmech.2014.02.051

Oak, P. S., Kopp, F., Thakur, C., Ellwart, J. W., Rapp, U. R., Ullrich, A., et al. (2012). Combinatorial treatment of mammospheres with trastuzumab and salinomycin efficiently targets HER2-positve cancer cells and cancer stem cells. *Int. J. Cancer* 131, 2808–2019. doi: 10.1002/ijc.27595

Orfao, A., and Ruiz-Arguelles, A. (1996). General concepts about cell sorting techniques. *Clin. Biochem.* 29, 5–9. doi: 10.1016/0009-9120(95)02017-9

Park, J. T., Li, M., Nakayama, K., Mao, T. L., Davidson, B., Zhang, Z., et al. (2006). Notch3 gene amplification in ovarian cancer. *Cancer Res.* 66, 6312–6318. doi: 10.1158/0008-5472.CAN-05-3610

Patterson, L. H., Craven, M. R., Fisher, G. R., and Teesdale-Spittle P. (1994). Aliphatic amine N-oxides of DNA binding agents as bioreductive drugs. *Oncol. Res.* 6, 533–538.

Patterson, L. H., McKeown, S. R., Ruparelia, K., Double, J. A., Bibby, M. C., Cole, S., et al. (2000). Enhancement of chemotherapy and radiotherapy of murine tumours by AQ4N, a bioreductively activated anti-tumour agent. *Br. J. Cancer* 82, 1984–1990. doi: 10.1054/bjoc.2000.1163

Perez-Tomas, R. (2006). Multidrug resistance: retrospect and prospects in anti-cancer drug treatment. *Curr. Med. Chem.* 13, 1859–1876. doi: 10.2174/092986706777585077

Perlia, C. P., Gubisch, N. J., Wolter, J., Edelberg, D., Dederick, M. M., and Taylor, S. G. 3rd. (1970). Mithramycin treatment of hypercalcemia. *Cancer* 25, 389–394. doi: 10.1002/1097-0142(197002)25:2<389::AID-CNCR2820250217>3.0.CO;2-X

Pharm, A. N., Penchala, S., Graf, R. A., Wang, J., and Huang, Y. (2008). "Pharmacogenomic characterization of ABC transporters involved in Multidrug Resistance," in *Multidrug Resistance: Biological and Pharmaceutical Advance in the Antitumour Treatment*, ed N. A. Colabufo (Kerala: Research Signpost), 19–62.

Phillips, R. M., Hendriks, H. R., and Peters, G. J. (2013). EO9 (Apaziquone): from the clinic to the laboratory and back again. *Br. J. Pharmacol.* 168, 11–18. doi: 10.1111/j.1476-5381.2012.01996.x

Pietras, A. (2011). Cancer stem cells in tumor heterogeneity. *Adv. Cancer Res.* 112, 255–281. doi: 10.1016/B978-0-12-387688-1.00009-0

Pollard, S. M., Yoshikawa, K., Clarke, I. D., Danovi, D., Stricker, S., Russell, R., et al. (2009). Glioma stem cell lines expanded in adherent culture have tumor-specific phenotypes and are suitable for chemical and genetic screens. *Cell Stem Cell* 4, 568–580. doi: 10.1016/j.stem.2009.03.014

Proske, D., Blank, M., Buhmann, R., and Resch, A. (2005). Aptamers-basic research drug development and clinical applications. *Appl. Microbiol. Biotechnol.* 69, 367–374. doi: 10.1007/s00253-005-0193-5

Rauth, A. M., Melo, T., and Misra, V. (1998). Bioreductive therapies: an overview of drugs and their mechanisms of action. *Int. J. Radiat. Oncol. Biol. Phys.* 42, 755–762. doi: 10.1016/S0360-3016(98)00302-2

Riccioni, R., Dupuis, M. L., Bernabei, M., Petrucci, E., Pasquini, L., Mariani, G., et al. (2010). The cancer stem cell selective inhibitor salinomycin is a P-glycoprotein inhibitor. *Blood Cells Mol. Dis.* 45, 16–92. doi: 10.1016/j.bcmd.2010.03.008

Ricci-Vitiani, L., Lombardi, D. G., Pilozzi, E., Biffoni, M., Todaro, M., Peschle, C., et al. (2007). Identification and expansion of human colon-cancer-initiating cells. *Nature* 445, 111–115. doi: 10.1038/nature05384

Riobo, N. A., Lu, K., Ai, X., Haines, G. M., and Emerson, C. P. Jr. (2006). Phosphoinositide 3-kinase and AKT are essential for Sonic Hedgehog signaling. *Proc. Natl. Acad. Sci. U.S.A.* 103, 4505–4510. doi: 10.1073/pnas.0504337103

Rischin, D., Peters, L. J., O'Sullivan, B., Giralt, J., Fisher, R., Yuen, K., et al. (2010). Tirapazamine, cisplatin, and radiation versus cisplatin and radiation for advanced squamous cell carcinoma of the head and neck (TROG 02.02, HeadSTART): a phase III trial of the Trans-Tasman Radiation Oncology Group. *J. Clin. Oncol.* 28, 2989–2995. 10.1200/JCO.2009.27.4449

Sagiv, E., Starr, A., Rozovski, U., Khosravi, R., Altevogt, P., Wang, T., et al. (2008). Targeting CD24 for treatment of colorectal and pancreatic cancer by monoclonal antibodies or small interfering RNA. *Cancer Res.* 68, 2803–2812. doi: 10.1158/0008-5472.CAN-07-6463

Sasaki, H., Nishizaki, Y., Hui, C., Nakafuku, M., and Kondoh, H. (1999). Regulation of Gli2 and Gli3 activities by an amino-terminal repression domain: implication of Gli2 and Gli3 as primary mediators of Shh signaling. *Development* 126, 3915–3924.

Saunders, M. P., Jaffar, M., Patterson, A. V., Nolan, J., Naylor, M. A., Phillips, R. M., et al. (2000). The relative importance of NADPH: cytochrome c (P450) reductase for determining the sensitivity of human tumour cells to the indolequinone EO9 and related analogues lacking functionality at the C-2 and C-3 positions. *Biochem. Pharmacol.* 59, 993–996. doi: 10.1016/S0006-2952(99)00405-0

Sefah, K., Shangguan, D., Xiong, X. L., O'Donoghue, M. B., and Tan, W. (2010). Development of DNA aptamers using Cell-SELEX. *Nat. Protoc.* 5, 1169–1185. doi: 10.1038/nprot.2010.66

Shangguan, D., Li, Y., Tang, Z. W., Cao, Z. C., Chen, H. W., Mallikaratchy, P., et al. (2006). Aptamers evolved from live cells as effective molecular probes for cancer study. *Proc. Natl. Acad. Sci. U.S.A.* 103, 11838–11843. doi: 10.1073/pnas.0602615103

Shank, J. J., Yang, K., Ghannam, J., Cabrera, L., Johnston, C. J., Reynolds, R. K., et al. (2012). Metformin targets ovarian cancer stem cells *in vitro* and *in vivo*. *Gynecol. Oncol.* 127, 390–397. doi: 10.1016/j.ygyno.2012.07.115

Shinde, S. S., Maroz, A., Hay, M. P., Patterson, A. V., Denny, W. A., and Anderson, R. F. (2010). Characterization of radicals formed following enzymatic reduction of 3-substituted analogues of the hypoxia-selective cytotoxin 3-amino-1,2,4-benzotriazine 1,4-dioxide (tirapazamine). *J. Am. Chem. Soc.* 132, 2591–2599. doi: 10.1021/ja908689f

Siemann, D. W., and Keng, P. C. (1986). Cell cycle specific toxicity of the Hoechst 33342 stain in untreated or irradiated murine tumor cells. *Cancer Res.* 46, 3556–3559.

Singh, S. K., Clarke, I. D., Terasaki, M., Bonn, V. E., Hawkins, C., Squire, J., et al. (2003). Identification of a cancer stem cell in human brain tumors. *Cancer Res.* 63, 5821–5828.

Singleton, R. S., Guise, C. P., Ferry, D. M., Pullen, S. M., Dorie, M. J., Brown, J. M., et al. (2009). DNA crosslinks in human tumor cells exposed to the prodrug PR-104A: relationships to hypoxia, bioreductive metabolism and cytotoxicity. *Cancer Res.* 69, 3884–3891. doi: 10.1158/0008-5472.CAN-08-4023

Smith, K. M., Datti, A., Fujitani, M., Grinshtein, N., Zhang, L., Morozova, O., et al. (2010). Selective targeting of neuroblastoma tumour-initiating cells by compounds identified in stem cell-based small molecule screens. *EMBO Mol. Med.* 2, 371–384. doi: 10.1002/emmm.201000093

Smith, L. M., Nesterova, A., Ryan, M. C., Duniho, S., Jonas, M., Anderson, M., et al. (2008). CD133/prominin-1 is a potential therapeutic target for antibodydrug conjugates in hepatocellular and gastric cancers. *Br. J. Cancer* 99, 100–109. doi: 10.1038/sj.bjc.6604437

Storms, R. W., Trujillo, A. P., Springer, J. B., Shah, L., Colvin, O. M., Ludeman, S. M., et al. (1999). Isolation of primitive human hematopoietic progenitors on the basis of aldehyde dehydrogenase activity. *Proc. Natl. Acad. Sci. U.S.A.* 96, 9118–9123. doi: 10.1073/pnas.96.16.9118

Stratford, E. W., Bostad, M., Castro, R., Skarpen, E., Berg, K., Høgset, A., et al. (2013). Photochemical internalization of CD133-targeting immunotoxins efficiently depletes sarcomacells with stem-like properties and reduces tumorigenicity. *Biochim. Biophys. Acta* 1830, 4235–4243. doi: 10.1016/j.bbagen.2013.04.033

Su, Y., Qiu, Q., Zhang, X., Jiang, Z., Leng, Q., Liu, Z., et al. (2010). Aldehyde dehydrogenase 1 A1-positive cell population is enriched in tumor-initiating cells and associated with progression of bladder cancer. *Cancer Epidemiol. Biomarkers Prev.* 19, 327–337. doi: 10.1158/1055-9965.EPI-09-0865

Takaishi, S., Okumura, T., Tu, S., Wang, S. S., Shibata, W., Vigneshwaran, R., et al. (2009). Identification of gastric cancer stem cells using the cell surface marker CD44. *Stem Cells* 27, 1006–1020. doi: 10.1002/stem.30

Takebe, N., Harris, P. J., Warren, R. Q., and Ivy, S. P. (2011). Targeting cancer stem cells by inhibiting Wnt, Notch, and Hedgehog pathways. *Nat. Rev. Clin. Oncol.* 8, 97–106. doi: 10.1038/nrclinonc.2010.196

Tanaka, K., Okabayashi, K., Asashima, M., Perrimon, N., and Kadowaki, T. (2000). The evolutionarily conserved porcupine gene family is involved in the processing of the Wnt family. *Eur. J. Biochem.* 267, 4300–4311. doi: 10.1046/j.1432-1033.2000.01478.x

Tang, Q. L., Zhao, Z. Q., Li, J. C., Liang, Y., Yin, J. Q., Zou, C. Y., et al. (2011). Salinomycin inhibits osteosarcoma by targeting its tumor stem cells. *Cancer Lett.* 311, 113–121. doi: 10.1016/j.canlet.2011.07.016

Teng, Y., Wang, X., Wang, Y., and Ma, D. (2010). Wnt/β-catenin signaling regulates cancer stem cells in lung cancer A549 cells. *Biochem. Biophys. Res. Commun.* 392, 373–379. doi: 10.1016/j.bbrc.2010.01.028

Teodori, E., Dei, S., Martelli, S., Scapecchi, F., and Gualtieri, F. (2006). The functions and structure of ABC transporters: implications for the design of new inhibitors of Pgp and MRP1 to control multidrug resistance (MDR). *Curr. Drug Targets* 7, 893–909. doi: 10.2174/138945006777709520

Thomas, T., Nowka, K., Lan, L., and Derwahl, M. (2006). Expression of endoderm stem cell markers: evidence for the presence of adult stem cells in human thyroid glands. *Thyroid* 16, 537–544. doi: 10.1089/thy.2006.16.537

Tomiyasu, S., Miyamoto, T., Mori, M., Yaguchi, T., Yakushiji, H., Ohno, S., et al. (2014). Isolation of side population cells from endometrial cancer cells using a violet laser diode. *Hum. Cell* 27, 36–42. doi: 10.1007/s13577-013-0079-2

Tuerk, C., and Gold, L. (1990). Systematic evolution of ligands by exponential enrichment—RNA ligands to bacteriophage-T4 DNA-polymerase. *Science* 249, 505–510. doi: 10.1126/science.2200121

Varjosalo, M., and Taipale, J. (2008). Hedgehog: functions and mechanisms. *Genes Dev.* 22, 2454–2472. doi: 10.1101/gad.1693608

Waaler, J., Machon, O., Tumova, L., Dinh, H., Korinek, V., Wilson, S. R., et al. (2012). A novel Tankyrase inhibitor decreases canonical Wnt signaling in colon carcinoma cells and reduces tumor growth in conditional APC mutant mice. *Cancer Res.* 72, 2822–2832. doi: 10.1158/0008-5472.CAN-11-3336

Waldron, N. N., Kaufman, D. S., Oh, S., Inde, Z., Hexum, M. K., Ohlfest, J. R., et al. (2011). Targeting tumor-initiating cancer cells with dCD133KDEL shows impressive tumor reductions in a xenotransplant model of human head and neck cancer. *Mol. Cancer Ther.* 10, 1829–1838. doi: 10.1158/1535-7163.MCT-11-0206

Wang, S., Huang, S., Zhao, X., Zhang, Q., Wu, M., Sun, F., et al. (2013a). Enrichment of prostate cancer stem cells from primary prostate cancer cultures of biopsy samples. *Int. J. Clin. Exp. Pathol.* 7, 184–193.

Wang, X., Moon, J., Dodge, M. E., Pan, X., Zhang, L., Hanson, J. M., et al. (2013b). The development of highly potent inhibitors for porcupine. *J. Med. Chem.* 56, 2700–2704. doi: 10.1021/jm400159c

Wang, Y. (2011). Effects of salinomycin on cancer stem cell in human lung adenocarcinoma A549 cells. *Med. Chem.* 7, 206–111. doi: 10.2174/15734061179 4859307

Wang, Z., Li, Y., Kong, D., Banerjee, S., Ahmad, A., Azmi, A. S., et al. (2009). Acquisition of epithelialmesenchymal transition phenotype of gemcitabine-resistant pancreatic cancer cells is linked with activation of the notch signaling pathway. *Cancer Res.* 69, 2400–2407. doi: 10.1158/0008-5472.CAN-08-4312

Whitworth, J. M., Londono-Joshi, A. I., Sellers, J. C., Oliver, P. J., Muccio, D. D., Atigadda, V. R., et al. (2012). The impact of novel retinoids in combination with platinum chemotherapy on ovarian cancer stem cells. *Gynecol. Oncol.* 125, 226–230. doi: 10.1016/j.ygyno.2011.12.425

Wintzell, M., Lofstedt, L., Johansson, J., Pedersen, A. B., Fuxe, J., and Shoshan, M. (2012). Repeated cisplatin treatment can lead to a multiresistant tumor cell population with stem cell features and sensitivity to 3-bromopyruvate. *Cancer Biol. Ther.* 13, 1454–1462. doi: 10.4161/cbt.22007

Wright, M. H., Calcagno, A. M., Salcido, C. D., Carlson, M. D., Ambudkar, S. V., and Varticovski, L. (2008). Brca1 breast tumors contain distinct CD44+/CD24- and CD133+ cells with cancer stem cell characteristics. *Breast Cancer Res.* 10:R10. doi: 10.1186/bcr1855

Xia, J., Zhang, Y., Qian, J., Zhu, X., Zhang, Y., Zhang, J., et al. (2013). Isolation, identification and expression of specific human CD133 antibodies. *Sci. Rep.* 3:3320. doi: 10.1038/srep03320

Xin, L. I., Lawson, D. A., and Witte, O. N. (2005). The Sca-1 cell surface marker enriches for a prostate-regenerating cell subpopulation that can initiate prostate tumorigenesis. *Proc. Natl. Acad. Sci. U.S.A.* 102, 6942–6947. doi: 10.1073/pnas.0502320102

Yang, X., Zheng, X., Cao, J., Xiang, H., Liu, F., and Lv, Y. (2010). 8-bromo-7-methoxychrysin-induced apoptosis of hepatocellular carcinoma cells involves ROS and JNK. *World J. Gastroenterol.* 16, 27385–23393. doi: 10.3748/wjg.v16.i27.3385

Yasmeen, A., Beauchamp, M. C., Piura, E., Segal, E., Pollak, M., and Gotlieb, W. H. (2011). Induction of apoptosis by metformin in epithelial ovarian cancer: involvement of the Bcl-2 family proteins. *Gynecol. Oncol.* 121, 492–498. doi: 10.1016/j.ygyno.2011.02.021

Yeung, J., Esposito, M. T., Gandillet, A., Zeisig, B. B., Griessinger, E., Bonnet, D., et al. (2010). β-catenin mediates the establishment and drug resistance of MLL leukemic stem cells. *Cancer Cell* 18, 606–618. doi: 10.1016/j.ccr.2010.10.032

Yin, J., Glaser, R., and Gates, K. S. (2012). On there action mechanism of tirapazamine reduction chemistry: unimolecular N-OH homolysis, stepwise dehydration, ortriazene ring-opening. *Chem. Res. Toxicol.* 25, 634–645. doi: 10.1021/tx200546u

Yo, Y. T., Lin, Y. W., Wang, Y. C., Balch, C., Huang, R. L., Chan, M. W., et al. (2012). Growth inhibition of ovarian tumor-initiating cells by niclosamide. *Mol. Cancer Ther.* 11, 1703–1712. doi: 10.1158/1535-7163.MCT-12-0002

Zeman, E. M., Brown, J. M., Lemmon, M. J., Hirst, V. K., and Lee, W. W. (1986). SR-4233: a new bioreductive agent with high selective toxicity for hypoxic mammalian cells. *Int. J. Radiat. Oncol. Biol. Phys.* 12, 1239–1242. doi: 10.1016/0360-3016(86)90267-1

Zhang, S., Balch, C., Chan, M. W., Lai, H. C., Matei, D., Schilder, J. M., et al. (2008). Identification and characterization of ovarian cancer-initiating cells from primary human tumors. *Cancer Res.* 68, 4311–4320. doi: 10.1158/0008-5472.CAN-08-0364

Zhao, C., Chen, A., Jamieson, C. H., Fereshteh, M., Abrahamsson, A., Blum, J., et al. (2009). Hedgehog signaling is essential for maintenance of cancer stem cells in myeloid leukaemia. *Nature* 458, 776–779. doi: 10.1038/nature07737

Zhi, Q. M., Chen, X. H., Ji, J., Zhang, J. N., Li, J. F., Cai, Q., et al. (2011). Salinomycin can effectively kill ALDH(high) stem-like cells on gastric cancer. *Biomed. Pharmacother.* 65, 509–515. doi: 10.1016/j.biopha.2011.06.006

Zhou, F., Mu, Y. D., Liang, J., Liu, Z. X., Chen, H. S., and Zhang, J. F. (2014). Expression and prognostic value of tumor stem cell markers ALDH1 and CD133 in colorectal carcinoma. *Oncol. Lett.* 7, 507–512. doi: 10.3892/ol.2013.1723

Zhou, J., Wulfkuhle, J., Zhang, H., Gu, P., Yang, Y., Deng, J., et al. (2007). Activation of the PTEN/mTOR/STAT3 pathway in breast cancer stem-like cells is required for viability and maintenance. *Proc. Natl. Acad. Sci. U.S.A.* 104, 16158–16163. doi: 10.1073/pnas.0702596104

Zhou, J., Zhang, H., Gu, P., Bai, J., Margolick, J. B., and Zhang, Y. (2008). NF-κB pathway inhibitors preferentially inhibit breast cancer stem-like cells. *Breast Cancer Res. Treat.* 111, 419–427. doi: 10.1007/s10549-007-9798-y

16

A practical approach to aid physician interpretation of clinically actionable predictive biomarker results in a multi-platform tumor profiling service

Kenneth Russell[1]*, Leonid Shunyakov[2], Karel A. Dicke[3], Todd Maney[4] and Andreas Voss[1]

[1] Caris Life Sciences, Basel, Switzerland
[2] Central Care Cancer Center, Bolivar, MO, USA
[3] Arlington Cancer Center, Arlington, TX, USA
[4] Caris Life Sciences, Phoenix, AZ, USA

Edited by:
Jan Trøst Jørgensen, Dx-Rx Institute, Denmark

Reviewed by:
James Kevin Hicks, Cleveland Clinic, USA
Rafael Rosell, Catalan Institute of Oncology – Hospital Germans Trias i Pujol, Spain

***Correspondence:**
Kenneth Russell, Caris Life Sciences, Saint Jakobstrasse 199, Basel 4052, Switzerland
e-mail: krussell@carisls.com

Patients in whom the standard of care has failed or who have uncommon tumors for which no standard of care exists are often treated with drugs selected based on the physician's best guess. The rate of success for this method is generally low. With the advent of fast, affordable tumor profiling technologies, and a growth in the understanding of predictive biomarkers, it is now possible to identify drugs potentially associated with clinical benefit for such patients. We present the Caris approach to evidence-based tumor profiling and two patients with advanced ovarian and prostate cancer in whom standard of care had failed and tumor profiling identified an effective treatment schedule. To establish Caris Molecular Intelligence^{TM} (CMI), over 120,000 clinical publications were screened and graded to characterize the predictive value of biomarkers that form the panel of tests. CMI includes multiple technologies to measure changes in proteins, ribonucleic acid, and deoxyribonucleic acid and proprietary software that matches the test results with the published evidence. The CMI results enable physicians to select drugs that are more likely to benefit the patients, avoid drugs that are not likely to work, and find treatment options that otherwise would not be considered. Worldwide, over 60,000 cancer patients have undergone evidence-based tumor profiling with CMI. In the cases reported in this article, CMI identified treatments that would not have been routinely used in the respective clinical setting. The clinical outcomes observed help to illustrate the utility of this approach.

Keywords: evidence-guided, personalized medicine, biomarkers, oncology

INTRODUCTION

Patients who reach the end of their guidelines-defined treatment options and are suitable and willing to receive further treatment, or who present with an uncommon cancer type where treatment options are limited, are among the most difficult to treat. In such cases, the treatment decision is based on the individual patient's clinical context, physician's experience and clinical judgment, local practice guidelines and the patient's medical and treatment history. While the overall rate of success for cancer drug treatment has been estimated at 35% (Jackson, 2009), treatment for these patients is less effective, e.g., the response rate to therapy in patients meeting the inclusion criteria for early clinical studies is around 10% (Olmos et al., 2012).

Advances in the discovery of prognostic and predictive biomarkers can provide oncologists with vital information which helps to stratify their patients for risk of tumor progression and identify potentially beneficial therapeutic agents based on biomarker expression patterns. For example, lung cancer has traditionally been viewed as difficult to treat and associated with poor prognosis. The last 5 years has seen epidermal growth factor receptor (EGFR) mutation testing become standard of care for selection of treatment with erlotinib or gefitinib in non-small cell lung cancer (NSCLC). Many companion diagnostics are now part of the approved drug label and clinical guidelines indicate which specific biomarker should be assessed in a consistent manner in all patients prior to treatment selection in certain tumor types in order to identify a defined subgroup for which the respective treatment is indicated.

While many new drugs received regulatory approval together with companion diagnostics in a limited, often lineage specific, clinical setting, the biological principles governing cancer growth can often be extrapolated to other indications as well. One example is the utility of human EGFR 2 (HER2)-directed treatments for patients with lung cancer that have a HER2 (encoded by the *ERBB2* gene) mutation. While this occurs in fewer than 2% of all patients with lung cancer HER2-directed targeted treatments led to disease control in 82% of patients with HER2 mutations (Mazières et al., 2013). This shows that for a patient with no available standard treatment options molecular profiling can reveal specific biomarkers that are associated with benefit from drugs that would typically not have been considered for treatment.

As the majority of individual mutations or other molecular changes are usually rare, a comprehensive profiling increases the chance that a valuable alteration is identified. Comprehensive profiling delivers all relevant information at once, rather than taking a stepwise approach where tests are ordered one by one dependent on the outcome of single biomarker results. This saves valuable time for the patient and confers an important advantage because the comprehensive overview of the patient's molecular changes provides the best support for rational treatment decisions.

Over recent years, tumor profiling has become a standard in many large university centers. Tsimberidou et al. (2012) published how tumor profiling guided recruitment of patients into clinical trials with targeted drugs at the MD Anderson Cancer Center. Patients enrolled in studies that required a matching genetic aberration had a clinical response rate of 27% whereas only 5% of patients that could not be assigned to a trial based on molecular profiling responded (Tsimberidou et al., 2012). In a similar approach undertaken at the Princess Margaret Cancer Centre in Toronto, six of twenty-one patients (29%) enrolled into ongoing clinical trials with a therapy matched to a genetic aberration had a confirmed partial response (Bedard et al., 2013). Both of these groups employed large, cross-functional teams of experts to interpret the results from molecular testing. The ability to dedicate experienced teams to guide tumor profiling-directed treatment is beyond the capabilities of most community practices. Therefore alternative methods had to be developed to allow patient's access to reliable and actionable tumor profiling results.

CMI: AN EVIDENCE-BASED APPROACH OF TUMOR PROFILING FOR CLINICAL DECISION-MAKING

Caris Life Sciences started to offer evidence-based molecular profiling over 8 years ago. The approach taken has been constantly refined, resulting in a service which is adapted to the latest scientific knowledge. Caris Molecular Intelligence™ (CMI) supports physicians in implementing actionable results from comprehensive tumor profiling in their routine practice. CMI is performed in a high-throughput laboratory that has been customized to accommodate large numbers of specimens for testing on multiple technology platforms. Comprehensive molecular testing is coupled with an evidence-based proprietary algorithm that translates complex biomarker results into a table of drugs that may provide benefit or lack of benefit for that patient. Caris has received accreditation from Clinical Laboratory Improvement Amendments (CLIAs), as well as an extensive list of certifications from the state of New York. Caris also has recently obtained the molecular profiling industry's first-ever accreditation to the International Standards Organization (ISO) 15189: 2012 "Medical laboratories – Requirements for quality and competence," by the American Association for Laboratory Accreditation (A2LA). The CMI service provides each treating physician with the relevant biomarker testing and current expert interpretation needed to make clinical treatment decisions for each patient.

The CMI service uses a variety of established technology platforms to measure a panel of carefully selected biomarkers including immunohistochemistry (IHC), fluorescent *in situ* hybridization (FISH), polymerase chain reaction (PCR), and direct gene sequencing. Taking an approach that is not reliant on a single technology is critical to perform clinically relevant biomarker testing. Proteins, gene expression, mutations, and gene rearrangements can all have utility as predictive biomarkers. For example, of the 93.5% of compounds predicted to be beneficial which were identified, 87.2% of them were driven by IHC and ISH results, 12.6% by IHC, ISH, and NGS results, and 0.2% driven by NGS results alone. Therefore, an assessment of the molecular profile of a tumor with just one technology will miss potential therapeutic options for the patient.

To keep the biomarker panel current, an ongoing review of the medical literature is performed to review the evidence of predictive associations of biomarkers with available therapeutics. The interpretation of the biomarker evidence is under the governance of a cross-functional group comprised of oncologists, molecular geneticists, pathologists, and research scientists. All biomarkers tested in the CMI service are included based on the strength of their supporting evidence according to a version of the United States Preventative Services Task Force (USPSTF) level of evidence methodology adapted from Harris et al. (2001). The content of each scientific paper is appraised for study design, study validity, and applicability of the biomarker in drug selection. Today, over 95% of drug/biomarker associations included in the service are supported by level 1 (randomized, controlled trials or meta-analyzes) or level 2 (non-randomized, controlled trials, single arm or cohort/case-control analytic studies) evidence. The evidence system used by Caris allows the service to evolve in response to new clinical data. As new markers are identified and vetted, they can be added to the panel quickly. An overview of the evidence process for CMI is shown in **Figure 1**.

The CMI report aligns the molecular profile of the patient's tumor to relevant therapeutic agents associated with potential benefit or potential lack of benefit for the purpose of serving as a decision support aid for the treating physician. The report results are provided to the treating physician and supported by the relevant references from the peer-reviewed literature as determined by the evidence review process. The report also enables the treating clinician to review in detail the biomarker testing that has been performed, as well as link directly to the clinical evidence supporting the biomarker-drug association.

CLINICAL EVIDENCE SUPPORTING USE OF CMI

A manuscript has been published with a number of independent accompanying abstracts which have reported how CMI was used in clinical practice. The Bisgrove study (Von Hoff et al., 2010) was the first clinical trial to assess the use of a multi-platform approach to molecular profiling to identify treatment targets in patients with refractory cancers. In this study, patients were profiled with the CMI panel and physicians chose a treatment regimen based on the results. Clinical benefit was defined as a 30% increase in progression-free-survival (PFS) with molecularly guided treatments, compared to the PFS under the most recent prior regimen. The majority of patients had molecularly identifiable targets and 18 of 66 patients (27%) treated on the basis of molecular profiling derived clinical benefit. A recent study in patients with refractory breast cancer showed that tumor profiling resulted in a revision of the original treatment decision for all patients. Tumor profiling based therapy resulted in a clinical benefit in 52% of heavily pretreated patients (Jameson et al., 2013). A review of all patients

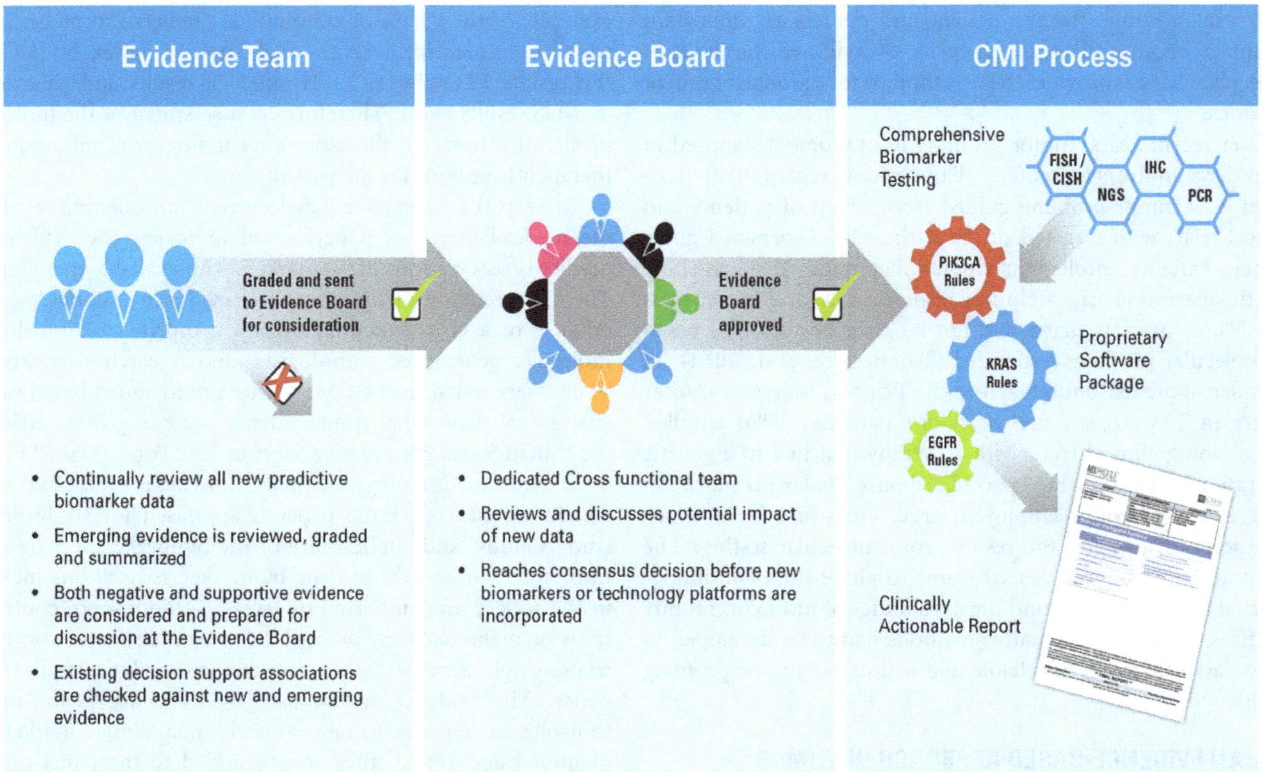

FIGURE 1 | Generating Molecular Intelligence: an extensive literature review is performed by a multi-disciplinary review team, which examines new research and relevant research, and grades it based on US Preventative Task Force methodology in the context of the biomarkers revealed through the profiling services. The output from this evidence review forms the basis of a proprietary software package which is used to translate the results of comprehensive biomarker testing to a clinically actionable report, providing physicians with meaningful biomarkers, actionable drug associations, and relevant clinical trials for their individual patient.

treated in a single center in Australia resulted in clinical and survival benefits in over half of the patients and confirmed the role of molecular profiling in a clinical practice setting (Dean and Wallace, 2013). Though preliminary evidence supports clinical utility, the degree to which CMI improves patient outcomes has not yet been demonstrated conclusively. Further evaluations of the approach are currently ongoing.

CASE STUDY: RESPONSE TO PEMETREXED IN A PATIENT WITH METASTATIC PROSTATE CANCER

A 63-year-old patient was diagnosed with metastatic prostate cancer in 2006 with a Gleason score of 9 and involvement of the pelvic lymph nodes. The patient initially received radiation therapy to the pelvis and the prostate followed by treatment with gonadotropin-releasing hormone (GnRH) analogs. After 4 years the disease progressed and metastasized to the bones, lung, and liver. Treatment with bisphosphonates, sipuleucel-T, abiraterone, enzalutamide, docetaxel, and cabazitaxel did not stop progression. The disease could never be controlled except for short transient partial responses under docetaxel and abiraterone. Embolization of the left liver lobe resulted in temporary local pain relief and as a last resort, the patient received carboplatin with etoposide, which resulted in a transient partial response followed by rapidly progressive disease.

As all guideline-recommended treatment options had failed, it was decided to perform CMI tumor profiling. At this time, the patient had extensive liver metastases with underlying cirrhosis, which caused considerable pain. He was wheelchair bound and unable to walk with an Eastern Cooperative Oncology Group (ECOG) performance status of 3, approaching 4. Within 6 weeks, his prostate specific antigen (PSA) had risen from 84 ng/ml to 177 ng/ml and lactate dehydrogenase (LDH) levels had risen from 569 to 2196 IU/L. All signs and symptoms pointed to a rapidly progressive decline of the patient's general condition.

The CMI report indicated that the tumor was not expressing thymidylate synthase (TS), a protein involved in generation of critical components for DNA synthesis and repair pathways. Published level II evidence from a study of 268 patients with advanced NSCLC who received treatment with pemetrexed after prior chemotherapy found that patients with low TS expression had a longer median PFS compared to those with high TS expression (Chen et al., 2011). The CMI report associated low TS expression with tumor sensitivity to fluoropyrimidines and other folate analogs with potential benefit from 5-fluorouracil, capecitabine or pemetrexed. Therefore, it was decided to begin treatment with single agent pemetrexed at the end of September 2013 based on the physician's choice. The patient's general condition improved rapidly and the intense right upper quadrant pain resolved completely. Within 5 weeks of starting pemetrexed treatment, a computed tomography (CT) scan showed decrease in size of multiple liver metastases (**Figure 2**). The tumor marker PSA dropped to 5.1 ng/mL and LDH returned to normal (423 IU/L). The patient can now care for himself and his ECOG performance status is 1. The treatment has been tolerated exceptionally well and no further admissions to the hospital became necessary. After 4 months, at this time of this report, the patient continues to receive 3 weekly cycles of pemetrexed, PSA (7.5 ng/mL) and LDH (539 IU/L) are indicating a continued response.

CASE STUDY: RESPONSE TO CETUXIMAB AND IRINOTECAN IN A PATIENT WITH METASTATIC OVARIAN CANCER

A 49-year-old woman was diagnosed with stage IV ovarian cancer in August 2009 after feeling abdominal pain. A CT scan revealed that she had a mass in her right ovary, which was diagnosed as a mixed high grade serous and endometrioid carcinoma. Surgery confirmed metastatic disease and the patient began standard treatment with a combination of intraveneous paclitaxel and carboplatin and intraperitoneal docetaxel/cisplatin. During the time on treatment, the patient had a partial response; her cancer antigen 125 (CA-125) level dropped from 475 to 70 U/mL but did not return to normal levels (less than 35 U/mL). A laparotomy revealed no obvious tumor masses but the persisting elevation of CA-125 indicated residual disease.

As the standard treatments had failed a portion of the initial biopsy material was sent for CMI testing to identify additional treatment options. Based on the findings of the report, the patient was treated with doxorubicin followed by topotecan but both treatments had to be discontinued due to intolerable toxicities. Doxorubicin was selected based on overexpression of topoisomerase 2A (TOP2A), which has been linked with level II evidence to doxorubicin response in breast cancer (Durbecq et al., 2004).

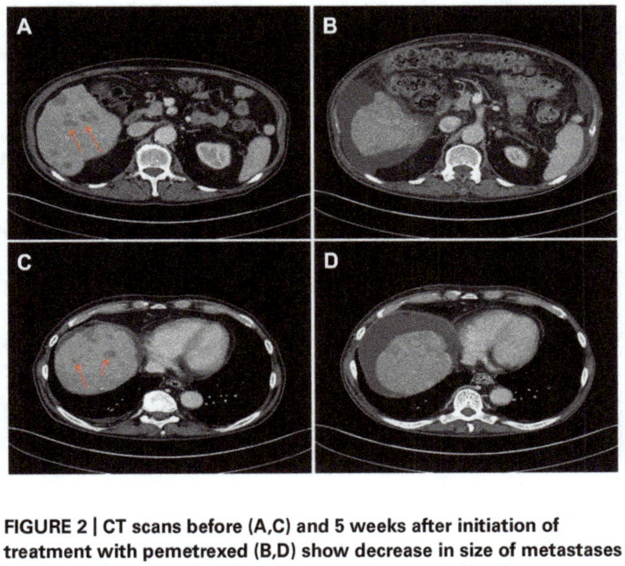

FIGURE 2 | CT scans before (A,C) and 5 weeks after initiation of treatment with pemetrexed (B,D) show decrease in size of metastases and liver sclerosis and ascites due to previous embolization.

In patients with ovarian cancer treated with topotecan, tumors with low or undetectable Topoisomerase 1 (TOPO1) protein levels had a median time to progression of 4.3 months, compared to 13.2 months in patients with high TOPO1 expressing tumors (Litzow et al., 2010). Although poorly tolerated, both treatments resulted in transient decreases in CA-125 to normal levels.

The CMI report also found overexpression of the *EGFR* gene and overexpression of the TOPO1 protein. EGFR gene overexpression along with high phosphatase and tensin homolog (PTEN) protein expression indicated potential efficacy from cetuximab, which is targeting the EGFR receptor (Personeni et al., 2008; Sartore-Bianchi et al., 2009). Irinotecan causes cell killing by blocking TOPO1. In addition to the topotecan evidence cited above, level II evidence in colorectal cancer (CRC) patients treated with irinotecan-containing adjuvant chemotherapy demonstrated that there was a significant improvement in survival in patients who expressed TOPO1 compared to those with low TOPO1 expression (Kostopoulos et al., 2009). These results indicated potential benefit from cetuximab and irinotecan and combination treatment with these drugs was started in late October 2010. After 2 months, bevacizumab was transiently added to this combination (based on overexpression of the hypoxia-inducible factor 1-alpha (*HIF1A*) gene) until it caused toxicity. Within 2 months of the starting the combination of cetuximab and irinotecan the patient's CA-125 level dropped from 64 to 10 and stayed normal over the course of the first 8 months of treatment. Although an attenuated dose was used, toxicities led to discontinuation of therapy. After discontinuation of cetuximab and irinotecan the patient developed progressive disease with pelvic and liver metastases. The patient was then put on treatment with cyclophosphamide, which was not included on the CMI report but resulted in a transient response. Currently the disease is slowly progressive and the patient is still on cyclophosphamide at an attenuated dose.

A significantly long remission after recurrence is unusual in ovarian cancer and irinotecan and cetuximab are rarely used in ovarian cancer. This observation is of significant importance as it justifies further exploration of treatments guided by tumor profiling instead of using histological diagnosis of the tumor alone.

CONCLUSION

Patients with metastatic cancer frequently arrive to a point in their clinical care when all standard of care options have been tried and they require further treatment. Although guidelines recommend that these patients enter either clinical trials or palliative care, they are often fit enough and willing to continue to receive further cytotoxic treatment. Comprehensive tumor profiling can identify active treatment options, help avoiding treatments which are likely not active, and find treatments that otherwise would not have been considered. Meaningful integration of the information generated by comprehensive biomarker testing requires cross-functional expertise to aid interpretation and determine which results are clinically relevant. As this level of support is rarely accessible, CMI provides a service which helps physicians to develop evidence-based treatment plans. CMI combines the results of tumor profiling with a thorough assessment of the published clinical evidence in a comprehensive report that includes drugs associated with benefit, lack of benefit as well clinical trials that may be relevant for the patient. The clinical experience with tumor profiling in routine clinical practice has been promising.

REFERENCES

Bedard, P. L., Ozo, A. M., Tsao, M. S., Leighl, N. B., Shepherd, F. A., Chen, E. X., et al. (2013). Princess Margaret Cancer Centre integrated molecular profiling in advanced cancers trial (IMPACT) using genotyping and targeted next-generation sequencing. *J. Clin. Oncol.* 31(suppl.), abstr. 11002.

Chen, C. Y., Yang, P. C., Shih, J. Y., Lin, J. W., Chen, K. Y., Yang, C. H., et al. (2011). Thymidylate synthase and dihydrofolate reductase expression in non-small cell lung carcinoma: the association with treatment efficacy of pemetrexed. *Lung Cancer* 74, 132–138. doi: 10.1016/j.lungcan.2011.01.024

Dean, A., and Wallace, R. (2013). Clinical application of molecular profiling in selecting treatment for advanced refractory and rare solid tumours: an Australian experience. Abstract 955 presented at ECCO. Available at: http://eccamsterdam2013.ecco-org.eu/Scientific-Programme/Abstract-search.aspx?abstractid = 5274 (accessed April 07, 2014).

Durbecq, V., Paesmans, M., Cardoso, F., Desmedt, C., Di Leo, A., Chan, S., et al. (2004). Topoisomerase-II alpha expression as a predictive marker in a population of advanced breast cancer patients randomly treated with either single-agent doxorubicin or single-agent docetaxel. *Mol. Cancer Ther.* 3, 1207–1214.

Harris, R. P., Helfand, M., Woolf, S. H., Lohr, K. N., Mulrow, C. D., Teutsch, S. M., et al. (2001). Current methods of the US Preventive Services Task Force: a review of the process. *Am. J. Prev. Med.* 20(3 Suppl.), 21–35. doi: 10.1016/S0749-3797(01)00261-6

Jackson, D. B. (2009). Clinical and economic impact of the non-responder phenomenon – implications for systems based discovery. *Drug Discov. Today* 14, 380–385. doi: 10.1016/j.drudis.2009.01.006

Jameson, G. S., Petricoin, E., Sachdev, J. C., Liotta, L. A., Loesch, D., Anthony, S. P., et al. (2013). A pilot study utilizing molecular profiling to find potential targets and select individualized treatments for patients with metastatic breast *Cancer. J. Clin. Oncol.* 31(suppl.), abstr. TPS11123.

Kostopoulos, I., Karavasilis, V., Karina, M., Bobos, M., Xiros, N., Pentheroudakis, G., et al. (2009). Topoisomerase I but not thymidylate synthase is associated with improved outcome in patients with resected colorectal cancer treated with irinotecan containing adjuvant chemotherapy. *BMC Cancer* 9:339. doi: 10.1186/1471-2407-9-339

Litzow, M. R., Peethambaram, P. P., Safgren, S. L., Keeney, G. L., Ansell, S. M., Dispenzieri, A., et al. (2010). Phase I trial of autologous hematopoietic SCT with escalating doses of topotecan combined with CY and carboplatin in patients with relapsed or persistent ovarian or primary peritoneal carcinoma. *Bone Marrow Transplant.* 45, 490–497. doi: 10.1038/bmt.2009.181

Mazières, J., Peters, S., Lepage, B., Cortot, A. B., Barlesi, F., Beau-Faller, M., et al. (2013). Lung cancer that harbors an HER2 mutation: epidemiologic characteristics and therapeutic perspectives. *J. Clin. Oncol.* 31, 1997–2003. doi: 10.1200/JCO.2012.45.6095

Olmos, D., A'Hern, R. P., Marsoni, S., Morales, R., Gomez-Roca, C., Verweij, J., et al. (2012). Patient selection for oncology phase I trials: a multi-institutional study of prognostic factors. *J. Clin. Oncol.* 30, 996–1004. doi: 10.1200/JCO.2010.34.5074

Personeni, N., Fieuws, S., Piessevaux, H., De Hertogh, G., De Schutter, J., Biesmans B., et al. (2008). Clinical usefulness of EGFR gene copy number as a predictive marker incolorectal cancer patients treated with cetuximab: a fluorescent in situ hybridization study. *Clin. Cancer Res.* 14, 5869–5876. doi: 10.1158/1078-0432.CCR-08-0449

Sartore-Bianchi, A., Di Nicolantonio, F., Nichelatti, M., Molinari, F., De Dosso, S., Saletti, P., et al. (2009). Multi-determinants analysis of molecular alterations for predicting clinical benefit to EGFR-targeted monoclonal antibodies in colorectal cancer. *PLoS ONE* 4:e7287. doi: 10.1371/journal.pone.0007287

Tsimberidou, A. M., Iskander, N. G., Hong, D. S., Wheler, J. J., Falchook, G. S., Fu, S., et al. (2012). Personalized medicine in a phase I clinical trials program: the M. D. Anderson Cancer Center Initiative. *Clin. Cancer Res.* 18, 6373–3683. doi: 10.1158/1078-0432.CCR-12-1627

Von Hoff, D. D., Stephenson, J. J. Jr., Rosen, P., Loesch, D. M., Borad, M. J., Anthony, S., et al. (2010). Pilot study using molecular profiling of patients' tumors to find potential targets and select treatments for their refractory cancers. *J. Clin. Oncol.* 28, 4877–4883. doi: 10.1200/JCO.2009.26.5983

17

Small and innovative molecules as new strategy to revert MDR

*Laura Zinzi, Elena Capparelli, Mariangela Cantore, Marialessandra Contino, Marcello Leopoldo and Nicola Antonio Colabufo**

Dipartimento di Farmacia – Scienze del Farmaco, Università degli Studi di Bari "A. Moro," Bari, Italy

Edited by:
Chiara Riganti, University of Turin, Italy

Reviewed by:
Chiara Riganti, University of Turin, Italy
Attilio Di Piero, UMR5086
CNRS-University of Lyon, France

Correspondence:
Nicola Antonio Colabufo,
Dipartimento di Farmacia – Scienze del Farmaco, Università degli Studi di Bari "A. Moro," Via Orabona 4, 70125 Bari, Italy
e-mail: nicolaantonio.colabufo@uniba.it

Multidrug resistance (MDR) is a complex phenomenon principally due to the overexpression of some transmembrane proteins belonging to the ATP binding cassette (ABC) transporter family. Among these transporters, P-glycoprotein (P-gp) is mostly involved in MDR and its overexpression is the major cause of cancer therapy failure. The classical approach used to overcome MDR is the co-administration of a P-gp inhibitor and the classic antineoplastic drugs, although the results were often unsatisfactory. Different classes of P-gp ligands have been developed and, among them, Tariquidar has been extensively studied both *in vitro* and *in vivo*. Although Tariquidar has been considered for several years as the lead compound for the development of P-gp inhibitors, recent studies demonstrated it to be a substrate and inhibitor, in a dose-dependent manner. Moreover, Tariquidar structure–activity relationship studies were difficult to carry out because of the complexity of the structure that does not allow establishing the role of each moiety for P-gp activity. For this purpose, SMALL molecules bearing different scaffolds such as tetralin, biphenyl, arylthiazole, furoxane, furazan have been developed. Many of these ligands have been tested both in *in vitro* assays and in *in vivo* PET studies. These preliminary evaluations lead to obtain a library of P-gp interacting agents useful to conjugate chemotherapeutic agents displaying reduced pharmacological activity and appropriate small molecules. These molecules could get over the limits due to the antineoplastic-P-gp inhibitor co-administration since pharmacokinetic and pharmacodynamic profiles are related to a dual innovative drug.

Keywords: MDR, P-gp, dual effect, multitarget drugs, MDR reverting activity

INTRODUCTION

Human ATP binding cassette (ABC) transporters belong to a family of 49 genes classified in seven subfamilies (A–G) (1, 2).

Some of these transporters are involved in multidrug resistance (MDR) such as ABC-B1 (P-glycoprotein, P-gp), ABC-G2 (breast cancer resistance protein, BCRP), and ABC-C1-6 (MDR associated proteins, MRP1-6) (3).

Multidrug resistance is a complex phenomenon that limits the efficacy of chemotherapeutic treatment. Some tumors are intrinsically resistant to pharmacological therapy, while others, initially sensitive to chemotherapy, become resistant during the treatment. Resistance to anticancer drugs is due to several factors such as pharmacokinetic, tumor micro-environmental changes, or cancer cell-specific factors that occur at different levels:

- increased drug efflux or decreased drug influx;
- drug inactivation;
- drug target modification;
- apoptosis evasion.

The first of these mechanisms is mediated by plasma membrane transporters such as P-gp.

Several strategies were suggested for reversing MDR and, among them, the co-administration of anticancer drugs with an ABC transporter inhibitor has been proposed to improve the bioavailability of chemotherapeutic agents (4, 5).

Among MDR pumps, P-gp is one of the most studied because of the broadest substrate specificity and the widest tissues and organs distribution such as liver, intestine, brain, and kidneys (6). This transporter actively effluxes several compounds from cells and, being overexpressed in tumor cells exerting a significant effect on the bioavailability, distribution, and activity of many drugs, especially those used in the cancer treatment (7).

P-glycoprotein is a 170-kDa phosphorylated glycoprotein encoded by MDR1 gene. Structurally, P-gp contains 12 transmembrane helices organized in 2 membrane spanning domains (MSDs), each containing 6 transmembrane helices and 2 nucleotide-binding domains (NBDs) responsible for ATP binding (3, 8) (**Figure 1**).

This protein uses ATP hydrolysis as the energy source for the translocation of several structurally unrelated molecules (9). This suggests the presence of different binding sites (10, 11). Indeed, four distinct interacting binding sites have been identified in P-gp structure (**Figure 2**). Sites I–II are assigned for the binding of substrates, site III is for the modulators, and site IV binds the inhibitors. It has been hypothesized that the binding site of inhibitors is folded to inhibit the ATP binding and so the pump, although binds the substrate, cannot extrude it. The four binding

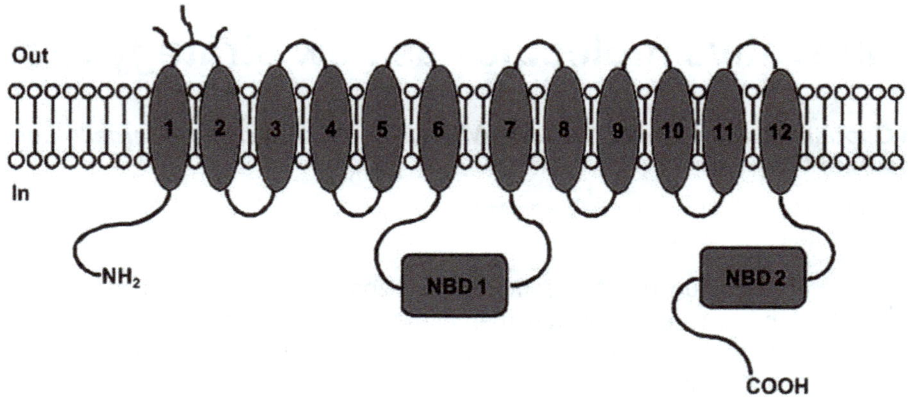

FIGURE 1 | P-gp structure: MSDs and NBDs. Picture reported in Ref. (6).

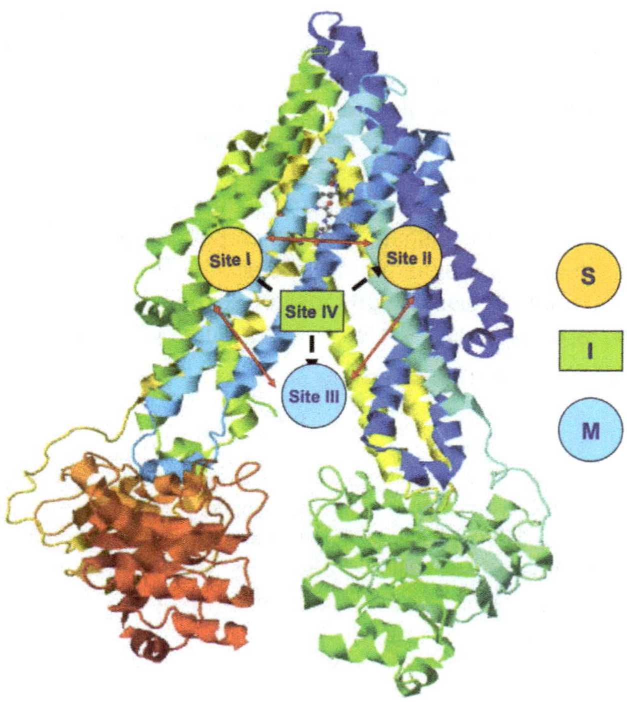

FIGURE 2 | P-gp binding sites (S: substrate, M: modulator, I: inhibitor).

sites are able to allosterically communicate in a negative heterotropic manner and the binding to one of these sites switches the other sites to a low-affinity conformation (9).

Several models have been proposed for P-gp efflux: (1) pore, (2) flippase, (3) hydrophobic vacuum cleaner, and (4) two-cylinder engine (12, 13).

In the pore model, drugs binding P-gp to the cytosol are transported out of cells through a channel created by protein.

In the flippase model, P-gp links the drugs that are transported from the inner to the outer compartment of the plasma membrane against a concentration gradient.

In the hydrophobic vacuum cleaner model, molecules, recognized by P-gp in the lipid bilayer, enter into the protein from the membranous site and exit through the central cavity.

In the two-cylinder engine model, it has been hypothesized that P-gp contains two drug-binding sites, in which each half-transporter has its own drug carrier (14).

The translocation mechanism of P-gp was blocked by inhibitors activity (12).

Indeed, the initial step of the translocation process is the binding of drugs to an high-affinity site and simultaneously the binding of ATP to the NBDs. Drug and ATP binding are coupled to the ATP hydrolysis and two ATP molecules are needed for the turnover; the first molecule is responsible for drug translocation and the second is needed to set the transporter in the basal state (**Figure 3**).

Compounds interacting with P-gp have been classified into three categories: substrates, inhibitors, and modulators (**Figure 4**).

Substrates are molecules that are actively transported by the protein and therefore have a higher concentration outside the cell with respect to the cytosol (10).

High substrate concentration causes a block of the pump by saturating the substrate-binding sites and in literature, this finding led to a mistake in terms of intrinsic P-gp-interacting mechanism (10).

Modulators modify substrate-binding site through a negative allosteric mechanism. Imaging studies with radiotracers demonstrated that modulators are able to alter the substrate-binding site in a non-competitive manner, modifying the maximal receptor density (B_{max}) but not the dissociation equilibrium constant (K_d). Therefore, it suggests that allosteric communication between substrate- and modulator-binding sites exists (10).

Inhibitors block the translocation activity of P-gp by interfering with the ATP binding to NBD. However, although different mechanisms, substrates, modulators, and inhibitors could exert the same final biological effect restoring cell sensitivity to chemotherapeutic agents.

BIOLOGICAL ASSAYS

The characterization of P-gp-interacting mechanism of drugs is an important task in the development of P-gp ligands and it is performed by specific biological *in vitro* assays (15) (**Figure 5**).

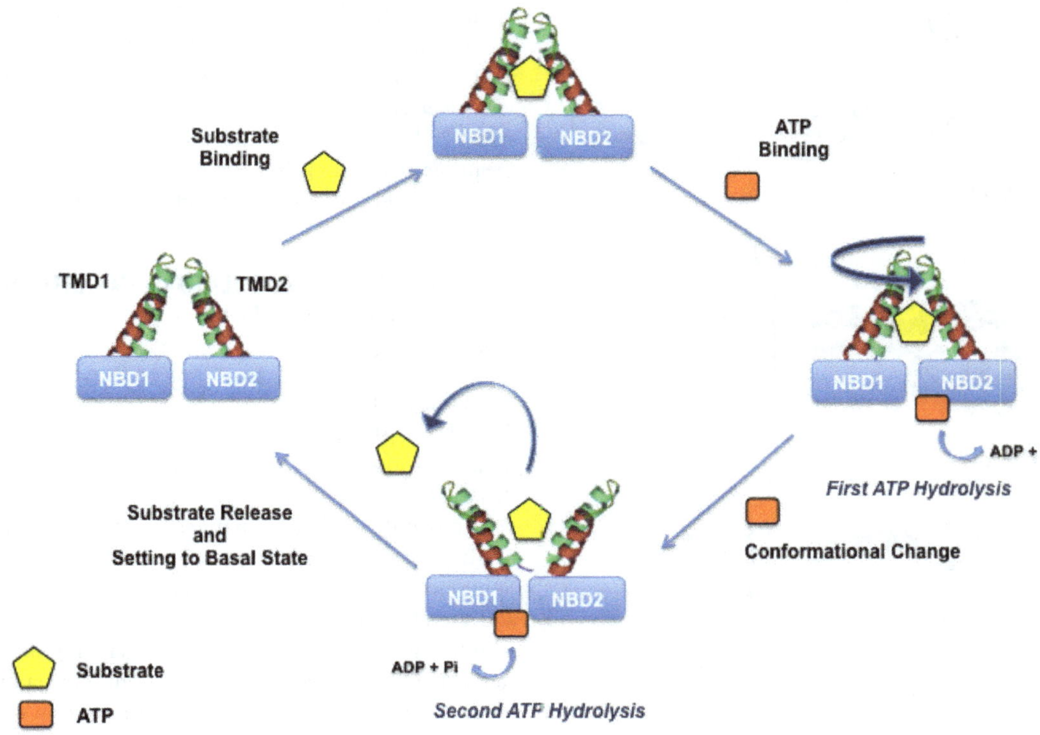

FIGURE 3 | P-gp translocation mechanism.

A wide range of methodologies has been used to characterize the P-gp interaction. These methods employ intact cells or purified protein and a combination of different approaches is often required to identify the mechanism of interaction.

The identification of the P-gp-interacting mechanism is performed by the combination of three biological assays:

- determination of the apparent permeability (P_{app});
- ATP cell depletion;
- inhibition of the P-gp-mediated transport of a fluorescent probe (Calcein or Rhodamine);
- everted gut sac model.

APPARENT PERMEABILITY DETERMINATION

Apparent permeability (P_{app}) is a pharmacokinetic parameter that is determined in Caco-2 cells system, a cell monolayer model suitable for the study of the passive and active transport through the biological membranes. Indeed, in this system the Basolateral–Apical flux (B → A), representative of passive diffusion, and Apical–Basolateral flux (A → B), representative of active P-gp-modulated transport, are determined.

The BA/AB ratio is useful to identify P-gp inhibitors (BA/AB <2), P-gp substrates (BA/AB from 18 to 20), or P-gp modulators (BA/AB ranging from 2 to 18).

ATP CELL DEPLETION

This assay, performed in Caco-2 cell monolayer and in Madin–Darby Canine Kidney cells (MDCK) overexpressing P-gp, permits to establish if the compound is able to deplete ATP. Substrates activate ATPase whereas inhibitors are not transported unchanging the ATP cell level.

INHIBITION OF CALCEIN-AM TRANSPORT

This assay is useful to determine the potency (EC_{50}) of P-gp ligands and is performed in MDCK cells, stably transfected for P-gp overexpression (MDCK-MDR1). The assay is carried out using a non-fluorescent prodrug, the acetoxymethyl ester of calcein (calcein-AM), which is a P-gp substrate. In the presence of a P-gp modulator, calcein-AM diffuses into the cytosol where it is hydrolyzed to the fluorescent dye calcein, that is not a P-gp substrate and since hydrophilic, it cannot diffuse through the membrane (17). In this assay also Rhodamine may be employed as a probe although calcein-AM is more useful because Rhodamine displays good cell permeability and therefore, its fluorescence determination at stationary state is more complex than calcein-AM.

THE EVERTED GUT SAC MODEL

This assay is an *ex vivo* method to study the P-gp-mediated intestinal absorption of drugs and their interactions with CYP450 enzymes (18, 19). This double information (the effect of P-gp-mediated transport and CYP450-metabolizing activity) is obtained since the everted gut sac assay is performed on isolated rat ileum where CYP450 enzymes and P-gp are present.

This combined study is needed because inhibitors and substrates may display overlapping activities toward CYP450 enzymes and the P-gp pump (20).

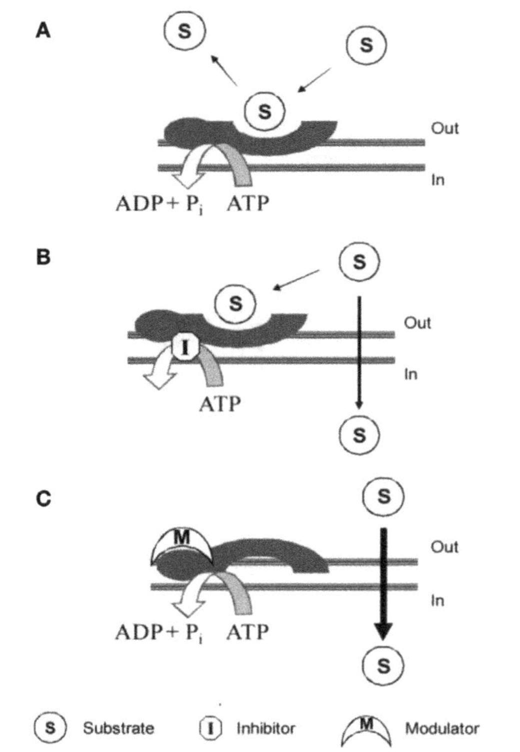

FIGURE 4 | P-gp interacting mechanism of: (A) substrate; (B) inhibitor; (C) modulator. Picture reported in *Journal of Medicinal Chemistry* (2010) 53:1883–97.

In this method, the transport of a known P-gp radiolabeled or fluorescent substrate, in the absence and presence of a P-gp-interacting agent, is evaluated. The flux of a P-gp substrate such as Rhodamine 125, from serosal to mucosal compartment and *vice versa*, is represented by the efflux ($k'2$) and influx rate constants ($k'1$), respectively. These determinations are carried out in the presence of a P-gp-interacting agent to determine $k''2$ and $k''1$, the efflux and influx constants of the tested substrate after P-gp interaction.

P-gp SUBSTRATES, MODULATORS, INHIBITORS

The most important studied P-gp ligands are classified in three different categories.

P-gp SUBSTRATES

This class is the most extensively studied and Verapamil and *N*-desmethyl-loperamide (**Chart 1**) are to date the gold standard of this class of compounds.

Verapamil, a calcium channel blocker, was found to reverse MDR (21) and it has become the reference compound for developing other P-gp substrates. It saturates the pump at high doses and therefore, it is a potential ligand for reversing MDR in co-administration with antineoplastic agent for different types of cancer (21, 22). However, verapamil cannot be employed because of toxic cardiovascular side effects. Despite this, the radiolabeled compound, ^{11}C-verapamil, has been developed to visualize P-gp function and to date, it is considered to be the reference substrate for imaging P-gp activity (23). However, verapamil is quickly metabolized by CYP450 enzymes giving radiometabolites, some of which are themselves P-gp substrates (24).

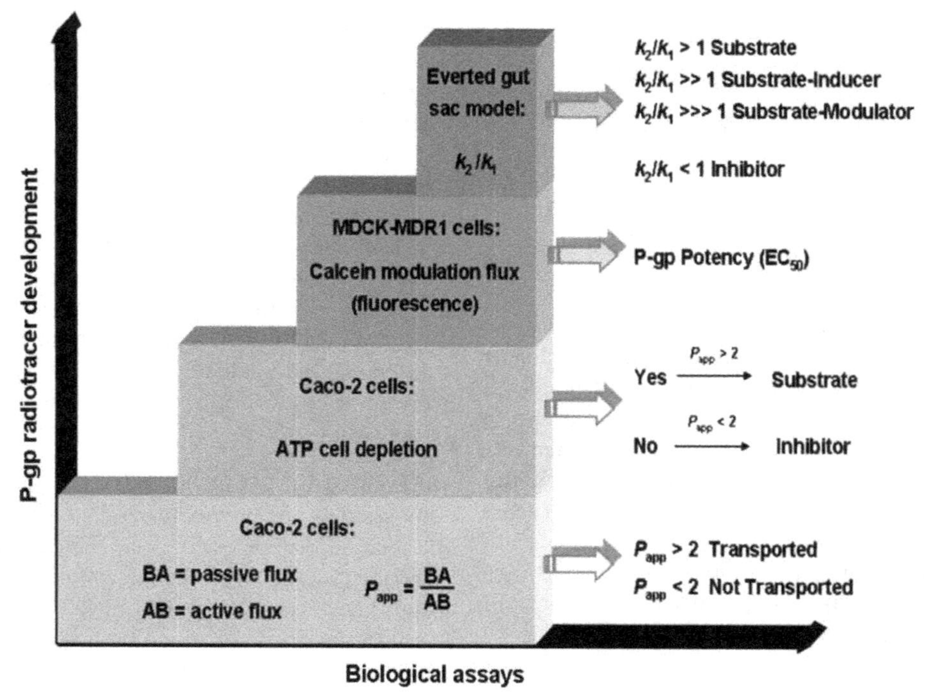

FIGURE 5 | Characterization of P-gp ligands (k_1: influx constant; k_2: efflux constant). Picture reported in Ref. (16).

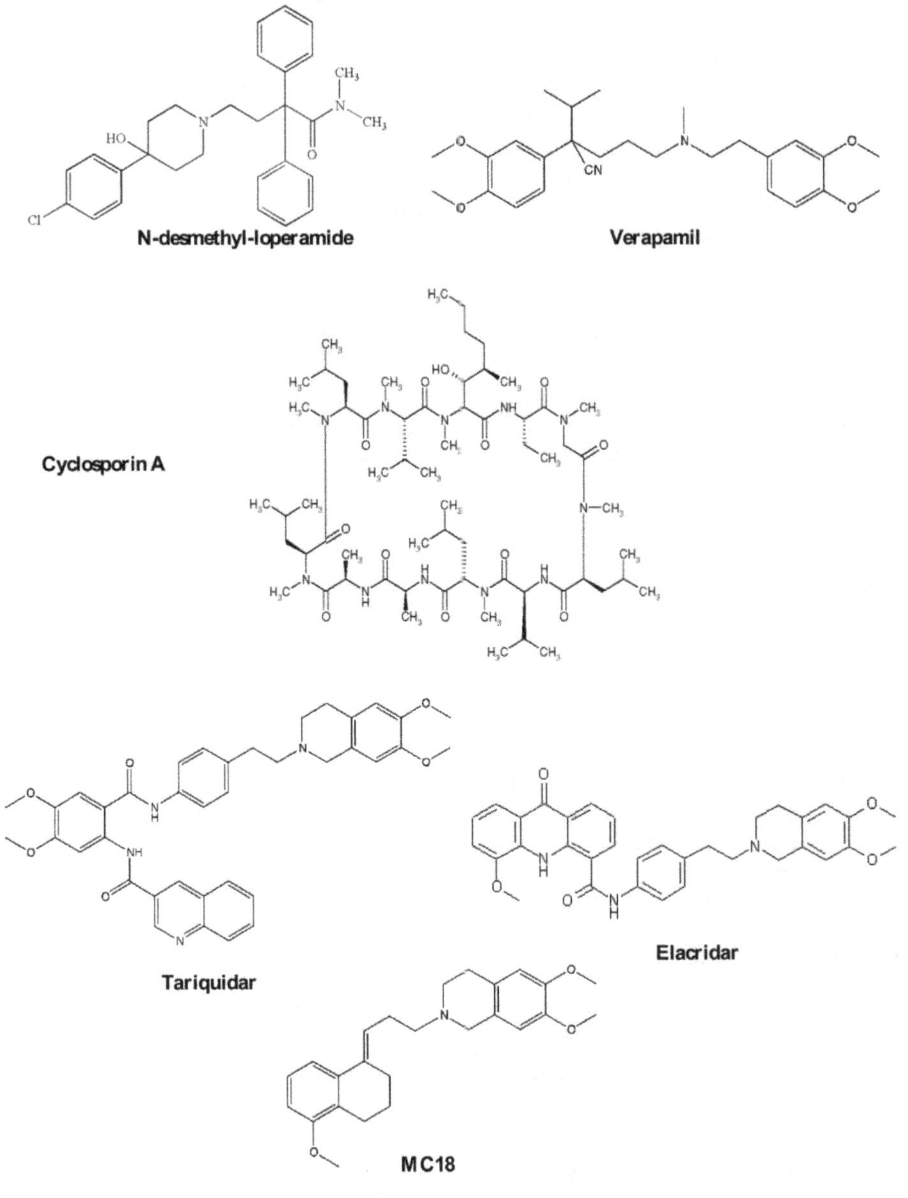

CHART 1 | P-gp ligands.

N-desmethyl-loperamide (dLop) is the major metabolite of Loperamide and at low concentrations it acts as substrate while at high concentrations, as reported for verapamil, dLop saturates the pump (25). Also, dLop has been radiolabeled and used for imaging P-gp *in vivo* by PET analysis (26).

P-gp MODULATORS

Cyclosporin A (CsA, **Chart 1**), an immunosuppressant agent, is a P-gp modulator, widely used *in vitro* as a tool to study MDR because it restores the cell concentration of chemotherapeutic agents. In imaging studies, the co-administration of CsA with a radiolabeled P-gp substrate (27) has been performed to visualize the P-gp activity because it increases radiotracer cell uptake by modulating the P-gp-binding sites. However, CsA treatment enhances the uptake of the radioligand in all regions where P-gp is present including targeted and non-targeted tissues (2–15, 17–30).

P-gp INHIBITORS

Elacridar (**Chart 1**) is a dual P-gp/BCRP ligand and can be orally administered. It was tested in combination with doxorubicin in patients with advanced solid tumors (31). At the recommended dose of doxorubicin, a pharmacologic hematologic toxicity was observed, mainly consisting of leukocytopenia and granulocytopenia.

Moreover, Elacridar was co-administrated with topotecan (32), a P-gp and BCRP substrate (Phase I) with unsatisfactory results (33). ^{11}C-Elacridar is tested *in vivo* to evaluate the overexpression of P-gp and BCRP in human colon adenocarcinoma (33, 34).

Tariquidar (**Chart 1**), an anthranilic derivative, is the most potent P-gp ligand in nanomolar range. It has been co-administrated in clinical trials with chemotherapeutic agents for restoring the efficacy of therapy (35–38). Results were quite unsatisfactory because of poor selectivity against other ABC transporters that are not involved in MDR. Tariquidar has been evaluated *in vivo* for diagnosing breast tumors in animal model using (R)-^{11}C-verapamil (35, 39, 40).

Recently, the suitability of ^{11}C-tariquidar and ^{11}C-elacridar for visualizing cerebral P-gp expression in healthy human subjects, in analogy to a previous preclinical study (16, 35), was investigated. However, ^{11}C-tariquidar and ^{11}C-elacridar displayed a "substrate-like *in vivo* behavior"; in particular, they are dual P-gp/BCRP substrates and these findings disagreed with *in vitro* results (41).

(*E*)-6,7-Dimethoxy-2-[3-(5-methoxy-3,4-dihydronaphthalen-1(2*H*)-ylidene)propyl]-1,2,3,4-tetrahydroisoquinoline, better known as MC18 (**Chart 1**), is a small molecule bearing tetralin moiety (42). To date, ^{11}C-MC18 is the first P-gp inhibitor studied *in vivo* in PET studies. It displayed fourfold higher uptake in the target organs compared with ^{11}C-tariquidar and ^{11}C-elacridar (43).

STRATEGIES TO REVERT MDR

The pivotal role of P-gp in MDR has stimulated the development of P-gp ligands able to reverse the resistance to a wide number of drugs. Hence, the need to design potent and selective P-gp inhibitors stimulated the development of small molecules on which structure–activity relationship (SAR) studies could be easily and better performed. The development of these compounds is depicted in **Figure 6** and it is based on the synthesis of bioisosteres obtained through subsequent lead optimization studies.

SMALL LIBRARIES FROM VERSATILE SCAFFOLDS

Tetralin derivatives

The *lead compound* of this class is MC18 (**Figure 6A**) ($EC_{50} = 1.50\,\mu M$), bearing an (*E*)-double bond, a potent P-gp inhibitor (42). When the double bond shifts into the tetralin ring, the ligands are less potent than MC18 and are P-gp substrates. Moreover, the presence and the position of methoxy substituent on tetralin nucleus are important in terms of the potency and intrinsic activity. The saturated derivative, MC266 ($EC_{50} = 6.35\,\mu M$), was the best P-gp substrate in this class. Therefore, the partial conformational restriction of spacer is involved in the P-gp-interacting mechanism. These two lead compounds, inhibitor and substrate respectively, have been ^{11}C-radiolabeled and tested *in vivo* PET studies leading to significant and coherent results in comparison with the *in vitro* data previously reported (43).

Biphenyl and naphthyl derivatives

The conformational restriction of MC18 seems to be a requirement for improving P-gp-inhibitory activity. In order to evaluate this statement, the restriction of the spacer linking the non-basic moiety was tested in a series of molecules bearing two different fragments: 1,4-biphenyl and 2-naphthyl moieties (**Figure 6A**) (44).

In the biphenyl series, 4-biphenyl derivatives displayed the best activity in P-gp-inhibitory activity and among these compounds, the best result was obtained for MC70 ($EC_{50} = 0.69\,\mu M$). In recent years, MC70 was extensively studied in order to confirm its P-gp-interacting activity considering its role to enhance the chemotherapeutic agent when co-administrated (45).

Although tetralin and biphenyl derivatives displayed high P-gp activity, they were active toward other ABC transporters such as BCRP and MRP1.

Aryloxazole and arylthiazole derivatives

Aryloxazole and arylthiazole derivatives (**Figure 6A**) were designed as cycloisosters to improve the P-gp-inhibitory activity and selectivity. The results demonstrated that aryloxazole and arylthiazole derivatives, designed as cycloisosteres of biphenyl derivative MC70, were found to be less potent than the reference compound in inhibiting P-gp (46). Indeed, these compounds were screened by SAR studies toward BCRP and MRP1 giving interesting structural determinants for these pumps as depicted (**Figure 7**). Finally, it was found that both aryloxazoles and arylthiazoles were P-gp substrates.

Furthermore, the aryl fragments were replaced by a naphthyl nucleus and three heteronuclei (oxazole, thiazole, and furyl) have been evaluated (47). The obtained results showed that the replacement of aryl nucleus with naphthyl moiety lead to obtain compounds with three different activity profiles:

1. P-glycoprotein inhibitors: unsubstituted oxazoles or bearing $-F$ and $-OH$ on the naphthyl fragment;
2. Unambiguous substrates (48): oxazole bearing $-OCH_3$ on the naphthyl fragment and thiazole bearing $-Br$ and $-OCH3$ on the naphthyl fragment.
3. Ambiguous substrates (48): oxazole bearing Br on the naphthyl fragment and unsubstituted thiazole or bearing Br on the naphthyl fragment.

Finally, all furyl derivatives were ambiguous substrates.

Galloyl-based derivatives

The 3,4,5-trihydroxybenzoyl and 3,4- and 3,5-dihydroxybenzoyl fragments (**Figure 6A**) have been employed as scaffolds for a set of ligands that are representative of pharmacophoric nucleus of tariquidar (49).

For this purpose, compounds have been divided into four different structural series that present:

1. variation at R,
2. variation at R1,
3. polyhydroxy derivatives,
4. pyrogallol 1-methyl ethers.

The benzamides of the first set showed good P-gp-inhibitory activity (IC_{50} ranging from 20 to $1.4\,\mu M$). These outcomes led to deepen the study with two approaches:

1. keeping fixed the 3,4,5-trimethoxy-*N*-(2-nitrophenyl)benzamide scaffold and introducing a series of R1 substituents in the 4-position of the aniline moiety;
2. desmethylating one or more methoxy groups belonging to A ring.

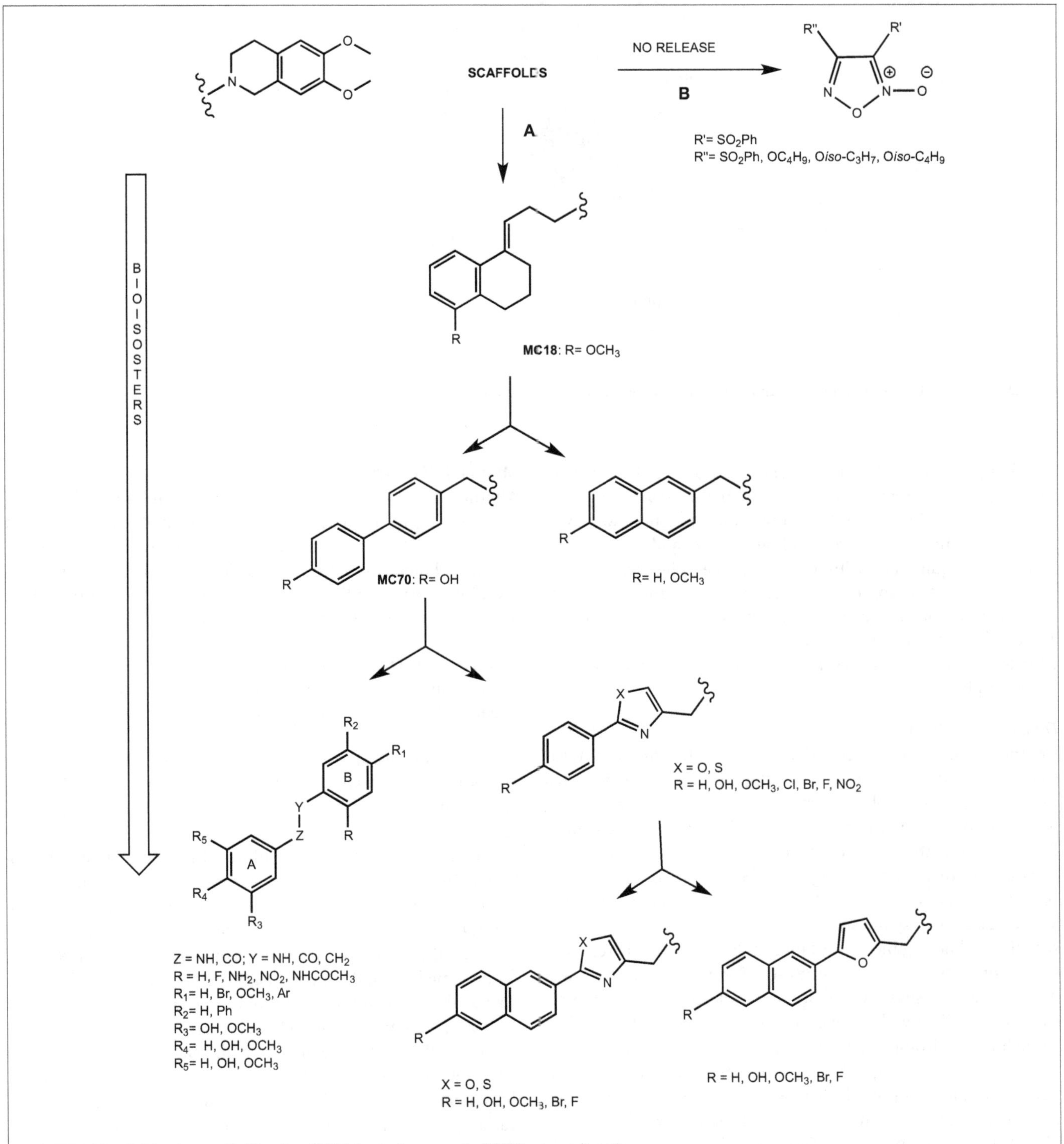

FIGURE 6 | Scaffolds of versatile libraries. (A) Bioisosteric approach; **(B)** NO release ligands.

The evaluation of data suggested that, with the exception of the 4-bromo and 4-methoxy congeners, all compounds of this second set were potent and selective P-gp inhibitors. In particular, molecules bearing $R = NO_2$ and in R1 H or benzo[1,3]dioxol-5-yl displayed submicromolar activity.

The screening of the gallamide derivatives indicated a moderate inhibitory potency for P-gp, independently with respect to the number and position of phenolic groups.

In the last series, all the pyrogallol-1-monomethyl ether derivatives showed moderate P-gp-inhibitory activity.

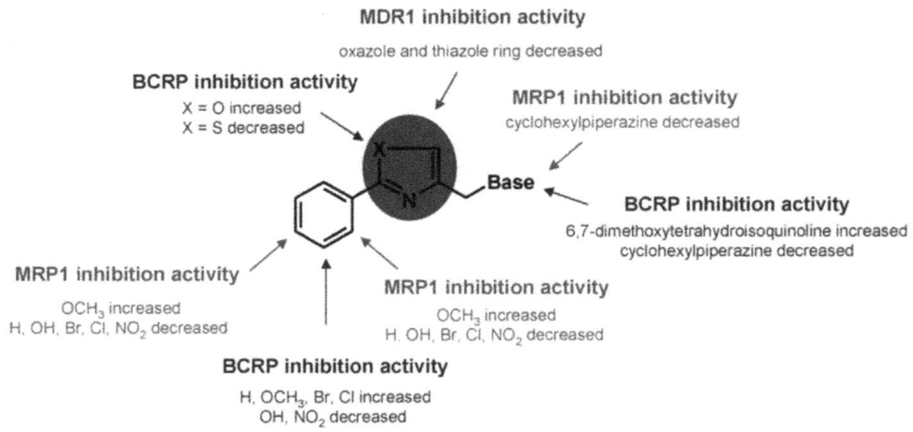

FIGURE 7 | SAR studies of aryloxazole and arylthiazole derivatives. Picture reported in Ref. (47).

Taking into account that the most important inhibitory activity changes were mainly concerned with the structural modifications on B ring, the role of the amide function was evaluated by testing the corresponding anilide and amine. The amine was equipotent with respect to the other tested compounds toward P-gp, despite the drastic change in terms of planarity and conformational flexibility. By contrast, the anilide showed no inhibitory activity toward P-gp. The 3,4,5-trimethoxyamide derivatives displayed moderate inhibitory activity toward P-gp.

Furoxan derivatives

Another strategy to reverse MDR is the nitration of a tyrosine present in TM6 domain of P-gp (50). It was reported that furoxans are able to produce *in situ* NO interacting with a thiol group. In fact, furoxans (**Figure 6B**) have been developed on the base of their properties to induce NO release and this pharmacological effect is the mechanism of coronary dilators (51–53). Moreover, the correlation between a decreased NO synthesis and MDR onset in doxorubicin-sensitive and doxorubicin-resistant cells has been widely reported (54). For this reason, a series of furoxan derivatives was designed and tested in activity and selectivity toward ABC transporters. Firstly, diphenylfuroxan derivatives and 3- and 4-phenylfuroxan isomer pairs, bearing different substituents with stereo-selective and lipophilic properties, were evaluated. In particular, the compounds having electron-withdrawing substituent and high lipophilic group such as phenylsulfonyl, displayed the best P-gp activity. The evaluation of phenylsulfonylfuroxan isomer pairs, bis(phenylsulfonyl)furoxan derivatives, and 3-phenylsulfonyl substituted furoxans, bearing alkoxy groups at position 4, displayed that 3-phenylsulfonyl substituted furoxans were found to be P-gp inhibitors, and the 4-substituted ligands showed the best activity and selectivity. Indeed, the best results were obtained both for 3,4-diphenylsulfonyl derivative ($EC_{50} = 3.0\,\mu M$) and for alkoxy derivatives such as *n*-Butoxy, *iso*-Propoxy, and *iso*-Butoxy ($EC_{50} = 2.26$, 2.15, and $2.23\,\mu M$, respectively) (55).

DUAL EFFECT DRUGS

Although the co-administration of a P-gp inhibitor and an antineoplastic agent could be considered a potential strategy to revert MDR, to date this approach was not clinically available because of pharmacokinetic limitations, in particular different apparent permeability, bioavailability, and metabolism. For this reason, others approaches were taken into account in the recent past:

- use of P-gp-targeted antibodies (56);
- encapsulation of anticancer drugs in liposomes (57);
- nanospheres able to circumvent MDR (58).

New innovative approaches to revert MDR could be: the development of molecules having a dual effect, potent cancer cell-killing agent and P-gp activity/expression inhibitor, and the collateral sensitivity (CS).

For example, some taxanes inhibited P-gp activity employing Rhodamine 123 as a fluorescent dye (59). These compounds could disclose new perspectives because they not only acted as cytotoxic agents but also inhibited the activity of P-gp efflux pump.

In another study (60), starting from Indirubin (a traditional Chinese medicine), the most potent derivative, PH II-7, has been evaluated. This compound showed antitumor activity inducing itself apoptosis and S phase cell cycle arrest, and in the meantime, it is not a P-gp substrate and so, high cell concentration of this compound was detected. The confocal microscopy displayed that this compound was not P-gp effluxed and significantly increased Adriamycin and Vincristine effect by reversing MDR.

MULTITARGET DRUGS

Another strategy could be the design of multitarget drugs bearing scaffolds depicted in **Figure 6**, having antitumor and P-gp inhibitory activities. An example is the hybridization of the NO-donor furoxan scaffold with the anilinopyrimidine moiety present in Gefitinib, leading to phenylsulfonylfuroxan-anilinopyrimidine derivative (**Figure 8**). This compound displayed epidermal growth factor receptor (EGFR) inhibitory activity in the treatment of non-small-cell lung cancer (NSCLC) (61). It induced apoptosis in

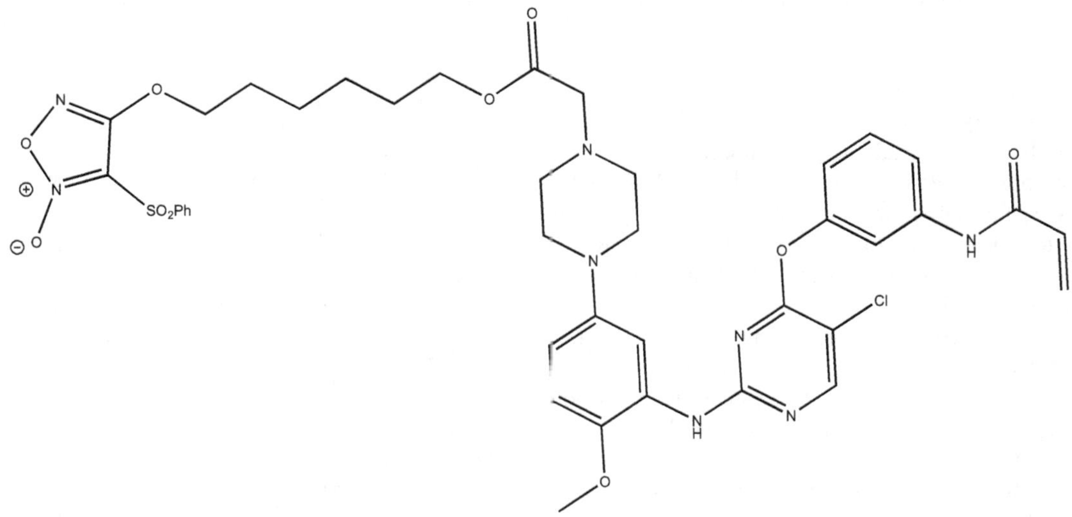

FIGURE 8 | NO-donor furoxan moiety linked to Gefitinib-like scaffold.

H1975 and HCC827 cells, inhibited EGFR downstream signaling in H1975 cells, and suppressed the nuclear factor-κB activation in H1975 cells. Furthermore, it released high levels of NO in H1975 cells but not in normal human cells, inducing apoptosis, inhibiting metastasis, and sensitizing tumor cells to chemotherapy by the inhibition of drug efflux transporters (51, 62). In this study, the two nuclei, furoxan and anilinopyrimidine, were separately evaluated for their effects. The activity showed by the two nuclei separately was lower than that exerted by the linked molecule. These results suggest that the antiproliferative activity of the compound might be attributed to the synergic effects of anilinopyrimidine and NO-donor moieties.

In another study, a class of 4-substituted methoxybenzoylarylthiazoles (SMART, **Figure 9**) was evaluated (63). These compounds exhibited great potency *in vitro* and broad spectrum cellular cytotoxicity. The *in vitro* and *in vivo* evaluation of the anticancer properties of three SMART compounds demonstrated that they potently bound to the colchicine-binding site in tubulin, inhibited tubulin polymerization, arrested cancer cells in G2/M phase, and induced apoptosis. Moreover, these compounds were able to overcome MDR since they were found equally cytotoxic in a parent cell line (OVCAR-8) and in a MDR-positive cell line (NCI/ADR-RES).

These findings demonstrated that some scaffolds such as furoxan and arylthiazole, already reported in our library as P-gp ligands, could be considered as the starting point to develop multitarget drugs. In these studies, the chemotherapeutic moiety is linked to furoxan (NO donor useful to revert MDR) or arylthiazole fragment (P-gp modulator), and the final effect was more potent that the single effect expected from each drug.

COLLATERAL SENSITIVITY

An alternative potential approach to treat drug-resistant tumors is the CS where several compounds selectively kill MDR cells without affecting the non-resistant parental cells (64).

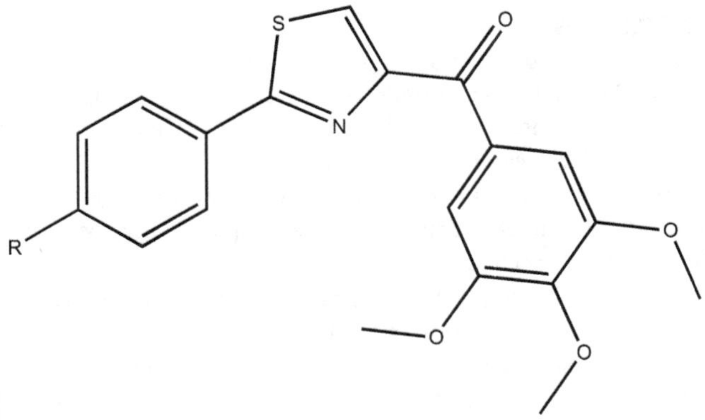

FIGURE 9 | SMART ligand.

Different hypotheses have been proposed to better explain this mechanism:

- production of reactive oxygen species (ROS);
- energetic level changes;
- extrusion of essential endogenous substrates for cell survival;
- perturbation of cell membranes.

The first hypothesis takes into account that several CS agents are substrates of P-gp, stimulating ATPase activity and in the meantime, the substrate extrusion from the plasma membrane into the extracellular environment (65). Once back in the extracellular environment, substrates repeat this cycle and P-gp performs a process known as futile cycling to increase the ATP hydrolysis inducing oxidative stress. MDR cells initiate apoptosis when ROS levels overcome a certain limit. Two reported ligands inducing CS are siramesine and the P-gp substrate and

σ_2 agonist 9-[4-(6,7-dimethoxy-1,2,3,4-tetrahydroisoquinolin-2-yl)butyl]-9*H*-carbazole that generate more ROS in the MCF7/Adr than in the MCF7 cell line (66).

Another hypothesis is that P-gp-expressing cells are more sensitive to changes in energy utilization. Indeed, several compounds that interfere with cellular metabolic pathways, such as glycolysis or oxidative phosphorylation, have been identified as MDR-selective agents. The glycolysis antimetabolite 2-deoxy-D-glucose (2-DG) seems to confirm this finding. Indeed, 2-DG activates apoptosis and selectively kills numerous MDR cell lines compared to drug-sensitive parental lines.

The extrusion hypothesis asserts that CS agents mediate cytotoxicity by stimulating, sensitizing, or facilitating the extrusion of endogenous essential components. This phenomenon is not reported in P-gp-expressing cells but it may be the case for MPR1-mediated CS.

Moreover, several CS agents alter membrane biophysical properties (67). Indeed, they induce membrane perturbation in P-gp-expressing cell lines, leading to the hypothesis that changes in membrane structure and fluidity contribute to CS (68). Pentazocine and verapamil are reported to reduce membrane fluidity in the colchicine-resistant B30 cell line.

CONCLUSION

To date the co-administration of a chemotherapeutic drug with a P-gp inhibitor, the encapsulation of anticancer drugs in liposomes, and the nanosphere formulation to reverse MDR failed for several reasons. This review aims to disclose new strategies in the design of multitarget drugs useful toward MDR. Interesting approaches are: (i) the development of drugs bearing a unique moiety responsible for the anticancer effect and MDR reversing activity; (ii) the design of molecules bearing different pharmacophores for multitarget activity; (iii) the evaluation of CS agents.

In the present review, we overviewed our P-gp ligands library to suggest new scaffolds that could be used to design multitarget drugs in accordance with the approaches already reported.

REFERENCES

1. Ross DD, Doyle LA. Mining our ABCs: pharmacogenomic approach for evaluating transporter function in cancer drug resistance. *Cancer Cell* (2004) **6**:105–7. doi:10.1016/j.ccr.2004.08.003
2. Pharm AN, Penchala S, Graf RA, Wang J, Huang Y. *Multidrug Resistance: Biological and Pharmaceutical Advance in the Antitumour Treatment.* Kerala: Research Signpost (2008). 19 p.
3. Gimenez-Bonafe P, Guillen Canovas A, Ambrosio S, Tortosa A, Perez-Tomas R. *Multidrug Resistance: Biological and Pharmaceutical Advance in the Antitumour Treatment.* Kerala: Research Signpost (2008). 63 p.
4. Nobili S, Landini I, Giglioni B, Mini E. Pharmacological strategies for overcoming multidrug resistance. *Curr Drug Targets* (2006) **7**:861–79. doi:10.2174/138945006777709593
5. Gottesman MM, Fojo T, Bates SE. Multidrug resistance in cancer: role of ATP-dependent transporters. *Nat Rev Cancer* (2002) **2**:48–58. doi:10.1038/nrc706
6. Colabufo NA, Berardi F, Contino M, Niso M, Perrone R. ABC pumps and their role in active drug transport. *Curr Top Med Chem* (2009) **9**:119–29. doi:10.2174/156802609787521553
7. German UA. P-glycoprotein – a mediator of multidrug resistance in tumour cells. *Eur J Cancer* (1996) **32A**:927–44. doi:10.1016/0959-8049(96)00057-3
8. Gottesman MM, Ambudkar SV, Xia D. Structure of a multidrug transporter. *Nat Biotechnol* (2009) **27**:546–7. doi:10.1038/nbt0609-546
9. Avendaño C, Menendez JC. Inhibitors of multidrug resistance to antitumor agents (MDR). *Curr. Med Chem* (2002) **9**:159–93. doi:10.2174/0929867023371175
10. Martin C, Berridge G, Mistry P, Higgins C, Charlton P, Callaghan R. Drug binding sites on P-glycoprotein are altered by ATP binding prior to nucleotide hydrolysis. *Biochemistry* (2000) **39**:11901–6. doi:10.1021/bi000559b
11. Aller SG, Yu J, Ward A, Weng Y, Chittaboina S, Zhuo R, et al. Structure of P-glycoprotein reveals a molecular basis for polyspecific drug binding. *Science* (2009) **323**:1718–22. doi:10.1126/science.1168750
12. Callaghan R, Ford RC, Kerr ID. The translocation mechanism of P-glycoprotein. *FEBS Lett* (2006) **580**:1056–63. doi:10.1016/j.febslet.2005.11.083
13. Constantinides PP, Wasan KM. Lipid formulation strategies for enhancing intestinal transport and absorption of P-glycoprotein (P-gp) substrate drugs: in vitro/in vivo case studies. *J Pharm Sci* (2007) **96**:235–48. doi:10.1002/jps.20780
14. vanVeen HW, Higgins CF, Konings WN. Multidrug transport by ATP binding cassette transporters: a proposed two-cylinder engine mechanism. *Res Microbiol* (2001) **152**:365–74. doi:10.1016/S0923-2508(01)01208-6
15. Sharom FJ, Siarheyeva A. *Multidrug Resistance: Biological and Pharmaceutical Advance in the Antitumour Treatment.* Kerala: Research Signpost (2008). 261 p.
16. Colabufo NA, Berardi F, Perrone MG, Capparelli E, Cantore M, Inglese C, et al. Substrates, inhibitors and activators of P-glycoprotein: candidates for radiolabeling and imaging perspectives. *Curr Top Med Chem* (2010) **10**:1703–14. doi:10.2174/156802610792928022
17. Feng B, Mills JB, Davidson RE, Mireles RJ, Janiszewski JS, Troutman MD, et al. *In vitro* P-glycoprotein assays to predict the *in vivo* interactions of P-glycoprotein with drugs in the central nervous system. *Drug Metab Dispos* (2008) **36**:268–75. doi:10.1124/dmd.107.017434
18. Arellano C, Philibert C, Vachoux C, Woodley J, Houin G. The metabolism of midazolam and comparison with other CYP enzyme substrates during intestinal absorption: *in vitro* studies with rat everted gut sacs. *J Pharm Pharm Sci* (2007) **10**:26–36.
19. Berruet N, Sentenac S, Auchere D, Gimenez F, Farinotti R, Fernandez C. Effect of efavirenz on intestinal p-glycoprotein and hepatic p450 function in rats. *J Pharm Pharm Sci* (2005) **8**:226–34.
20. Benet LZ, Cummins CL, Wu CY. Unmasking the dynamic interplay between efflux transporters and metabolic enzymes. *Int J Pharm* (2004) **277**:3–9. doi:10.1016/j.ijpharm.2002.12.002
21. Cano-Gauci DF, Riordan JR. Action of calcium antagonists on multidrug resistant cells. Specific cytotoxicity independent of increased cancer drug accumulation. *Biochem Pharmacol* (1987) **36**:2115–23. doi:10.1016/0006-2952(87)90139-0
22. Teodori E, Dei S, Martelli C, Scapecchi S, Gualtieri F. *Multidrug Resistance: Biological and Pharmaceutical Advance in the Antitumour Treatment.* Kerala: Research Signpost (2008). 141 p.
23. Luurtsema G, Molthoff CF, Schuit RC, Windhorst AD, Lammertsma AA, Franssen EJ. Evaluation of (R)-[^{11}C]verapamil as PET tracer of P-glycoprotein function in the blood-brain barrier: kinetics and metabolism in the rat. *Nucl Med Biol* (2005) **32**(1):87–93. doi:10.1016/j.nucmedbio.2004.06.007
24. Pauli-Magnus C, von Richter O, Burk O, Ziegler A, Mettang T, Eichelbaum M, et al. Characterization of the major metabolites of verapamil as substrates and inhibitors of P-glycoprotein. *J Pharmacol Exp Ther* (2000) **293**:376–82.
25. Zoghbi SS, Liow JS, Yasuno F, Hong J, Tuan E, Lazarova N, et al. ^{11}C-loperamide and its N-desmethylradiometabolite are avid substrates for brain permeability-glycoprotein efflux. *J Nucl Med* (2008) **49**:649–56. doi:10.2967/jnumed.107.047308
26. Kreisl WC, Liow JS, Kimura N, Seneca N, Zoghbi SS, Morse CL, et al. P-glycoprotein function at the blood-brain barrier in humans can be quantified with the substrate radiotracer 11C-N-desmethyl-loperamide. *J Nucl Med* (2010) **51**:559–66. doi:10.2967/jnumed.109.070151
27. Muzi M, Mankoff DA, Link JM, Shoner S, Collier AC, Sasongko L, et al. Imaging of cyclosporine inhibition of P-glycoprotein activity using 11C-verapamil in the brain: studies of healthy humans. *J Nucl Med* (2009) **50**:1267–75. doi:10.2967/jnumed.108.059162
28. Ishiwata K, Kawamura K, Yanai K, Hendrikse NH. *In vivo* evaluation of P-glycoprotein modulation of 8 PET radioligands used clinically. *J Nucl Med* (2007) **48**:81–7.
29. Syvänen S, Blomquist G, Sprycha M, Höglund AU, Roman M, Eriksson O, et al. Duration and degree of cyclosporin induced P-glycoprotein inhibition in the rat blood-brain barrier can be studied with PET. *Neuroimage* (2006) **32**:1134–41. doi:10.1016/j.neuroimage.2006.05.047

30. Syvänen S, Hooker A, Rahman O, Wilking H, Blomquist G, Långström B, et al. Pharmacokinetics of P-glycoprotein inhibition in the rat blood-brain barrier. *J Pharm Sci* (2008) **97**:5386–400. doi:10.1002/jps.21359
31. Planting AS, Sonneveld P, van der Gaast A, Sparreboom A, van der Burg ME, Luyten GP, et al. A phase I and pharmacologic study of the MDR converter GF120918 in combination with doxorubicin in patients with advanced solid tumors. *Cancer Chemother Pharmacol* (2005) **55**:91–9. doi:10.1007/s00280-004-0905-z
32. De Bruin M, Miyake K, Litman T, Robey R, Bates SE. Reversal of resistance by GF120918 in cell lines expressing the ABC half-transporter, MXR. *Cancer Lett* (1999) **146**:117–26. doi:10.1016/S0304-3835(99)00182-2
33. De Vries NA, Zhao J, Kroon E, Buckle T, Beijnen JH, van Tellingen O. P-glycoprotein and breast cancer resistance protein: two dominant transporters working together in limiting the brain penetration of topotecan. *Clin Cancer Res* (2007) **13**:6440–9. doi:10.1158/1078-0432.CCR-07-1335
34. Dörner B, Kuntner C, Bankstahl JP, Bankstahl M, Stanek J, Wanek T, et al. Synthesis and small-animal positron emission tomography evaluation of [^{11}C]-elacridar as a radiotracer to assess the distribution of P-glycoprotein at the blood-brain barrier. *J Med Chem* (2009) **52**: 6073–82. doi:10.1021/jm900940f
35. Yamasaki T, Kawamura K, Hatori A, Yui J, Yanamoto K, Yoshida Y, et al. PET study on mice bearing human colon adenocarcinoma cells using [11C]GF120918, a dual radioligand for P-glycoprotein and breast cancer resistance protein. *Nucl Med Commun* (2010) **31**(11):985–93. doi:10.1097/MNM.0b013e32833fbf87
36. Wanek T, Kuntner C, Bankstahl JP, Bankstahl M, Stanek J, Sauberer M, et al. A comparative small-animal PET evaluation of [11C]tariquidar, [11C]elacridar and (R)-[11C]verapamil for detection of P-glycoprotein-expressing murine breast cancer. *Eur J Nucl Med Mol Imaging* (2012) **39**:149–59. doi:10.1007/s00259-011-1941-7
37. Stewart AJ, Mistry P, Dangerfield W, Bootle D, Baker M, Kofler B, et al. Antitumor activity of XR5944, a novel and potent topoisomerase poison. *Anticancer Drugs* (2001) **12**:359–67. doi:10.1097/00001813-200104000-00009
38. Mistry P, Stewart AJ, Dangerfield W, Okiji S, Liddle C, Bootle D, et al. In vitro and in vivo reversal of P-glycoprotein mediated multidrug resistance by a novel potent modulator, XR9576. *Cancer Res* (2001) **61**:749–58.
39. Stewart A, Steiner J, Mellows G, Laguda B, Norris D, Bevan P. Phase I trial of XR9576 in healthy volunteers demonstrates modulation of P-glycoprotein in CD56+ lymphocytes after oral and intravenous administration. *Clin Cancer Res* (2000) **6**:4186–91.
40. Bankstahl JP, Kuntner C, Abrahim A, Karch R, Stanek J, Wanek T, et al. Tariquidar-induced P-glycoprotein inhibition at the rat blood-brain barrier studied with (R)-11C-verapamil and PET. *J Nucl Med* (2008) **49**:1328–35. doi:10.2967/jnumed.108.051235
41. Müllauer J, Karch R, Bankstahl JP, Bankstahl M, Stanek J, Wanek T, et al. Assessment of cerebral P-glycoprotein expression and function with PET by combined [11C]inhibitor and [11C]substrate scans in rats. *Nucl Med Biol* (2013) **40**:755–63. doi:10.1016/j.nucmedbio.2013.05.005
42. Bauer M, Karch R, Zeitlinger M, Stanek J, Philippe C, Wadsak W, et al. Interaction of 11C-tariquidar and 11C-elacridar with P-glycoprotein and breast cancer resistance protein at the human blood-brain barrier. *J Nucl Med* (2013) **54**(8):1181–7. doi:10.2967/jnumed.112.118232
43. Colabufo NA, Berardi F, Cantore M, Perrone MG, Contino M, Inglese C, et al. Small P-gp modulating molecules: SAR studies on tetrahydroisoquinoline derivatives. *Bioorg Med Chem* (2008) **16**:362–73. doi:10.1016/j.bmc.2007.09.039
44. Van Waarde A, Ramakrishnan NK, Rybczynska AA, Elsinga PH, Berardi F, de Jong JR, et al. Synthesis and preclinical evaluation of novel PET probes for P-glycoprotein function and expression. *J Med Chem* (2009) **52**:4524–32. doi:10.1021/jm900485a
45. Colabufo NA, Berardi F, Cantore M, Perrone MG, Contino M, Inglese C, et al. 4-Biphenyl and 2-naphthyl substituted 6,7-dimethoxytetrahydroisoquinoline derivatives as potent P-gp modulators. *Bioorg Med Chem* (2008) **16**:3732–43. doi:10.1016/j.bmc.2008.01.055
46. Azzariti A, Quatrale AE, Porcelli L, Colabufo NA, Cantore M, Cassano G, et al. MC70 potentiates doxorubicin efficacy in colon and breastcancer in vitro treatment. *Eur J Pharmacol* (2011) **670**:74–84. doi:10.1016/j.ejphar.2011.08.025
47. Colabufo NA, Berardi F, Perrone MG, Cantore M, Contino M, Inglese C, et al. Multi-drug-resistancereverting agents: 2-aryloxazole and 2-arylthiazole derivatives as potent BCRP or MRP1 inhibitors. *ChemMedChem* (2009) **4**:188–95. doi:10.1002/cmdc.200800329
48. Colabufo NA, Contino M, Cantore M, Capparelli E, Perrone MG, Cassano G, et al. Naphthalenyl derivatives for hitting P-gp/MRP1/BCRP transporters. *Bio Med Chem* (2013) **21**:1324–32. doi:10.1016/j.bmc.2012.12.021
49. Wanek T, Kuntner C, Banksthahl JP, Stanek J, Sauberer M, Mairinger S, et al. A comparative small-animal PET evaluation of [11C]tariquidar, [11C]elacridar and (R)-[11C]verapamil for detection of P-glycoprotein-expressing murine breast cancer. *Eur J Nucl Med Mol Imaging.* (2012) **39**:149–59. doi:10.1007/s00259-011-1941-7
50. Pellicani RZ, Stefanachi A, Niso M, Carotti A, Leonetti F, Nicolotti O, et al. Potent galloyl-based selective modulators targeting multidrug resistance associated protein 1 and P-glycoprotein. *J Med Chem* (2012) **55**:424–36. doi:10.1021/jm201305y
51. Feelisch M, Schonafinger K, Noack E. Thiol-mediated generation of nitric oxide accounts for the vasodilator action of furoxans. *Biochem Pharmacol* (1992) **44**:1149–57. doi:10.1016/0006-2952(92)90379-W
52. Riganti C, Miraglia E, Viarisio D, Costamagna C, Pescarmona G, Ghigo D, et al. Nitric oxide reverts the resistance to doxorubicin in human colon cancer cells by inibhiting the drug efflux. *Cancer Res* (2005) **65**:516–25.
53. Medana C, Ermondi G, Fruttero R, Di Stilo A, Ferretti C, Gasco A. Furoxans as nitric oxide donors. 4-Phenyl-3-furoxancarbonitrile: thiol-mediated nitric oxide release and biological evaluation. *J Med Chem* (1994) **37**:4412–6. doi:10.1021/jm00051a020
54. Sorba G, Medana C, Fruttero R, Cena C, Di Stilo A, Galli U, et al. Water soluble furoxan derivatives as NO prodrugs. *J Med Chem* (1997) **40**:463–9. doi:10.1021/jm970281u
55. Fruttero R, Crosetti M, Chegaev K, Guglielmo S, Gasco A, Berardi F, et al. Phenylsulfonylfuroxans as modulators of multidrug-resistance-associated protein-1 and P-glycoprotein. *J Med Chem* (2010) **53**:5467–75. doi:10.1021/jm100066y
56. Mechetner E, Roninson IB. Efficient innhibition of P-glycoprotein-mediated multidrug resistance with a monoclonal antibody. *Proc Natl Acad Sci USA* (1992) **89**:5824–8. doi:10.1073/pnas.89.13.5824
57. Thierry AR, Vige D, Coughlin SS, Belli JA, Dritschillo A, Rahman A. Modulation of doxorubicin resistance in multidrug-resistent cells by liposomes. *FASEB J* (1993) **7**:572–9.
58. Cuvier C, Roblot-treupel L, Millot JM, Lizard G, Chevillard S, Manfait M, et al. Doxorubicin-loaded nanospheres bypass tumor cell multidrug resistance. *Biochem Pharmacol* (1992) **44**:509–17.
59. Ferlini C, Distefano M, Pignatelli F, Lin S, Riva A, Bombardelli E, et al. Antitumour activity of novel taxanes that act at the same time as cytotoxic agents and P-glycoprotein inhibitors. *Br J Cancer* (2000) **83**(12):1762–8. doi:10.1054/bjoc.2000.1500
60. Su Y, Cheng X, Tan Y, Hu Y, Zhou Y, Liu J, et al. Synthesis of a dual functional anti-MDR tumor agent PH II-7 with elucidations of anti-tumor effects and mechanisms. *PLoS One* (2012) **7**(3):e32782. doi:10.1371/journal.pone.0032782
61. Han C, Huang Z, Zheng C, Wan L, Zhang L, Peng S, et al. Novel hybrids of (phenylsulfonyl)furoxan and anilinopyrimidine as potent and selective epidermal growth factor receptor inhibitors for intervention of non-small-cell lung cancer. *J Med Chem* (2013) **56**:4738–48. doi:10.1021/jm400463q
62. Sullivan R, Graham CH. Chemosensitization of cancer bynitric oxide. *Curr Pharm Des* (2008) **14**:1113–23. doi:10.2174/138161208784246225
63. Li CM, Wang Z, Lu Y, Ahn S, Narayanan R, Kearbey JD, et al. Biological activity of 4-substituted methoxybenzoyl-aryl-thiazole: an active microtubule inhibitor. *Cancer Res* (2011) **71**:216–24. doi:10.1158/0008-5472.CAN-10-1725
64. Hall MD, Handley MD, Gottesman MM. Is resistance useless? Multidrug resistance and collateral sensitivity. *Trends Pharmacol Sci* (2009) **30**:546–56. doi:10.1016/j.tips.2009.07.003
65. Laberge RM, Ambadipudi R, Georges E. P-glycoprotein (ABCB1) modulates collateral sensitivity of a multidrug resistant cell line to verapamil. *Arch Biochem Biophys* (2009) **491**:53–60. doi:10.1016/j.abb.2009.09.012
66. Niso M, Abate C, Contino M, Ferorelli S, Azzariti A, Perrone R, et al. Sigma-2 receptor agonists as possible antitumor agents in resistant tumors: hints for collateral sensitivity. *ChemMedChem* (2013) **8**:2026–2035. doi:10.1002/cmdc.201300291
67. Bech-Hansen NT, Till JE, Ling V. Pleiotropic phenotype of colchicines resistant CHO cells: cross-resistance and collateral sensitivity. *J Cell Physiol* (1976) **8**:23–31. doi:10.1002/jcp.1040880104
68. Callaghan R, Riordan JR. Collateral sensitivity of multidrug resistant cells to narcotic analgesics is due to effects on the plasma membrane. *Biochim Biophys Acta* (1995) **1236**:155–62. doi:10.1016/0005-2736(95)00042-2

18

ABCG2 is not able to catalyze glutathione efflux and does not contribute to GSH-dependent collateral sensitivity

Charlotte Gauthier[1], Csilla Ozvegy-Laczka[2], Gergely Szakacs[3], Balazs Sarkadi[4] and Attilio Di Pietro[1]*

[1] Drug Resistance Mechanism and Modulation Group, Ligue 2013 Certified, Bases Moléculaires et Structurales des Systèmes Infectieux, UMR5086, Centre National de la Recherche Scientifique, Université de Lyon, Institut de Biologie et Chimie des Protéines, University of Lyon, Lyon, France

[2] Research Group of Active Transport Proteins, Institute of Enzymology, Research Centre for Natural Sciences, Hungarian Academy of Sciences, Budapest, Hungary

[3] Institute of Enzymology, Research Centre for Natural Sciences, Hungarian Academy of Sciences, Budapest, Hungary

[4] Molecular Biophysics Research Group, Hungarian Academy of Sciences, Semmelweiss University, Budapest, Hungary

Edited by:
Chiara Riganti, University of Turin, Italy

Reviewed by:
Chiara Riganti, University of Turin, Italy
Joanna Kopecka, University of Turin, Italy

***Correspondence:**
Attilio Di Pietro, Drug Resistance Mechanism and Modulation Group, Ligue 2013 Certified, Bases Moléculaires et Structurales des Systèmes Infectieux, UMR5086, Centre National de la Recherche Scientifique, Université de Lyon, Institut de Biologie et Chimie des Protéines, University of Lyon, 7 Passage du Vercors, 69367 Lyon Cedex 07, France
e-mail: a.dipietro@ibcp.fr

ABCG2 is a key human ATP-binding cassette (ABC) transporter mediating cancer cell chemoresistance. In the case of ABCC1, another multidrug transporter, earlier findings documented that certain modulators greatly increase ABCC1-mediated glutathione (GSH) efflux and, upon depletion of intracellular GSH, induce "collateral sensitivity" leading to the apoptosis of multidrug resistant cells. Recently, it has been suggested that ABCG2 may mediate an active GSH transport. In order to explore if ABCG2-overexpressing cells may be similarly targeted, we first looked for the effects of ABCG2 expression on cellular GSH levels, and for an ABCG2-dependent GSH transport in HEK293 and MCF7 cells. We found that, while ABCG2 overexpression altered intracellular GSH levels in these transfected or drug-selected cells, ABCG2 inhibitors or transport modulators did not influence GSH efflux. We then performed direct measurements of drug-stimulated ATPase activity and ^{3}H-GSH transport in inside-out membrane vesicles of human ABC transporter-overexpressing Sf9 insect cells. Our results indicate that ABCG2-ATPase is not modulated by GSH and, in contrast to ABCC1, ABCG2 does not catalyze any significant GSH transport. Our data suggest no direct interaction between the ABCG2 transporter and GSH, although a long-term modulation of cellular GSH by ABCG2 cannot be excluded.

Keywords: breast cancer resistance protein ABCG2, collateral sensitivity, glutathione efflux, intracellular glutathione depletion, multidrug resistance protein ABCC1, selective apoptosis, modulators

INTRODUCTION

The development of multidrug resistance (MDR) constitutes a major issue in cancer treatment. Overexpression of the three human ATP-binding cassette (ABC) transporters, ABCB1 (P-glycoprotein/P-gp; Juliano and Ling, 1976), ABCC1 (multidrug resistance protein 1/MRP1; Cole et al., 1992), and ABCG2 (breast cancer resistance protein, BCRP; Allikmets et al., 1998; Doyle et al., 1998; Miyake et al., 1999) has been proposed as one of the main causes of the MDR phenotype in resistant cancer cells. These proteins use ATP hydrolysis as energy source to catalyze the efflux of multiple structurally and functionally diverse chemotherapeutics from cancer cells.

Research has mainly focused on inhibitors development, in order to block this efflux mechanism and then restore chemotherapeutics efficacy. Unfortunately, scientists had to face clinical failures of third-generation ABCB1 inhibitors optimized *in vitro*, such as Zosuquidar (Cripe et al., 2010) or valspodar (Kolitz et al., 2010). In addition to improving clinical trials conducted with efflux inhibitors (Robey et al., 2010), alternative strategies to overcome the MDR phenotype need to be explored. Recently, a new strategy, so called collateral sensitivity (CS), characterized by hypersensitivity to small molecules triggering a preferential cytotoxicity, has been studied (Szakacs et al., 2006; Hall et al., 2009), and four different mechanisms have been hypothesized to underlie the hypersensitivity of ABCB1- and ABCC1-overexpressing cancer cells. CS agents may (i) produce reactive oxygen species by depleting intracellular ATP; (ii) exploit energetic sensitivities caused by ATP depletion; (iii) induce the extrusion of vital endogenous substrates; or (iv) perturb the plasma membrane (Pluchino et al., 2012).

A screening study identified two compounds as potential ABCG2-related CS agents in HEK293 transfected cells, one of them (NSC103054) directly interacting with the transporter (Deeken et al., 2009), and very recently an ABCG2 inhibitor (NP-1250) was reported to induce CS in mitoxantrone-selected MCF7 cancer cells (Ito et al., 2013). Although a mechanism based on extracellular vesicles photodestruction have been shown for another ABCG2-dependent CS (Goler-Baron and Assaraf, 2012), no direct mechanisms have yet been demonstrated; however, these different studies indicate that CS agents, specific for ABCG2, could be developed.

Reduced glutathione (GSH, γ-glutamyl-cysteinyl-glycine) is a tripeptide ubiquitously expressed in cells and involved in many

Abbreviations: ABC, ATP-binding cassette; BCRP (ABCG2), breast cancer resistance protein; CS, collateral sensitivity; 2′,5′-DHC, 2′,5′-dihydroxychalcone; DNP-SG, S-(2,4-dinitrophenyl)glutathione; GSH, reduced glutathione; MDR, multidrug resistance; MRP1 (ABCC1), multidrug resistance protein 1; P-gp (ABCB1), P-glycoprotein signaling pathways. It has been shown that ABCC1-overexpressing cells were hypersensitive to verapamil through a sharp GSH depletion due to an ABCC1-mediated efflux (Trompier et al., 2004). This phenomenon was further investigated in order to target resistant cancer cells in the frame of a new strategy to overcome the MDR phenotype in cancer (Barattin et al., 2010; Genoux-Bastide et al., 2011). ABCC1 is also known to transport oxidized glutathione disulfide (GSSG) which is however present in low amounts (Keppler et al., 1997). Based on our experience with ABCC1-specific CS and on recent reports in which ABCG2 was proposed as a new GSH transporter (Brechbuhl et al., 2009, 2010) we aimed at developing new ABCG2-specific modulators able to induce ABCG2-mediated GSH extrusion in order to induce a drastic intracellular GSH depletion leading to cell death.

In this study, we focused on searching inducers of ABCG2-dependent depletion of intracellular GSH among known death inducers of ABCC1-overexpressing cells, such as verapamil and xanthones (Genoux-Bastide et al., 2011), or known ABCG2 inhibitors (Ahmed-Belkacem et al., 2005; Valdameri et al., 2012). To ascertain the direct role of ABCG2 in GSH efflux, we measured direct transport of radioactive GSH in membrane vesicles.

MATERIALS AND METHODS

COMPOUNDS

Verapamil, Ko143, apigenin, ATP, chrysin, ditiothreitol (DTT), galangin, 5,5′-dithiobis(2-nitrobenzoic acid; DTNB), β-nicotinamide adenine dinucleotide 2′-phosphate reduced tetrasodium salt hydrate (NADPH), quercetin, glutathione (GSH), glutathione reductase, and bicinchoninic acid (BCA) were purchased from Sigma Aldrich (Saint-Quentin Fallavier, France). Acivicin was purchased from CliniSciences (Montrouge, France). ^{3}H-methotrexate and ^{3}H-GSH were purchased from Moravek Biochemicals and PerkinElmer, respectively. All other tested compounds were kindly provided by Prof. Ahcène Boumendjel (UJF Grenoble, France) and prepared as previously described (Genoux-Bastide et al., 2011; Valdameri et al., 2012). Tested compounds were dissolved in DMSO and stored at −20°C; they were warmed to 25°C and diluted in Dulbecco's modified Eagle's medium (DMEM) just before use (0.5% DMSO final concentration).

CELL CULTURE

The cell lines were kindly provided by Drs Susan Bates and Robert Robey, NCI, Bethesda, MD, USA. The selected human breast cancer cell line (MCF7-MX100) and the human fibroblast HEK293 cell line transfected with either *ABCG2* (HEK-*ABCG2*) or the empty vector (HEK-pcDNA3.1) were prepared as respectively reported (Honjo et al., 2001; Robey et al., 2003). The HEK293 and MCF7 cells were maintained in DMEM (high glucose, PAA) and in Roswell Park Memorial Institute medium (RPMI-1640, PAA) respectively, supplemented with 10% fetal bovine serum (FBS, PAA), 1% penicillin/streptomycin (PAA) and with 0.75 mg/ml G418 (for HEK-pcDNA3.1 and HEK-*ABCG2* cells) or 100 nM mitoxantrone (for MCF7-MX100 cells). Cells were cultured at 37°C, 5% CO_2 in a humid atmosphere. Sf9 insect cells were cultured at 27°C in TNM-FH insect medium supplemented with 10% fetal calf serum (FCS) and penicillin (100 U/ml)–streptomycin (100 μg/ml; Sigma Aldrich, Hungary).

INTRACELLULAR GLUTATHIONE ASSAY

HEK293 and MCF7 cells were seeded in 96-well plates at respective densities of 1×10^4 and 2×10^4 cells/well. After 24 h in culture, cells were exposed to the different compounds during 6 or 24 h under normal culture conditions. They were then washed with 200 μl PBS 1X (PAA), stirred during 1 h at 4°C with 100 μl of 10 mM HCl and freezed at −20°C overnight, to be lysed. The intracellular total glutathione (reduced GSH and oxidized GSSG) was measured using the method described by Tietze (1969) as modified by Anderson (1985). About 70 μl of the lysate were used to measure intracellular total glutathione and 20 μl for protein quantitation, both being performed in 96-well plates. Total glutathione was assessed by adding 100 μl of a reaction buffer containing 266 μM NADPH, *GSH reductase* at 10 U/ml and 555 μM DTNB, and the absorbance was read at 412 nm in a microplate reader (PowerWave 340, Biotek) every 30 s during 2 min. The slope for each sample and glutathione standard range was determined to quantify sample glutathione. Protein quantitation was performed using the BCA assay. The results were expressed in nmol glutathione/mg protein and intracellular total glutathione percentages were calculated using the 0 μM samples as 100%.

EXTRACELLULAR GLUTATHIONE ASSAY

HEK293 cells were seeded in 24-well plates at a density of 1.5×10^5 cells/well. After 24 h in culture, cells were co-treated with the compound and 0.5 mM acivicin (to block GSH degradation out of the cells) during the 24-h incubation time. Supernatants were collected and cells were washed with 200 μl PBS 1× and treated as for intracellular total glutathione measurement. About 70 μl of the supernatant were used to assess total extracellular glutathione, and protein titration was performed with cell lysate, by the same method as described for intracellular glutathione measurement.

CELL PROLIFERATION AS DETERMINED BY MTT ASSAY

The MTT colorimetric assay, as previously described (Mosmann, 1983), was used to assess the sensitivity of cells to compounds toxicity. HEK293 cells were seeded in 96-well plates at a density of 1×10^4 cells/well. After 24 h under normal culture conditions, cells were treated with compounds at increasing concentrations. After 72-h incubation under normal culture conditions a 3-(4,5-dimethyl-2-thiazoyl)-2,5-diphenyl-2*H*-tetrazolium Bromide (MTT) solution was added (0.5 mg/ml final concentration) in wells, and cells were incubated for 4 h at 37°C. Thereafter, supernatants were carefully withdrawn and 100 μl/well of the buffer ethanol/DMSO (50/50, v/v) were added to solubilize the reduced formazan dye under stirring. Absorbance at 570 and 690 nm were determined by using a microplate reader (PowerWave 340, Biotek). Results were expressed as the difference between OD_{570} and OD_{690}; cell survival percentage was calculated using 0 μM sample OD as 100%.

MEMBRANE PREPARATION

For obtaining membrane vesicles insect cells were infected with recombinant baculoviruses containing the cDNA of wtABCG2 or ABCG2-K86M (Ozvegy-Laczka et al., 2005) or of ABCC1 (Bakos et al., 1996). Membrane preparation and cholesterol enrichment of ABCG2-containing membranes was then performed as described earlier (Ozvegy et al., 2001; Telbisz et al., 2007).

ATPase ACTIVITY ASSAY

The ATP hydrolytic activity of ABCG2 has been determined as described in Ozvegy et al. (2001) and Telbisz et al. (2007). When the effect of GSH was investigated a minor modification in the assay buffer was introduced. About 10 mM DTT was used instead of 2 mM to prevent the oxidation of GSH.

^{3}H-METHOTREXATE AND ^{3}H-GSH TRANSPORT ASSAY

Sf9 membrane vesicles containing 90 μg protein were incubated in the presence or absence of 4 mM MgATP (or 4 mM MgATP + 1 μM Ko143 or 4 μM MK571) in a buffer containing 40 mM 3-(*N*-morpholino) propanesulfonic acid–Tris (pH 7.0), 56 mM KCl, 6 mM $MgCl_2$, and 10 mM DTT, in a final volume of 140 μl, at 37°C for 5–10 min as indicated on the figure legends. The measurement was started by the addition of 50 μM [^{3}H]methotrexate (Moravek Biochemicals) or 0.1–1 mM ^{3}H-GSH and carried out as described earlier (Ozvegy-Laczka et al., 2005).

STATISTICAL ANALYSIS

Statistic t-test analyses were performed using the SigmaPlot 12 software with $^*p < 0.05$, $^{**}p < 0.01$, $^{***}p < 0.001$.

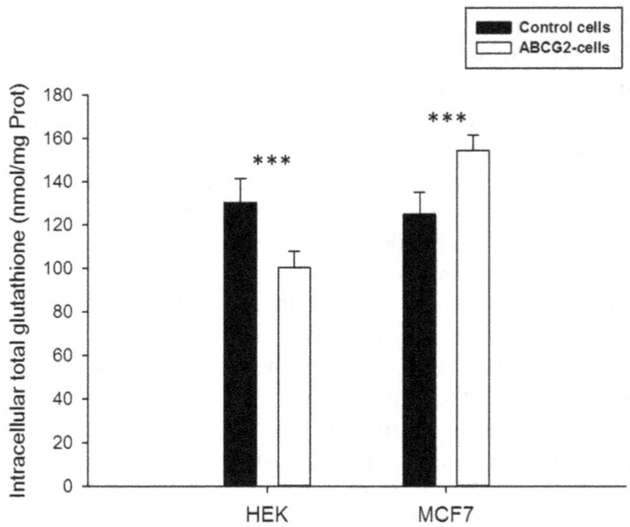

FIGURE 1 | Basal total intracellular glutathione levels in HEK293 or MCF7 cells. The values of either ABCG2-overexpressing cells (white bars) or control cells (black bars) represent means ± SD corresponding to at least three independent experiments performed in triplicates. The differences observed between both cell line pairs were significantly different. t-test analysis: $^{***}p < 0.001$.

RESULTS

INTRACELLULAR GLUTATHIONE CONCENTRATION IN ABCG2-OVEREXPRESSING CELLS

In order to determine the influence of ABCG2 on cellular glutathione levels, we used two different cell lines overexpressing this transporter. The high level of ABCG2 expression and functionality, through ability to transport a number of substrate drugs, were previously described, in both transfected HEK-ABCG2 cells (Robey et al., 2003) and drug-selected MCF7-MX100 cancer cells (Honjo et al., 2001). Moreover, we performed western blot analyses which revealed that all cell lines did not express the ABCC1 protein (data not shown). The intracellular concentration of total glutathione (free GSH + oxidized GSSG) appeared to be significantly modulated by the presence of overexpressed ABCG2 (**Figure 1**). The glutathione level was lower in ABCG2-transfected HEK293 cells by comparison to the same cells transfected by the pcDNA3.1 empty vector (100 ± 8 versus 130 ± 11 nmol glutathione/mg protein). Interestingly, in drug-selected MCF7 cancer cells, which also overexpress ABCG2, the intracellular glutathione content was significantly higher than in the parental MCF7 cells (154 ± 7 versus 125 ± 10 nmol glutathione/mg protein). These data may indicate a long-term modulation of glutathione levels in various ABCG2-overexpressing cell types. Since total glutathione is known to be essentially constituted of free GSH and low amounts of oxidized GSSG, we measured both components separately in the different cell lines, upon incubation with 2-vinylpiridine behaving as a thiol scavenger. In all cases, the remaining oxidized GSSG was too low to be detected (not shown here), indicating no evidence of any change in the ratio between reduced and oxidized forms of glutathione.

INABILITY OF MODULATORS TO STIMULATE AN ACTIVE ABCG2-MEDIATED GLUTATHIONE EFFLUX

Since the 2′,5′-DHC chalcone was reported to stimulate ABCG2-dependent GSH efflux (Brechbuhl et al., 2010), the effects produced by addition of 2′,5′-DHC at increasing concentrations (up to 40 μM) were analyzed here on the intracellular glutathione levels of both transfected and drug-selected cells. A weak concentration-dependent decrease appeared in ABCG2-transfected cells after 6-h incubation with 2′,5′-DHC (**Figure 2A**), but not after 24-h incubation where an increase in intracellular glutathione content was observed in both cell lines (**Figure 2B**). By contrast, in drug-selected MCF7 cells, no decrease in glutathione content appeared after 6-h incubation (**Figure 2C**); a significant difference in glutathione level was observed after 24-h incubation, which was however essentially due to a higher increase in control cells than in ABCG2-overexpressing cells (**Figure 2D**). The extracellular glutathione content increased after 24-h incubation of ABCG2-transfected cells with increasing 2′,5′-DHC concentrations (around 40% at 10 μM), but the increase was at least as high in control cells indicating that it was not dependent on ABCG2 (**Figure 2E**).

We then studied the effects of verapamil which is known to strongly stimulate GSH efflux in ABCC1-overexpressing cells, leading to a fast and massive intracellular glutathione depletion able to trigger apoptosis (Trompier et al., 2004; Perrotton et al., 2007). A significant decrease of intracellular glutathione was indeed observed in ABCG2-transfected cells with increasing verapamil concentrations, up to 40 μM, which was 25–30% higher than in control HEK293 cells (**Figure 3A**). However, no decrease in glutathione content was observed under the same conditions with the ABCG2-overexpressing drug-selected cells,

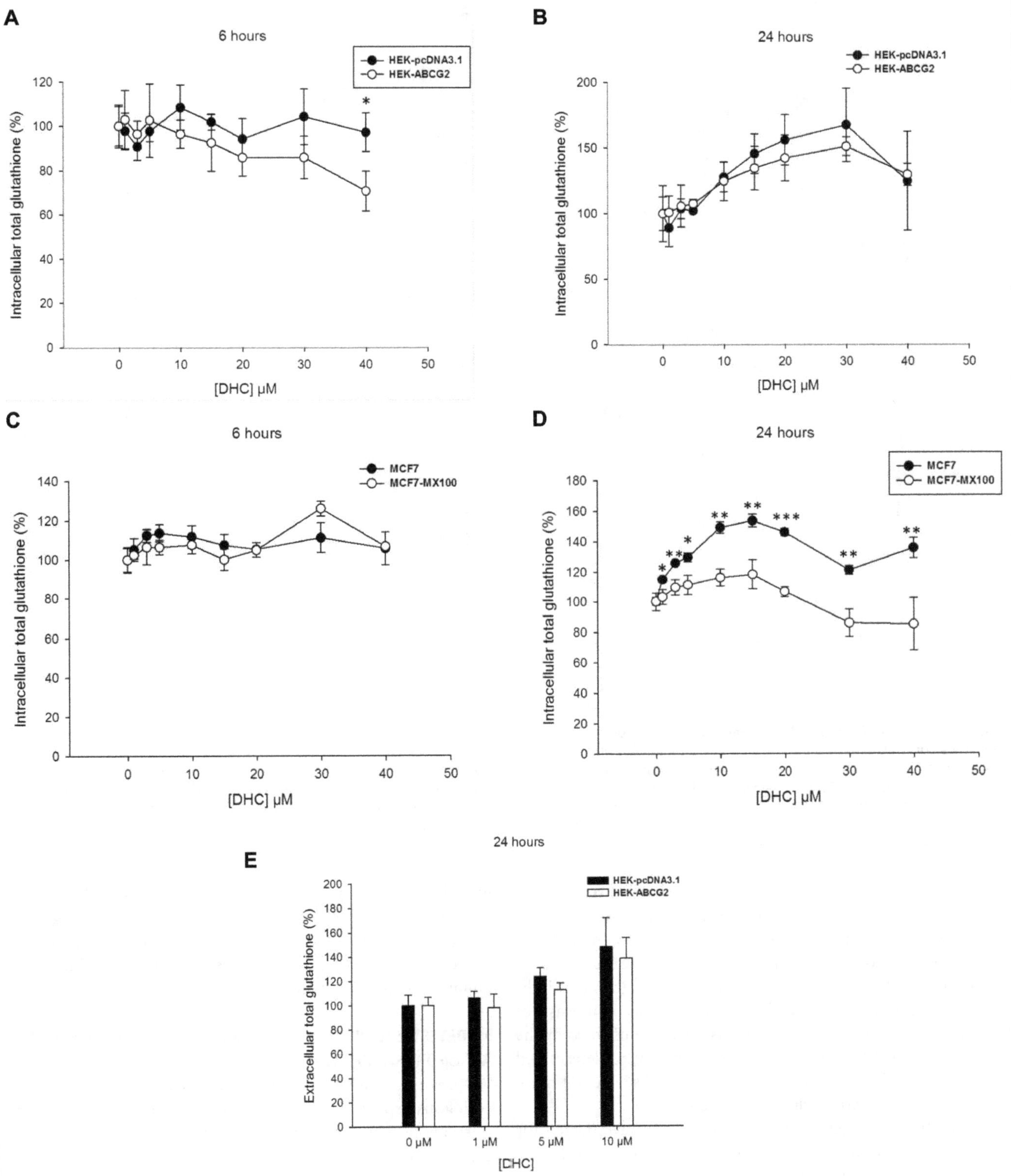

FIGURE 2 | Effects of 2′,5′-DHC increasing concentrations on total intracellular and extracellular glutathione levels. 2′,5′-DHC did not induce intracellular GSH depletion in ABCG2 cells (white circles) by comparison to control cells (black circles) in either HEK293 transfected cells during 6 **(A)** or 24 h **(B)**, or MCF7 cancer cells during 6 **(C)** or 24 h **(D)**. Moreover, there was no net ABCG2-dependent increase in extracellular GSH **(E)** induced by 2′,5′-DHC when comparing HEK-ABCG2 (white bars) and HEK-pcDNA3.1 (black bars) cells after 24-h incubation. The values represent means ± SD corresponding to at least two independent experiments performed in triplicates. Only the differences observed in **(D)**, between MCF7 and MCF7-MX100 cell lines at 24 h, were significant. *t*-test analysis: $*p < 0.05$, $**p < 0.01$, and $***p < 0.001$.

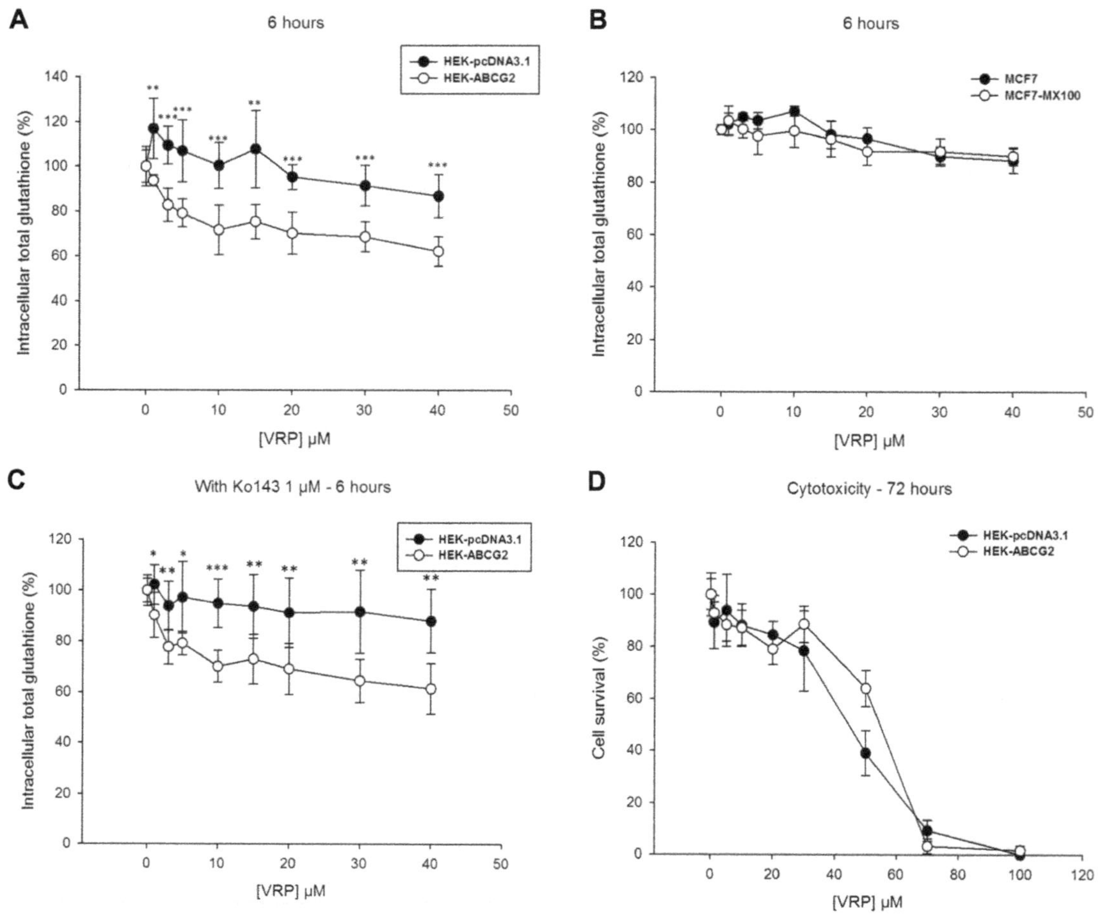

FIGURE 3 | Effects of verapamil on intracellular glutathione depletion and cells survival. Verapamil induced a significant intracellular GSH depletion in HEK293 transfected cells during 6-h incubation **(A)**, but not in the MCF7 selected cells **(B)** when comparing ABCG2-overexpressing cells (white circles) to control cells (black circles). This weak effect was not inhibited by Ko143 **(C)**, the difference in intracellular glutathione remaining unchanged. It was not either correlated to any ABCG2-specific collateral sensitivity in MTT cell survival assays **(D)** with ABCG2-overexpressing cells (white circles) and control cells (black circles). The values represent means ± SD corresponding to at least two independent experiments performed in triplicates. *t*-test analysis: $*p < 0.05$, $**p < 0.01$, and $***p < 0.001$.

which behaved similarly to control MCF7 cells (**Figure 3B**). The ABCG2-related decrease of intracellular glutathione was therefore further characterized in the presence of Ko143, a potent and specific inhibitor of ABCG2 transport activity. **Figure 3C** shows no significant alteration by comparison to **Figure 3A**, therefore indicating that such a decrease in intracellular glutathione was not dependent on ABCG2 activity. This was further confirmed by the absence of any CS toward verapamil cytotoxicity, as determined by MTT assays, since the ABCG2-transfected cells were not more sensitive than the control cells (**Figure 3D**).

Finally, two other series of compounds were investigated for their ability to modify the intracellular glutathione level. The first series included xanthones (X8, 9, 10, 18, 22, 23) known to induce, similarly as verapamil, a strong depletion in intracellular glutathione in ABCC1-overexpressing cells (Genoux-Bastide et al., 2011), and the second series contained chalcones (C27, 37, 38, 40; Valdameri et al., 2012) and 6-prenylchrysin (6-Pc; Ahmed-Belkacem et al., 2005) known as ABCG2 inhibitors. **Figure 4** shows that some xanthones induced a significant decrease in intracellular glutathione, up to around 30% for X8 and X9 and 20% for X23, similarly to the effect observed with verapamil in **Figure 3A**. By contrast, the ABCG2 inhibitory chalcones, except for C27, and 6-prenylchrysin did not induce any decrease of intracellular glutathione in ABCG2-transfected cells.

NO DETECTABLE INTERACTION BETWEEN GSH AND ABCG2 IN EITHER ATPase OR TRANSPORT ASSAY

We previously demonstrated that the baculovirus-insect cell heterologous expression system is a useful tool for the detection of interactions between a given test compound and ABCG2 (Szakács et al., 2008). Briefly, compounds modifying the ATP hydrolytic activity of ABCG2 interact with the transporter, and can be either transported substrates or inhibitors of the protein. In order to define whether GSH is able to interact with ABCG2, we have tested its effect in the ATPase assay using cholesterol-loaded Sf9 vesicles ensuring higher ABCG2 activity. We found that the ATPase activity of ABCG2 was not affected by GSH addition up to 10 mM, by contrast to a transported substrate such as 1 μM quercetin which

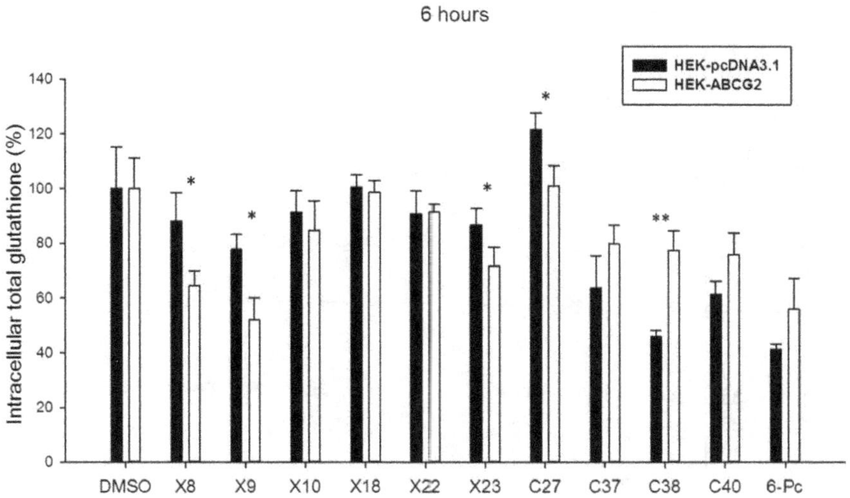

FIGURE 4 | Effects of other modulators on ABGC2-specific intracellular glutathione depletion. Screening of Xanthones (Genoux-Bastide et al., 2011), Chalcones (Valdameri et al., 2012), and 6-Prenylchrysin (Ahmed-Belkacem et al., 2005) reveal a significant ABCG2-dependent intracellular glutathione depletion in 6-h incubation for some compounds, as indicated. The values represent means ± SD corresponding to at least two independent experiments performed in triplicates. *t*-test analysis: $*p < 0.05$, $**p < 0.01$.

stimulated twofold the basal ATPase activity, and the ABCG2-specific inhibitor Ko143 which fully inhibited (**Figures 5A,B**). GSH did not alter the quercetin-stimulated ATPase activity either. Moreover, no effect was produced by the glutathione-conjugate *S*-(2,4-dinitrophenyl)glutathione (DNP-SG; **Figure 5B**) known to be actively transported by ABCC1 (Leier et al., 1994).

As the ATPase assay did not give any proof of interaction between GSH and ABCG2, we investigated the ability of GSH to modify the transport of ^{3}H-methotrexate. As shown in **Figure 6**, the ABCG2-mediated transport of tritiated methotrexate was not significantly inhibited by GSH addition, up to a 10 mM concentration, by difference with 1 μM Ko143 leading to the low background level observed with inactive mutant ABCG2. This contrasts with the reported prevention by 10 μM methotrexate against the increased extracellular GSH level observed in transformed yeast expressing human ABCG2 (Brechbuhl et al., 2010).

INABILITY OF ABCG2 TO CATALYZE AN ACTIVE TRANSPORT OF GSH

Finally, we measured the direct transport of ^{3}H-GSH into ABCG2-containing membrane vesicles. We found that, in contrast to ABCC1 serving as a positive control, no direct, ATP-dependent and specific inhibitor-sensitive, transport of tritiated GSH by ABCG2 could be detected in insect-cell membrane vesicles (**Figure 7**). Any ABCG2-mediated GSH transport could not be either determined at other ^{3}H-GSH concentrations (0.1 or 1 mM, data not shown).

DISCUSSION

The key results of this paper strongly suggest that human ABCG2 is unable to transport GSH. This has been demonstrated by direct measurement of ATP-dependent tritiated GSH uptake in inverted vesicles of insect-cell membranes overexpressing human ABCG2. In contrast, human ABCC1 catalyzed a high level of ATP-dependent and MK571-sensitive GSH transport under the same conditions. There was a low level of GSH accumulation in the presence of ABCG2 observed without ATP, which was also observed in the presence of the selective ABCG2 inhibitor Ko143 (Allen et al., 2002), or when the catalytically inactive K86M ABCG2 mutant was expressed. Thus, this background GSH binding could not be attributed to any ABCG2-mediated active transport.

This result is fully consistent with the lack of effect of GSH, even at high concentrations, on both basal and quercetin-stimulated ABCG2-ATPase activity of the insect cell membrane vesicles. Indeed, transported substrates such as prazosin, quercetin, or nilotinib (Telbisz et al., 2012) strongly stimulate the basal ATPase activity, then enhancing "coupled" ATPase activity. Our present results also show the lack of any effect by DNP-SG on the ABCG2 transporter, suggesting that glutathione conjugates are not transported by ABCG2. This is in contrast to various compounds conjugated with either sulfate (Suzuki et al., 2003) or glucuronate (Chen et al., 2003), whereas DNP-SG is actively transported by ABCC1 (Leier et al., 1994). The lack of ABCG2-mediated GSH transport is also consistent with the lack of any antagonism by GSH addition against ABCG2-mediated tritiated-methotrexate transport in inverted vesicles. These results, however disagree with the methotrexate-induced inhibition of GSH efflux reported in transformed yeast cells, expressing human ABCG2 (Brechbuhl et al., 2010).

Our results from experiments using membrane vesicles are quite consistent with those obtained with either transfected or drug-selected ABCG2-overexpressing cells where we did not observe any sharp and rapid decrease of intracellular GSH stimulable by modulators (such as 2′,5′-DHC, verapamil, or xanthones), or alterable by ABCG2 inactivation (such as using the potent Ko143 inhibitor). In addition, there was no inverse correlation between the observed decrease of intracellular GSH and increase of extracellular GSH, as also noticed in other drug-selected cancer cells overexpressing ABCG2 (Brechbuhl et al.,

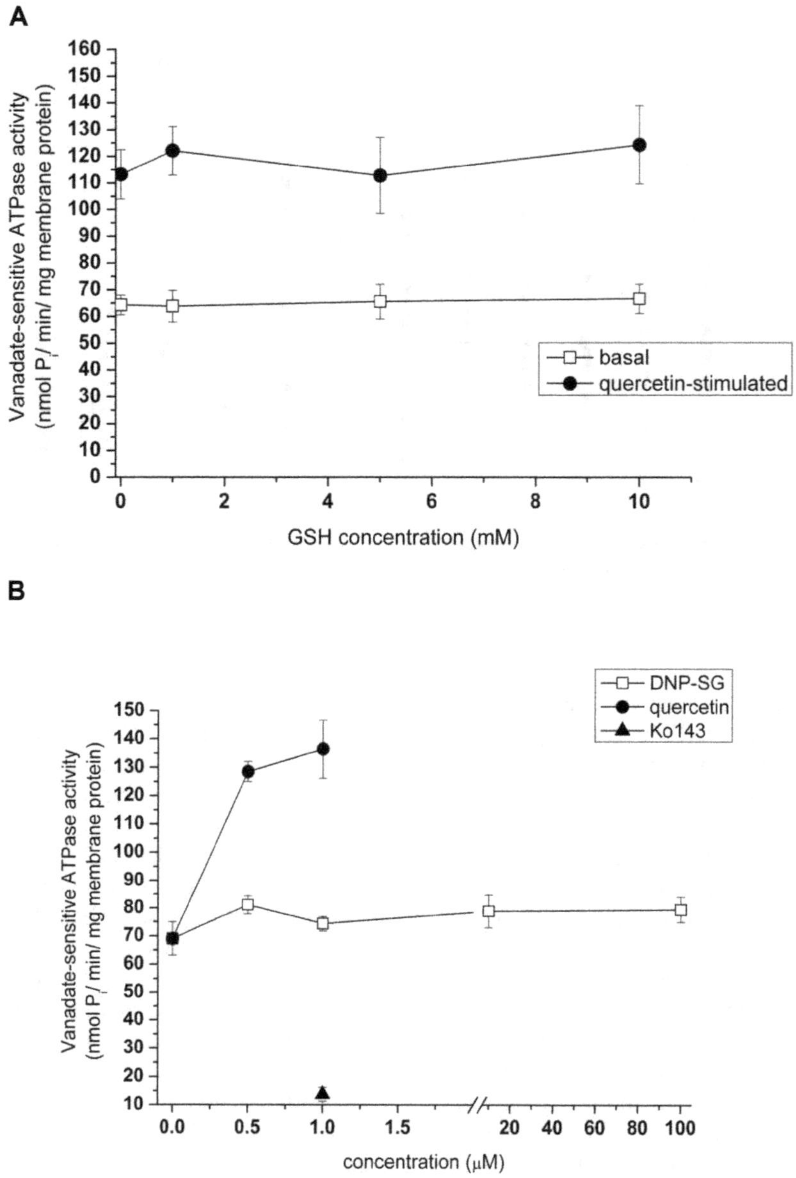

FIGURE 5 | Effects of GSH and DNP-SG on the ATP hydrolytic activity of ABCG2. Sodium orthovanadate-dependent ATP cleavage by wtABCG2 in 2 mM cholesterol-loaded Sf9 membrane vesicles was determined in the presence of increasing concentrations of GSH **(A)** both in the absence ("basal") and in the presence of a known transported substrate (1 μM quercetin, "quercetin-stimulated") without producing any significant effect. It was also assayed with increasing concentrations of DNP-SG or quercetin or with 1 μM Ko143 **(B)**. Data points represent the average ± SD values of two independent measurements.

2010). This contrasts with the strong effects clearly observed with ABCC1-overexpressing cells (Trompier et al., 2004; Perrotton et al., 2007; Barattin et al., 2010; Genoux-Bastide et al., 2011).

Nevertheless, the intracellular total glutathione concentration appeared to be modulated by overexpressed ABCG2 since, for unknown reasons possibly resulting from different signaling pathways, glutathione was lower in HEK293 transfected cells and higher in the drug-selected MCF7 cancer cells by comparison to their respective control cells. In addition, a significant decrease of intracellular glutathione was actually observed, either in some cases with 2′,5′-DHC, as previously reported (Brechbuhl et al., 2010), or with known ABCC1 modulators such as verapamil and xanthones. Such a decrease of intracellular glutathione however displayed special characteristics, such as being slow, requiring at least 6–24 h incubation, and not depending on ABCG2 activity since it was not altered by Ko143 inhibition. These results are more likely compatible with the induction of associated signaling pathways, leading to changes in intracellular GSH, than with a direct GSH transport.

ABCG2 is known to be regulated by a number of signaling pathways including NF-KB (Shen et al., 2010), RAR/RXR (Hessel and Lampen, 2010), hedgehog (Singh et al., 2011),

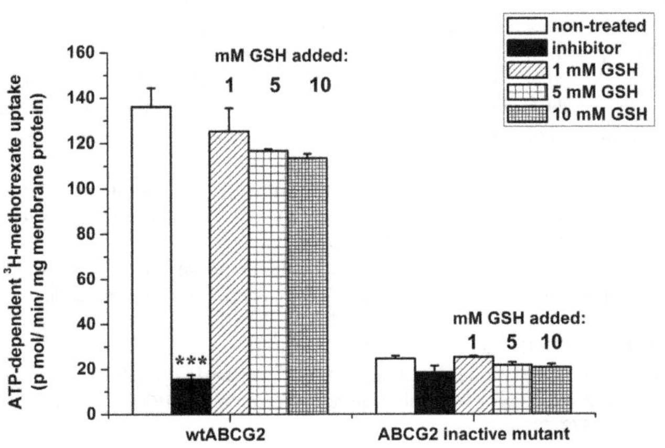

FIGURE 6 | Effect of GSH on the transport of methotrexate by ABCG2. ATP-dependent transport of ^{3}H-methotrexate in 2 mM cholesterol-loaded insect-cell membranes expressing ABCG2 (either wild-type or the inactive K86M mutant) was measured for 10 min at 37°C. Transport was determined in the absence or presence of an ABCG2-specific inhibitor (1 μM Ko143) or 1–10 mM GSH. Bars represent the average ± SD values of at least two measurements. *t*-test analysis: $***p < 0.001$.

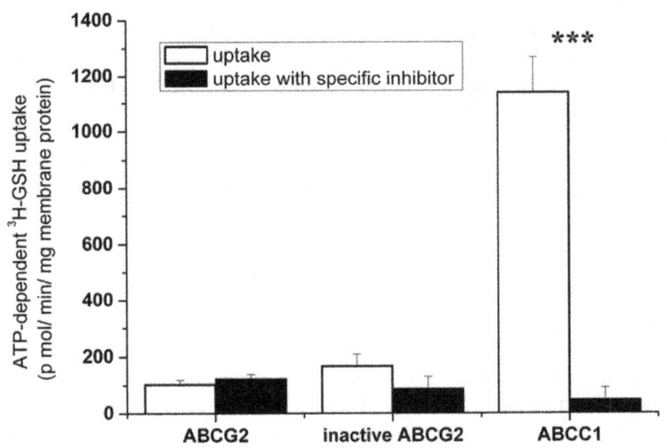

FIGURE 7 | Investigation of the transport of ^{3}H-GSH into wtABCG2-containing insect vesicles. Uptake of 500 μM ^{3}H-GSH was measured in Sf9 vesicles expressing ABCC1, wtABCG2, or inactive ABCG2, for 5 min at 37°C. ATP-dependent transport with or without the ABCC1- or ABCG2-specific inhibitor, 4 μM MK-571 or 1 μM Ko143 respectively, is shown. Bars represent the average of three independent measurements ± SD values. *t*-test analysis: $***p < 0.001$.

P13K/AKT (Nakanishi and Ross, 2012), JNK1/c-jun (Zhu et al., 2012), HER2 and EGFR/HER1 (Gilani et al., 2012), and ERK1/2 (de Boussac et al., 2012). Some signaling pathways, such as notch (Battacharya et al., 2007), CXCL12-CXCR4 (Katoh and Katoh, 2010), Oct4-TCL1-AKT (Wang et al., 2010), PTEN/P13K/Akt (Li et al., 2011), β-catenin/Tcf (Usongo and Farookhi, 2012), AhR (Dubrovska et al., 2012), and HIF-2α with TGF-β/Smad2 (Cui et al., 2013) are related to the ABCG2 status as a marker of stem cells or stem-like cancer cells. Nrf2, a critical transcription factor that regulates antioxidants, detoxification enzymes, and drug efflux proteins in response to oxidative stress (Hong et al., 2010; Singh et al., 2010; Chen et al., 2012; Zhang et al., 2012; Ishikawa et al., 2013; Shelton and Jaiswal, 2013), may provide a link between cellular GSH homeostasis and ABCG2 expression. Whatever the mechanism(s) involved, changes in intracellular GSH are evidently too slow and too low to induce a sufficient cellular GSH depletion susceptible to trigger CS-induced cell apoptosis, as observed for ABCC1. It is still an important question if, and how, an ABCG2-dependent CS can effectively be produced. Indeed, the few known examples report very low selectivity ratio values, limited to 2.5–3 (Deeken et al., 2009), by comparison with the values, at least one order of magnitude higher, reported for both ABCB1- (Ludwig et al., 2006; Hall et al., 2009; Türk et al., 2009; Pluchino et al., 2012) and ABCC1- (Trompier et al., 2004; Barattin et al., 2010; Genoux-Bastide et al., 2011) overexpressing cells. Such a difference may be at least partly related to the complex involvement of ABCG2 in many signaling pathways. Further identification and characterization of mechanisms directly connecting ABCG2 to CS-associated apoptosis and signaling are mandatory for establishing a new therapeutic strategy, selectively targeting and eliminating resistant cancer cells.

ACKNOWLEDGMENTS

Drs. S. E. Bates and R. W. Robey from the NCI at Bethesda, MD, are acknowledged for providing the different cell lines, and Drs. H. Baubichon-Cortay and D. Lorendeau for critical discussion about ABCC1-related CS. Charlotte Gauthier was recipient of a doctoral fellowship from the Ligue Nationale Contre le Cancer. Financial support was provided by the CNRS and Université Lyon 1 (UMR 5086), the Ligue Nationale Contre le Cancer (Equipe labellisée Ligue 2013), the Région Rhône-Alpes (CIBLE 2010), the Hungarian OTKA (83533), ERC Stg 260572, and an international grant from French ANR and Hungarian NIH (2010-INT-1101-01; NIH-ANR 10-1-2011-0401). Gergely Szakacs was supported by a Momentum Grant of the Hungarian Academy of Sciences.

REFERENCES

Ahmed-Belkacem, A., Pozza, A., Munoz-Martinez, F., Bates, S. E., Castanys, S., Gamarro, F., et al. (2005). Flavonoid structure–activity studies identify 6-prenylchrysin and tectochrysin as potent and specific inhibitors of breast cancer resistance protein ABCG2. *Cancer Res.* 65, 4852–4860. doi: 10.1158/0008-5472.CAN-04-1817

Allen, J. D., van Loevezijn, A., Lakhai, J. M., van der Valk, M., van Tellingen, O., Reid, G., et al. (2002). Potent and specific inhibition of the breast cancer resistance protein multidrug transporter in vitro and in mouse intestine by a novel analogue of fumitremorgin C. *Mol. Cancer Ther.* 1, 417–425.

Allikmets, R., Schriml, L. M., Hutchinson, A., Romano-Spica, V., and Dean, M. (1998). A human placenta-specific ATP-binding cassette gene (ABCP) on chromosome 4q22 that is involved in multidrug resistance. *Cancer Res.* 58, 5337–5339.

Anderson, M. E. (1985). Determination of glutathione and glutathione disulfide in biological samples. *Methods Enzymol.* 113, 548–555. doi: 10.1016/S0076-6879(85)13073-9

Bakos, E., Hegedüs, T., Hollo, Z., Welker, E., Tusnàdy, G. E., Zaman, G. F., et al. (1996). Membrane topology and glycosylation of the human multidrug resistance-associated protein. *J. Biol. Chem.* 271, 12322–12326. doi: 10.1074/jbc.271.21.12322

Barattin, R., Perrotton, T., Trompier, D., Lorendeau, D., Di Pietro, A., du Moulinet d'Hardemare, A., et al. (2010). Iodination of verapamil for a stronger induction of death, through GSH efflux, of cancer cells overexpressing MRP1. *Bioorg. Med. Chem.* 18, 6265–6274. doi: 10.1016/j.bmc.2010.07.031

Battacharya, S., Das, A., Mallya, K., and Ahmad, I. (2007). Maintenance of retinal stem cells by Abcg2 is regulated by notch signaling. *J. Cell Sci.* 120(Pt 15), 2652–2662. doi: 10.1242/jcs.008417

Brechbuhl, H. M., Gould, N., Kachadourian, R., Riekhof, W. R., Voelker, D. R., and Day, B. J. (2010). Glutathione transport is a unique function of the ATP-binding cassette protein ABCG2. *J. Biol. Chem.* 285, 16582–16587. doi: 10.1074/jbc.M109.090506

Brechbuhl, H. M., Min, E., Kariya, C., Frederick, B., Raben, D., and Day, B. J. (2009). Select cyclopentenone prostaglandins trigger glutathione efflux and the role of ABCG2 transport. *Free Radic. Biol. Med.* 47, 722–730. doi: 10.1016/j.freeradbiomed.2009.06.005

Chen, Q., Li, W., Wan, Y., Xia, X., Wu, Q., Chen, Y., et al. (2012). Amplified in breast cancer 1 enhances human cholangiocarcinoma growth and chemoresistance by simultaneous activation of Akt and Nrf2 pathways. *Hepatology* 55, 1820–1829. doi: 10.1002/hep.25549

Chen, Z. S., Robey, R. W., Belinsky, M. G., Shchaveleva, I., Ren, X. Q., Sugimoto, Y., et al. (2003). Transport of methotrexate, methotrexate polyglutamates and 17 beta-estradiol 17-(beta-D-glucuronide) by ABCG2: effects of acquired mutations at R482 on methotrexate transport. *Cancer Res.* 63, 4048–4054.

Cole, S. P., Bhardwaj, G., Gerlach, J. H., Mackie, J. E., Grant, C. E., Almquist, K. C., et al. (1992). Overexpression of a transporter gene in a multidrug-resistant human lung cancer cell line. *Science* 258, 1650–1654. doi: 10.1126/science.1360704

Cripe, L. D., Uno, H., Paietta, E. M., Litzow, M. R., Ketterling, R. P., Bennett, J. M., et al. (2010). Zosuquidar, a novel modulator of P-glycoprotein, does not improve the outcome of older patients with newly diagnosed acute myeloid leukemia: a randomized, placebo-controlled trial of the Eastern Cooperative Oncology Group 3999. *Blood* 116, 4077–4085. doi: 10.1182/blood-2010-04-277269

Cui, X. Y., Skretting, G., Jing, Y., Sun, H., Sandset, P. M., and Sun, L. (2013). Hypoxia influences stem cell-like properties in multidrug resistant K562 leukemic cells. *Blood Cells Mol. Dis.* 51, 177–184. doi: 10.1016/j.bcmd.2013.05.003

de Boussac, H., Orban, T. I., Varady, G., Tihanyi, B., Bacquet, C., Brozik, A., et al. (2012). Stimulus-induced expression of the ABCG2 multidrug transporter in HepG2 hepatocarcinoma model cells involves the ERK1/2 cascade and alternative promoters. *Biochem. Biophys. Res. Commun.* 426, 172–176. doi: 10.1016/j.bbrc.2012.08.046

Deeken, J. F., Robey, R. W., Shukla, S., Steadman, K., Chakraborty, A. R., Poonkuzhali, B., et al. (2009). Identification of compounds that correlate with ABCG2 transporter function in the National Cancer Institute Anticancer Drug Screen. *Mol. Pharmacol.* 76, 946–956. doi: 10.1124/mol.109.056192

Doyle, L. A., Yang, W., Abruzzo, L. V., Krogmann, T., Gao, Y., Rishi, A. K., et al. (1998). A multidrug resistance transporter from human MCF-7 breast cancer cells. *Proc. Natl. Acad. Sci. U.S.A.* 95, 15665–15670. doi: 10.1073/pnas.95.26.15665

Dubrovska, A., Hartung, A., Bouchez, L. C., Walker, J. R., Reddy, V. A., Cho, C. Y., et al. (2012). CXCR4 activation maintains a stem cell population in tamoxifen-resistant breast cancer cells through AhR signaling. *Br. J. Cancer* 107, 43–52. doi: 10.1038/bjc.2012.105

Genoux-Bastide, E., Lorendeau, D., Nicolle, E., Yahiaoui, S., Magnard, S., Di Pietro, A., et al. (2011). Identification of xanthones as selective killers of cancer cells overexpressing the ABC transporter MRP1. *ChemMedChem* 6, 1478–1484. doi: 10.1002/cmdc.201100102

Gilani, R. A., Kazi, A. A., Shah, P., Schech, A. J., Chumsri, S., Sabnis, G., et al. (2012). The importance of HER2 signaling in the tumor-initiating cell population in aromatase inhibitor-resistant breast cancer. *Breast Cancer Res. Treat.* 135, 681–692. doi: 10.1007/s10549-012-2148-8

Goler-Baron, V., and Assaraf, Y. G. (2012). Overcoming multidrug resistance via photodestruction of ABCG2-rich extracellular vesicles sequestering photosensitive chemotherapeutics. *PLoS ONE* 7:e35487. doi: 10.1371/journal.pone.0035487

Hall, M. D., Handley, M. D., and Gottesman, M. M. (2009). Is resistance useless? Multidrug resistance and collateral sensitivity. *Trends Pharmacol. Sci.* 30, 546–556. doi: 10.1016/j.tips.2009.07.003

Hessel, S., and Lampen, A. (2010). All-trans retinoic acid enhances the transport of phase II metabolites of benzo[a]pyrene by inducing the breast cancer resistance protein expression in Caco-2 cells. *Toxicol. Lett.* 197, 151–155. doi: 10.1016/j.toxlet.2010.05.018

Hong, Y. B., Kang, H. J., Kwon, S. Y., Kim, H. J., Kwon, K. Y., Cho, C. H., et al. (2010). Nuclear factor (erythroid-derived 2)-like 2 regulates drug resistance in pancreatic cancer cells. *Pancreas* 39, 463–472. doi: 10.1097/MPA.0b013e3181c31314

Honjo, Y., Hrycyna, C. A., Yan, Q. W., Medina-Perez, W. Y., Robey, R. W., van de Laar, A., et al. (2001). Acquired mutations in the MXR/BCRP/ABCP gene alter substrate specificity in MXR/BCRP/ABCP-overexpressing cells. *Cancer Res.* 61, 6635–6639.

Ishikawa, T., Kajimoto, Y., Sun, W., Nakagawa, H., Inoue, Y., Ikegami, Y., et al. (2013). Role of Nrf2 in cancer photodynamic therapy: regulation of human ABC transporter ABCG2. *J. Pharm. Sci.* 102, 3058–3069. doi: 10.1002/jps.25563

Ito, M., Kajino, K., Abe, M., Fujimura, T., Mineki, R., Ikegami, T., et al. (2013). NP-1250, an ABCG2 inhibitor, induces apoptotic cell death in mitoxantrone-resistant breast carcinoma MCF7 cells via a caspase-independent pathway. *Oncol. Rep.* 29, 1492–1500. doi: 10.3892/or.2013.2249

Juliano, R. L., and Ling, V. (1976). A surface glycoprotein modulating drug permeability in Chinese hamster ovary cell mutants. *Biochim. Biophys. Acta* 455, 152–162. doi: 10.1016/0005-2736(76)90160-7

Katoh, M., and Katoh, M. (2010). Integrative genomic analyses of CXCR4: transcriptional regulation of CXCR4 based on TGFbeta, Nodal, activin signaling and POU5F1, FOXA2, FOXC2, FOXH1, SOX17, and GFI1 transcription factors. *Int. J. Oncol.* 36, 415–420. doi: 10.3892/ijo_00000514

Keppler, D., Leier, I., and Jedlitschky, G. (1997). Transport of glutathione conjugates and glucuronides by the multidrug resistance proteins MRP1 and MRP2. *Biol. Chem.* 378, 787–791.

Kolitz, J. E., George, S. L., Marcucci, G., Vij, R., Powell, B. L., Allen, S. L., et al. (2010). P-glycoprotein inhibition using valspodar (PSC-833) does not improve outcomes for patients younger than age 60 years with newly diagnosed acute myeloid leukemia: cancer and leukemia group B study 19808. *Blood* 116, 1413–1421. doi: 10.1182/blood-2009-07-229492

Leier, I., Jedlitschki, G., Buchholz, U., Cole, S. P., Deeley, R. G., and Keppler, D. (1994). The MRP gene encodes an ATP-dependent export pump for leukotriene C4 and structurally related conjugates. *J. Biol. Chem.* 269, 27807–27810.

Li, H., Gao, Q., Guo, L., and Lu, S. H. (2011). The PTEN/P13K/AKT pathway regulates stem-like cells in primary esophageal carcinoma cells. *Cancer Biol. Ther.* 11, 950–958. doi: 10.4161/cbt.11.11.15531

Ludwig, J. A., Szakács, G., Martin, S. E., Chu, B. F., Cardarelli, C., Sauna, Z. E., et al. (2006). Selective toxicity of NSC73306 in MDR1-positive cells as a new strategy to circumvent multidrug resistance in cancer. *Cancer Res.* 66, 4808–4815. doi: 10.1158/0008-5472.CAN-05-3322

Miyake, K., Mickley, L., Litman, T., Zhan, Z., Robey, R., Cristensen, B., et al. (1999). Molecular cloning of cDNAs which are highly overexpressed in mitoxantrone-resistant cells: demonstration of homology to ABC transport genes. *Cancer Res.* 59, 8–13.

Mosmann, T. (1983). Rapid colorimetric assay for cellular growth and survival: application to proliferation and cytotoxicity assays. *J. Immunol. Methods* 65, 55–63. doi: 10.1016/0022-1759(83)90303-4

Nakanishi, T., and Ross, D. D. (2012). Breast cancer resistance protein (BCRP/ABCG2): its role in multidrug resistance and regulation of its gene expression. *Chin. J. Cancer* 31, 73–99. doi: 10.5732/cjc.011.10320

Ozvegy, C., Litman, T., Szakacs, G., Nagy, Z., Bates, S. E., Varadi, A., et al. (2001). Functional characterization of the human multidrug transporter, ABCG2, expressed in insect cells. *Biochem. Biophys. Res. Commun.* 285, 111–117. doi: 10.1006/bbrc.2001.5130

Ozvegy-Laczka, C., Köblös, G., Sarkadi, B., and Varadi, A. (2005). Single amino acid (482) variants of the ABCG2 multidrug transporter: major differences in transport capacity and substrate recognition. *Biochim. Biophys. Acta* 1668, 53–63. doi: 10.1016/j.bbamem.2004.11.005

Perrotton, T., Trompier, D., Chang, X-B., Di Pietro, A., and Baubichon-Cortay, H. (2007). S- and R-verapamil differentially modulate the multidrug resistance protein MRP1. *J. Biol. Chem.* 282, 31542–31548. doi: 10.1074/jbc.M703964200

Pluchino, K. M., Hall, M. D., Goldsborough, A. S., Callaghan, R., and Gottesman, M. M. (2012). Collateral sensitivity as a strategy against cancer multidrug resistance. *Drug Resist. Updat.* 15, 98–105. doi: 10.1016/j.drup.2012.03.002

Robey, R. W., Honjo, Y., Morisaki, K., Nadjem, T. A., Runge, S., Risbood, M., et al. (2003). Mutations at amino-acid 482 in the ABCG2 gene affect substrate and antagonist specificity. *Br. J. Cancer* 89, 1971–1978. doi: 10.1038/sj.bjc.6601370

Robey, R. W., Massey, P. R., Amiri-Kordestani, L., and Bates, S. E. (2010). ABC transporters: unvalidated therapeutic targets in cancer and the CNS. *Anticancer Agents Med. Chem.* 10, 625–633. doi: 10.2174/187152010794473957

Shelton, P., and Jaiswal, A. K. (2013). The transcription factor NF-E2-related factor 2 (Nrf2): a protooncogene? *FASEB J.* 27, 414–423. doi: 10.1096/fj.12-217257

Shen, S., Callaghan, D., Juzwik, C., Xiong, H., Huang, P., and Zhang, W. (2010). ABCG2 reduces ROS-mediated toxicity and inflammation: a potential role in Alzheimer's disease. *J. Neurochem.* 114, 1590–1604. doi: 10.1111/j.1471-4159.2010.06887.x

Singh, A., Wu, H., Zhang, P., Happel, C., Ma., J., and Biswal, S. (2010). Expression of ABCG2 (BCRP) is regulated by Nrf2 in cancer cells that confers side population and chemoresistance phenotype. *Mol. Cancer Ther.* 9, 2365–2376. doi: 10.1158/1535-7163.MCT-10-0108

Singh, R. R., Kunkalla, K., Qu, C., Schlette, E., Neelapu, S. S., Samaniego, F., et al. (2011). Abcg2 is a direct transcriptional target of hedgehog signaling and involved in stroma-induced drug tolerance in diffuse large B-cell lymphoma. *Oncogene* 30, 4874–4886. doi: 10.1038/onc.2011.195

Suzuki, M., Suzuki, H., Sugimoto, Y., and Sugiyama, Y. (2003). ABCG2 transports sulfated conjugates of steroids and xenobiotics. *J. Biol. Chem.* 278, 22644–22649. doi: 10.1074/jbc.M212399200

Szakacs, G., Paterson, J. K., Ludwig, J. A., Booth-Genthe, C., and Gottesman, M. M. (2006). Targeting multidrug resistance in cancer. *Nat. Rev. Drug Discov.* 5, 219–234. doi: 10.1038/nrd1984

Szakács, G., Varadi, A., Ozvegy-Laczka, C., and Sarkadi, B. (2008). The role of ABC transporters in drug absorption, distribution, metabolism, excretion and toxicity (ADME-tox). *Drug Discov. Today* 13, 379–393. doi: 10.1016/j.drudis.2007.12.010

Telbisz, A., Hegedus, C., Ozvegy-Laczka, C., Goda, K., Varady, G., Takats, Z., et al. (2012). Antibody binding shift assay for rapid screening of drug interactions with the human ABCG2 multidrug transporter. *Eur. J. Pharm. Sci.* 45, 101–109. doi: 10.1016/j.ejps.2011.10.021

Telbisz, A., Müller, M., Ozvegy-Laczka, C., Homolya, L., Szente, L., Varadi, A., et al. (2007). Membrane cholesterol selectively modulates the activity of the human ABCG2 multidrug transporter. *Biochim. Biophys. Acta* 1768, 2698–2713. doi: 10.1016/j.bbamem.2007.06.026

Tietze, F. (1969). Enzymic method for quantitative determination of nanogram amounts of total and oxidized glutathione: applications to mammalian blood and other tissues. *Anal. Biochem.* 27, 502–522. doi: 10.1016/0003-2697(69)90064-5

Trompier, D., Chang, X. B., Barattin, R., du Moulinet d'Hardemare, A., Di Pietro, A., and Baubichon-Cortay, H. (2004). Verapamil and its derivative trigger apoptosis through glutathione extrusion by multidrug resistance protein MRP1. *Cancer Res.* 64, 4950–4956. doi: 10.1158/0008-5472.CAN-04-0143

Türk, D., Hall, M. D., Chu, B. F., Ludwig, J. A., Fales, H. M., Gottesman, M. M., et al. (2009). Identification of compounds selectively killing multidrug-resistant cancer cells. *Cancer Res.* 69, 8293–8301. doi: 10.1158/0008-5472.CAN-09-2422

Usongo, M., and Farookhi, R. (2012). β-Catenin/Tcf-signaling appears to establish the murine ovarian surface epithelium (OSE) and remains active in selected postnatal OSE cells. *BMC Dev. Biol.* 12:17. doi: 10.1186/1471-213X-12-17

Valdameri, G., Gauthier, C., Terreux, R., Kachadourian, R., Day, B. J., Winnischofer, S. M., et al. (2012). Investigation of chalcones as selective inhibitors of the breast cancer resistance protein: critical role of methoxylation in both inhibition potency and cytotoxicity. *J. Med. Chem.* 55, 3193–3200. doi: 10.1021/jm2016528

Wang, X. Q., Ongkeko, W. M., Chen, L., Yang, Z. F., Lu, P., Chen, K. K., et al. (2010). Octamer 4 (Oct4) mediates chemotherapeutic drug resistance in liver cancer cells through a potential Oct4-AKT-ATP-binding cassette G2 pathway. *Hepatology* 52, 528–539. doi: 10.1002/hep.23692

Zhang, M., Mathur, A., Zhang, Y., Xi, S., Atay, S., Hong, J. A., et al. (2012). Mithramycin represses basal and cigarette smoke-induced expression of ABCG2 and inhibits stem cell signaling in lung and esophageal cancer cells. *Cancer Res.* 72, 4178–4192. doi: 10.1158/0008-5472.CAN-11-3983

Zhu, M. M., Tong, J. L., Xu, Q., Nie, F., Xu, X. T., Xia, S. D., et al. (2012). Increased JNK1 signaling pathway is responsible for ABCG2-mediated multidrug resistance in human colon cancer. *PLoS ONE* 7:e41763. doi: 10. 1371/journal.pone.0041763

19

Biomarker-guided repurposing of chemotherapeutic drugs for cancer therapy: a novel strategy in drug development

***Jan Stenvang*[1,2]*, Iben Kümler*[3]*, Sune Boris Nygård*[1]*, David Hersi Smith*[1,4]*, Dorte Nielsen*[3]*, Nils Brünner*[1,2]** *and José M. A. Moreira*[1,2]**

[1] *Faculty of Health and Medical Sciences, Department of Veterinary Disease Biology, Section for Molecular Disease Biology and Sino-Danish Breast Cancer Research Centre, University of Copenhagen, Copenhagen, Denmark*

[2] *Danish Centre for Translational Breast Cancer Research, Copenhagen, Denmark*

[3] *Department of Oncology, Center for Cancer Research, Herlev Hospital, University of Copenhagen, Copenhagen, Denmark*

[4] *DAKO A/S, Glostrup, Denmark*

Edited by:
Jan Trøst Jørgensen, Dx-Rx Institute, Denmark

Reviewed by:
Marc Poirot, Institut national de la santé et de la recherche médicale, France
Hardik J. Patel, Memorial Sloan-Kettering Cancer Center, USA

****Correspondence:***
Nils Brünner, Faculty of Health and Medical Sciences, Department of Veterinary Disease Biology, Section for Molecular Disease Biology and Sino-Danish Breast Cancer Research Centre, University of Copenhagen, Strandboulevarden 49, Copenhagen 2100, Denmark
e-mail: nbr@sund.ku.dk

Cancer is a leading cause of mortality worldwide and matters are only set to worsen as its incidence continues to rise. Traditional approaches to combat cancer include improved prevention, early diagnosis, optimized surgery, development of novel drugs, and honing regimens of existing anti-cancer drugs. Although discovery and development of novel and effective anti-cancer drugs is a major research area, it is well known that oncology drug development is a lengthy process, extremely costly and with high attrition rates. Furthermore, those drugs that do make it through the drug development mill are often quite expensive, laden with severe side-effects and unfortunately, to date, have only demonstrated minimal increases in overall survival. Therefore, a strong interest has emerged to identify approved non-cancer drugs that possess anti-cancer activity, thus shortcutting the development process. This research strategy is commonly known as drug repurposing or drug repositioning and provides a faster path to the clinics. We have developed and implemented a modification of the standard drug repurposing strategy that we review here; rather than investigating target-promiscuous non-cancer drugs for possible anti-cancer activity, we focus on the discovery of novel cancer indications for already approved chemotherapeutic anti-cancer drugs. Clinical implementation of this strategy is normally commenced at clinical phase II trials and includes pre-treated patients. As the response rates to any non-standard chemotherapeutic drug will be relatively low in such a patient cohort it is a pre-requisite that such testing is based on predictive biomarkers. This review describes our strategy of biomarker-guided repurposing of chemotherapeutic drugs for cancer therapy, taking the repurposing of topoisomerase I (Top1) inhibitors and Top1 as a potential predictive biomarker as case in point.

Keywords: drug repurposing, irinotecan, TOP1, breast cancer, biomarker

INTRODUCTION

Despite the significant improvements in diagnosis and treatment experienced in the past few decades, cancer remains the leading cause of death worldwide, and deaths from cancer are forecasted to reach a staggering 13.2 million deaths by 2030 (1). What's more, these numbers are only set to worsen, as a result of population aging and growth. Assuming that the estimated cancer-specific and sex-specific trends continue, it is expected that the incidence of all-cancer cases will rise from 12.7 million new cases in 2008 to 22.2 million by 2030 (2). Until now this unremitting increase has been offset by significant improvements in prognosis, as a result of earlier diagnosis, advances in surgical therapy, and the use of radiation therapy and adjuvant systemic treatments; as a consequence the survival rates for most cancers have increased significantly in the past few decades. But, unless novel and dramatically improved therapies are introduced, this compensation is unlikely to persist (2, 3). This is particularly crucial for metastatic disease as, for the large majority of cancers, it presents the biggest problem to medical management, being the main cause of death of cancer patients. In recent years our understanding of cancer biology has improved significantly, and resulted in the development of new targeted anti-cancer therapies such as targeting of the EGF-receptor or VEGF. In spite of the initial hope that agents targeting molecular alterations underlying cancer genesis and progression would provide unparalleled therapeutic benefit, reality proved otherwise. Overall, targeted therapies have shown relatively modest clinical benefit, presumably due to intrinsic resistance of tumors to inhibition of signaling intermediates, due mainly to redundancy in signaling pathways in cancer cells (4–8). As a consequence, these novel treatment modalities are not single-agent treatments as they, most often, are combined with conventional cytotoxic drugs. In short, many of the currently available molecular targeted cancer drugs are very costly, provide modest improvements in overall survival, and have significant side-effects.

REPURPOSING OF CANCER DRUGS AS A DRUG DEVELOPMENT STRATEGY

Although there is an acute need for developing new and better anti-cancer drugs, the lengthy time and astronomical high costs associated with cancer drug development, together with high failure rates and limited efficacy of targeted drugs have necessitated alternative approaches to cancer drug discovery (9). Drug repurposing or repositioning is a promising approach to identify suitable drug candidates for treatment of cancer; essentially it entails finding novel therapeutic indications for already approved drugs (10–14). Departing from this drug development strategy, our laboratory developed a simplified variant to identify novel therapeutic indications for chemotherapeutic agents. Our approach differs from the traditional view of drug repurposing in that we do not investigate established target-promiscuous non-cancer drugs for anti-cancer activity (10, 15, 16), but rather try to find new cancer indications for conventional chemotherapeutic agents. Most types of conventional chemotherapy are considered to kill cancer cells not by one single mechanism but by affecting several pivotal pathways/mechanisms with the sum of cellular effects resulting in cancer cell death. Accordingly, the efficacy of any given chemotherapeutic agent may be difficult to foretell using a single molecular predictor. On the other hand, some key molecules have been identified as major targets for chemotherapy drugs. With the above in mind, one could initiate systematic analyses of gene aberrations, mRNA expression, and/or protein determinations of known key target molecules for given chemotherapeutic drugs, specifically in those cancer types that are not conventionally offered these drugs – a knowledge-driven repurposing strategy.

As the response rates to a specific chemotherapeutic drug might be relatively low in an unselected pre-treated patient population, it is a pre-requisite, that the repurposing strategy includes preselection of those patients with a favorable molecular profile in their cancer cells, i.e., those patients with the highest likelihood of obtaining benefit from the treatment. One reasonable assumption would be that one and the same molecule would be both a major target for a chemotherapeutic drug and a predictive biomarker, a hypothesis that is supported by recent evidence. For example, two meta-analyses recently concluded that breast cancer patients with amplification of the topoisomerase 2A (*TOP2A*) gene have more clinical benefit from treatment with topoisomerase II inhibitors than patients with normal *TOP2A* gene number in their cancer cells (17–19). In the present review, we first describe and discuss experiences with topoisomerase I (Top1) measurements in colorectal cancer (CRC). We then turn to a discussion of the repurposing of DNA Top1 inhibitors for treatment of breast cancer.

REPURPOSING OF TOP1 INHIBITORS – IRINOTECAN

Several classes of cytotoxic agents, such as Top1 inhibitors (irinotecan, topotecan), topoisomerase II inhibitors (etoposide), anthracyclines (epirubicin, doxorubicin, mitoxantrone), taxanes (docetaxel, paclitaxel), anti-mitotics (vinorelbine, eribulin), antimetabolites (capecitabine, gemcitabine), or platinum analogs (cisplatin, carboplatin) can be used for the treatment of cancer, be it in the adjuvant, neoadjuvant, or metastatic setting. Each drug class, in addition to a specific therapeutic profile, has its own characteristic toxicity profile. The interplay of these two parameters determines the clinical use of any given drug class, which in many cases is disease specific. As a consequence, in current clinical practice, various drugs are used following evidence-based recommendations for each cancer type; for instance, drugs such as taxanes and anthracyclines are commonly used for standard treatment of breast cancer but not CRC (20). Conversely, camptothecins are used for standard treatment of CRC but not breast cancer (21). These differences in standard clinical use of chemotherapeutic agents essentially reflect the magnitude of clinical benefit attained by the different drugs in clinical trials for each specific disease. One class of anti-cancer drugs of particular interest to us is that of Top1 inhibitors, in particular irinotecan. Irinotecan is a derivative of camptothecin, and it has a unique pharmacological profile, as Top1 is its only target (22), and therefore an obvious candidate for our knowledge-driven repurposing strategy.

Irinotecan is a prodrug, 7-ethyl-10-[4-(1-piperidino)-1-piperidino] carbonyloxycamptothecin (CPT-11), which is converted by carboxylesterases into its active metabolite, 7-ethyl-10-hydroxycamptothecin (SN-38), a potent Top1 inhibitor (23, 24). SN-38 functions by inhibiting the Top1 enzyme, which plays an essential role in alleviating the topological stresses that arise during DNA replication and transcription by nicking, relaxing, and re-ligating the double-stranded DNA structure (22). The current model for anti-cancer activity by irinotecan revolves around the stabilization of (normally) transient DNA-Top1 complexes (termed "cleavage complexes" or Top1cc) by SN-38, thereby inhibiting subsequent re-ligation of the nicked DNA strand. Following the collision of DNA or RNA polymerases into the SN-38-stabilized Top1cc, DNA damage occurs. It has been suggested that upon collision with a DNA polymerase, double-strand breaks are formed, whereas RNA polymerase collision causes the formation of irreversible Top1cc-associated single strand breaks (22, 25, 26). Unless repaired, this DNA damage can lead to cell death [reviewed in (27)].

TOP1 INHIBITORS IN ROUTINE CANCER TREATMENT

Irinotecan and topotecan are the two Top1 inhibitors routinely used in cancer treatment (**Table 1**). In both Europe and the United States (US) irinotecan is recommended by national guidelines as first or second line treatment for metastatic CRC (28, 29). Recently, the combination of 5 FU, irinotecan, and oxaliplatin (FOLFIRINOX) has been recommended in European guidelines on pancreatic cancer, for patients with metastatic disease, $\leq$75 years of age with a good performance status (30). American guidelines, however, do not recommend the use of irinotecan for the treatment of advanced pancreatic cancer (31). A new liposomal formulation of irinotecan (MM-398) has recently been tested in a large phase II study in patients with metastatic pancreatic cancer. Patient recruitment has been completed, however, no results have been published yet (32).

Topotecan is recommended for later line treatment of metastatic ovarian cancer in both Europe and the US (33, 34). Also in both Europe and the US topotecan in combination with cisplatin is approved for the treatment of recurrent cervical cancer (35, 36). Although European guidelines refer an overall survival

Table 1 | Approved and recommended indications for the use of irinotecan and topotecan.

	Europe	United States
IRINOTECAN		
Metastatic colorectal cancer	X	X
Metastatic pancreatic cancer	X	
Metastatic small-cell lung cancer	X	X
TOPOTECAN		
Metastatic ovarian cancer	X	X
Metastatic cervical cancer	X[a]	X
Metastatic small-cell lung cancer	X	

[a]*Approved by authorities but not recommended in clinical guidelines.*

advantage with topotecan in combination with cisplatin compared to monotherapy, combination therapy with topotecan is not recommended for the treatment of metastatic cervical cancer (37). European guidelines on small-cell lung cancer (SCLC) recommend combinations of irinotecan–cisplatin, or topotecan–cisplatin as alternative treatment options for metastatic disease in the case of contraindications to etoposide (a topoisomerase II inhibitor) (38). US guidelines recommend irinotecan combined with cisplatin (among other regimens) as first line treatment for metastatic SCLC and irinotecan monotherapy as second line therapy (39).

A search on clinicaltrials.gov revealed that irinotecan and topotecan alone or in combination with other drugs, currently are being investigated for numerous other indications including various brain tumors, sarcomas, non-small-cell lung cancer (NSCLC), triple negative breast cancer, and gastric, esophageal, and gastroesophageal junction cancers (32). Finally, etirinotecan is a new polymer conjugate of irinotecan (NKTR-102). This drug formulation has a half-life of approximately 50 days compared to 5 days for irinotecan and has shown a lower maximum concentration resulting in greater systemic exposure to SN-38 compared to irinotecan (40). It is currently investigated for the indications SCLC, NSCLC, glioblastomas, and breast cancer (32, 41, 42).

TOPOISOMERASE I GENE STRUCTURE, EXPRESSION, AND ACTIVITY IN CANCER

The topoisomerase I (*TOP1*) gene is located at 20q12, a region that frequently undergoes copy-number alterations across cancer types, including melanoma, breast, colorectal, ovarian, and gastric cancer (43–47). These copy-number alterations have been reported to occur as either gains of chromosome 20, 20q, or as amplification of smaller chromosomal regions, termed "amplicons." Research suggests that in CRC, *TOP1* copy number increases occur predominately in conjunction with the rest of 20q (44–48). Amplification of the *TOP1* gene is observed in a subset of *TOP1* gains, and interestingly, these two types of copy number increases appear to have differential prognostic effects in stage III CRC patients (49). We have recently applied a *TOP1*/CEN-20 fluorescence *in situ* hybridization (FISH) probe mixture to explore the *TOP1* gene copy numbers in stage III CRC (44, 48). The *TOP1* and CEN-20 signals from unaffected epithelial mucosa ($n = 50$) located adjacent to the tumor cells were applied to determine the diploid copy numbers in non-cancer cells. Based on these non-cancer signals we found that 84% of the tumor samples demonstrated an increased *TOP1* gene copy number and 64% had an increased *TOP1*/CEN-20 ratio compared with the non-affected mucosa (44). Of the 50 stage III CRC patients, 13 (26%) had more than 4 *TOP1* copies/cells and 16 (32%) had a *TOP1*/CEN-20 ratio above 1.5 (44). In another study we included 154 stage III CRC chemonaïve patients and found that 55 (35.7%) of the tumors had an increased *TOP1* copy number above $4n$ gene copies per cell and 44 (28.6%) had a *TOP1*/CEN-20 ratio above 1.5 (48). There was no significant correlation between the *TOP1* copy number and proliferation, while multivariate analyses demonstrated a prognostic value since the *TOP1* copy number was significantly associated with overall survival (48). In gastric cancer, several amplicons have been observed on 20q, including one encompassing the *TOP1* gene (43). In malignant melanoma, high level amplifications of the *TOP1* locus can be detected by FISH, indicating the presence of an amplicon, which includes *TOP1* (45). In breast cancer, several amplicons mapped to 20q have been identified, including one covering the 20q12-q13 region (46). By FISH analyses we have established the normal range of *TOP1* copy numbers and found that 31% of primary breast cancer patients have *TOP1* copy number gains (≥ 4 copies) (50). However, it does not appear that *TOP1* is part of the minimal common region of amplification, indicating that its amplification may occur as a passenger to events involving of an amplicon located at 20q13.1–q13.2 (51). A similar finding has been made in ovarian cancer (47). Taken together, the *TOP1* locus appears to undergo frequent copy number increases in several cancer types. These aberrations are either focal in nature, i.e., amplicon-driven, or may involve larger chromosomal regions, such as 20q. Numerous candidate oncogenes located on 20q have been suggested as the targets of these copy-number alterations. Putative targets include *BCL2L1* (20q11.21), *AIB1* (20q12), and *AURKA* (20q13.2), which have all been implicated in cancer (43, 52, 53). Whether *TOP1* is truly the target of these copy number increases, or whether these increases occur as passenger-related events targeting alternative oncogenes, remains to be elucidated.

Beyond the *TOP1* copy-number alterations at the genomic level, there is also frequent over-expression of *TOP1* mRNA, Top1 protein or enzyme activity level in various cancer types compared to normal adjacent non-cancerous tissue (54–56). Generally, there appears to be a positive correlation between gene expression level, protein level, and activity in cancer tissues (54–56).

COLORECTAL CANCER

Colorectal cancer is the most thoroughly examined cancer with regard to Top1 expression and several studies have found increased Top1 protein in CRC tissues compared to non-cancerous tissues. Already in 1989, immunoblot analyses were applied to show that Top1 protein levels were 14- to 16-fold higher in primary colon adenocarcinoma tissue ($n = 38$) than in normal colonic mucosa (57). Approximately 20–30% of the tumors presented with very high levels of Top1 expression, whereas all normal tissue samples had low levels. Subsequent studies have largely confirmed these data finding 2- to 40-fold increases of *TOP1* mRNA, Top1 protein, or activity (55, 58) in cancer tissue. Copy-number analyses showed that *TOP1* was amplified in 23% of Dukes' C CRC patients ($n = 52$) when compared to paired normal colon tissue and these *TOP1* amplified tumors had approximately two-times higher RNA level and protein expression level than did the diploid tumors (56). The enzyme activity of Top1 has also been evaluated in crude nuclear extracts from CRC and normal tissue. These data showed that the Top1 activity was significantly higher in primary tumor tissue compared to normal tissue ($n = 53$) (59). In concordance with Giovanella et al. (57), it was found that 20–30% of the tumors possessed very high Top1 activity although the coefficients of variations in these analyses were about 75–80% indicating that these data may be somewhat ambiguous.

Studies have also compared the Top1 protein levels and activity in metastatic CRC tissue to normal tissue and to primary CRC tissue. These data are so far inconclusive. Apparently, the Top1 activity was significantly lower in liver metastases than in the normal liver ($n = 8$) (59). The *TOP1* mRNA levels in FFPE samples did not show significant changes when comparing primary CRC tumor and liver metastasis ($n = 33$) (60) whereas the levels of Top1 protein expression were higher in malignant cells from tumor recurrences compared to primary tumors ($n = 40$) (61) and $n = 25$ (62). Yet another study found concordance between Top1 protein levels in paired primary CRC and lymph node metastases in 33 of 42 cases (63).

Other studies have investigated the protein levels of Top1 in primary tumor CRC tissue by Immunohistochemistry (IHC). These studies have found high Top1 expression in 45% ($n = 62$) of metastatic CRC patients that received a first line 5 FU/CPT-11 chemotherapy (64), 86% ($n = 29$) of primary colon cancers (65), 31% ($n = 13$) among patients with recurrent CRC (66), 17% ($n = 1{,}313$) in metastatic CRC patients (67), and a study comprising 498 Dukes' stage B and C patients reported positive/high Top1 protein expression in 48% of the cases (68). These differences may be due to differences among the studied patient cohorts, choice of antibodies, tissue micro arrays (TMAs) versus full section analyses and scoring systems. In brief, *TOP1* mRNA, Top1 protein, and activity are increased in CRC tissues in comparison to non-cancerous tissues and a substantial subgroup of CRC patients has high levels of Top1.

OTHER CANCERS

Elevated levels of Top1 have also been reported in various other cancers. In poorly differentiated ovarian carcinomas the activity of Top1 was found to be much higher than in non-cancerous tissue or benign tumors (54, 69). In support of this, IHC analyses demonstrated that Top1 protein is primarily associated with tumor cells and much less to normal infiltrating cells (70) and increased Top1 protein expression was found in 43% of ovarian carcinomas (71). Prostate tumors also possessed increased levels of Top1 protein levels and Top1 activity compared to matched non-cancerous tissues, whereas no difference between malignant and normal tissue was found in kidney tumors (55). Similar over-expression of Top1 protein have been reported in urinary bladder carcinomas (77%) (72), gastric carcinomas (68%) (73), testicular tumors (74), renal cell carcinomas (36–100%) (75), malignant melanomas (42%) (76), squamous cell carcinomas (92%) (77), and sarcomas (13%) (78). In metastatic breast cancer (mBC) the Top1 protein expression has been evaluated by IHC in FFPE tissue from 22 primary breast cancer. It was found that 41% over-expressed Top1 (79). Interestingly, the expression of Top1 protein varies from undetectable to strongly positive among the analyzed samples, which indicate that Top1 expression may be a suitable biomarker in a subgroup of mBC patients.

CLINICAL STUDIES EVALUATING THE PREDICTIVE ROLE OF TOP1

Until now the association between Top1 assessed in tumor tissue and irinotecan efficacy has only been investigated retrospectively and with focus on CRC. Top1 levels have been determined by IHC where protein expression was assessed (64, 67, 68) and by RT-PCR where gene expression (mRNA) was analyzed (60). Tumor samples were obtained from patients who were originally enrolled in randomized phase III trials or from patients routinely treated in accordance with current local clinical guidelines.

Two small single-cohort biomarker studies investigated patients with advanced CRC who were all treated with different regimens of 5 FU/leucovorin + irinotecan (60, 64, 67, 68). These studies did not identify any significant association between *TOP1* gene expression or Top1 protein expression and objective response rates or survival endpoints. However, both studies were methodologically flawed as Top1 data was only available from 62 to 33 patients, respectively, and due to the consequent inherent lack of sufficient statistical power, this makes it almost impossible to obtain statistically significant results even though the association in question was in fact true. Additionally, a true distinction between a predictive and a prognostic component of a biomarker will not be identified when survival analysis is performed in a single-cohort study without a relevant control group (80, 81).

Biomarker studies designed to obtain Level of Evidence (LoE) 1 as proposed by Simon et al. (81) have been conducted where material from randomized clinical phase III trials was used in order to conduct a so-called prospective-retrospective biomarker evaluation according to a stringent analysis plan. In a study by Braun et al. (67) primary tumor material from patients originally accrued in the UK MRC FOCUS study (82) was used. The UK MRC FOCUS study was a randomized clinical trial investigating different combinations of chemotherapy for patients with advanced CRC. In first line 1,628 patients were randomized between 5 FU/levofolinate, 5 FU/levofolinate + irinotecan or 5 FU/levofolinate + oxaliplatin. As patients in the 5 FU/levofolinate arm could be used as relevant controls to correct for potential concurrent prognostic qualities of the biomarkers in question, this clinical design was ideal when investigating putative predictive biomarkers of either irinotecan or oxaliplatin efficacy. In the biomarker study, Top1 protein expression was assessed by IHC using a murine monoclonal antibody (clone 1D6, Novocastra), and the staining intensity was graded as low, moderate, or high. Due to inadequate tumor material or failed IHC analysis 315 cases were excluded, which resulted in available Top1 data from 1,313 tumor samples (81%). The authors reported a significant association between staining intensity and progression free survival where patients with tumors showing moderate or high expression benefited from the addition of irinotecan compared to 5 FU/levofolinate therapy alone. In contrast, patients with Top1 low classified tumors did not benefit more from the irinotecan combination than from the 5 FU/levofolinate treatment alone.

The interaction between Top1 and the irinotecan combination was reported to be statistically significant ($P = 0.001$). An attempt to validate these results was performed in tumor material from the CAIRO trial (83). In the CAIRO trial, 820 patients with advanced CRC were originally randomized between capecitabine, a prodrug of 5 FU, or capecitabine + irinotecan as first line treatment. In the following biomarker study (84), which was only published in abstract form, tumor samples from 545 patients were included and the same methodologies as in the study by Braun et al. (67) were applied. The study failed to confirm the positive association between Top1 protein expression and irinotecan efficacy. There are several explanations to why confirmation failed. First, the hypothesis may not be correct, and second, potential methodological bias may have been introduced unintentionally. Assessment of IHC staining intensity can be problematic and inter-observer variability due to staining heterogeneity and the somewhat subjective nature of the evaluation is a challenge to this methodology. Additionally, information on analytical validation of the applied antibody is essential to ensure prober sensitivity and specificity, and to our knowledge this is lacking for the 1D6 clone, which was used in both the CAIRO and the UK MRC FOCUS trials – as a result we cannot objectively determine which trial, if any, may be at fault. However, as stated previously, both the CAIRO and the UK MRC FOCUS trials fulfill the requirements set by Simon et al. (81) in order to obtain LoE 1 for a predictive biomarker of irinotecan efficacy, and the trials still represent the best available option to retrospectively assess the association between other biomarkers or Top1 analyzed by techniques other than IHC and irinotecan in the advanced setting of CRC.

The association between Top1 protein expression and irinotecan efficacy has also been investigated in the adjuvant setting of CRC, and results from a retrospective biomarker study suggested a positive predictive role of Top1 protein expression (68). The study did not use material from one randomized clinical trial but included material from several clinical trials, which resulted in two cohorts of patients who were either treated with 5 FU/leucovorin alone or 5 FU/leucovorin + irinotecan. However, this methodology was intrinsically flawed as the original clinical trials spanned almost two decades, a time frame in where great surgical improvements in the managements of CRC have taken place.

Based on negative results from several phase III trials, i.e., the PETACC-3 (85) and the CALGB 89803 (86), the 5 FU/leucovorin + irinotecan combination is today not recommended in the adjuvant setting of colon cancer. However, as patients in these trials were randomized between 5 FU/leucovorin and 5 FU/leucovorin + irinotecan, tumor tissue from these trials is highly appropriate for retrospective biomarker research in relation to prediction of irinotecan efficacy. The main challenge with such an approach is the availability of a sufficient number of tumor samples to obtain the necessary statistical power.

DESIGN OF CLINICAL STUDIES TO VALIDATE PREDICTIVE BIOMARKERS

Repurposing often involves drugs where the mechanisms of action are fully or partly known. Thus, clinical repurposing trials may take the advantage of such knowledge and from early phase development/testing include predictive biomarkers. Such biomarkers will often be found among molecules known to be mechanistically involved in sensitivity/resistance to the drug. The use of predictive biomarkers in early drug testing may increase the therapeutic index of the drug in question by increasing the efficacy of the drug in the selected biomarker favorable population and at the same time avoid drug-induced toxicity in the biomarker unfavorable population as these patients will not be exposed to the drug. Looking ahead, future drug indications might be limited to small subgroups of patients based on predictive biomarkers. Targeted drug selection is already in routine use e.g., estrogen receptor and human epidermal growth factor receptor (HER) 2 in breast cancer, *KRAS* in CRC and *BRAF* in malignant melanomas. The status of the relevant marker is frequently based only on analysis of the primary tumor. However, in e.g., breast cancer accumulating evidence suggests that tumor characteristics, including ER and HER2 might change through tumor progression (87). Thus, the treatment strategy may require readiness to perform serial biopsies, including biopsies from metastatic lesions. The statistical considerations and principles for repurposing an old drug accompanied by a biomarker are exactly the same as for the development of a new (targeted) drug.

PHASE I

Most often, repurposing of an old drug will not involve a phase I trial. However, new knowledge concerning relevant biomarkers might encourage the clinicians to try new drug combinations and thus perform a phase I trial.

The goal of incorporating biomarkers in this stage of development is a better characterization of the biomarker and the assay performance in human samples (88). In this context the present EMA guidelines urge investigators of non-cytotoxic products to analyze not only biopsies from the primary tumor and metastasis but also normal tissue to understand the molecular background for efficacy (89). More recently, molecular pre-screening has been suggested for selecting patients for early drug development. Thus, it is envisioned that academic institutions establish molecular pre-screening programs in order to select patients for phase I trials (90).

PHASE II

The biomarker should be included for hypothesis testing and early indications for proof-of concept. There are two types of clinical trial designs effective in evaluating the role of a potential predictive biomarker in phase II: the adaptive parallel two stage design and the tandem two-step predictor biomarker evaluation trial design. The designs and rational behind them have been reviewed by McShane et al. (88).

PHASE III

Phase III studies designed to repurpose an old drug will most often involve late stage cancer patients in order to compare monotherapy with a test drug versus best supportive care. Alternatively, the test drug might be evaluated as an add-on to a known treatment.

Prospectively designed clinical trials are regarded as the gold standard for evaluating a predictive biomarker. In many instances, however, due to time and expenses required for these trials, a retrospective testing of predictive biomarkers is more feasible.

Retrospective validation of biomarkers is regarded as an acceptable strategy in selected circumstances. The strategy requires data from well-designed prospective phase III, randomized trials, sample availability from on a large majority of patients to avoid bias due to patient selection, a prospectively stated hypothesis, a predefined and standardized assay, and upfront sample size and power justification (91). Optimally, evidence should be provided from two independent randomized trials. *KRAS* as a predictor for efficacy of cetuximab and panitumumab in CRC is an example of a biomarker which has successfully been validated using a retrospective strategy.

In general there are four types of clinical trial designs to evaluate a potentially predictive biomarker: (1) the all-comers design with a "biomarker end point" as second objective, (2) a targeted design that restricts the study population to patients who have a favorable predictive biomarker profile, (3) a strategy design which randomizes patients to receive biomarker-based or non-biomarker-based (standard) treatment, and (4) a multiple hypothesis design, which combines the targeted design and the all-comers design. The latter design addresses the multiple hypotheses by having co-primary objectives (91, 92). Each of the designs has potential advantages and disadvantages. The all-comers design requires validation in a separate trial while the other designs prospectively evaluate the biomarker. Choice of design should depend upon knowledge on the biomarker and disease setting (91–94).

The REporting recommendations for tumor MARKer prognostic studies (REMARK) guidelines were developed in order to standardize and improve the quality of cancer biomarker studies. Reporting of results should follow these guidelines (95). More recently, guidelines for conducting experiments using tissue microarrays have been published (96). This checklist should be used in addition to the REMARK guidelines. With a more rational drug development including biomarker driven trials, researchers might ultimately yield greater benefits for patients.

REPURPOSING IRINOTECAN TO BREAST CANCER

Breast cancer is the most common kind of cancer among women. Improved adjuvant treatment in early breast cancer has resulted in better prognosis, but still approximately 20% of women, initially diagnosed with regional disease will develop systemic recurrence within 5 years.

Two major, still unresolved, medical problems are that almost all patients with mBC who obtain an objective response to chemotherapy will eventually experience disease recurrence and death from their disease. Secondly, a large fraction of the patients with mBC who receive first line systemic chemotherapy will not gain any beneficial effects from the treatment. In contrast, they may suffer from drug-induced side-effects and in addition, initiation of a potential effective second line treatment may be delayed until lack of response to the first line treatment is evidenced.

In current treatment of mBC, the main first line cytotoxic drugs are anthracyclines, and/or taxanes combined with cyclophosphamide. Second line treatment may include 5 FU, gemcitabine, platin derivatives, or vinorelbine. Unfortunately, very few options are available as third line treatment. It is thus clear that there is an urgent need for new and effective drugs in this setting. On the other hand, such drugs should be used with caution as they may be associated with significant side-effects with severe influence on the quality of life of the patients. If possible, such drugs should be used in combination with predictive biomarkers, allowing for a personalized treatment approach in which only patients with a high likelihood of an objective response should be offered the treatment in question. A number of publications have demonstrated some benefit from irinotecan treatment in patients with mBC being refractory to current breast cancer treatment (21). However, with a relatively small group of patients obtaining benefit from the treatment and the rather serious side-effects associated with irinotecan treatment, there will be a need for a predictive biomarker profile when introducing irinotecan in the treatment of mBC. We describe here, using the example of repurposing of Top1 inhibitors for the treatment of breast cancer, our approach to identify novel therapeutic indications for standard chemotherapeutic agents, based on prior knowledge of the pharmacology of these agents and exploratory studies for biomarker establishment.

The gene expression level of *TOP1* may not always predict response to camptothecin (97, 98) and the currently available antibodies to the Top1 protein have not yet been sufficiently validated. FISH is a validated clinical method to be used on FFPE tissue and it provides a direct measure of cancer cell gene aberrations on a cell to cell basis and may therefore provide more specific information than global genomics techniques. Therefore, we have used a *TOP1*/CEN-20 FISH probe mix to determine the *TOP1* gene aberration frequency in clinical breast cancer biopsies ($n = 100$) and compared to findings in normal breast tissue ($n = 100$). These data demonstrated that *TOP1* gene copy numbers of normal breast tissues were all in the diploid range, whereas 31% of the breast cancer samples had *TOP1* copy number gain (≥4 copies) (50). In breast cancer tissue we have observed a significant association between the *TOP1* copy numbers and the *TOP1* mRNA expression (50) which in combination with the frequent amplification of the *TOP1* gene suggest that *TOP1* gene copy numbers may be clinically relevant as a potential predictive biomarker for irinotecan sensitivity in breast cancer. Based on our FISH data and published reports on the response rates of irinotecan in mBC (21), we have initiated two clinical phase II trials with mBC patients being refractory to anthracyclines and taxanes. Patients with *TOP1* copy number gain (≥4 copies) are offered treatment with irinotecan. The patients are stratified according to HER2 levels being either HER2-positive (POSIRI; EudraCT 2012-002347-23) or HER2-negative (NEGIRI; EudraCT and 2012-002348-26). The main goal is to get objective response rate according to RECIST 1.1. In **Figure 1** we have exemplified our approach to biomarker-guided repurposing of irinotecan in breast cancer by picturing two individual ER-positive and HER2-neutral breast cancer patients. These patients possess either *TOP1* copy numbers in the normal range (**Figure 1A**) or increased *TOP1* copy numbers (**Figure 1B**) and only the latter would therefore be eligible for irinotecan therapy. If these studies and a subsequent phase III trial are positive, the *TOP1* copy number may be applied as a predictive biomarker for irinotecan treatment in anthracycline and/or taxane refractory mBC. Additionally, an association between *TOP1* copy numbers and irinotecan effect should subsequently be tested in the other cancer types not currently being treated with irinotecan. We believe that the workflow described here can be applied to

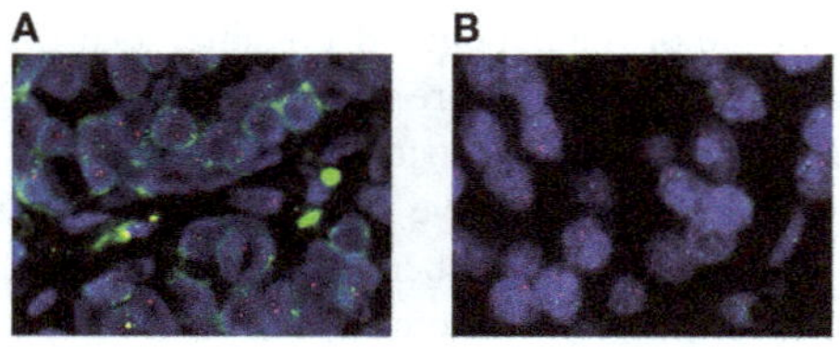

FIGURE 1 | Microscope photographs of two different primary breast cancer specimens stained with a fluorescent *TOP1*/CEN-20 fluorescence *in situ* hybridization (FISH) probe mix. Red spots visualize the *TOP1* gene and green spots represent CEN-20. **(A)** A breast cancer specimen with diploid *TOP1* copy number of 2.97, CEN-20 copy number of 1.90, and a ratio of 1.56. **(B)** A breast cancer specimen with amplified *TOP1* copy number of 6.35, CEN-20 copy number of 1.90, and a ratio of 3.34.

other chemotherapeutic drugs and/or other indications, providing a viable shortcut to novel effective treatments.

CONCLUSION

Currently, few people would argue against that the future of drug development in oncology lies with the identification of predictive biomarkers capable of identifying those subsets of patients who will benefit from a given therapy. The use of biomarkers to pinpoint those with a favorable response profile, normally a small subgroup of patients, within a large population is at the heart of the concept of personalized medicine. Also, the use of companion molecular diagnostics promise to minimize the size, costs, and failure rates of cancer agents in clinical trials.

We describe here our strategy of biomarker-guided repurposing of chemotherapeutic drugs for cancer therapy, exemplified with the repurposing of Top1 inhibitors and Top1 as a potential predictive biomarker. This approach can conceivably be implemented to a substantial number of currently used chemotherapeutic drugs, since their mechanisms of action are well studied with thousands of studies available in the literature. We believe that this strategy is valuable and can, potentially, add new tools to the armamentarium of drugs at the disposal of oncologists.

ACKNOWLEDGMENTS

DAKO A/S, Denmark for providing the *TOP1* probe mix. This work was supported by Danish National Research Foundation: Sino-Danish Breast Cancer Research Centre; A Race Against Breast Cancer; Danish Center for Translational Breast Cancer Research; the IMK Almene Fond and the Danish Cancer Society.

REFERENCES

1. Ferlay J, Shin HR, Bray F, Forman D, Mathers C, Parkin DM. Estimates of worldwide burden of cancer in 2008: GLOBOCAN 2008. *Int J Cancer* (2010) **127**(12):2893–917. doi:10.1002/ijc.25516
2. Bray F, Jemal A, Grey N, Ferlay J, Forman D. Global cancer transitions according to the human development index (2008-2030): a population-based study. *Lancet Oncol* (2012) **13**(8):790–801. doi:10.1016/S1470-2045(12)70211-5
3. Soerjomataram I, Lortet-Tieulent J, Parkin DM, Ferlay J, Mathers C, Forman D, et al. Global burden of cancer in 2008: a systematic analysis of disability-adjusted life-years in 12 world regions. *Lancet* (2012) **380**(9856):1840–50. doi:10.1016/S0140-6736(12)60919-2
4. Workman P, Clarke PA. Resisting targeted therapy: fifty ways to leave your EGFR. *Cancer Cell* (2011) **19**(4):437–40. doi:10.1016/j.ccr.2011.03.020
5. Engelman JA, Zejnullahu K, Mitsudomi T, Song Y, Hyland C, Park JO, et al. MET amplification leads to gefitinib resistance in lung cancer by activating ERBB3 signaling. *Science* (2007) **316**(5827):1039–43. doi:10.1126/science.1141478
6. De Palma M, Hanahan D. The biology of personalized cancer medicine: facing individual complexities underlying hallmark capabilities. *Mol Oncol* (2012) **6**(2):111–27. doi:10.1016/j.molonc.2012.01.011
7. Poulikakos PI, Persaud Y, Janakiraman M, Kong X, Ng C, Moriceau G, et al. RAF inhibitor resistance is mediated by dimerization of aberrantly spliced BRAF(V600E). *Nature* (2011) **480**(7377):387–90. doi:10.1038/nature10662
8. Nazarian R, Shi H, Wang Q, Kong X, Koya RC, Lee H, et al. Melanomas acquire resistance to B-RAF(V600E) inhibition by RTK or N-RAS upregulation. *Nature* (2010) **468**(7326):973–7. doi:10.1038/nature09626
9. DiMasi JA, Grabowski HG. Economics of new oncology drug development. *J Clin Oncol* (2007) **25**(2):209–16. doi:10.1200/JCO.2006.09.0803
10. Gupta SC, Sung B, Prasad S, Webb LJ, Aggarwal BB. Cancer drug discovery by repurposing: teaching new tricks to old dogs. *Trends Pharmacol Sci* (2013) **34**(9):508–17. doi:10.1016/j.tips.2013.06.005
11. Patel MN, Halling-Brown MD, Tym JE, Workman P, Al-Lazikani B. Objective assessment of cancer genes for drug discovery. *Nat Rev Drug Discov* (2013) **12**(1):35–50. doi:10.1038/nrd3913
12. Weir SJ, DeGennaro LJ, Austin CP. Repurposing approved and abandoned drugs for the treatment and prevention of cancer through public-private partnership. *Cancer Res* (2012) **72**(5):1055–8. doi:10.1158/0008-5472.CAN-11-3439
13. Nair P. Second act: drug repurposing gets a boost as academic researchers join the search for novel uses of existing drugs. *Proc Natl Acad Sci USA* (2013) **110**(7):2430–2. doi:10.1073/pnas.201300188
14. Mullard A. Drug repurposing programmes get lift off. *Nat Rev Drug Discov* (2012) **11**(7):505–6. doi:10.1038/nrd3776
15. Peters JU. Polypharmacology – foe or friend? *J Med Chem* (2013) **56**(22):8955–71. doi:10.1021/jm400856t
16. Ekins S, Williams AJ. Finding promiscuous old drugs for new uses. *Pharm Res* (2011) **28**(8):1785–91. doi:10.1007/s11095-011-0486-6
17. Di Leo A, Desmedt C, Bartlett JM, Piette F, Ejlertsen B, Pritchard KI, et al. HER2 and TOP2A as predictive markers for anthracycline-containing chemotherapy regimens as adjuvant treatment of breast cancer: a meta-analysis of individual patient data. *Lancet Oncol* (2011) **12**(12):1134–42. doi:10.1016/S1470-2045(11)70231-5
18. Knoop AS, Knudsen H, Balslev E, Rasmussen BB, Overgaard J, Nielsen KV, et al. Retrospective analysis of topoisomerase IIa amplifications and deletions as predictive markers in primary breast cancer patients randomly assigned to cyclophosphamide, methotrexate, and fluorouracil or cyclophosphamide, epirubicin, and fluorouracil: Danish Breast Cancer Cooperative Group. *J Clin Oncol* (2005) **23**(30):7483–90. doi:10.1200/JCO.2005.11.007
19. Ejlertsen B, Jensen MB, Nielsen KV, Balslev E, Rasmussen BB, Willemoe GL, et al. HER2, TOP2A, and TIMP-1 and responsiveness to adjuvant anthracycline-containing chemotherapy in high-risk breast cancer patients. *J Clin Oncol* (2010) **28**(6):984–90. doi:10.1200/JCO.2009.24.1166
20. Cardoso F, Harbeck N, Fallowfield L, Kyriakides S, Senkus E, Group EGW. Locally recurrent or metastatic breast cancer: ESMO clinical practice guidelines for diagnosis, treatment and follow-up. *Ann Oncol* (2012) **23**(Suppl 7):vii11–9. doi:10.1093/annonc/mds232
21. Kumler I, Brunner N, Stenvang J, Balslev E, Nielsen DL. A systematic review on topoisomerase 1 inhibition in the treatment of metastatic breast cancer. *Breast Cancer Res Treat* (2013) **138**(2):347–58. doi:10.1007/s10549-013-2476-3
22. Pommier Y. Topoisomerase I inhibitors: camptothecins and beyond. *Nat Rev Cancer* (2006) **6**(10):789–802. doi:10.1038/nrc1977
23. Xu G, Zhang W, Ma MK, McLeod HL. Human carboxylesterase 2 is commonly expressed in tumor tissue and is correlated with activation of irinotecan. *Clin Cancer Res* (2002) **8**(8):2605–11.
24. Khanna R, Morton CL, Danks MK, Potter PM. Proficient metabolism of irinotecan by a human intestinal carboxylesterase. *Cancer Res* (2000) **60**(17):4725–8.
25. Wu J, Liu LF. Processing of topoisomerase I cleavable complexes into DNA damage by transcription. *Nucleic Acids Res* (1997) **25**(21):4181–6. doi:10.1093/nar/25.21.4181
26. Pommier Y, Redon C, Rao VA, Seiler JA, Sordet O, Takemura H, et al. Repair of and checkpoint response to topoisomerase I-mediated DNA damage. *Mutat Res* (2003) **532**(1-2):173–203. doi:10.1016/j.mrfmmm.2003.08.016
27. Roos WP, Kaina B. DNA damage-induced cell death by apoptosis. *Trends Mol Med* (2006) **12**(9):440–50. doi:10.1016/j.molmed.2006.07.007

28. Benson AB III, Bekaii-Saab T, Chan E, Chen YJ, Choti MA, Cooper HS, et al. Metastatic colon cancer, version 3.2013: featured updates to the NCCN guidelines. *J Natl Compr Canc Netw* (2013) **11**(2):141–52.quiz 52,
29. Schmoll HJ, Van Cutsem E, Stein A, Valentini V, Glimelius B, Haustermans K, et al. ESMO consensus guidelines for management of patients with colon and rectal cancer. A personalized approach to clinical decision making. *Ann Oncol* (2012) **23**(10):2479–516. doi:10.1093/annonc/mds236
30. Seufferlein T. Systemic treatment of advanced pancreatic cancer – step by step progress. *Gut* (2013) **62**(5):660–1. doi:10.1136/gutjnl-2012-303129
31. Tempero MA, Arnoletti JP, Behrman SW, Ben-Josef E, Benson AB III, Casper ES, et al. Pancreatic adenocarcinoma, version 2.2012: featured updates to the NCCN guidelines. *J Natl Compr Canc Netw* (2012) **10**(6):703–13.
32. Available from: http://www.clinicaltrials.gov/
33. Morgan RJ Jr, Alvarez RD, Armstrong DK, Burger RA, Castells M, Chen LM, et al. Ovarian cancer, version 3.2012. *J Natl Compr Canc Netw* (2012) **10**(11):1339–49.
34. Colombo N, Peiretti M, Parma G, Lapresa M, Mancari R, Carinelli S, et al. Newly diagnosed and relapsed epithelial ovarian carcinoma: ESMO clinical practice guidelines for diagnosis, treatment and follow-up. *Ann Oncol* (2010) **21**(Suppl 5):v23–30. doi:10.1093/annonc/mdq244
35. Available from: http://www.cancer.gov/cancertopics/druginfo/fda-topotecan-hydrochloride/print
36. Available from: http://www.ema.europa.eu/ema/index.jsp?curl=pages/medicines/human/medicines/000123/human_med_000823.jsp&mid=WC0b01ac058001d124
37. Colombo N, Carinelli S, Colombo A, Marini C, Rollo D, Sessa C. Cervical cancer: ESMO clinical practice guidelines for diagnosis, treatment and follow-up. *Ann Oncol* (2012) **23**(Suppl 7):vii27–32.
38. Fruh M, De Ruysscher D, Popat S, Crino L, Peters S, Felip E. Small-cell lung cancer (SCLC): ESMO clinical practice guidelines for diagnosis, treatment and follow-up. *Ann Oncol* (2013) **24**(Suppl 6):vi99–105.
39. Kalemkerian GP, Akerley W, Bogner P, Borghaei H, Chow LQ, Downey RJ, et al. Small cell lung cancer. *J Natl Compr Canc Netw* (2013) **11**(1):78–98.
40. Jameson GS, Hamm JT, Weiss GJ, Alemany C, Anthony S, Basche M, et al. A multicenter, phase I, dose-escalation study to assess the safety, tolerability, and pharmacokinetics of etirinotecan pegol in patients with refractory solid tumors. *Clin Cancer Res* (2013) **19**(1):268–78. doi:10.1158/1078-0432.CCR-12-1201
41. Awada A, Garcia AA, Chan S, Jerusalem GHM, Coleman RE, Huizing MT, et al. Two schedules of etirinotecan pegol (NKTR-102) in patients with previously treated metastatic breast cancer: a randomised phase 2 study. *Lancet Oncol* (2013) **14**(12):1216–25. doi:10.1016/S1470-2045(13)70429-7
42. Von Hoff DD, Jameson GS, Borad MJ, Rosen LS, Utz J, Basche M, et al. First phase I trial of NKTR-102 (Peg-irinotecan) reveals early evidence of broad anti-tumor activity in three different schedules. *EORTC-NCI-AACR Symposium on "Molecular Targets and Cancer Therapeutics"* Poster No.: 595 (2008).
43. Fan B, Dachrut S, Coral H, Yuen ST, Chu KM, Law S, et al. Integration of DNA copy number alterations and transcriptional expression analysis in human gastric cancer. *PLoS One* (2012) **7**(4):e29824. doi:10.1371/journal.pone.0029824
44. Rømer MU, Jensen NF, Nielsen SL, Müller S, Nielsen KV, Nielsen HJ, et al. TOP1 gene copy numbers in colorectal cancer samples and cell lines and their association to in vitro drug sensitivity. *Scand J Gastroenterol* (2012) **47**(1):68–79. doi:10.3109/00365521.2011.638393
45. Ryan D, Rafferty M, Hegarty S, O'Leary P, Faller W, Gremel G, et al. Topoisomerase I amplification in melanoma is associated with more advanced tumours and poor prognosis. *Pigment Cell Melanoma Res* (2010) **23**(4):542–53. doi:10.1111/j.1755-148X.2010.00720.x
46. Tanner MM, Tirkkonen M, Kallioniemi A, Collins C, Stokke T, Karhu R, et al. Increased copy number at 20q13 in breast cancer: defining the critical region and exclusion of candidate genes. *Cancer Res* (1994) **54**(16):4257–60.
47. Tanner MM, Grenman S, Koul A, Johannsson O, Meltzer P, Pejovic T, et al. Frequent amplification of chromosomal region 20q12-q13 in ovarian cancer. *Clin Cancer Res* (2000) **6**(5):1833–9.
48. Rømer MU, Nygård SB, Christensen IJ, Nielsen SL, Nielsen KV, Müller S, et al. Topoisomerase 1 (TOP1) gene copy number in stage III colorectal cancer patients and its relation to prognosis. *Mol Oncol* (2012) **7**(1):101–11. doi:10.1016/j.molonc.2012.09.001
49. Smith DH, Christensen IJ, Jensen NF, Markussen B, Rømer MU, Nygård SB, et al. Mechanisms of topoisomerase I (TOP1) gene copy number increase in a stage III colorectal cancer patient cohort. *PLoS One* (2013) **8**(4):e60613. doi:10.1371/journal.pone.0060613
50. Stenvang J, Smid M, Nielsen S, Balslev E, Timmermans M, Rømer M, et al. *Topoisomerase 1 Gene Copy Aberration is a Frequent Finding in Clinical Breast Cancer Sample.* San Antonio: San Antonio Breast Cancer Symposium (2012).
51. Tanner MM, Tirkkonen M, Kallioniemi A, Isola J, Kuukasjärvi T, Collins C, et al. Independent amplification and frequent co-amplification of three nonsyntenic regions on the long arm of chromosome 20 in human breast cancer. *Cancer Res* (1996) **56**(15):3441–5.
52. Carvalho B, Postma C, Mongera S, Hopmans E, Diskin S, van de Wiel MA, et al. Multiple putative oncogenes at the chromosome 20q amplicon contribute to colorectal adenoma to carcinoma progression. *Gut* (2009) **58**(1):79–89. doi:10.1136/gut.2007.143065
53. Beroukhim R, Mermel CH, Porter D, Wei G, Raychaudhuri S, Donovan J, et al. The landscape of somatic copy-number alteration across human cancers. *Nature* (2010) **463**(7283):899–905. doi:10.1038/nature08822
54. Bronstein IB, Vorobyev S, Timofeev A, Jolles CJ, Alder SL, Holden JA. Elevations of DNA topoisomerase I catalytic activity and immunoprotein in human malignancies. *Oncol Res* (1996) **8**(1):17–25.
55. Husain I, Mohler JL, Seigler HF, Besterman JM. Elevation of topoisomerase I messenger RNA, protein, and catalytic activity in human tumors: demonstration of tumor-type specificity and implications for cancer chemotherapy. *Cancer Res* (1994) **54**(2):539–46.
56. Yu J, Miller R, Zhang W, Sharma M, Holtschlag V, Watson MA, et al. Copy-number analysis of topoisomerase and thymidylate synthase genes in frozen and FFPE DNAs of colorectal cancers. *Pharmacogenomics* (2008) **9**(10):1459–66. doi:10.2217/14622416.9.10.1459
57. Giovanella BC, Stehlin JS, Wall ME, Wani MC, Nicholas AW, Liu LF, et al. DNA topoisomerase I – targeted chemotherapy of human colon cancer in xenografts. *Science* (1989) **246**(4933):1046–8. doi:10.1126/science.2555920
58. Horisberger K, Erben P, Muessle B, Woernle C, Stroebel P, Kaehler G, et al. Topoisomerase I expression correlates to response to neoadjuvant irinotecan-based chemoradiation in rectal cancer. *Anticancer Drugs* (2009) **20**(6):519–24. doi:10.1097/CAD.0b013e32832b53ff
59. Guichard S, Terret C, Hennebelle I, Lochon I, Chevreau P, Fretigny E, et al. CPT-11 converting carboxylesterase and topoisomerase activities in tumour and normal colon and liver tissues. *Br J Cancer* (1999) **80**(3-4):364–70. doi:10.1038/sj.bjc.6690364
60. Vallbohmer D, Iqbal S, Yang DY, Rhodes KE, Zhang W, Gordon M, et al. Molecular determinants of irinotecan efficacy. *Int J Cancer* (2006) **119**(10):2435–42. doi:10.1002/ijc.22129
61. Tsavaris N, Lazaris A, Kosmas C, Gouveris P, Kavantzas N, Kopterides P, et al. Topoisomerase I and IIalpha protein expression in primary colorectal cancer and recurrences following 5-fluorouracil-based adjuvant chemotherapy. *Cancer Chemother Pharmacol* (2009) **64**(2):391–8. doi:10.1007/s00280-008-0886-4
62. Gouveris P, Lazaris AC, Papathomas TG, Nonni A, Kyriakou V, Delladetsima J, et al. Topoisomerase I protein expression in primary colorectal cancer and recurrences after 5-FU-based adjuvant chemotherapy. *J Cancer Res Clin Oncol* (2007) **133**(12):1011–5. doi:10.1007/s00432-007-0253-6
63. Boonsong A, Curran S, McKay JA, Cassidy J, Murray GI, McLeod HL. Topoisomerase I protein expression in primary colorectal cancer and lymph node metastases. *Hum Pathol* (2002) **33**(11):1114–9. doi:10.1053/hupa.2002.129202
64. Paradiso A, Xu J, Mangia A, Chiriatti A, Simone G, Zito A, et al. Topoisomerase-I, thymidylate synthase primary tumour expression and clinical efficacy of 5-FU/CPT-11 chemotherapy in advanced colorectal cancer patients. *Int J Cancer* (2004) **111**(2):252–8. doi:10.1002/ijc.20208
65. Staley BE, Samowitz WS, Bronstein IB, Holden JA. Expression of DNA topoisomerase I and DNA topoisomerase II-alpha in carcinoma of the colon. *Mod Pathol* (1999) **12**(4):356–61.
66. Mukai M, Sato S, Ninomiya H, Wakui K, Komatsu N, Matsui N, et al. Sensitivity to CPT-11 and platinum derivatives of stage II/Dukes' B colorectal cancer with occult neoplastic cells in lymph node sinuses. *Oncol Rep* (2007) **17**(5):1045–50.
67. Braun MS, Richman SD, Quirke P, Daly C, Adlard JW, Elliott F, et al. Predictive biomarkers of chemotherapy efficacy in colorectal cancer: results from the UK MRC FOCUS trial. *J Clin Oncol* (2008) **26**(16):2690–8. doi:10.1200/JCO.2007.15.5580
68. Kostopoulos I, Karavasilis V, Karina M, Bobos M, Xiros N, Pentheroudakis G, et al. Topoisomerase I but not thymidylate synthase is associated with improved outcome in patients with resected colorectal cancer treated with irinotecan containing adjuvant chemotherapy. *BMC Cancer* (2009) **9**:339. doi:10.1186/1471-2407-9-339

69. van der Zee AG, Hollema H, de Jong S, Boonstra H, Gouw A, Willemse PH, et al. P-glycoprotein expression and DNA topoisomerase I and II activity in benign tumors of the ovary and in malignant tumors of the ovary, before and after platinum/cyclophosphamide chemotherapy. *Cancer Res* (1991) **51**(21):5915–20.
70. Codegoni AM, Castagna S, Mangioni C, Scovassi AI, Broggini M, D'Incalci M. DNA-topoisomerase I activity and content in epithelial ovarian cancer. *Ann Oncol* (1998) **9**(3):313–9. doi:10.1023/A:1008207125986
71. Holden JA, Rahn MP, Jolles CJ, Vorobyev SV, Bronstein IB. Immunohistochemical detection of DNA topoisomerase I in formalin fixed, paraffin wax embedded normal tissues and in ovarian carcinomas. *Mol Pathol* (1997) **50**(5):247–53. doi:10.1136/mp.50.5.247
72. Monnin KA, Bronstein IB, Gaffney DK, Holden JA. Elevations of DNA topoisomerase I in transitional cell carcinoma of the urinary bladder: correlation with DNA topoisomerase II-alpha and p53 expression. *Hum Pathol* (1999) **30**(4):384–91. doi:10.1016/S0046-8177(99)90112-0
73. Coleman LW, Bronstein IB, Holden JA. Immunohistochemical staining for DNA topoisomerase I, DNA topoisomerase II-alpha and p53 in gastric carcinomas. *Anticancer Res* (2001) **21**(2A):1167–72.
74. Coleman LW, Perkins SL, Bronstein IB, Holden JA. Expression of DNA topoisomerase I and DNA topoisomerase II-alpha in testicular seminomas. *Hum Pathol* (2000) **31**(6):728–33. doi:10.1053/hupa.2000.8462
75. Gupta D, Bronstein IB, Holden JA. Expression of DNA topoisomerase I in neoplasms of the kidney: correlation with histological grade, proliferation, and patient survival. *Hum Pathol* (2000) **31**(2):214–9. doi:10.1016/S0046-8177(00)80222-1
76. Lynch BJ, Komaromy-Hiller G, Bronstein IB, Holden JA. Expression of DNA topoisomerase I, DNA topoisomerase II-alpha, and p53 in metastatic malignant melanoma. *Hum Pathol* (1998) **29**(11):1240–5. doi:10.1016/S0046-8177(98)90251-9
77. Hafian H, Venteo L, Sukhanova A, Nabiev I, Lefevre B, Pluot M. Immunohistochemical study of DNA topoisomerase I, DNA topoisomerase II alpha, p53, and Ki-67 in oral preneoplastic lesions and oral squamous cell carcinomas. *Hum Pathol* (2004) **35**(6):745–51. doi:10.1016/j.humpath.2004.02.004
78. Coleman LW, Rohr LR, Bronstein IB, Holden JA. Human DNA topoisomerase I: an anticancer drug target present in human sarcomas. *Hum Pathol* (2002) **33**(6):599–607. doi:10.1053/hupa.2002.124911
79. Lynch BJ, Bronstein IB, Holden JA. Elevations of DNA topoisomerase I in invasive carcinoma of the breast. *Breast J* (2001) **7**(3):176–80. doi:10.1046/j.1524-4741.2001.007003176.x
80. Nielsen KV, Brunner N. Re: topoisomerase II alpha and responsiveness of breast cancer to adjuvant chemotherapy. *J Natl Cancer Inst* (2011) **103**(4):352–3. doi:10.1093/jnci/djq528
81. Simon RM, Paik S, Hayes DF. Use of archived specimens in evaluation of prognostic and predictive biomarkers. *J Natl Cancer Inst* (2009) **101**(21):1446–52. doi:10.1093/jnci/djp335
82. Seymour MT, Maughan TS, Ledermann JA, Topham C, James R, Gwyther SJ, et al. Different strategies of sequential and combination chemotherapy for patients with poor prognosis advanced colorectal cancer (MRC FOCUS): a randomised controlled trial. *Lancet* (2007) **370**(9582):143–52. doi:10.1016/S0140-6736(07)61087-3
83. Koopman M, Antonini NF, Douma J, Wals J, Honkoop AH, Erdkamp FL, et al. Sequential versus combination chemotherapy with capecitabine, irinotecan, and oxaliplatin in advanced colorectal cancer (CAIRO): a phase III randomised controlled trial. *Lancet* (2007) **370**(9582):135–42. doi:10.1016/S0140-6736(07)61086-1
84. Koopman M, Knijn N, Richman S, Seymour M, Quirke P, van Tinteren H, et al. The correlation between topoisomerase-I (Topo1) expression and outcome of treatment with capecitabine and irinotecan in advanced colorectal cancer (ACC) patients (pts) treated in the CAIRO study of the Dutch Colorectal Cancer Group (DCCG). *Eur J Cancer Suppl* (2009) **7**(2):321–2. doi:10.1016/S1359-6349(09)71098-5
85. Van Cutsem E, Labianca R, Bodoky G, Barone C, Aranda E, Nordlinger B, et al. Randomized phase III trial comparing biweekly infusional fluorouracil/leucovorin alone or with irinotecan in the adjuvant treatment of stage III colon cancer: PETACC-3. *J Clin Oncol* (2009) **27**(19):3117–25. doi:10.1200/JCO.2008.21.6663
86. Saltz LB, Niedzwiecki D, Hollis D, Goldberg RM, Hantel A, Thomas JP, et al. Irinotecan fluorouracil plus leucovorin is not superior to fluorouracil plus leucovorin alone as adjuvant treatment for stage III colon cancer: results of CALGB 89803. *J Clin Oncol* (2007) **25**(23):3456–61. doi:10.1200/JCO.2007.11.2144
87. Foukakis T, Astrom G, Lindstrom L, Hatschek T, Bergh J. When to order a biopsy to characterise a metastatic relapse in breast cancer. *Ann Oncol* (2012) **23**(Suppl 10):x349–53. doi:10.1093/annonc/mds297
88. McShane LM, Hunsberger S, Adjei AA. Effective incorporation of biomarkers into phase II trials. *Clin Cancer Res* (2009) **15**(6):1898–905. doi:10.1158/1078-0432.CCR-08-2033
89. Bergh J. Quo vadis with targeted drugs in the 21st century? *J Clin Oncol* (2009) **27**(1):2–5. doi:10.1200/JCO.2008.18.8342
90. Rodon J, Saura C, Dienstmann R, Vivancos A, Ramon y Cajal S, Baselga J, et al. Molecular prescreening to select patient population in early clinical trials. *Nat Rev Clin Oncol* (2012) **9**(6):359–66. doi:10.1038/nrclinonc.2012.48
91. Mandrekar SJ, Sargent DJ. Clinical trial designs for predictive biomarker validation: theoretical considerations and practical challenges. *J Clin Oncol* (2009) **27**(24):4027–34. doi:10.1200/JCO.2009.22.3701
92. Hoering A, Leblanc M, Crowley JJ. Randomized phase III clinical trial designs for targeted agents. *Clin Cancer Res* (2008) **14**(14):4358–67. doi:10.1158/078-0432.CCR-08-288
93. Freidlin B, McShane LM, Korn EL. Randomized clinical trials with biomarkers: design issues. *J Natl Cancer Inst* (2010) **102**(3):152–60. doi:10.1093/jnci/djp477
94. Redman MW, Crowley JJ, Herbst RS, Hirsch FR, Gandara DR. Design of a phase III clinical trial with prospective biomarker validation: SWOG S0819. *Clin Cancer Res* (2012) **18**(15):4004–12. doi:10.1158/078-0432.CCR-12-167
95. Altman DG, McShane LM, Sauerbrei W, Taube SE. Reporting Recommendations for Tumor Marker Prognostic Studies (REMARK): explanation and elaboration. *PLoS Med* (2012) **9**(5):e1001216. doi:10.1371/journal.pmed.1001216
96. Ilyas M, Grabsch H, Ellis IO, Womack C, Brown R, Berney D, et al. Guidelines and considerations for conducting experiments using tissue microarrays. *Histopathology* (2013) **62**(6):827–39. doi:10.1111/his.12118
97. Perego P, Capranico G, Supino R, Zunino F. Topoisomerase I gene expression and cell sensitivity to camptothecin in human cell lines of different tumor types. *Anticancer Drugs* (1994) **5**(6):645–9. doi:10.1097/00001813-199412000-00006
98. Jansen WJ, Zwart B, Hulscher ST, Giaccone G, Pinedo HM, Boven E. CPT-11 in human colon-cancer cell lines and xenografts: characterization of cellular sensitivity determinants. *Int J Cancer* (1997) **70**(3):335–40. doi:10.1002/(SICI)1097-0215(19970127)70:3<335::AID-IJC15>3.3.CO;2-B

20

P-glycoprotein mediated efflux limits substrate and drug uptake in a preclinical brain metastases of breast cancer model

Chris E. Adkins[1], Rajendar K. Mittapalli[1], Vamshi K. Manda[1], Mohamed I. Nounou[1], Afroz S. Mohammad[1], Tori B. Terrell[1], Kaci A. Bohn[1], Celik Yasemin[2], Tiffany R. Grothe[2], Julie A. Lockman[2] and Paul R. Lockman[1]*

[1] Department of Pharmaceutical Sciences, School of Pharmacy, Texas Tech University Health Sciences Center, Amarillo, TX, USA
[2] Department of Life, Earth and Environmental Sciences, West Texas A&M University, Canyon, TX, USA

Edited by:
Chiara Riganti, University of Torino, Italy

Reviewed by:
Laura Annovazzi, Policlinico di Monza Foundation, Italy
Valentina Caldera, Neuro-Bio-Oncology Center, Policlinico di Monza Foundation, Italy

***Correspondence:**
Paul R. Lockman, Department of Pharmaceutical Sciences, School of Pharmacy, Texas Tech University Health Sciences Center, Amarillo Research Building, 1406 South Coulter, Amarillo, TX 79106-1712, USA
e-mail: paul.lockman@ttuhsc.edu

The blood–brain barrier (BBB) is a specialized vascular interface that restricts the entry of many compounds into brain. This is accomplished through the sealing of vascular endothelial cells together with tight junction proteins to prevent paracellular diffusion. In addition, the BBB has a high degree of expression of numerous efflux transporters which actively extrude compounds back into blood. However, when a metastatic lesion develops in brain the vasculature is typically compromised with increases in passive permeability (blood-tumor barrier; BTB). What is not well documented is to what degree active efflux retains function at the BTB despite the changes observed in passive permeability. In addition, there have been previous reports documenting both increased and decreased expression of P-glycoprotein (P-gp) in lesion vasculature. Herein, we simultaneously administer a passive diffusion marker (^{14}C-AIB) and a tracer subject to P-gp efflux (rhodamine 123) into a murine preclinical model of brain metastases of breast cancer. We observed that the metastatic lesions had similar expression ($p > 0.05$; $n = 756$–1214 vessels evaluated) at the BBB and the BTB. Moreover, tissue distribution of R123 was not significantly ($p > 0.05$) different between normal brain and the metastatic lesion. It is possible that the similar expression of P-gp on the BBB and the BTB contribute to this phenomenon. Additionally we observed P-gp expression at the metastatic cancer cells adjacent to the vasculature which may also contribute to reduced R123 uptake into the lesion. The data suggest that despite the disrupted integrity of the BTB, efflux mechanisms appear to be intact, and may be functionally comparable to the normal BBB. The BTB is a significant hurdle to delivering drugs to brain metastasis.

Keywords: drug resistance, chemotherapy, autoradiography, fluorescence microscopy, tumor

INTRODUCTION

The successful treatment of central nervous system (CNS) tumors and metastases using chemotherapy depends on the ability of therapeutic concentrations of drug to cross the blood–brain barrier (BBB). More than 98% of potential CNS active anti-cancer drugs fail in preclinical work and or clinical trials because of inadequate BBB penetration (Pardridge, 2007). Clinically this results in many anticancer agents failing to substantially reduce tumor burden and or significantly prolong survival (Deeken and Loscher, 2007).

The microvasculature of the brain is a unique anatomical structure which serves as a homeostatic and regulatory barrier between the blood and the brain parenchyma (Hawkins and Davis, 2005). Specifically, endothelial cells that line the blood vessels of the brain capillaries are fused together by numerous tight junction protein complexes, which restrict blood components from passively diffusing between the cell margins to gain entry into brain. The tight junction protein complexes consist of a number of proteins such as zonula occludins, junctional adhesion molecules, and claudins which function as a unit to seal the endothelia margins. Further the outside of the brain capillary is surrounded by astrocytic foot processes and pericytes that also contribute to the restriction of paracellular diffusion (Abbott et al., 2010).

Further restricting the brain entry of a large number of drugs and drug classes are efflux transporters at the BBB. Efflux transporters are richly expressed in the brain vasculature and have been shown to restrict the accumulation of antiepliptics, antidepressants, and antipsychotics (Schinkel et al., 1995; Loscher and Potschka, 2005). Multiple efflux transporters at the BBB act to actively extrude or prevent drug accumulation into brain, these include P-glycoprotein (P-gp; ABCB1) (Schinkel et al., 1996), breast cancer resistant protein (BCRP; ABCG2; Polli et al., 2009), multidrug resistance associated proteins (MRP; ABCC1-6; Breedveld et al., 2005), and organic anion transporters (OATs; Hagenbuch and Meier, 2004).

The net effect of the anatomical and molecular features of the BBB is that to a large degree it restricts drug movement from blood into brain. But some drugs are able to penetrate the BBB. Drug and/or solute permeation across the BBB is mostly limited to low molecular weight lipid-soluble molecules. Molecules that are large (typically >700 Da), protein bound or are hydrophilic will have difficulty crossing the BBB and accumulating in brain to a sufficient degree (Lipinski et al., 2001).

However, the vasculature within a brain tumor is different from the normal BBB. Previously it has been shown that the blood-tumor barrier (BTB) vasculature has disrupted integrity compared to the intact BBB. This disruption can allow small molecule to accumulate into lesions up to 30–100-fold more than the accumulation of the molecule in normal brain (Lockman et al., 2010; Taskar et al., 2012). While the degree of breakdown at the BTB does correlate with increases in drug uptake it is not clearly defined whether efflux pumps continue to limit drug uptake into metastatic lesions (Gallo et al., 2003). It has been previously shown that the BTB expresses P-gp (Cordon-Cardo et al., 1990); however, the expression of P-gp may be variable among different tumors types (Henson et al., 1992). In addition to P-gp expression at the BTB, many cancers have been shown to express functional P-gp *in vivo* which may restrict the cellular accumulation of chemotherapeutics.

Herein we set out to determine the expression and function of P-gp in a preclinical model of brain metastases of breast cancer using quantitative fluorescence microscopy and autoradiography. We observed that P-gp is expressed at the BTB in brain metastases at nearly similar levels to the BBB. In addition, P-gp is highly functional in limiting the lesion accumulation of the P-gp substrate, Rhodamine 123 (R123) despite significant passive permeability increases.

MATERIALS AND METHODS

CHEMICALS

R123 was purchased from Molecular Probes Invitrogen (Eugene, OR, USA). Verapamil was purchased from Sigma (St. Louis, MO, USA). Cyclosporine A was purchased from Tocris Biochemicals (St. Louis, MO, USA). ^{14}C-labeled aminoisobutyric acid (AIB) was purchased from American Radiolabelled Chemicals (St. Louis, MO, USA). All other chemicals used were of analytical grade and were used as supplied.

ANIMALS

Female NuNu mice (~24 g; 8 weeks of age) were purchased from Charles River Laboratories (Kingston, NY, USA) and were used for all the perfusion experiments done in this study. All studies were approved by the Animal Care and Use Committee and were performed in accordance with the NIH Guidelines for the Care and Use of Laboratory Animals.

IN SITU MOUSE HEART PERFUSION TECHNIQUE

The *in situ* mouse heart perfusion technique was utilized to evaluate brain uptake of R123 (Takasato et al., 1984; Lockman et al., 2003a) Mice were anesthetized with ketamine/xylazine (100 and 8 mg/kg, respectively) and the heart exposed. Body temperature was monitored and maintained at 37°C using a heating pad attached to a feedback device (YSI Indicating Controller, Yellow Springs, OH, USA). Prior to insertion of the cannula, the right cardiac atrium was cut to prevent venous return. Cannulation of the left cardiac ventricle was done using butterfly syringe (28G) attached to a perfusion apparatus. Perfusion fluid was pumped into the left cardiac ventricle by a cannula at a constant rate of 2.5 mL/min (Dagenais et al., 2000) using a Harvard Model 944 dual channel pump (Harvard Apparatus, South Natick, MA).

The perfusion fluid consisted of HCO_3 buffered physiological saline, containing 128 mM NaCl, 24 mM $NaHCO_3$, 4.2 mM KCl, 2.4 mM NaH_2PO_4, 1.5 mM $CaCl_2$, 0.9 mM $MgSO_4$, and 9 mM glucose (pH ~7.35; [Na] = 154.4 mM). All solutions were filtered, oxygenated, warmed to 37° C, and adjusted to pH 7.35 prior to perfusion. To determine initial brain uptake of R123, perfusion fluid containing R123 (50 μg/mL) was infused into the systemic circulation for 30–120 s. At the end of each experiment, mice were sacrificed, and the brain was rapidly removed (<60 s) from the skull. The brain was flash frozen in isopentane (−65°C). Concentration of the fluorophore (R123) in brain was determined using fluorescent microscopy and regional permeability was expressed by the unidirectional transfer constants, K_{in} (mL/s/g) derived from Eq. 1.

QUANTIFICATION OF R123 USING FLUORESCENCE MICROSCOPY

Fluorescence was observed with an Olympus MVX10 stereomicroscope (objective: 2×, NA 0.5) with an optical zoom range from 0.63 to 12.6. The excitation and emission of R123 was obtained using a GFP filter (excitation/band pass filter of 470/40, emission/band pass filter of 525/50 and dichromatic mirror at 495 nm; Chroma Technology, Bellow Falls, VT, USA). Tissue sections of 20 μm were obtained at −23°C using a cryotome (Leica CM3050S, Leica Microsystems, Buffalo Grove, IL, USA), mounted on charged glass slides, and kept at −23°C. Data were analyzed using quantitative fluorescence microscopy and all images were obtained with 15 ms exposures, though a 2.0 objective at 4× magnification (Olympus MVX10) with a monochromatic cooled CCD scientific camera (Retiga 4000R, QImaging, Surrey, BC, Canada). Slidebook® 5 software (Intelligent Imaging Innovations, Denver, CO, USA) was utilized to determine sum intensity per gram of brain which then converted into concentration of dye per gram of brain using the brain homogenate standards. The voxel by voxel sum intensity of fluorescence for brain homogenate samples was obtained with the 2× objective. The optical zoom range was maintained at 4× for a total optical magnification of 8×. The sum intensity per gram of brain homogenate was obtained using a set exposure time of 15 ms with camera gain settings of 615. The total fluorescence intensity signal for each concentration was then plotted as a function of grams of brain which was calculated using the area in microns squared multiplied by the thickness of the brain sample (20 μm) to obtain a total brain volume that was analyzed. The brain volume (μm^3) was multiplied by the density of brain tissue (1.04 g/cm^3) as similarly reported by (Tengvar et al., 1983) to obtain a weight of brain tissue that was analyzed.

PREPARATION OF BRAIN STANDARDS

To calculate the concentration of the R123 in brain, standard curves were generated in rat brain homogenates. Briefly, 100 μL of standard solution of the dye was added to each of 500 mg of the brain and homogenized. The homogenized mass was flash frozen in isopentane (−80°C) and sliced into 20 μm sections using a cryostat −23°C and mounted onto glass, superfrost slides. The slices were analyzed using quantitative fluorescence microscopy and the sum intensity per gram of brain homogenate was plotted against concentration of the dye.

KINETIC ANALYSIS

Unidirectional uptake transfer constants (K_{in}) were calculated from the following relationship to the linear portion of the uptake curve:

$$Q^*/C^* = K_{in}T + V_0 \quad (1)$$

where Q^* is the quantity of fluorophore (R123) in brain (μg/g) at the end of perfusion, C^* is the perfusion fluid concentration of fluorophore (μg/mL), T is the perfusion time (s) and V_0 is the extrapolated intercept ($T = 0$ s; "vascular volume" in mL/g). After determination of a perfusion time that allowed adequate amount of fluorescent marker to pass into brain and yet remained in the linear uptake zone, K_{in} was determined in single time-point experiments as:

$$K_{in} = [Q^* - V_0C^*]/C^*T]$$

(Takasato et al., 1984; Smith and Takasato, 1986).

ANTIBODY STAINING

Tissues were rehydrated in PBS and then fixed in 4% paraformaldehyde (PFA) for P-gp (Abcam, Cambridge, MA), cytokeratin (Abcam) and CD31 (BD Pharmingen, San Jose, CA), ice-cold methanol for ABCB1 (Santa Cruz Biotechnology), CD31 (BD Pharmingen). After three PBS washings (5 min), slides were blocked with 4% goat serum and 0.2% Triton-X 100 (1 h). After blocking, primary antibodies were added, followed by overnight incubation at 4°C. The next day, the slides were washed and secondary antibodies and DAPI (1 mg/mL) were added (1 h). Slides were again washed, DAKO mounting medium was added, and coverslips were applied.

RESULTS

To determine if P-gp expression is present in the vasculature of brain metastases, we analyzed the brains of tumor bearing mice using immunofluorescence staining for both P-gp and the vascular marker CD31 to quantify the amount of colocalization (**Figure 1**). There was significant expression of P-gp at the BBB and BTB (**Figure 1B**). Overall there was no difference between the fluorescent intensity of P-gp staining in the CD-31 defined regions in tumor vasculature (22.9 ±0.4 A.U.; $n = 756$ vessels) and in the normal brain vasculature (22.6 ±0.3 A.U.; $n = 1214$). In addition, there was positive P-gp staining that did not co-localize to the vasculature, but surrounded metastasis cells suggesting that P-gp may also be present on the metastatic cancer cells.

We measured P-gp function by the time dependent accumulation of the fluorescence P-gp substrate R123 according to previous methodology (Mittapalli et al., 2013). Using fluorescent brain standards we determined the blood to brain unidirectional transfer coefficient (K_{in}) of R123 in normal brain and in metastatic lesions by calculating the concentration of R123 divided by the concentration in the perfusate and plotted this over time (30–120 s; **Figure 2A**). We then applied a previously calculated correction to the vascular volume by perfusion of non-permeable [^{14}C]-sucrose and measuring its vascular space (0.015 ± 0.002 mL/g). We observed that the uptake of R123 was linear within the perfusion time with a K_{in} of 0.12 ± 0.03 μL/s/g. To determine if we could inhibit P-gp mediated efflux of R123, we added P-gp inhibitors verapamil and cyclosporine A (Choi and Li, 2005; Breedveld et al., 2006; Baumert and Hilgeroth, 2009) at various concentrations to the R123 perfusate in separate experiments (**Figure 2A**). Upon co-perfusion of R123 and each inhibitor, there was an increase in R123 permeability; Cyclosporin A (2.4 ± 0.5 μL/s/g); and Verapamil (2.2 ± 0.2 μL/s/g)] indicating that R123 uptake into brain is limited by the efflux function of P-gp at the BBB.

We then plotted R123's LogD (octanol/water coefficient; pH = 7.4) and observed K_{in} in comparison to known passive

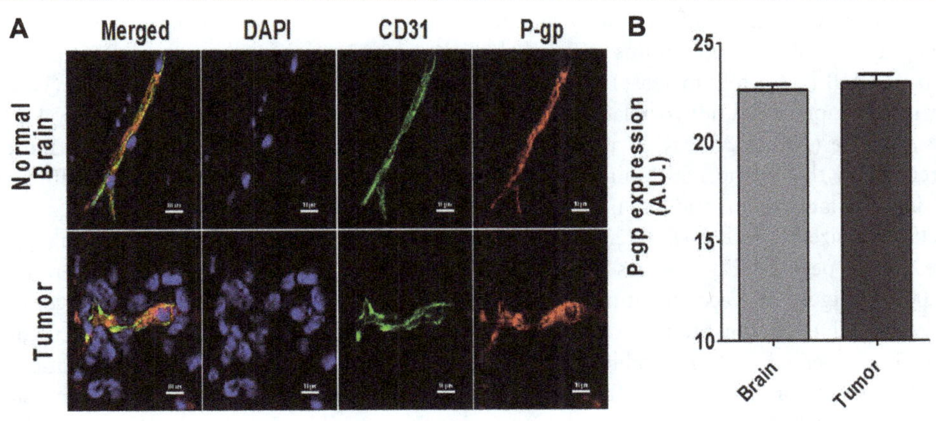

FIGURE 1 | (A) Representative images of the co-localized expression of P-gp (red) in a capillary in normal brain (top row) and a blood vessel in a 231Br brain metastasis (bottom row) are shown. Endothelial nuclei as well as the nuclei of the 231Br lesions are shown in blue (DAPI). Blood vessels (CD-31 expression) in both sections are shown in green (Alexa Fluor 488). P-gp expression is shown in red (Alexa Fluor 594). **(B)** The bar graph shows the relative P-gp expression per vessel as defined by CD31 stained regions. Mean ±SEM; BTB; $n = 756$ vessels and BBB $n = 1214$ vessels).

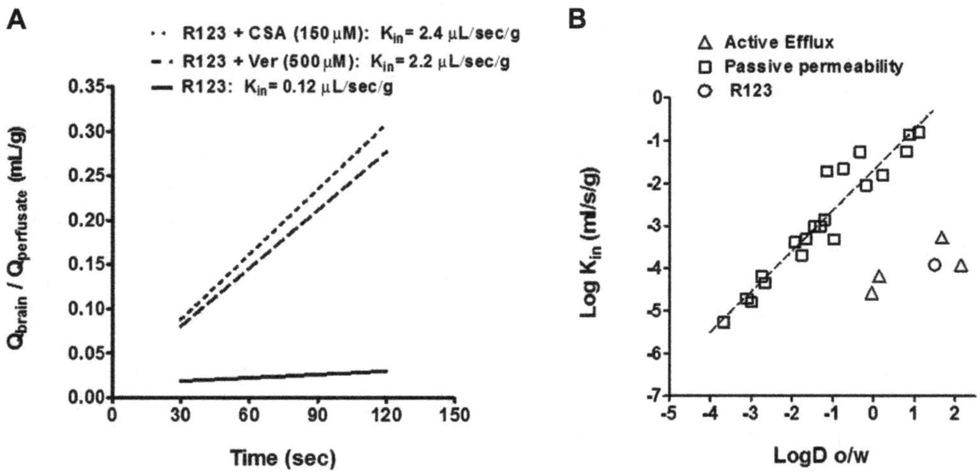

FIGURE 2 | (A) The K_{in} of R123 in the presence of the known P-gp inhibitors, cyclosporin A and verapamil, increases brain distribution (as reported by the K_{in}) by >10-fold. All data represent mean ± S.E.M for total brain; $n = 3–5$ for all groups. Statistics: one-way ANOVA; Dunnett's. **(B)** The relationship between LogD (octanol/water coefficient; pH = 7.4) and observed K_{in} is used to profile a molecule or drug's mechanism of distribution into brain. Compounds that are known to cross the BBB via passive diffusion are plotted using gray squares and those subject to efflux are plotted with gray triangles. R123 (open circle) falls below ~3 log units the line of identity for passive permeability indicating it may be subject to efflux.

permeability compounds (Begley, 1996) and efflux substrates (Summerfield et al., 2007; **Figure 2B**). Molecules and drugs that passively diffuse into brain exhibit a linear relationship between their LogD (octanol/water coefficient) and their observed Log K_{in} while molecules which are subject to efflux will exhibit observed Log K_{in} values well below the value predicted by its LogD (**Figure 2B**). R123 has a LogD of 1.51 (Forster et al., 2012) and Log K_{in} of −3.93 (calculated from observed K_{in}; **Figure 2A**) which places R123 several orders of magnitude below a passively diffusing molecule's profile which supports the evidence of R213's restriction from brain via an efflux transporter.

To determine BTB passive permeability and whether P-gp influences R123 uptake into brain metastases of breast cancer, tumor-bearing mice were injected with ^{14}C-AIB (passive permeability tracer) which was allowed to circulate for 10 min before a 2 min R123 perfusion, which was followed by sacrifice (**Figure 3**). Autoradiography analysis of the brains revealed elevated permeability to ^{14}C-AIB (~4.9-fold increase). The passive permeability marker tracer's uptake did not correlate ($r^2 = 0.17$ for AIB) with metastases size (**Figure 3A**). R123 uptake, however, was not different from that of normal brain on average (~0.98-fold change) in metastatic lesions and had no correlation ($r^2 = 0.033$) to metastasis size (**Figure 3B**). R123 permeability did not correlate passive permeability changes as measured by ^{14}C-AIB ($r^2 = 0.0008$) (**Figure 3C**) accumulation suggesting that R123 remains restricted from the brain parenchyma via P-gp mediated efflux. The observed R123 K_{in} value for normal brain (BDT; brain distant to tumor) regions of metastases bearing mice ($K_{in} = 0.11 \pm 0.06 \times 10^{-1}$ μL/s/g) (**Figures 4A–C**) was consistent with previous K_{in} measurements in tumor-free mice (**Figure 1B**). And, the K_{in} of R123 in the BTB (within metastases) was 0.12 ± 0.003 μL/s/g which was not different than that of normal brain ($p > 0.05$).

DISCUSSION AND CONCLUSION

In the current study, we present data suggesting P-gp retains its efflux function at the BTB despite a disruption in the integrity of the BBB induced by the presence of a metastatic lesion. Of notable methodology, to the best of our knowledge we are the first to combine quantitative fluorescence microscopy to measure R123 P-gp mediated efflux and quantitative autoradiography to measure changes in BTB passive permeability (^{14}C-AIB) in the same brain slice. This method is able to directly shed light on two independent processes occurring at the BTB.

The utilization of R123 to evaluate P-gp function is well established (Hegmann et al., 1992). However, there is less evidence regarding R123's affinity and efflux transport to other transporters that contribute to drug restriction to brain. R123 has been reported to be subject to transport by BCRP (Doyle et al., 1998), and OCT 1 & 2 (Jouan et al., 2012), and MRP2 (Munic et al., 2011). Though studies using specific transporter inhibitors at correct concentrations show P-gp primarily transports R123 and restricts accumulation into brain (Wang et al., 1995). Moreover, the magnitude of R123 efflux by P-gp is greater than that of BCRP and MRP1 (Chopra, 2004) and therefore should represent the major pathway of active efflux transport at the BBB and BTB.

Due to the difficulty in performing the *in situ* brain perfusion in mice, we modified the *in situ* brain perfusion to a cardiac perfusion method in female Nu/Nu mice bearing brain metastases of breast cancer to characterize P-gp function *in vivo*. This method has similar advantages to the *in situ* brain perfusion method in that we may control aspects of the perfusion to determine both influx and efflux kinetics, transporter inhibition coefficients, and BTB or BBB permeability (Smith and Allen, 2003). This control helps determine accurate apparent permeability coefficients (Lockman et al., 2005a), the degree to what a substrate is efflux back into blood (Lockman et al., 2003b), inhibition constants for

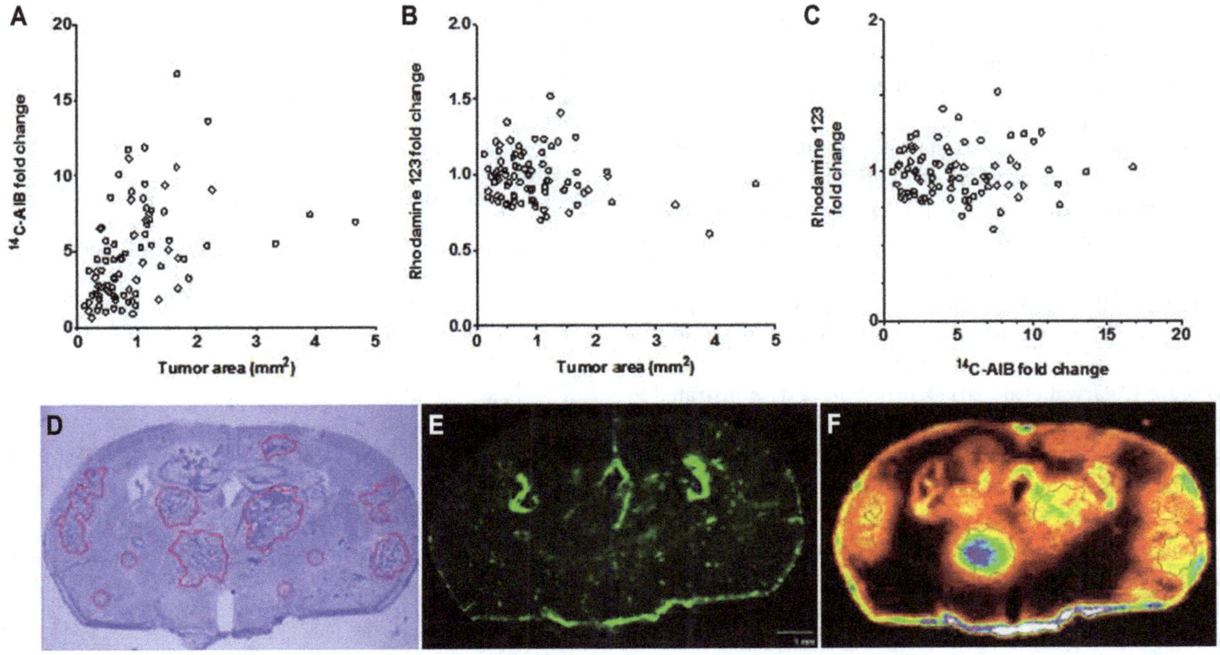

FIGURE 3 | The BTB is variably compromised for compounds entering via passive diffusion but retains P-gp mediated efflux. The passive permeability marker ^{14}C-AIB fold change in brain metastases did not correlate ($r^2 = 0.167$) with metastasis size (mm^2) **(A)**. R123 fold change in brain metastases did not correlate ($r^2 = 0.033$) with metastasis size **(B)**. There was no observed relationship ($r^2 = 0.0009$) between the fold increase in brain metastases of ^{14}C-AIB (passive permeability marker) and R123 (P-gp substrate) **(C)**. One representative brain slice showing metastases location (**D**, cresyl violet), R123 fluorescence distribution (**E**, fluorescence microscopy), and ^{14}C-AIB brain uptake (**F**, quantitative autoradiography).

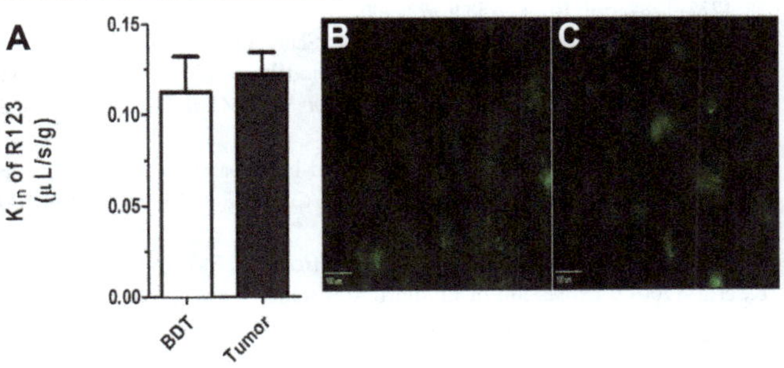

FIGURE 4 | (A) No difference ($p > 0.05$; student t-test, $n = 3$–5) was seen between R123 blood to brain transfer constant K_{in} between values measured in normal brain ($K_{in} = 0.11 \pm 0.01$ μL/s/g) and metastases ($K_{in} = 0.12 \pm 0.02$ μL/s/g). Representative R123 fluorescence images in normal brain **(B)** and within a metastasis **(C)** (scale bar = 100 μm).

transporters (Lockman et al., 2001) and a direct measurement of BBB and BTB integrity (Lockman et al., 2003a, 2004, 2005b)

Using the cardiac perfusion method, R123 accumulated in brain linearly over 2 min of perfusion time. Our observed blood to brain transfer constant (K_{in}) was ~10-fold less than what would be the calculated K_{in} based on values of similar molecules in terms of their octanol/water coefficient and molecular weight. The lower observed K_{in}, is typically seen when the compound is actively extruded by the BBB back into blood (Begley, 1996). Further confirmation that R123 is extruded by an efflux mechanism at the BBB was suggested by the significantly increased uptake of R123 from blood to brain after the addition of verapamil or cyclosporine A to the perfusate (Mittapalli et al., 2013).

Of importance to this study, the simultaneous administration of a passive permeability marker and a tracer subject to P-gp mediated efflux allowed us to measure BTB integrity and functional efflux. Both parameters have been shown to significantly impact drug uptake into metastases (Lockman et al., 2010) but have not been simultaneously measured directly in metastatic lesions. Our initial hypothesis prior to the experiment was that since we have seen increased permeability at the BTB in metastases (Lockman et al., 2010), we would also see a similar increase in R123 distribution into the lesion. However we did not observe R123 accumulation within metastases.

There are two possible explanations that may provide insight to the lack of increased R123 permeability in the lesion. First, it is known that P-gp is expressed in the vasculature of human brain tumors and metastases (Guo et al., 2010). Although, P-gp expression at the BTB has been shown to be variable among different types of tumors within the CNS (Cordon-Cardo et al., 1990; Toth et al., 1996; Tews et al., 2000) as well as different between separate intracranial metastases (Demeule et al., 2001; Lockman et al., 2010). We observed some variability of P-gp expression in the vessels of our metastases, but overall P-gp expression was not significantly different in the over 2,000 vessels we analyzed between the BTB and the BBB. Accordingly, this may be a reason why there was little overall difference in tissue accumulation of R123 between the two tissue types. Another possible explanation is that we observed tumor cells directly adjacent or proximal to the vasculature also express P-gp, which may also contribute to the restriction of R123 in the lesions. Overall, the pattern of distribution for each tracer suggests that the BTB is disrupted yet its efflux transport mechanisms are intact and can limit brain and or tumor uptake of P-gp substrates.

This work does have translational value to human drug distribution to brain. The expression of BCRP at human BBB is ~2 fold higher as compared to the expression levels at mouse BBB. The P-gp expression is 3 fold higher at mouse BBB as compared to the expression levels at human BBB. So BCRP still plays a major role at human BBB (Hoshi et al., 2013) suggesting P-gp plays a major functional role in the human BBB. While some studies have supported little efflux contribution for various anti-cancer drug to brain (Agarwal et al., 2011), others have demonstrated P-gp at the BBB and BTB restricts the uptake of many anti-cancer agents; such as paclitaxel, docetaxel, vemurafenib, erlotinib, axitinib, and tamoxifen (Gallo et al., 2003; Kemper et al., 2004; Wang et al., 2010; Iusuf et al., 2011; Poller et al., 2011; Mittapalli et al., 2012; Taskar et al., 2012; Agarwal et al., 2013). Attempts to modify P-gp using inhibitors have shown promise in preclinical settings (Kemper et al., 2004; Mittapalli et al., 2012; Agarwal et al., 2013).

Although we, and others, have observed variably elevated accumulations of small molecules across the BTB in brain metastases, the data herein provide evidence that P-gp retains much of its residual function. Thus, BTB function in this preclinical model may be viewed as only partially compromised and retains significant ability to impede uptake of therapeutic compounds. Given the large list of drugs, particularly anticancer agents such as paclitaxel and doxorubicin, which are subject to P-gp mediated efflux, the clinical impact of this retained function suggests the BTB remains a significant barrier in delivering chemotherapeutics into metastatic lesions.

AUTHORS' CONTRIBUTIONS

1. Concept and design – Chris E. Adkins, Rajendar K. Mittapalli, Vamshi K. Manda, Paul R. Lockman
2. Development of methodology Chris E. Adkins, Rajendar K. Mittapalli, Vamshi K. Manda, Kaci A. Bohn, Paul R. Lockman
3. Acquisition of data (provided animals, acquired and managed patients, provided facilities, etc) Chris E. Adkins, Rajendar K. Mittapalli, Vamshi K. Manda, Tori B. Terrell, Kaci A. Bohn, Celik Yasemin, Tiffany R. Grothe, Julie A. Lockman, Paul R. Lockman
4. Analysis and interpretation of data (e.g., statistical analysis, biostatistics, computational analysis) Chris E. Adkins, Rajendar K. Mittapalli, Vamshi K. Manda, Mohamed I. Nounou, Afroz S. Mohammad, Tori B. Terrell, Julie A. Lockman, Paul R. Lockman
5. Writing, review, and/or revision of the manuscript Chris E. Adkins, Mohamed I. Nounou, Afroz S. Mohammad, Tori B. Terrell, Paul R. Lockman
6. Study supervision Paul R. Lockman

ACKNOWLEDGMENT

Funding for this study was provided by the Department of Defense Breast Cancer Research Program Grant W81 XWH-062-0033 and National Cancer Institute, National Institutes of Health, Bethesda, MD. 1R01CA166067-01A1 to Paul R. Lockman.

REFERENCES

Abbott, N. J., Patabendige, A. A., Dolman, D. E., Yusof, S. R., and Begley, D. J. (2010). Structure and function of the blood-brain barrier. *Neurobiol. Dis.* 37, 13–25. doi: 10.1016/j.nbd.2009.07.030

Agarwal, S., Hartz, A. M., Elmquist, W. F., and Bauer, B. (2011). Breast cancer resistance protein and P-glycoprotein in brain cancer: two gatekeepers team up. *Curr. Pharm. Des.* 17, 2793–2802. doi: 10.2174/138161211797440186

Agarwal, S., Manchanda, P., Vogelbaum, M. A., Ohlfest, J. R., and Elmquist, W. F. (2013). Function of the blood-brain barrier and restriction of drug delivery to invasive glioma cells: findings in an orthotopic rat xenograft model of glioma. *Drug Metab. Dispos.* 41, 33–39. doi: 10.1124/dmd.112.048322

Baumert, C., and Hilgeroth, A. (2009). Recent advances in the development of P-gp inhibitors. *Anticancer Agents Med. Chem.* 9, 415–436. doi: 10.2174/1871520610909040415

Begley, D. J. (1996). The blood-brain barrier: principles for targeting peptides and drugs to the central nervous system. *J. Pharm. Pharmacol.* 48, 136–146. doi: 10.1111/j.2042-7158.1996.tb07112.x

Breedveld, P., Beijnen, J. H., and Schellens, J. H. (2006). Use of P-glycoprotein and BCRP inhibitors to improve oral bioavailability and CNS penetration of anticancer drugs. *Trends Pharmacol. Sci.* 27, 17–24. doi: 10.1016/j.tips.2005.11.009

Breedveld, P., Pluim, D., Cipriani, G., Wielinga, P., van Tellingen, O., Schinkel, A. H., et al. (2005). The effect of Bcrp1 (Abcg2) on the in vivo pharmacokinetics and brain penetration of imatinib mesylate (Gleevec): implications for the use of breast cancer resistance protein and P-glycoprotein inhibitors to enable the brain penetration of imatinib in patients. *Cancer Res.* 65, 2577–2582. doi: 10.1158/0008-5472.CAN-04-2416

Choi, J. S., and Li, X. (2005). The effect of verapamil on the pharmacokinetics of paclitaxel in rats. *Eur. J. Pharm. Sci.* 24, 95–100. doi: 10.1016/j.ejps.2004.10.002

Chopra, A. (2004). "11C-Labeled rhodamine-123," in *Molecular Imaging and Contrast Agent Database (MICAD)* (Bethesda:National Center for Biotechnology Information).

Cordon-Cardo, C., O'Brien, J. P., Boccia, J., Casals, D., Bertino, J. R., and Melamed, M. R. (1990). Expression of the multidrug resistance gene product (P-glycoprotein) in human normal and tumor tissues. *J. Histochem. Cytochem.* 38, 1277–1287. doi: 10.1177/38.9.1974900

Dagenais, C., Rousselle, C., Pollack, G. M., and Scherrmann, J. M. (2000). Development of an in situ mouse brain perfusion model and its application to mdr1a P-glycoprotein-deficient mice. *J. Cereb. Blood Flow Metab.* 20, 381–386. doi: 10.1097/00004647-200002000-00020

Deeken, J. F., and Loscher, W. (2007). The blood-brain barrier and cancer: transporters, treatment, and Trojan horses. *Clin. Cancer Res.* 13, 1663–1674. doi: 10.1158/1078-0432.CCR-06-2854

Demeule, M., Shedid, D., Beaulieu, E., Del Maestro, R. F., Moghrabi, A., Ghosn, P. B., et al. (2001). Expression of multidrug-resistance P-glycoprotein (MDR1) in human brain tumors. *Int. J. Cancer* 93, 62–66. doi: 10.1002/ijc.1306

Doyle, L. A., Yang, W., Abruzzo, L. V., Krogmann, T., Gao, Y., Rishi, A. K., et al. (1998). A multidrug resistance transporter from human MCF-7 breast cancer cells. *Proc. Natl. Acad. Sci. U.S.A.* 95, 15665–15670. doi: 10.1073/pnas.95.26.15665

Forster, S., Thumser, A. E., Hood, S. R., and Plant, N. (2012). Characterization of rhodamine-123 as a tracer dye for use in in vitro drug transport assays. *PLoS ONE* 7:e33253. doi: 10.1371/journal.pone.0033253

Gallo, J. M., Li, S., Guo, P., Reed, K., and Ma, J. (2003). The effect of P-glycoprotein on paclitaxel brain and brain tumor distribution in mice. *Cancer Res.* 63, 5114–5117.

Guo, Z., Zhu, J., Zhao, L., Luo, Q., and Jin, X. (2010). Expression and clinical significance of multidrug resistance proteins in brain tumors. *J. Exp. Clin. Cancer Res.* 29, 122. doi: 10.1186/1756-9966-29-122

Hagenbuch, B., and Meier, P. J. (2004). Organic anion transporting polypeptides of the OATP/ SLC21 family: phylogenetic classification as OATP/ SLCO superfamily, new nomenclature and molecular/functional properties. *Pflugers Arch.* 447, 653–665. doi: 10.1007/s00424-003-1168-y

Hawkins, B. T., and Davis, T. P. (2005). The blood-brain barrier/neurovascular unit in health and disease. *Pharmacol. Rev.* 57, 173–185. doi: 10.1124/pr.57.2.4

Hegmann, E. J., Bauer, H. C., and Kerbel, R. S. (1992). Expression and functional activity of P-glycoprotein in cultured cerebral capillary endothelial cells. *Cancer Res.* 52, 6969–6975.

Henson, J. W., Cordon-Cardo, C., and Posner, J. B. (1992). P-glycoprotein expression in brain tumors. *J. Neurooncol.* 14, 37–43. doi: 10.1007/BF00170943

Hoshi, Y., Uchida, Y., Tachikawa, M., Inoue, T., Ohtsuki, S., and Terasaki, T. (2013). Quantitative atlas of blood-brain barrier transporters, receptors, and tight junction proteins in rats and common marmoset. *J. Pharm. Sci.*102, 3343–3355. doi: 10.1002/jps.23575

Iusuf, D., Teunissen, S. F., Wagenaar, E., Rosing, H., Beijnen, J. H., and Schinkel, A. H. (2011). P-glycoprotein (ABCB1) transports the primary active tamoxifen metabolites endoxifen and 4-hydroxytamoxifen and restricts their brain penetration. *J. Pharmacol. Exp. Ther.* 337, 710–717. doi: 10.1124/jpet.110.178301

Jouan, E., Le Vee, M., Denizot, C., Da Violante, G., and Fardel, O. (2012). The mitochondrial fluorescent dye rhodamine 123 is a high-affinity substrate for organic cation transporters (OCTs) 1 and 2. *Fundam. Clin. Pharmacol.* doi: 10.1111/j.1472-8206.2012.01071.x [Epub ahead of print].

Kemper, E. M., Verheij, M., Boogerd, W., Beijnen, J. H., and van Tellingen, O. (2004). Improved penetration of docetaxel into the brain by co-administration of inhibitors of P-glycoprotein. *Eur. J. Cancer* 40, 1269–1274. doi: 10.1016/j.ejca.2004.01.024

Lipinski, C. A., Lombardo, F., Dominy, B. W., and Feeney, P. J. (2001). Experimental and computational approaches to estimate solubility and permeability in drug discovery and development settings. *Adv. Drug Deliv. Rev.* 46, 3–26. doi: 10.1016/S0169-409X(00)00129-0

Lockman, P. R., Koziara, J. M., Mumper, R. J., and Allen, D. D. (2004). Nanoparticle surface charges alter blood-brain barrier integrity and permeability. *J. Drug Target.* 12, 635–641. doi: 10.1080/10611860400015936

Lockman, P. R., Koziara, J., Roder, K. E., Paulson, J., Abbruscato, T. J., Mumper, R. J.,et al. (2003a). In vivo and in vitro assessment of baseline blood-brain barrier parameters in the presence of novel nanoparticles. *Pharm. Res.* 20, 705–713. doi: 10.1023/A:1023492015851

Lockman, P. R., Mumper, R. J., and Allen, D. D. (2003b). Evaluation of blood-brain barrier thiamine efflux using the in situ rat brain perfusion method. *J. Neurochem.* 86, 627–634. doi: 10.1046/j.1471-4159.2003.01888.x

Lockman, P. R., McAfee, G., Geldenhuys, W. J., Van der Schyf, C. J., Abbruscato, T. J., and Allen, D. D. (2005a). Brain uptake kinetics of nicotine and cotinine after chronic nicotine exposure. *J. Pharmacol. Exp. Ther.* 314, 636–642. doi: 10.1124/jpet.105.085381

Lockman, P. R., Van der Schyf, C. J., Abbruscato, T. J., and Allen, D. D. (2005b). Chronic nicotine exposure alters blood-brain barrier permeability and diminishes brain uptake of methyllycaconitine. *J. Neurochem.* 94, 37–44. doi: 10.1111/j.1471-4159.2005.03162.x

Lockman, P. R., Mittapalli, R. K., Taskar, K. S., Rudraraju, V., Gril, B., Bohn, K. A., et al. (2010). Heterogeneous blood-tumor barrier permeability determines drug efficacy in experimental brain metastases of breast cancer. *Clin. Cancer Res.* 16, 5664–5678. doi: 10.1158/1078-0432.CCR-10-1564

Lockman, P. R., Roder, K. E., and Allen, D. D. (2001). Inhibition of the rat blood-brain barrier choline transporter by manganese chloride. *J. Neurochem.* 79, 588–594. doi: 10.1046/j.1471-4159.2001.00589.x

Loscher, W., and Potschka, H. (2005). Role of drug efflux transporters in the brain for drug disposition and treatment of brain diseases. *Prog. Neurobiol.* 76, 22–76. doi: 10.1016/j.pneurobio.2005.04.006

Mittapalli, R. K., Manda, V. K., Bohn, K. A., Adkins, C. E., and Lockman, P. R. (2013). Quantitative fluorescence microscopy provides high resolution imaging of passive diffusion and P-gp mediated efflux at the in vivo blood-brain barrier. *J. Neurosci. Methods* 219, 188–195. doi: 10.1016/j.jneumeth.2013.07.001

Mittapalli, R. K., Vaidhyanathan, S., Sane, R., and Elmquist, W. F. (2012). Impact of P-glycoprotein (ABCB1) and breast cancer resistance protein (ABCG2) on the brain distribution of a novel BRAF inhibitor: vemurafenib (PLX4032). *J. Pharmacol. Exp. Ther.* 342, 33–40. doi: 10.1124/jpet.112.192195

Munic, V., Hlevnjak, M., and Erakovic Haber, V. (2011). Characterization of rhodamine-123, calcein and 5(6)-carboxy-2',7'-dichlorofluorescein (CDCF) export via MRP2 (ABCC2) in MES-SA and A549 cells. *Eur. J. Pharm. Sci.* 43, 359–369. doi: 10.1016/j.ejps.2011.05.003

Pardridge, W. M. (2007). Blood-brain barrier delivery. *Drug Discov. Today,* 12, 54–61. doi: 10.1016/j.drudis.2006.10.013

Poller, B., Iusuf, D., Sparidans, R. W., Wagenaar, E., Beijnen, J. H., and Schinkel, A. H. (2011). Differential impact of P-glycoprotein (ABCB1) and breast cancer resistance protein (ABCG2) on axitinib brain accumulation and oral plasma pharmacokinetics. *Drug Metab. Dispos.* 39, 729–735. doi: 10.1124/dmd.110.037317

Polli, J. W., Olson, K. L., Chism, J. P., John-Williams, L. S., Yeager, R. L., Woodard, S. M., et al. (2009). An unexpected synergist role of P-glycoprotein and breast cancer resistance protein on the central nervous system penetration of the tyrosine kinase inhibitor lapatinib (N-{3-chloro-4-[(3-fluorobenzyl)oxy]phenyl}-6-[5-({[2-(methylsulfonyl)ethyl]amino }methyl)-2-furyl]-4-quinazolinamine; GW572016). *Drug Metab. Dispos.* 37, 439–442. doi: 10.1124/dmd.108.024646

Schinkel, A. H., Wagenaar, E., Mol, C. A., and van Deemter, L. (1996). P-glycoprotein in the blood-brain barrier of mice influences the brain penetration and pharmacological activity of many drugs. *J. Clin. Invest.* 97, 2517–2524. doi: 10.1172/JCI118699

Schinkel, A. H., Wagenaar, E., van Deemter, L., Mol, C. A., and Borst, P. (1995). Absence of the mdr1a P-Glycoprotein in mice affects tissue distribution and pharmacokinetics of dexamethasone, digoxin, and cyclosporin A. *J. Clin. Invest.* 96, 1698–1705. doi: 10.1172/JCI118214

Smith, Q. R., and Allen, D. D., (2003). In situ brain perfusion technique. *Methods Mol. Med.* 89, 209–218.

Smith, Q. R., and Takasato, Y. (1986). Kinetics of amino acid transport at the blood-brain barrier studied using an in situ brain perfusion technique. *Ann. N. Y. Acad. Sci.* 481, 186–201. doi: 10.1111/j.1749-6632.1986.tb27150.x

Summerfield, S. G., Read, K., Begley, D. J., Obradovic, T., Hidalgo, I. J., Coggon, S., et al. (2007). Central nervous system drug disposition: the relationship between in situ brain permeability and brain free fraction. *J. Pharmacol. Exp. Ther.* 322, 205–213. doi: 10.1124/jpet.107.121525

Takasato, Y., Rapoport, S. I., and Smith, Q. R. (1984). An in situ brain perfusion technique to study cerebrovascular transport in the rat. *Am. J. Physiol.* 247,(Pt 2), H484–H493.

Taskar, K. S., Rudraraju, V., Mittapalli, R. K., Samala, R., Thorsheim, H. R., Lockman, J., et al. (2012). Lapatinib distribution in HER2 overexpressing experimental brain metastases of breast cancer. *Pharm. Res.* 29, 770–781. doi: 10.1007/s11095-011-0601-8

Tengvar, C., Hultstrom, D., and Olsson, Y. (1983). An improved Percoll density gradient for measurements of experimental brain edema. Addition of sucrose to an isotonic gradient in an attempt to balance osmotic conditions during density determinations. *Acta Neuropathol.* 61, 201–206. doi: 10.1007/BF00691986

Tews, D. S., Nissen, A., Külgen, C., and Gaumann, A. K. (2000). Drug resistance-associated factors in primary and secondary glioblastomas and their precursor tumors. *J. Neurooncol.* 50, 227–237. doi: 10.1023/A:1006491405010

Toth, K., Vaughan, M. M., Peress, N. S., Slocum, H. K., and Rustum, Y. M. (1996). MDR1 P-glycoprotein is expressed by endothelial cells of newly formed capillaries in human gliomas but is not expressed in the neovasculature of other primary tumors. *Am. J. Pathol.* 149, 853–858.

Wadhwani, K. C., Caspers-Velu, L. E., Murphy, V. A., Smith, Q. R., Kador, P. F., and Rapoport, S. I. (1989). Prevention of nerve edema and increased blood-nerve barrier permeability-surface area product in galactosemic rats by aldose reductase or thromboxane synthetase inhibitors. *Diabetes* 38, 1469–1477. doi: 10.2337/diab.38.11.1469

Wang, F., Zhou, F., Kruh, G. D., and Gallo, J. M. (2010). Influence of blood-brain barrier efflux pumps on the distribution of vincristine in brain and brain tumors. *Neuro Oncol.* 12, 1043–1049. doi: 10.1093/neuonc/noq056

Wang, Q., Yang, H., Miller, D. W., and Elmquist, W. F. (1995). Effect of the p-glycoprotein inhibitor, cyclosporin A, on the distribution of rhodamine-123 to the brain: an in vivo microdialysis study in freely moving rats. *Biochem. Biophys. Res. Commun.* 211, 719–726. doi: 10.1006/bbrc.1995.1872

Permissions

All chapters in this book were first published in DDCDO, by Frontiers; hereby published with permission under the Creative Commons Attribution License or equivalent. Every chapter published in this book has been scrutinized by our experts. Their significance has been extensively debated. The topics covered herein carry significant findings which will fuel the growth of the discipline. They may even be implemented as practical applications or may be referred to as a beginning point for another development.

The contributors of this book come from diverse backgrounds, making this book a truly international effort. This book will bring forth new frontiers with its revolutionizing research information and detailed analysis of the nascent developments around the world.

We would like to thank all the contributing authors for lending their expertise to make the book truly unique. They have played a crucial role in the development of this book. Without their invaluable contributions this book wouldn't have been possible. They have made vital efforts to compile up to date information on the varied aspects of this subject to make this book a valuable addition to the collection of many professionals and students.

This book was conceptualized with the vision of imparting up-to-date information and advanced data in this field. To ensure the same, a matchless editorial board was set up. Every individual on the board went through rigorous rounds of assessment to prove their worth. After which they invested a large part of their time researching and compiling the most relevant data for our readers.

The editorial board has been involved in producing this book since its inception. They have spent rigorous hours researching and exploring the diverse topics which have resulted in the successful publishing of this book. They have passed on their knowledge of decades through this book. To expedite this challenging task, the publisher supported the team at every step. A small team of assistant editors was also appointed to further simplify the editing procedure and attain best results for the readers.

Apart from the editorial board, the designing team has also invested a significant amount of their time in understanding the subject and creating the most relevant covers. They scrutinized every image to scout for the most suitable representation of the subject and create an appropriate cover for the book.

The publishing team has been an ardent support to the editorial, designing and production team. Their endless efforts to recruit the best for this project, has resulted in the accomplishment of this book. They are a veteran in the field of academics and their pool of knowledge is as vast as their experience in printing. Their expertise and guidance has proved useful at every step. Their uncompromising quality standards have made this book an exceptional effort. Their encouragement from time to time has been an inspiration for everyone.

The publisher and the editorial board hope that this book will prove to be a valuable piece of knowledge for researchers, students, practitioners and scholars across the globe.

List of Contributors

Saumya Pant, RussellWeiner and Matthew J. Marton
Merck Research Laboratories, Molecular Biomarkers and Diagnostics, Rahway, NJ, USA

Dong Fu
Faculty of Pharmacy, The University of Sydney, Sydney, NSW, Australia

Martina McDermott
National Institute for Cellular Biotechnology, Dublin City University, Dublin, Ireland
Department of Drug Discovery and Biomedical Sciences, South Carolina College of Pharmacy, University of South Carolina, Columbia, SC, USA

Alex J. Eustace
National Institute for Cellular Biotechnology, Dublin City University, Dublin, Ireland
Department of Medical Oncology, Beaumont Hospital, Royal College of Surgeons in Ireland, Dublin, Ireland

Steven Busschots
Department of Histopathology, St James' Hospital, Trinity College Dublin, Dublin, Ireland

Laura Breen, Martin Clynes and Norma O'Donovan
National Institute for Cellular Biotechnology, Dublin City University, Dublin, Ireland

John Crown
National Institute for Cellular Biotechnology, Dublin City University, Dublin, Ireland
Department of Medical Oncology, St Vincent's University Hospital, Dublin, Ireland

Britta Stordal
National Institute for Cellular Biotechnology, Dublin City University, Dublin, Ireland
Department of Histopathology, St James' Hospital, Trinity College Dublin, Dublin, Ireland

Nicholas C. Nicolaides, Daniel J. O'Shannessy, Earl Albone and Luigi Grasso
Department of Translational Medicine and Diagnostics, Morphotek Inc., Exton, PA, USA

Richard Simon
Biometric Research Branch, National Cancer Institute, Bethesda, MD, USA

Dana Olsen
Regulatory Affairs, Dako Denmark A/S, an Agilent Technologies Company, Glostrup, Denmark

JanTrøst Jørgensen
Dx-Rx Institute, Fredensborg, Denmark

Sanjoy Paul and W. Scott Moye-Rowley
Department of Molecular Physiology and Biophysics, Carver College of Medicine, University of Iowa, Iowa City, IA, USA

Frances Jane Sharom
Department of Molecular and Cellular Biology, University of Guelph, Guelph, ON, Canada

Sai-Hong Ignatius Ou
Chao Family Comprehensive Cancer Center, University of California Irvine School of Medicine, Orange, CA, USA

Ross A. Soo
National University Health System and Cancer Science Institute of Singapore, Singapore

Akihito Kubo
Aichi Medical University School of Medicine, Nagakute, Japan

Tomoya Kawaguchi
National Hospital Organization Kinki-Chuo Chest Medical Center, Sakai City, Japan

Myung-Ju Ahn
Division of Hematology-Oncology, Department of Medicine, Samsung Medical Center, Sungkyunkwan University School of Medicine, Seoul, South Korea

Sonali Kapse-Mistry
Department of Pharmaceutics, SVKM's Dr. Bhanuben Nanavati College of Pharmacy, University of Mumbai, Mumbai, India

Thirumala Govender
Discipline of Pharmaceutical Sciences, School of Health Sciences, University of KwaZulu-Natal, Durban, South Africa

Rohit Srivastava
Department of Biosciences and Bioengineering, Indian Institute of Technology Bombay, Mumbai, India

Mayur Yergeri
Department of Pharmaceutical Chemistry, SVKM's Dr. Bhanuben Nanavati College of Pharmacy, University of Mumbai, Mumbai, India

Alexey Goltsov and James Bown
Centre for Research in Informatics and Systems Pathology (CRISP), University of Abertay Dundee, Dundee, UK

Simon P. Langdon
Division of Pathology, Institute of Genetics and Molecular Medicine,Western General Hospital, University of Edinburgh, Edinburgh, UK

Gregory Goltsov
Touch Surgery, London, UK

David J. Harrison
School of Medicine, University of St Andrews, St Andrews, UK

Gabriela Gremel, Karin Grannas, Lesley Ann Sutton, Fredrik Pontén and Agata Zieba
Science for Life Laboratory, Department of Immunology, Genetics and Pathology, Uppsala University, Uppsala, Sweden

Boye Schnack Nielsen, Trine Møller and Kim Holmstrøm
Bioneer A/S, Hørsholm, Denmark

Eva Balslev, Tim Svenstrup Poulsen and Estrid Høgdall
Department of Pathology, Herlev Hospital, University of Copenhagen, Herlev, Denmark

Dorte Nielsen and Christiane Ehlers Mortensen
Department of Oncology, Herlev Hospital, University of Copenhagen, Herlev, Denmark

Laura Zinzi, Marialessandra Contino and Elena Capparelli
Dipartimento di Farmacia-Scienze del Farmaco, Università degli Studi di Bari "A. Moro," Bari, Italy

Mariangela Cantore
Dipartimento di Farmacia-Scienze del Farmaco, Biofordrug srl, Spin-off of University of Bari, Bari, Italy

Marcello Leopoldo and Nicola A. Colabufo
Dipartimento di Farmacia-Scienze del Farmaco, Università degli Studi di Bari "A. Moro," Bari, Italy
Dipartimento di Farmacia-Scienze del Farmaco, Biofordrug srl, Spin-off of University of Bari, Bari, Italy

Kenneth Russell and AndreasVoss
Caris Life Sciences, Basel, Switzerland

Leonid Shunyakov
Central Care Cancer Center, Bolivar, MO, USA

Karel A. Dicke
Arlington Cancer Center, Arlington, TX, USA

Todd Maney
Caris Life Sciences, Phoenix, AZ, USA

Charlotte Gauthier and Attilio Di Pietro
Drug Resistance Mechanism and Modulation Group, Ligue 2013 Certified, Bases Moléculaires et Structurales des Systèmes Infectieux, UMR5086, Centre National de la Recherche Scientifique, Université de Lyon, Institut de Biologie et Chimie des Protéines, University of Lyon, Lyon, France

Csilla Ozvegy-Laczka
Research Group of Active Transport Proteins, Institute of Enzymology, Research Centre for Natural Sciences, Hungarian Academy of Sciences, Budapest, Hungary

Gergely Szakacs
Institute of Enzymology, Research Centre for Natural Sciences, Hungarian Academy of Sciences, Budapest, Hungary

Balazs Sarkadi
Molecular Biophysics Research Group, Hungarian Academy of Sciences, Semmelweiss University, Budapest, Hungary

Jan Stenvang, Nils Brünner and José M. A. Moreira
Faculty of Health and Medical Sciences, Department of Veterinary Disease Biology, Section for Molecular Disease Biology and Sino-Danish Breast Cancer Research Centre, University of Copenhagen, Copenhagen, Denmark
Danish Centre for Translational Breast Cancer Research, Copenhagen, Denmark

Iben Kümler and Dorte Nielsen
Department of Oncology, Center for Cancer Research, Herlev Hospital, University of Copenhagen, Copenhagen, Denmark

Sune Boris Nygård
Faculty of Health and Medical Sciences, Department of Veterinary Disease Biology, Section for Molecular Disease Biology and Sino-Danish Breast Cancer Research Centre, University of Copenhagen, Copenhagen, Denmark

David Hersi Smith
Faculty of Health and Medical Sciences, Department of Veterinary Disease Biology, Section for Molecular Disease Biology and Sino-Danish Breast Cancer Research Centre, University of Copenhagen, Copenhagen, Denmark
DAKO A/S, Glostrup, Denmark

Chris E. Adkins, Rajendar K. Mittapalli, Vamshi K. Manda, Mohamed I. Nounou, Afroz S. Mohammad, Tori B.Terrell, Kaci A. Bohn and Paul R. Lockman
Department of Pharmaceutical Sciences, School of Pharmacy, Texas Tech University Health Sciences Center, Amarillo, TX, USA

Celik Yasemin, Tiffany R. Grothe and Julie A. Lockman
Department of Life, Earth and Environmental Sciences,West Texas A&M University, Canyon, TX, USA

Jan Trøst Jørgensen
Dx-Rx Institute, Fredensborg, Denmark

Index

www.ingramcontent.com/pod-product-compliance
Lightning Source LLC
LaVergne TN
LVHW060554210926
848485LV00005B/1314